Pharmacogenomics in Clinical Practice

Dragan Primorac · Wolfgang Höppner ·
Lidija Bach-Rojecky

Editors

Pharmacogenomics in Clinical Practice

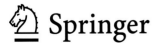 Springer

Editors
Dragan Primorac
St. Catherine Specialty Hospital
Zagreb, Croatia

Universities of Split
Osijek and Rijeka, Croatia

Eberly College of Science
The Pennsylvania State University
University Park
State College, PA, USA

The Henry C. Lee College of Criminal
Justice and Forensic Sciences
University of New Haven
West Haven, CT, USA

Regiomed Kliniken
Coburg, Germany

National Forensic Sciences University
Gandhinagar
Gandhinagar, India

Lidija Bach-Rojecky
University of Zagreb Faculty of Pharmacy
and Biochemistry
Zagreb, Croatia

Wolfgang Höppner
Bioglobe GmbH
Hamburg, Hamburg, Germany

ISBN 978-3-031-45905-4   ISBN 978-3-031-45903-0 (eBook)
https://doi.org/10.1007/978-3-031-45903-0

This Springer imprint is published by the registered company Springer Nature Switzerland AG
The registered company address is: Gewerbestrasse 11, 6330 Cham, Switzerland

Paper in this product is recyclable.

Contents

Principles of Pharmacogenetics

Ron H. N. van Schaik, Lidija Bach-Rojecky, and Dragan Primorac

Abstract

There is no doubt that pharmacogenetics represents the backbone of personalized medicine. While pharmacogenomics investigates how multiple variants across the genome affect drug response or reflect the combination of genetic variants and gene expression profiles, pharmacogenetics typically refers to effects involving inherited variants in a limited number of genes. Despite a number of excellent medicines that improved therapeutic outcomes for some

R. H. N. van Schaik
Erasmus MC University Medical Hospital, 3015 CE Rotterdam, The Netherlands

L. Bach-Rojecky
University of Zagreb Faculty of Pharmacy and Biochemistry, 10000 Zagreb, Croatia

D. Primorac (✉)
St. Catherine Specialty Hospital, 10000 Zagreb, Croatia
e-mail: dragan.primorac@svkatarina.hr; draganprimorac2@gmail.com

University of Split School of Medicine, 21000 Split, Croatia

Josip Juraj Strossmayer University of Osijek Faculty of Medicine Osijek, 31000 Osijek, Croatia

University of Rijeka School of Medicine, 51000 Rijeka, Croatia

Josip Juraj Strossmayer University of Osijek Faculty of Dental Medicine and Health, 31000 Osijek, Croatia

Eberly College of Science, Penn State University, 517 Thomas St, State College, PA 16803, USA

The Henry C. Lee College of Criminal Justice and Forensic Sciences, University of New Haven, West Haven, CT, USA

National Forensic Science University, Gandhinagar, Gujarat, India

College of Medicine and Forensics, Xi'an Jiaotong University, Xi'an, China

Medical School REGIOMED, 96450 Coburg, Germany

International Center For Applied Biological Sciences, 10000, Zagreb, Croatia

dangerous illnesses, contemporary medicine faces significant challenges. For example, statistics show that in the USA, only around 50% of drugs show the expected therapeutic efficacy. Also, their side effects, among which some might cause serious health issues potentially leading to death, represent a challenge because they are a direct or indirect cause for up to 7% of all hospital admissions and up to 20% of re-admissions, with the annual estimated cost of $136 billion. The striking fact is that ADRs are the fourth leading cause of death. The best predictors of variability in therapeutic response and ADRs are DNA variants in genes encoding drug-metabolizing enzymes, transporter proteins, receptors (drug targets), human leukocyte antigen (HLA) loci, some cytokines, and other proteins. In order to increase treatment efficacy, the Clinical Pharmacogenetics Implementation Consortium (CIPC), the Dutch Pharmacogenetics Working Group (DPWG), and the Canadian Pharmacogenomics Network for Drug Safety (CPNDS) provide freely available, evidence-based, peer-reviewed, and updated pharmacogenetic clinical practice guidelines for gene/drug pairs to help physicians select and optimize the treatment of each patient.

Keywords

Gene polymorphisms • Pharmacogenetics • Pharmacogenomics • Drug–gene interaction • CPIC • Guidelines

1   Introduction

Traditional therapy based on the concept of "one drug fits all" is replaced with a patient-oriented treatment, which encompasses a more predictive, preventive, participatory, and personalized approach to patients, health, and diseases [1, 2]. Pharmacogenetics reflects a scientific field of medical sciences with rapid advancement in clinical care in the last two decades. It studies the relationship between an individual's genetic predisposition and the response to a particular drug. While pharmacogenomics investigates how multiple variants across the genome affect drug effect and may also include a genetic profile of tumors and/or gene expression profiles, pharmacogenetics typically refers to inherited variants that influence a limited number of genes in relation to response to medicines. In that way, pharmacogenetics can represent a subgroup of pharmacogenomics [3].

After the completion of the Human Genome Project (HGP) in 2001, the knowledge of human sequence variations influenced drug discovery and prediction of drug efficacy. Genetic differences identification helps to understand interindividual variability in drug response, i.e., why some people with the same disease respond differently to drugs. Additionally, it may indicate the risk of therapeutic failure and adverse drug reactions (ADRs) [4]. According to statistical data, only half of the prescribed medicines show the expected therapeutic efficacy. The other striking fact is that ADRs are a direct or indirect cause of up to 7% of all hospital admissions and up to 20% of re-admissions, thus representing the fourth leading cause of death, with an annual estimated cost of $136 billion. Genetic factors can account for as much as 20% of the total reported ADRs [5].

The results of a meta-analysis of 39 prospective studies in American hospitals conducted by Lazaro et al. [6] showed that an average of 6.7% (5.2–8.2%) of patients were hospitalized due to ADRs, and 0.32% (0.23–0.41%) completed lethally. These figures put the ADRs between the fourth and sixth leading causes of death in US hospitals, after heart diseases, cancer, stroke, lung disease, and accidents [6]. The high incidence of ADRs and variability in the therapeutic success might be related to patient characteristics such as age, renal function, liver function, drug-drug interactions with individual genetic factors known to play a role in the therapeutic success of many drugs (genetic factors can account for up to 95% of an individual drug response) [5, 7].

Robust genome-wide association studies during the last decade have revealed many polymorphisms that could underlie variations in therapeutic success. Over 400 genes are clinically relevant in drug efficacy and safety, and ≈200 are associated with ADRs [7]. Besides genes encoding drug-metabolizing enzymes, those encoding transporter proteins, receptors (drug targets), human leukocyte antigen (HLA) loci, some cytokines, and other proteins are predictors of variability in therapeutic response and ADRs as well [1]. During the last two decades, there is a significant increase in the addition of pharmacogenomics data (PGx) in drug labels in all areas of medicine. Pharmacogenomics Knowledgebase (PharmGKB), funded by the US National Institute of Health (NIH), is dedicated to the dissemination of PGx information [8]. Drug labels containing PGx information are approved by regulatory agencies worldwide, including the US Food and Drug Administration (FDA), the European Medicine Agency (EMA), and the Pharmaceuticals and Medical Devices Agency of Japan. By March 2022, PGx information is included on the labels of more than 400 FDA-approved drugs, where the largest proportion (75.5%) of biomarker–drug pairs for which PGx testing is required account for antineoplastic drugs [9].

With the development and application of pharmacogenetics, support for clinical decision-making can be significantly improved. The use of genetic information, which is unchangeable throughout a lifetime, would help predict the response to the drug to enable safer, more effective, and cost-effective treatment [1].

2 The Significance of Pharmacogenetics in the Context of Personalized (Precision) Medicine

Contemporary medicine strives for cutting-edge methods of early diagnosis and individually designed treatment to provide better therapeutic outcomes. Unfortunately, millions of people every day are taking drugs that do not elicit a therapeutic response or even suffer from more or less severe ADRs. In contrast to the "one size fits all" approach, personalized (precise) medicine considers individuals' biological and genetic profiles to determine the predisposition to certain diseases and tailor the right preventive and/or therapeutic strategy to the right person at the right time [1]. Personalized medicine includes, among others, the identification of genes associated with diseases and those relevant to drug action (pharmacogenes). Therefore, pharmacogenetics represents an inseparable part of personalized medicine because it relies on accurate, precise, and evidence-based information, which would allow prescribing the right drug in the optimal dose for each patient. Such an approach enables the transformation of medicine from reactive to proactive and improves the achievement of positive therapeutic outcomes.

In 2016, the EU Commission included the concept of personalized medicine among its key health priorities and established the International Consortium of Personalized Medicine (ICPerMed). Its task is the synchronization of the work of all EU member states on the standardization of diagnostic and therapeutic procedures related to personalized medicine [10]. Despite all benefits of PGx testing implementation in clinical practice, there are some barriers and challenges to its broader acceptance, like financial aspects, lack of specific knowledge among clinicians, lack of decision support tools, and limited evidence from well-designed clinical studies [11]. In 2005, the Dutch Pharmacogenetics Working Group (DPWG) started providing evidence-based dosing guidelines and therapeutic recommeendations [12]. An international Clinical Pharmacogenetics Implementation Consortium (CPIC) was established in 2009 as a shared project between the PharmGKB and the US NIH. The CPIC aims to facilitate pharmacogenomic research data translation into clinical actions for gene/drug pairs with sufficient evidence [13]. The CPIC collects published data and delivers guidelines for gene/drug pairs based on the highest level of clinical evidence, with free access under a Creative Commons public domain license. These peer-reviewed guidelines facilitate PGx knowledge implementation in the clinical setting and help clinicians select and optimize treatment for their patients [13, 14].

Translation of pharmacogenetics in clinical practice during the past two decades relies on the new technologies developed for assessing genetic variants. Over the years, advanced and sophisticated technologies allowed the identification of genomic loci associated with inter-individual variability in drug response [15]. Efficient and low-cost single nucleotide polymorphisms (SNPs) or single nucleotide variants (SNV) panel testing remains the most used technology. However, it will not detect rare and structural variants. The multiple high-throughput whole-genome sequencing techniques can yield plenty of genetic information but are not yet incorporated into everyday practice [16]. In particular, the CYP2D6 analysis using novel genome sequencing (NGS) gives problematic issues due to gene deletions, multiplications, *CYP2D6/2D7* hybrids, and the very homologous *CYP2D7* pseudogene.

SNV panel testing employs commercially available micro-array platforms or custom arrays. Polymerase Chain Reaction (PCR), sequencing by synthesis, and nanospheres or beads combined with fluorescence or chemiluminescence detection are commonly used, in addition to mass spectrometry [16]. Several ready-to-use target panels are available today and have preselected genetic variants with evidence-based well-defined drug associations and recommendations. One of the first PGx platforms was the drug-metabolizing enzymes and Transporters (DMET) Plus panel designed by Affymetrix (nowadays known as Thermo Fisher Scientific). It can simultaneously analyze 1936 SNPs and five copy number variants

(CNV) in 231 pharmacogenes [17]. In addition, the Illuminin Veracode ADME panel tested 184 variants in 34 pharmacogenes [18], whereas the recent gene-set analysis (GSA) v3 array detects even more pharmacogenetic variants. The NeuroIDgenetix® gene panel allows for the simultaneous analysis of 10 genes and provides recommendations for 40 drugs used to treat depression and anxiety [19]. The RightMed® panel (OneOme Spin-off Company of the Mayo Clinic) analyzes 25 genes plus Factor V Leiden, Factor II, and MTHFR genes. It provides recommendations for more than 300 drugs used for 30 different medical conditions, including those with a high prevalence in the population, such as depression, cancer, and cardiovascular disease [1, 20]. St. Catherine Specialty Hospital from Croatia brought this system to routine clinical practice [1]. A more extensive panel is the ThermoFisher Pharmacoscan, which can test 4627 variants in 1191 genes, covering all genes and variants with clinical annotations in CPIC and PharmGKB [21]. Genotyping by selecting commercial ready-made relevant PGx panels may miss newly identified but potentially clinically significant alleles. Therefore, it is important to regularly update panel sequences by recognizing new relevant alleles or supplementing the PGx panel with an updated SNP test. On the other hand, different test designs can make a comparison of the results of several genotyping panels challenging, leading to discrepancies in estimates of copy number variants and misidentified phenotypes [15]. In line with the rapid advancement of technology and more accessible pharmacogenomics investigations, the use of genome sequencing could overcome the mentioned deficiencies.

The development of pharmacogenetics has occurred in parallel with the implementation of electronic health records (EHR)—a digital system for the storage of a whole range of personal and medical, including genomic data about a patient, and may also include a decision support system (DSS). This concept will increase healthcare quality by reducing medication errors and improving therapeutic efficacy and safety [22]. PGx results can improve the design of clinical trials, where specific genomic biomarkers can affect patients' selection and recruitment. Moreover, PGx knowledge has a significant impact on every step of new drug research and development processes as well. Genomics provides a tool for the accurate identification of proteins that play a role in a certain disease and are amenable to targeting by drugs [23].

3   Influence of Genetic Inter-individual Variations on Therapeutic Outcomes

To achieve a pharmacological activity, the majority of drugs should undergo passage through cell membranes from the site of application, transport to cell compartments, biotransformation to active or inactive metabolites, elimination from the body, and finally bind to specific biological macromolecules (drug targets). These molecules include enzymes, transporters, cell membrane receptors, ion channels, and other intra- or extracellular proteins. The genetic polymorphisms of the genes encoding these proteins can lead to changes in the drug's pharmacological effect

[1, 24]. Variations in pharmacokinetic genes involved in absorption, distribution, metabolism, and elimination can alter drug's pharmacokinetic profile, influencing systemic exposure and concentration at the site of action. The human genome consists of between 19,000 to 21,000 protein-coding genes. Within them, multiple types of variations can occur [25].

The most important family of enzymes involved in the metabolism of many different drugs in the first phase of biotransformation is the enzymes of the Cytochrome P450 family (CYP 450). At least five enzymes (CYP3A5, CYP2B6, CYP2C9, CYP2C19, and CYP2D6) encoded by a different gene are particularly important for pharmacogenomics [26]. Based on the ability to metabolize a drug substrate, the genetic polymorphism of these enzymes is associated with several types of metabolic phenotypes. The physiologically normal or extensive phenotype (NM/EM) reflects physiologically normal (or population average) drug biotrans-formation. Reduced or non-existent enzyme activity represents a phenotype of an intermediate (IM) or poor metabolizer (PM), respectively and results in the accumulation of a drug substrate in the body. It is a typical autosomal reces-sive trait caused by mutation and/or deletion of one or both alleles responsible for phenotypic expression. The phenotype of ultra-extensive (UE) or ultra-rapid metabolizer (UM) results in accelerated drug-substrate degradation and is found for the CYP2D6 gene (gene duplication) or the CYP2C19 gene (two alleles with the CYP2C19*17 hyperactivity allele due to a promotor polymorphism causing increased expression). Also, for CYP2C19, a rapid metabolizer (RM) pheno-type is recognized, as caused by having just one hyperactive CYP2C19*17 allele (CYP2C19*1/*17 genotype) [27].

Experts suggested the activity score system (AS) to facilitate the translation of genotype into phenotype. The AS of a genotype is the sum of the functional values of both alleles. Each allele, depending on the functional status, is assigned a value of 0 (no function), 0.5 (decreased function), or 1 (normal function). For example, regarding the CYP2D6 there is consensus to define AS = 0 as PM, AS = 0.5 as IM, AS = 1.5 and 2 as NM, and those with an AS $\geq$ 3 as UM, although there are some inconsistencies regarding certain AS that need elucidation [28]. Based on a high level of clinical evidence for CYP3A5, CYP2B6, CYP2C9, CYP2C19, and CYP2D6 enzymes, CPIC has developed evidence-based guidelines for the PGx testing before the prescription of some substrate drugs, as listed in Table 1 [1, 14].

Gene polymorphisms of transporters and drug receptors are associated with the phenotype of slow or rapid drug absorption and poor or effective interac-tion with receptors, respectively. Thus, polymorphisms in genes of transport and receptor molecules result in three types of phenotypes, normal, enhanced, and decreased function [26]. For now, numerous polymorphisms of genes that alter the activity and physiological function of both transporters and receptors were dis-covered; however, their importance for clinical practice has not been sufficiently investigated and adequately evidenced. Only a few gene-drug pairs have available evidence-based clinical practice guidelines [14].

Table 1 Examples of genes-drugs pairs with the highest level of clinical relevance (according to CPIC publicly available data)

Classification of genes	Example of genes	Drug examples	Effect
I. Genes involved in the first phase of drug metabolism—cytochrome P450 enzymes	CYP2C9	Phenytoin Warfarin NSAIDs	Certain genotype may influence drug-substrate metabolism—consequent
	CYP2C19	Amitriptyline (Es)citalopram, sertraline Clopidogrel[a] Voriconazole Proton pump inhibitors	
	CYP2D6	TCA Atomoxetine Codeine[a], tramadol[a] Fluvoxamine, paroxetine Ondansetron, tropisetron Tamoxifen[a]	
	CYP3A5	Tacrolimus	
	CYP4F2	Warfarin	
II. Genes involved in the second phase of drug metabolism	UGT1A1	Atazanavir	Safety–risk of hyperbilirubinemia
III. Other genes involved in drug metabolism	TPMT/NUDT15	Azathioprine** Mercaptopurine** Thioguanine**	Efficacy and safety
	DPYD	Capecitabine Tegafur Fluorouracil	Safety—increased drug toxicity
IV. Genes for drug transporters	SLCO1B1	Simvastatin	Safety – risk of myopathy
V. Genes for drug targets	VKORC1	Warfarin	Efficacy
	CFTR	Ivacaftor*	Efficacy
VI. Genes for other proteins important for drug action and	HLA-A	(Ox)carbamazepine	Safety—increased risk of SJS/TEN
	HLA-B	(Ox)carbamazepine* Abacavir* Phenytoin Allopurinol	Safety—increased risk of SJS/TEN
	IFNL3	Peginterferon-alfa2A and 2B Ribavirin	Efficacy

(continued)

Table 1 (continued)

Classification of genes	Example of genes	Drug examples	Effect
	G6PD	Rasburicase*	Toxicity—risk of hemolysis
	CACNA1S/ RyR1	Inhalational anesthetics Suxamethonium	Toxicity—increased risk of malignant hyperthermia
	mtRNR1	Aminoglycosides	Toxicity—risk of hearing loss

TCA tricyclic antidepressants; *NSAID* non-steroidal anti-inflammatory drugs; *SJS/TEN* Steven-Johnson syndrome/toxic epidermal necrolysis
*Testing required (according to FDA); **testing recommended (according to FDA)
^aEnzyme involved in activation of the drug

4   Gene/Drug Interaction—Level of Evidence for the Development of Pharmacotherapeutic Guidelines

The application of pharmacogenetics in clinical practice confronts several challenges and obstacles. They include, but are not limited to difficulties in the interpretation of the pharmacogenetic test results, pricing/reimbursement, unavailability of the genetic tests, low level of education in pharmacogenomics, or unclear guidelines. Therefore, experts from different professions working together on the systematic collection of results of pharmacogenomic studies and meta-analyses develop guidelines that provide a basis for applying evidence-based PGx results in clinical practice and help clinicians to understand, interpret, and transform the information obtained by genetic testing into clinical decision.

CPIC publishes the latest evidence-based data and develops guidelines for the use of drugs following the results of PGx tests [14]. The level of significance of clinical evidence is presented in several categories. Categories derive from clear criteria depending on the number and quality of scientific papers, the size of groups of subjects, the results of meta-analyses that confirmed the importance of pharmacogenetic testing of gene/drug interaction, and clinical utility after testing. According to the CPIC, four categories of recommendations have been established; A, B, C, and D, and means the following [13, 29]:

- *Category A*—genetic information should be used to change the prescription of a drug (adjusted dose or use of an alternative drug) with strong or moderate evidence.
- *Category B*—genetic information can be used to change the prescription of a drug; however, with weaker and conflicting evidence.

- *Categories C and D* of the gene/drug relationship do not have sufficient evidence for pharmacogenetic testing; therefore, there are no recommendations for changes in drug prescribing.

PharmaGKB evidence levels for gene-drug pairs are divided into six categories: 1A, 1B, 2A, 2B, 3, 4 [30]:

- *1A*—the highest clinical level of evidence—before starting therapy, it is indicated to take a genetic test and to follow the guidelines of relevant sources.
- *1B*—clinical level of evidence—genetic testing is recommended as there is clinical evidence of at least one cohort study with statistically relevant significance. The recommendation may apply to all or only a specific subset of patients, and the clinical benefit of testing is likely.
- *2A*—clinical level of evidence—available research information indicates that genetic testing is not necessary, but information obtained from testing may be relevant to treatment efficacy, dosing, or toxicity in all or some patients.
- *2B*—clinical level of evidence—available research information suggests that the polymorphic gene is involved in drug metabolism or pharmacodynamics, but without suggestions on a possible effect on the therapeutic response.
- *3 and 4*—clinical levels of evidence—available information is insufficient to issue a pharmacogenetic testing proposal.

The CPIC suggested a three-layer scheme that assesses the quality of the evidence, linking drug-related phenotypes and certain genetic variations, as follows [13]:

- *"Level 1* evidence contains consistent results from well-designed, well-conducted studies" (CPIC A, PharmaGKB 1A, 1B)—a strong recommendation;
- *"Level 2* evidence is sufficient to determine the effects, but the strength of the evidence is limited by the number, quality, or consistency of individual studies, the inability to generalize to routine practice, or the indirect nature of evidence" (CPIC B; PharmaGKB 2A, 2B)—moderate recommendation;
- *"Level 3* evidence is insufficient to assess effects on treatment outcomes due to a limited number of studies, low strength of studies, deficiencies in their design, gaps in the evidence collected, etc." (CPIC C and D; PharmaGKB 3 and 4)—the recommendation for application is optional.

To date, CPIC guidelines have been published for about 80 gene/drug pairs with a high level of clinical evidence and a strong recommendation [14].

5 Conclusion

Undoubtedly, in the last twenty years, pharmacogenetics has attracted attention as a discipline that can contribute to the quality of patient health care and present an important part of the personalized medicine concept. Research has shown that many health professionals consider pharmacogenomics as relevant in clinical practice, but also showed the need for additional educational activities to help interpret PGx results and raise the overall competence of all involved in providing care to patients [31]. These could result in more comprehensive implementation of pharmacogenomics into everyday clinical practice, better treatment efficacy, and lower ADRs, which would lead to lower health system costs. Current pharmacogenetic implementation programs already offer a variety of educational resources. Consortia, such as CPIC, DPWG, and the CPNDS, provide guidelines for gene/drug pairs that clearly define which genetic profiles or haplotypes need testing for a drug of interest, how to translate pharmacogenomic results into a phenotype, and how to apply data to clinical decision-making [32].

The application of pharmacogenetics in advancing the concept of personalized medicine also depends on the ability of clinical laboratories to provide accurate, applicable, and timely PGx information [1]. Systematic implementation of preventive pharmacogenomic testing requires greater standardization of the tested gene variants by setting simple instructions for using genotype translation tables in a clinical phenotype and results interpretation.

Pharmacogenetics efficacy assessments provide evidence of the economic benefits of genotype-driven treatment. Currently, the prices of a single pharmacogenetic test are acceptable, but the cost of pharmacogenomic panels is still relatively high. With their more comprehensive application, accompanied by the advancement of technology, the implementation of PGx will be more cost-effective in the future. Wider implementation must be accompanied with robust cost-effectiveness analyses to inform policymakers on how to allocate resources effectively [33]. Implementation of pharmacogenetics in clinical decision-making, along with other "omics", like transcriptomics, proteomics, epigenomics, and metabolomics, will change the face of modern medicine.

References

1. Primorac D, Bach-Rojecky L, Vađunec D, Juginović A, Žunić K, Matišić V, et al. Pharmacogenomics at the center of precision medicine: challenges and perspective in an era of Big Data. Pharmacogenomics. 2020;21(2):141–56. https://doi.org/10.2217/pgs-2019-0134.
2. Hood L, Friend SH. Predictive, personalized, preventive, participatory (P4) cancer medicine. Nat Rev Clin Oncol. 2011;8(3):184–7.
3. International Conference on Harmonisation. Guidance on E15 pharmacogenomics definitions and sample coding; availability. Notice Fed Regist. 2008;73:19074–76.
4. Carrasco-Ramiro F, Peiró-Pastor R, Aguado B. Human genomics projects and precision medicine. Gene Ther. 2017;24(9):551–61.

5. Plumpton CO, Roberts D, Pirmohamed M, Hughes DA. A systematic review of economic evaluations of pharmacogenetic testing for prevention of adverse drug reactions. Pharmacoeconomics. 2016;34(8):771–93. https://doi.org/10.1007/s40273-016-0397-9.

6. Lazarou J, Pomeranz BH, Corey PN. Incidence of adverse drug reactions in hospitalized patients: a meta-analysis of prospective studies. JAMA. 1998;279(15):1200–5. https://doi.org/10.1001/jama.279.15.1200

7. Cacabelos R, Cacabelos N, Carril JC. The role of pharmacogenomics in adverse drug reactions. Expert Rev Clin Pharmacol. 2019;12(5):407–42. https://doi.org/10.1080/17512433.2019.1597706.

8. Thorn CF, Klein TE, Altman RB. PharmGKB: the pharmacogenomics knowledge base. Methods Mol Biol. 2013;1015:311–20. https://doi.org/10.1007/978-1-62703-435-7_20.

9. FDA. https://www.fda.gov/drugs/science-and-research-drugs/table-pharmacogenomic-biomarkers-drug-labeling. Accessed 2 Apr 2022

10. ICPERMED International Consortium. https://www.icpermed.eu/. Accessed 2 Apr 2022

11. Johnson JA, Cavallari LH. Pharmacogenetics and cardiovascular disease–implications for personalized medicine. Pharmacol Rev. 2013;65(3):987–1009. https://doi.org/10.1124/pr.112.007252.

12. Swen JJ, Wilting I, de Goede AL, Grandia L, Mulder H, Touw DJ, et al. Pharmacogenetics: from bench to byte. Clin Pharmacol Ther. 2008;83(5):781–7. https://doi.org/10.1038/sj.clpt.6100507.

13. Relling MV, Klein TE. CPIC: Clinical pharmacogenetics implementation consortium of the pharmacogenomics research network. Clin Pharmacol Ther. 2011;89(3):464–7. https://doi.org/10.1038/clpt.2010.279.

14. CPIC-Guideliines. https://cpicpgx.org/guidelines/. Accessed 2 Apr 2022

15. Arbitrio M, Di Martino MT, Scionti F, Barbieri V, Pensabene L, Tagliaferri P. Pharmacogenomic profiling of ADME gene variants: current challenges and validation perspectives. High Throughput. 2018;7(4):40. https://doi.org/10.3390/ht7040040.

16. van der Lee M, Kriek M, Guchelaar HJ, Swen JJ. Technologies for Pharmacogenomics: A Review. Genes (Basel). 2020;11(12):1456. https://doi.org/10.3390/genes11121456.

17. Arbitrio M, Di Martino MT, Scionti F, Agapito G, Hiram Guzzi P, Cannataro M, et al. DMETTM (Drug Metabolism Enzymes and Transporters): a pharmacogenomic platform for precision medicine. Oncotarget. 2016;7:54028–50. https://doi.org/10.18632/oncotarget.9927

18. Lin CH, Yeakley JM, McDaniel TK, Shen R. Medium- to high-throughput SNP genotyping using VeraCode microbeads. Methods Mol Biol. 2009;496:129–42. https://doi.org/10.1007/978-1-59745-553-4_10.

19. Maciel A, Cullors A, Lukowiak AA, Garces J. Estimating cost savings of pharmacogenetic testing for depression in real-world clinical settings. Neuropsychiatr Dis Treat. 2018;14:225–30. https://doi.org/10.2147/NDT.S145046.

20. Personalized Prescriptions with the RightMed® Solution. https://oneome.com/home-international/ Accessed 2 Apr 2022

21. ThermoFisher Scientific. Pharmacoscan Assay. https://www.thermofisher.com/order/catalog/product/903010TS. Accessed 2 Apr 2022

22. Campanella P, Lovato E, Marone C, Fallacara L, Mancuso A, Ricciardi W, Specchia ML. The impact of electronic health records on healthcare quality: a systematic review and meta-analysis. Eur J Public Health. 2016;26(1):60–4. https://doi.org/10.1093/eurpub/ckv122.

23. Hingorani AD, Kuan V, Finan C. Improving the odds of drug development success through human genomics: modelling study. Sci Rep. 2019;9:18911. https://doi.org/10.1038/s41598-019-54849-w

24. Rollinson V, Turner R, Pirmohamed M. Pharmacogenomics for primary care: an overview. Genes (Basel). 2020;11(11):1337. https://doi.org/10.3390/genes11111337.

25. Gray KA, Yates B, Seal RL, Wright MW, Bruford EA. Genenames.org: the HGNC resources in 2015. Nucleic Acids Res. 2015; 43(Database issue):D1079–85. https://doi.org/10.1093/nar/gku1071

26. Zanger UM, Schwab M. Cytochrome P450 enzymes in drug metabolism: regulation of gene expression, enzyme activities, and impact of genetic variation. Pharmacol Therapy. 2013;138:103–41. https://doi.org/10.1016/j.pharmthera.2012.12.007.
27. Caudle KE, Dunnenberger HM, Freimuth RR, Peterson JF, Burlison JD, Whirl-Carrillo M, et al. Standardizing terms for clinical pharmacogenetic test results: consensus terms from the Clinical Pharmacogenetics Implementation Consortium (CPIC). Genet Med. 2017;19(2):215–23. https://doi.org/10.1038/gim.2016.87.
28. Gaedigk A, Dinh JC, Jeong H, Prasad B, Leeder JS. Ten years' experience with the CYP2D6 activity score: a perspective on future investigations to improve clinical predictions for precision therapeutics. J Pers Med. 2018;8(2):15. https://doi.org/10.3390/jpm80200.
29. Prioritization. https://cpicpgx.org/prioritization/#leveldef. Accessed 2 Apr 2022
30. Whirl-Carrillo M, McDonagh EM, Hebert JM, et al. Pharmacogenomics knowledge for personalized medicine. Clin Pharmacol Ther. 2012;92(4):414–7. https://doi.org/10.1038/clpt.201 2.96.
31. Just KS, Steffens M, Swen JJ, Patrinos GP, Guchelaar HJ, Stingl JC. Medical education in pharmacogenomics-results from a survey on pharmacogenetic knowledge in healthcare professionals within the European pharmacogenomics clinical implementation project Ubiquitous Pharmacogenomics (U-PGx). Eur J Clin Pharmacol. 2017;73(10):1247–52. https://doi.org/10. 1007/s00228-017-2292-5.
32. Primorac D, Höppner W, editors. Pharmacogenetics in clinical practice: experience with 55 commonly used drugs. Zagreb, Hamburg, Philadelphia: St. Catherine Specialty Hospital, Bioglobe GmbH, ISABS; 2022. https://www.stcatherine.com/centre-of-excellence/10/ind ividualized-and-preventive-medicine/pharmacogenomics/69. Accessed 2 Apr 2022
33. Turongkaravee S, Jittikoon J, Rochanathimoke O, Boyd K, Wu O, Chaikledkaew U. Pharmacogenetic testing for adverse drug reaction prevention: systematic review of economic evaluations and the appraisal of quality matters for clinical practice and implementation. BMC Health Serv Res. 2021;21(1):1042. https://doi.org/10.1186/s12913-021-07025-8.

Principles of Xenobiotic Metabolism (Biotransformation)

Mirza Bojić, Željko Debeljak, and F. Peter Guengerich

Abstract

This chapter provides a general overview of metabolic reactions and their significance. Basic concepts and terminology related to biotransformation, activity, and toxicity are explained and discussed. Major enzymes involved in oxidation, reduction, hydrolytic, and conjugation are covered including enzyme nomenclature, localization, catalytic cycle, coenzymes, relevance of individual enzymes, types of reactions, substrates and metabolites, influence of metabolic reactions on the activity/toxicity of xenobiotics, enzyme inhibition, and relevance if applicable.

Keywords

Oxidation · Reduction · Conjugation · Metabolic enzymes · Drug metabolism

M. Bojić
Department of Medicinal Chemistry, University of Zagreb Faculty of Pharmacy and Biochemistry, Zagreb, Croatia

Ž. Debeljak
Clinical Institute of Laboratory Diagnostics, Clinical Hospital Center Osijek, Osijek, Croatia

Department of Pharmacology, Josip Juraj Strossmayer University of Osijek Faculty of Medicine, Osijek, Croatia

F. P. Guengerich (✉)
Department of Biochemistry, Vanderbilt University School of Medicine, Nashville, TN, USA
e-mail: f.guengerich@vanderbilt.edu

© The Author(s), under exclusive license to Springer Nature Switzerland AG 2023
D. Primorac et al. (eds.), *Pharmacogenomics in Clinical Practice*,
https://doi.org/10.1007/978-3-031-45903-0_2

1 Introduction

Humans are continuously exposed to xenobiotics. Xenobiotics are substances foreign to an organism, i.e., substances that are not needed for the maintenance of normal physiological processes; the opposite term is endogenous agent or endobiotic, which includes proteins and amino acids, carbohydrates, fats, vitamins, and minerals. The role and destiny of endobiotics are usually studied as a part of biochemistry, while xenobiotics are of interest primarily due to their biological, beneficial, or toxic effects and are studied as a part of pharmacology (pharmacodynamics, pharmacokinetics) and toxicology. Consequently, some of the most studied xenobiotics are drugs (both medicinal and illicit), pesticides, and organic solvents.

Organisms have developed two major mechanisms, on the cellular level, to prevent systemic exposure to xenobiotics—transport proteins and metabolic enzymes. Transport proteins or transporters prevent absorption or facilitate excretion of xenobiotics or their metabolites, while the metabolic enzymes generally convert lipophilic xenobiotics to hydrophilic products (metabolites) that are consequently easier to eliminate through urine or bile. The reaction in which organism transforms xenobiotic into a metabolite is called biotransformation or metabolic reaction [1].

Metabolic reactions are divided into two major groups: oxidoreductions and conjugations. Previously, these were referred to as Phase 1 (oxidations, reductions, hydrolysis) and Phase 2 (conjugations, reactions with glutathione) reactions. This terminology is still in use. However, we stress that its use is discouraged [2], for the following reasons:

– Phase terminology was introduced to differentiate bioactivation reactions that could produce a toxic substance (Phase 1) for conjugations (phase 2) that were regarded reactions of detoxication. There are numerous examples that show the opposite, such as 2-aminofluorene, which induces tumors in animal models. 2-Aminofluorene is toxic due to conjugation reactions (glucuronidation, sulfoconjugation, and acetylation) that result in generation of a nitrenium ion;
– Although Phase 1 reactions are regarded as activations, they can also result in inactive products, while the Phase 2 reactions can produce metabolites that are more potent compared to parent compound, e.g., morphine 6-O-glucuronide is more potent than morphine itself;
– Phase 2 reactions were regarded to follow Phase 1 reactions in sequence. However, some xenobiotics do not necessarily go through Phase 1 reactions at all, e.g., acetaminophen (paracetamol) used in normal doses undergoes glucuronidation and sulfoconjugation (Fig. 1) or when glucuronidation precedes oxidation as it is the case with gemfibrozil;
– Not all metabolic reactions fit the concept. Phase 1 reactions introduce new functional groups to the substrate, but in the case of hydrolysis a group is not

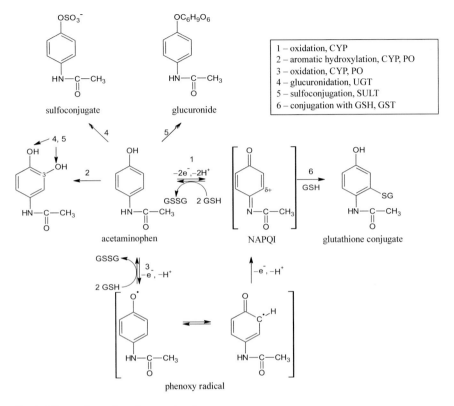

Fig. 1 Biotransformation of acetaminophen

introduced, rather liberated. Phase 2 reactions require activation of the conjugating agent; however, that is not the case in conjugation reactions with
glutathione.

As the role of the metabolism is to minimize the exposure of the body to the xenobiotic, major metabolic enzymes are located in the liver and gut. On the cellular
level, metabolic enzymes are either situated on intracellular membranes or in the
cytoplasm. In principle, the membrane enzymes process more lipophilic and the
cytoplasmic enzymes process more hydrophilic substrates.

Metabolic enzymes are proteins that catalyze metabolic reactions. The active
site can be part of protein (e.g., carboxylesterase) or a prosthetic group that is
bound to the apoprotein (e.g., heme in cytochromes P450). Prosthetic groups
catalyze the transfer of electrons or activated conjugating group. A good example is the cofactor nicotinamide adenine dinucleotide phosphate (NADPH), which
represents a source of electrons required for the oxidation by cytochromes P450
(cofactors are distinguished from prosthetic groups in that they appear in the overall reaction stoichiometry). Uridine 5′-diphosphoglucuronic acid (UDPGA) is an

example of activated form of glucuronic acid (a cofactor) in conjugation reactions that are termed glucuronidations.

Metabolic enzymes are susceptible to induction and inhibition, which, respectively, result in elevation or reduction of enzyme activity. Induction is achieved through ligand (xenobiotic) binding to a nuclear receptor, whose activation frequently results in increased expression of group of enzymes. Often xenobiotics (as well as endobiotics) are autoinducers, i.e., they induce their own metabolism. In hyperbilirubinemia, bilirubin is an autoinducer of UGT1A1 enzyme. The majority of anticonvulsants (antiepileptics) also cause autoinduction. Since the liver is the major metabolic organ, antiepileptics consequently require monitoring of hepatic function (liver function tests). Inhibition of metabolic enzymes can cause accumulation of drug in systemic circulation and consequently increased side/toxic effects or lack of pharmacological effect (prodrugs). Warfarin is a good example of such interactions if used with a CYP2C9 inhibitor (fluconazole) [3]. Due to the inhibition of CYP2C9, metabolic elimination of warfarin is blocked, and the pharmacological effect of warfarin is prolonged, increasing the risk of bleeding. Reversible inhibition can be resolved by simple discontinuation of treatment with the drug causing inhibition, while irreversible inhibition requires enzyme biosynthesis.

Some metabolic enzymes exhibit genetic polymorphism—variation in gene sequence that is present in at least 1% of the population and influences enzyme activity. "Extensive" metabolizers have enzyme activity in the majority of population, "poor" metabolizers have reduced enzyme activity, and "rapid" and "ultrarapid" metabolizers have increased enzyme activity. CYP2D6 and CYP2C19 are well-known examples of cytochromes P450 susceptible to clinically significant polymorphism [4].

Biotransformation of xenobiotics can include non-enzymatic reactions, such as hydrolysis or conjugation of glutathione with reactive substrates. Some xenobiotics undergo biotransformation catalyzed by enzymes involved in physiological processes. Examples are antimetabolites (i.e., enzyme inhibitors), nucleoside cytostatics, and immunosuppressants.

In this chapter, we will focus on metabolic enzymes involved in oxidation, reduction, hydrolytic, and conjugation reactions.

2   Oxidations

Biotransformation of over 90% of drugs in humans involves oxidation reactions [5]. Major enzymes involved in oxidations are cytochrome P450, alcohol dehydrogenase, aldehyde dehydrogenase, peroxidase, xanthine oxidoreductase, aldehyde oxidase, flavin-containing monooxygenase, and monoamine oxidase (Table 1). Each (super)family involved in oxidation reactions will be discussed: nomenclature, localization, catalytic cycle, coenzymes and prosthetic groups, relevance of individual enzymes, types of reactions, substrates and metabolites, influence of

Table 1 Overview of enzymes involved in oxidation reactions

Enzyme	Oxygen source/ Coenzyme	Reaction	Substrate
Cytochrome P450 (CYP)	O_2, NADPH	Oxidations, reductions, deaminations, dealkylations, aliphatic and aromatic hydroxylations, oxidation of heteroatoms, etc	Numerous xenobiotics including drugs
Alcohol dehydrogenase (ADH)	Substrate, NADH	Oxidation of simple alcohols and reduction of simple aldehydes	Ethanol, ethambutol, and vitamin B6
Aldehyde dehydrogenase (ALDH)	H_2O, NADH	Oxidation of simple aldehydes	Chloral hydrate
Xanthine oxidoreductase (XOR)	OH^-	Purine oxidations	Hypoxanthine, alopurinol, and mercaptopurine
Aldehyde oxidase (AO)	OH^-	Purine oxidations	Nicotine, 6-methylpurin
Flavin monooxygenase (FMO)	O_2, NADPH	Oxidations of heteroatom	Xenobiotics containing heteroatoms
Monoamine oxidase (MAO)	H_2O	Deamination of primary amines	Tyramine, sumatriptan, and primaquine

metabolic reactions on the activity/toxicity of xenobiotics, and enzyme inhibition and its relevance if applicable.

2.1   Cytochrome P450

Cytochromes P450 were discovered and characterized during period 1950/1960 [6]. The name was derived from their properties; structurally they contain heme as prosthetic group, which is characteristic of cytochromes, are red-colored pigments, and have an absorption maximum in reduced difference spectra at 450 nm. Cytochromes P450 contain iron that is tightly bound to heme (four bonds) and a cysteine residue of the apoprotein, while the sixth coordination site is used for the activation of molecular oxygen, which will usually be incorporated into the substrate. These enzymes are located on intracellular membranes, most notably the smooth endoplasmic reticulum (ER) and mitochondria. There are some significant differences between enzyme systems located in mitochondria and the ER, and further discussion in this chapter will focus on the latter one as it is more generally involved in metabolism of drugs.

Although cytochromes P450 can catalyze a plethora of reactions, they are primarily monooxygenases, i.e., they incorporate one oxygen atom into substrate from molecular oxygen:

$$RH + O_2 + NADPH + H^+ \xrightarrow{CYP} ROH + H_2O + NADP^+$$

NADPH serves as a source of electrons that enables reduction of iron from the ferric to ferrous form. Transfer of electrons is facilitated by the NADPH reductase and sometimes cytochrome b_5.

At first cytochromes P450 were named by the substrate and reaction they catalyze, e.g., CYP3A4 was named nifedipine oxidase when first discovered. Over the years, as the number of cytochromes P450 expanded, their substrates and reactions catalyzed also grew, prompting the need for the introduction of cytochrome P450 nomenclature [7]. The cytochrome P450 superfamily was abbreviated CYP, and further division was into families, subfamilies, and individual enzymes based on genetic similarity/amino acid sequence, e.g., CYP2D6:

CYP	Superfamily
CYP2	Family ($\geq$40% similarity)
CYP2D	Subfamily ($\geq$55% similarity)
CYP2D6	Enzyme ($\geq$98% similarity of variants)

Obviously, cytochromes P450 (as well as other metabolic enzymes) do not fit the lock-and-key model as they have large number of substrates susceptible to different types of reactions. Quite often scientific literature will refer to CYP2D6 as an isoform or isoenzyme. These terms may go well with the lock-and-key model (i.e., different enzymes that catalyze the same reaction), but in light of the cytochrome P450 nomenclature, this should be avoided, and each cytochrome P450 should be referred as an individual enzyme.

When the human genome sequence was delineated 20 years ago, the exact number of cytochrome P450 genes was determined to be 57, although the roles (substrates and reaction types) are not known for all of them. In these cases, the enzymes are often referred to as orphans. Not all cytochromes P450 are equally involved in drug metabolism. CYP3A4 is the most important enzyme, catalyzing biotransformation of roughly one-third of registered drugs. Together, CYP3A4, CYP2D6, CYP2C19, CYP2C8, and CYP2C9 are involved in oxidative metabolism of over 90% of drugs [5].

Two of the major characteristics of cytochromes P450 can be described by two terms—promiscuity and laziness. Cytochromes P450 are promiscuous in that they have numerous partners, i.e., metabolize numerous drugs. Consequently, drugs that are metabolized by the same cytochrome P450 can interact with each other and sometimes cause clinically significant interactions if used concomitantly. Laziness refers to relatively slow metabolic reactions, which is a preferable characteristic for once-a-day dosed medications. As an alternative in this anthropomorphic description, one could consider the drug-metabolizing cytochrome P450 enzymes as "yeoman-like," in that they are present to do many hard, general tasks without grudging.

The CYP3A subfamily includes CYP3A4, CYP3A5, CYP3A7, and CYP3A43. CYP3A4 and CYP3A5 are involved in metabolism of xenobiotics in adults. Their substrate selection mostly overlaps, i.e., substrates of CYP3A4 are usually substrates of CYP3A5 and vice versa. However, catalytic efficacy is usually higher in case of CYP3A4. The list of CYP3A4 substrates is extensive and among others includes antihyperlipidemic statins (atorvastatin, lovastatin, and simvastatin), antihypertensives, and antiarrhythmics like calcium channel blockers (amiodarone, amlodipine, diltiazem, nifedipine, and verapamil), opioid analgesics (hydrocodone, oxycodone, and tramadol), HIV antiretrovirals (atazanavir, efavirenz, ritonavir, and saquinavir), immunosuppressants (cyclosporine, tacrolimus, and sirolimus), and phosphodiesterase 5 (PDE5) inhibitors used for treatment of erectile dysfunction (sildenafil and tadalafil) [3].

CYP3A4 is induced by anticonvulsants (carbamazepine, oxcarbazepine, phenobarbitone, and phenytoin), the tuberculostatic rifampin, and the herbal antidepressant St. John's wort [3]. If a CYP3A4 inducer is used with CYP3A4 opioid substrates, the metabolism of opioids will increase and lead to decrease or lack of analgesic effect. If dose augmentation is necessary, caution is needed as opioids can cause respiratory depression.

Common inhibitors of CYP3A4 are macrolide antibiotics (clarithromycin and erythromycin, but not azithromycin), azole antifungals, calcium channel blockers, and HIV antiretrovirals, as well as grapefruit juice [3]. If CYP3A4 inhibitors are used with PDE5 inhibitors (substrates of CYP3A4), the dose of the PDE5 inhibitor should be half of normal starting dose, in that the decreased metabolism can increase side effects such as headache, dizziness, and risk of falls and injury. Ritonavir is a low potency protease inhibitor that is used as a booster in HIV therapy; it is a stronger CYP3A4 inhibitor compared to other protease inhibitors. Consequently, it can be used as a booster in triple therapy even in fixed combinations (e.g., with lopinavir).

CYP2D6 is involved in the metabolism of opioid analgesics (codeine, hydrocodone, meperidine, oxycodone, and tramadol), antipsychotics, and antidepressants such as aripiprazole, doxepin, fluoxetine, haloperidol, risperidone, trazadone, and tricyclic antidepressants. Amiodaron, paroxetine, and quinidine are inhibitors of CYP2D6. Some of the substrates (doxepin and fluoxetine) are inhibitors of metabolism of other drug substrates of this enzyme. Contrary to most other cytochromes P450 involved in drug metabolism, CYP2D6 is not inducible [3]. CYP2D6 is a highly polymorphic enzyme, and ultrarapid metabolizers have greater pharmacological effects of analgesic prodrugs (codeine and tramadol). This can have fatal consequences on neonates of breastfeeding mothers who are CYP2D6 ultrarapid metabolizers, as exemplified by a fatal case in Canada. Due to rapid conversion of codeine to morphine, the risk of opioid toxicity increases. On the other hand, in the case of poor metabolizers, the analgesic prodrugs lack efficacy.

CYP2C19 is involved in the metabolism of clopidogrel (activation of the prodrug), omeprazole, and voriconazole, among others. Its expression can be induced by anticonvulsants and rifampin, while the substrates omeprazole and its S-enantiomer (esomeprazole) also act as inhibitors. CYP2C19 is also highly polymorphic, and patients with variants *2 and *3 who are poor metabolizers and have higher incidence of cardiovascular events, in that clopidogrel fails to undergo oxidation of its thiophen ring [8]. Alternative therapy ought to be considered.

CYP2C9 is the major enzyme involved in metabolism of the anti-coagulant warfarin. It is induced by many common inducers of CYP3A4. Clinically relevant inhibitors include amiodarone, fluconazole, metronidazole, and trimethoprim/sulfamethoxazole. A combination of amiodarone and warfarin results in decreased metabolism of warfarin, and the risk of bleeding increases. Depending on the international normalized ratio (INR), the adjustment of warfarin dose is required. As CYP2C9 is polymorphic, patients with *2 and *3 alleles require dose reduction at the initiation of the warfarin pharmacotherapy [9].

2.2   Alcohol and Aldehyde Dehydrogenases

Alcohol dehydrogenase (ADH) is a dimer, and each polypeptide chain contains zinc in the active site. These enzymes are mainly located in liver, where they are cytosolic enzymes. ADH oxidizes primary alcohols to aldehydes, and this reaction is reversible:

$$RCH_2OH + NAD^+ \overset{ADH}{\longleftrightarrow} RCHO + NADH + H^+$$

Aldehyde dehydrogenase (ALDH) oxidizes aldehydes to carboxylic acids. There are 19 ALDH enzymes in human genome. ALDH2 is a polymorphic enzyme, especially in East Asian populations. ALDHs are mainly located in in the cytosol and mitochondria, as well as tumor tissues. Oxidation reactions catalyzed by ADH are irreversible:

$$RCHO + NAD^+ + H_2O \overset{ALDH}{\longrightarrow} RCOOH + NADH + H^+$$

When the concentration of ethanol is low, ADH metabolizes ethanol to acetaldehyde which is further converted to acetic acid by ALDH. If the concentration of ethanol is high, other enzymes such as CYP2E1 and catalase can also be involved in its oxidation. Oxidation of ethanol by ADH is pH dependent: if the pH is high, oxidation is preferred, while reduction of acetaldehyde is preferred at physiological pH. However, as oxidation of acetaldehyde to acetic acid is fast, oxidation of ethanol by ADH is favored [1].

ADH and ALDH are involved in the oxidation of the tuberculostatic ethambutol, as well as vitamin B6 (pyridoxine). Fomepizole is an ADH inhibitor, used as antidote in case of methanol or ethylene glycol poisoning. Disulfiram is an ALDH inhibitor used in aversion therapy for alcoholism. In presence of disulfiram, acetaldehyde starts accumulating and causing toxic effects when even small quantities of ethanol have been ingested. The uroantiseptic metronidazole also inhibits ALDH, causing disulfiram like effect in presence of alcohol. Thus, use of alcohol with metronidazole is contraindicated [10].

2.3　Peroxidases

Peroxidases (PO) are enzymes that reduce peroxides (note that R1 can be H, so that the substrate is a hydroperoxide):

$$R_1OOR_2 + 2H^+ + 2e^- \xrightarrow{PO} R_1OH + R_2OH$$

They show diversity as well as specificity, based on the active site structure and accessibility. Some peroxidases are heme-containing enzymes that enable oxidation of substrates; the source of oxygen is peroxide and catalytic cycle by electron transfer from to iron as well protoporphyrin. Although the extent of oxidations catalyzed by peroxidases is not comparable to cytochromes P450, peroxidases are well distributed extrahepatically where they can cause toxic effects. One of the enzymes involved in the extrahepatic metabolism of acetaminophen (paracetamol) is a peroxidase, prostaglandin H synthase, that also metabolizes acetaminophen into *N*-acetyl-*p*-benzoquinone imine (NAPQI, Fig. 1). NAPQI generated by peroxidases is responsible for nephrotoxicity, while the enzyme involved in hepatotoxicity is CYP2E1. Peroxidases are also involved in toxicity of phenylbutazone, diethylstilbestrol, phenytoin, thalidomide, and cyclophosphamide [1].

2.4　Xanthine Oxidoreductase and Aldehyde Oxidase

Xanthine oxidoreductase (XOR) and aldehyde oxidase (AO) are molybdenum-containing hydroxylases:

$$RH + OH^- \xrightarrow{XOR/AO} ROH + H^+ + 2e^-$$

XOR and AO are involved in oxidation of electron-deficient carbon atoms within nitrogen-containing heterocycles such as pyrroles, pyridines, pyrimidines, purines, and pteridines. AO is involved in metabolism of aromatic cyclic substrates (e.g., 6-methylpurine, nicotine), while aliphatic aldehydes are substrates of aldehyde dehydrogenase (ALDH).

XOR is mainly involved in the catabolism of purine bases. It oxidizes cyclic carbon atoms bound to nitrogen, producing lactam metabolites. Substrates include purines (alopurinol, 6-mercaptopurine), xanthines (hypoxanthine, xanthines, and monomethylated xanthines), pyridoxal, and *N*-methyl nicotinamide.

Allopurinol is a substrate and inhibitor of XOR that is used for treatment of gout. The metabolite, oxypurinol, also acts as an irreversible inhibitor of XOR. It inhibits oxidation of xanthines and hypoxanthines to uric acid, decreasing the concentration of urates that accumulate and crystalize in joints causing inflammation [11]. Azathioprine and 6-mercapropurine can be combined with allopurinol to reduce their dose and toxicity. However, caution is needed because other polymorphic enzymes (thiopurine methyltransferase) are involved in metabolism.

2.5   Flavin-Containing Monooxygenase

Flavin monooxygenases (FMOs) are, along with cytochromes P450, major enzymes involved in metabolism of amines. FMO is monomer containing flavin adenine dinucleotide (FAD) as a prosthetic group. The reaction stoichiometry is similar to that of most cytochromes P450:

$$RX + O_2 + NADPH + H^+ \xrightarrow{FMO} RXO + H_2O + NADP^+$$

FMO catalyzes oxidations of cyclic and acyclic amines at physiological pH. Cytochromes P450 preferentially oxidize nitrogen in aromatic heterocycles. Tertiary amines are oxidized to N-oxides (e.g., imipramine and chlorpromazine), secondary amines are converted to hydroxylamines and nitrones (e.g., methamphetamine), and primary amines are metabolized to hydroxylamines and oximes (e.g., amphetamine and phentermine).

FMO3 is one of the major FMOs involved in metabolism of drugs and is polymorphic. Trimethylamine is a degradation product of amino acids present in fish, as well as a FMO3 substrate. It is one of the chemicals that humans can sense in low ppm concentrations and has a characteristic fish odor. The N-oxide metabolite is less volatile and odorless. If a patient has reduced FMO3 activity, trimethylamine will accumulate in excretes (trimethylaminuria), and the patient will produce a characteristic fish odor [12].

2.6   Monoamine Oxidase

Monoamine oxidase (MAO) catalyzes cleavage of C-N bonds, i.e., oxidative deamination, another type of reactions that is preferentially catalyzed by cytochromes P450.

$$RCH_2NH_2 + H_2O + FAD \xrightarrow{MAO} RCHO + NH_3 + FADH_2$$

MOAs are mitochondrial membrane enzymes, located primarily in brain. Xenobiotics, metabolized by MAO, includes β-blockers and metabolites, sumatriptan, phenelzine, almotriptan, bicifadine, citalopram, and its active metabolite desmethylcitalopram, rizatriptan, ozanimod, and zolmitriptan. However, the major significance of MAO is in the biotransformation of biogenic amines, in that MAO inhibitors are used as antidepressants. MAO inhibition increases the concentrations of epinephrine, norepinephrine, dopamine, and serotonin. If MAO inhibitors are used with serotonin-norepinephrine reuptake inhibitors, tricyclic antidepressants, or stimulants (amphetamines), increased concentrations of epinephrine, norepinephrine, and dopamine can cause hypertensive crisis or serotonin syndrome [13]. The aforementioned combinations should be avoided.

3   Reductions

The primary metabolic reactions in aerobic organism are oxidations. Reductions require reduced partial oxygen pressure and negative redox potential. Thus, the gut microflora plays an important role in reductive reactions. Xenobiotics such as polyhalogenated carbohydrates, organic compounds containing an aldehyde, keto, nitro, nitroso, disulfide, sulfoxide, quinone, N-oxide, and hydroxylamine are susceptible to reduction [1].

Reductions usually include several electron transfers that generate reactive intermediary radicals. These radicals are toxic to the cell as they react with macromolecules especially with unsaturated fatty and nucleic acids. This approach is used in therapeutic purposes, e.g., metronidazole is used for treatment of anaerobic urinary infections. Under reduced oxygen partial pressure, a nitro group is reduced to an amine, which is not inherently toxic. However, sequential reduction generates nitroanion radicals, nitroso compounds, hydroxylamine radicals, and hydroxylamines, many of which are regarded as toxic.

The carbonyl group in aldehydes and ketones containing xenobiotics is reduced to an alcohol:

$$R_1C(=O)R_2 \xrightarrow{reductase} R_1CH(OH)R_2$$

Some of the enzymes involved in reductions of xenobiotics are carbonyl reductases (CBR), aldo-ketoreductases (AKR), and NAD(P)H quinone oxidoreductase (NQO), located in cytosol. Previously mentioned enzymes, the alcohol dehydrogenases and aldehyde dehydrogenases, can catalyze reductions under favorable conditions. Hydroxysteroid dehydrogenases (HSD) that are involved in conversion of endogenous oxo to hydroxy forms of steroids (and vice versa) can also reduce xenobiotics. One of the examples is enzyme 11β-HSD, which converts cortisone to cortisol and vice versa. This enzyme is involved in the reduction of metyrapone; however, it does not catalyze oxidation of the product.

Reductions are part of the metabolism of ethacrynic acid, haloperidol, daunorubicin, doxorubicin, ketotifen, ketoprofen, menadione, and some other drugs. Warfarin reduction is catalyzed by CBR to produce dihydrowarfarin and is characterized by stereoselectivity toward substrate (R) and product (R- and S-enantiomers). Reduction of testosterone into the more potent metabolite dihydrotestosterone is a bioactivation reaction. This reaction is catalyzed by the steroid

5α-reductase, and 5α-reductase inhibitors (finasteride and dutasteride) are used for treatment of benign prostate hyperplasia [14].

Reduction of azo bonds is catalyzed by gut microflora and is important for the metabolism of azo dyes. Sulfasalazine is activated in the similar manner into sulphapyridine and mesalamine (mesalazine or 5-aminosalicylic acid), which are active forms used for management of Crohn's disease [15].

4 Hydrolysis and Conjugations

Conjugations are metabolic reactions of xenobiotics and their oxidized metabolites with endogenous substances: glucuronic acid (the reaction is termed glucuronidation), sulfate (sulfoconjugation), acetyl (acetylation), methyl (methylation), α-amino acids, glutathione, and water (hydrolysis). In principle conjugations are catalyzed by transferases, except for hydrolysis, which is catalyzed by hydrolases (Table 2). Enzymes are mainly located in the cytosol, except for glucuronidases and epoxide hydrolase that are situated in the endoplasmic reticulum. Functional groups that are conjugated (glucuronidation) are hydroxyls, amines, thiols, and carboxylic acids.

Conjugation reactions are generally faster than oxidations and result in metabolites that are usually inactive, more hydrophilic, and water-soluble, with some exceptions. Consequently, they are eliminated by kidneys or liver.

4.1 Hydrolysis

Hydrolysis is reaction of an endogenous or exogenous substrate with a nucleophilic water molecule. Quite often this reaction can be spontaneous (nonenzymatic). However, the majority of xenobiotics are hydrolyzed by enzymes called hydrolases. Hydrolases are classified based on a specific substrate, e.g., carboxylesterases, choline esterases, aryl esterases, sterol esterases, epoxide hydrolases, phosphatases, and peptidases (amidases).

In most cases, hydrolysis will result in an inactive metabolite if the parent drug is active. However, hydrolysis can also result in an active metabolite from an inactive drug. These drugs are termed prodrugs and often serves as modifiers of ADMET properties of a drug. The most common substrates for hydrolysis are esters and amides, resulting in carboxylic acids, alcohols, and amines as metabolites.

Carboxylesterases are serine hydrolases, i.e., the amino acid serine is located in the active site and is responsible for the hydrolysis. The superfamily of carboxylesterases is abbreviated CES, and the enzymes follow nomenclature similar to the cytochromes P450. CES1 family is selective for substrates with small alcohols and larger acyl groups such as methylphenidate and meperidine (pethidine), while CES2 hydrolyzes substrates with smaller acyl groups and larger alcohol moieties present in procaine, aspirin (Fig. 2), heroin, and irinotecan [1].

Table 2 Overview of conjugation reactions: reactions, enzymes, conjugating agent, and typical substrates

Reaction	Enzyme	Conjugating agent	Substrate
Hydrolysis	Carboxylesterase (CES)	H_2O	Irinotecan, aspirin, lidocaine
Methylation	Methyl transferase (MT)	S-Adenosylmethionine (SAM)	Catechol, thiopurine
Acetylation	N-Acetyl transferase (NAT)	Acetyl coenzyme A (AcCoA)	Procaine, iscniazid, sulfametoxazole
Conjugation with amino acid	Acyltransferase (AT)	Amino acid (e.g., Gly, Glu, taurine)	Salicylic acid, benzoic acid
Sulfoconjugation	Sulfotransferase (SULT)	3'-Phosphoadenosine-5'-phosphosulfate (PAPS)	Acetaminophen, estrogens
Glucuronidation	UDP-Glucuronyltransferase (UDPGA)	Uridine 5'-diphosphoglucuronic acid (UDPGA)	Acetaminophen, irinotecan, bilirubin
Conjugation with glutathione	Glutathione transferase (GST)	Glutathione (GSH)	Halogenated hydrocarbons, aflatoxin epoxides

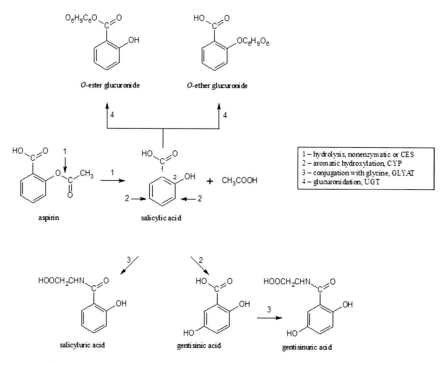

Fig. 2 Biotransformation of aspirin

Epoxide hydrolases (EPH) are enzymes that hydrolyze epoxide metabolites into *trans*-diols. Epoxides are reactive species associated with the toxic effects of xenobiotics. Benzo[*a*]pyrene and aflatoxin are substrates of CYP enzymes that are oxidized to corresponding epoxides. Some of these epoxides are poor substrates of EPH due to steric hindrance. As they are susceptible to hydrolysis, they persist in the cell causing toxic effects by covalently binding to nucleic acids [16].

Prodrugs are primarily used to facilitate patient compliance by extending dosing intervals. There are numerous examples. Propranolol undergoes extensive glucuronidation after first passage through liver, which can be avoided if propranolol is used as a hemisuccinate prodrug. Acyclovir is a frequently dosed antivirotic (five times a day), but conjugation with valine forms the prodrug valacyclovir which has higher bioavailability and a longer half-life. Testosterone has a rather short half-life that can be extended in a form of prodrug with fatty acids.

Another use of prodrugs is to prevent drug abuse. Lisdexamfetamine is a lysine-amphetamine conjugate that requires hydrolysis after oral ingestion. This prevents missuses of drug by crushing a tablet and inhaling the drug through the nose [17].

4.2   Glucuronidation

Glucuronidations are major metabolic reactions in the majority of mammals. In these reactions, a glycosyl group is transferred from uridine $5'$-diphosphoglucuronic acid (UDPGA) to endogenous and exogenous substances and their metabolites. Enzymes catalyzing glucuronidation are named uridine $5'$-diphosphoglucuronosyltransferase, and the superfamily is abbreviated UGT. UGT nomenclature is similar to the cytochrome P450 nomenclature.

The majority of steroids and bile acids are conjugated by the UGT2B subfamily except for 17α-ethynylestradiol, which is conjugated by UGT1A1. The later enzyme catalyzes the glucuronidation of bilirubin and is related to neonatal jaundice. Exogenous substrates are phenols and alcohols that result in ether O-glucuronide metabolites, carboxylic acids that produce O-glucuronide esters, amines that produce N-glucuronides, thiols that produce S-glucuronides, and a limited number of carbon compounds that result in formation of C-glucuronides [18].

UDPGA is synthetized from α-D-glucose-1-phosphate in a reaction catalyzed by UDP-glucose pyrophosphorylase, resulting in uridine-diphosphoglucose which is further oxidized by UDP-glucose-dehydrogenase. In the next step, the glucuronyl group is transferred by nucleophilic substitution to the substrate in a reaction catalyzed by UGT. The last step is characterized by inversion of stereochemical configuration: all resulting metabolites are β-glucuronides while the glucuronic acid in UDPGA is of the α configuration.

Glucuronides are acids that are ionized at physiological pH. They are preferentially eliminated depending on the molecular weight; smaller molecules are eliminated in urine (molecular weight lower than 300 Da) and larger glucuronides in bile. Glucuronides generally lose the biological activity of the parent compounds, except for morphine whose metabolite morphine O^6-glucuronide has higher pharmacological effect [19].

A significant number of xenobiotics undergo O-glucuronidation: benzodiazepines (oxazepam, temazepam), steroid hormones, morphine, acetaminophen (Fig. 1), chloramphenicol, salicylic acid, trimethoprim, etc. Chloramphenicol, acetaminophen, and salicylic acid are xenobiotics that are preferentially metabolized in conjugation reactions (glucuronidations).

Many glucuronides extend the half-life of xenobiotics through enterohepatic circulation. Irinotecan, a cytostatic agent, is a prodrug that is activated by hydrolysis. The active compound SN-38 is glucuronidated in liver and eliminated through bile. β-Glucuronidase in bacteria present in the gut liberates SN-38, which is reabsorbed and again glucuronidated in liver to complete the cycle. SN-38 is also responsible for side effects observed, in that delayed diarrhea is reported in high number of patients [20].

4.3   Sulfoconjugation

Sulfoconjugations are transfer reactions in which sulfate is transferred from 3'-phosphoadenosine-5'-phosphosulfate (PAPS) onto a substrate. Substrates are phenols, alcohols, steroids, hydroxylamines, and acryl-aryl amines. Reactions are catalyzed by sulfotransferases that are located in cytosol.

The sulfoconjugations cycle includes three steps. The sulfate group is activated with ATP in a reaction catalyzed by ATP-sulfurylase. In the second step, adenosine 5'-phosphosulfate (APS) is phosphorylated with ATP to form 3'-phosphoadenosine-5'-phosphosulfate (PAPS) in a reaction catalyzed by APS-phosphokinase. In the last step, a phosphate group from PAPS is transferred to a substrate in a reaction catalyzed by sulfotransferase.

$$SO_4^{2-} + ATP \xrightarrow{\text{ATP-sulfurylase}} APS + PP_i$$

$$APS + ATP \xrightarrow{\text{APS-phosphokinase}} PAPS + ADP$$

$$RXH + PAPS \xrightarrow{\text{sulfotransferase}} RXSO_3^- + PAP$$

Sulfoconjugations are competitive reactions with glucuronidations, but their K_m values are generally lower and rates (V_{max} or k_{cat}) are lower due to low concentrations of PAPS in comparison with UDPGA. Sulfoconjugates are more dominant metabolites when the dose of xenobiotic is low and the xenobiotic has a simple structure and is liposoluble. Products are ionized at physiological pH, are eliminated in urine, and pharmacologically inactive.

Acetaminophen (paracetamol) undergoes conjugation reactions under normal dosing regimes. Acetaminophen glucuronides are dominant metabolites in adults, and sulfoconjugates are major metabolites in neonates until the third month after birth, when glucuronidation enzymes develop (Fig. 1) [21].

4.4   Methylation

Methylations are conjugation reactions in which a methyl group is transferred to a heteroatom of a xenobiotic. Donors of the methyl group are S-adenosylmethionine (SAM) for xenobiotics and some endogenous compounds, as well as tetrahydrofolic acid derivatives and biotin which serve as C1 donors for some endogenous substrates. Substrates in these reactions are xenobiotics that contain a phenol, thiol, amine, or azide. Enzymes are named based on the heteroatom that is being methylated, e.g., O-methyltransferase, N-methyltransferase, and S-methyltransferase. Methylations do not share a common characteristic of conjugation reaction, as methylated metabolites are lipophilic (except for N-methylations of a pyridine ring in xenobiotic structures).

Methylation requires activation of a methyl group in the form of the SAM cofactor. Methionine adenosyl transferase catalyzes the biosynthesis of SAM from methionine and ATP. An activated methyl group is transferred from SAM to a substrate in a reaction catalyzed by methyltransferase. Liberated S-adenosylhomocysteine (SAH) is then hydrolyzed, and homocysteine (HCys) is methylated to methionine, completing the catalytic cycle. The donor of the methyl group in the last step is N^5-methyltetrahydrofolic acid (N^5MeTHF), and the enzyme that enables transfer is homocysteine methyltransferase:

$$Met + ATP \xrightarrow{\text{methionine adenosyl transferase}} SAM + PP_i + P_i$$

$$RXH + SAM \xrightarrow{\text{methyltransferase}} RXCH_3 + SAH$$

$$SAH + H_2O \xrightarrow{\text{adenosylhomocysteinase}} HCys + A$$

$$HCys + N^5MeTHF \xrightarrow{\text{homocysteine methyltransferase}} Met + THF$$

Estrogens are involved in the initiation and progression of (estrogen receptor-positive) breast cancer. Initiation is related to hydroxylation of vicinal C-atoms catalyzed by cytochromes P450 that can result in further oxidation to semiquinones and quinones. Production of these reactive metabolites can be prevented by catechol O-methyltransferase (COMT), e.g., estradiol hydroxylated at C-2 is a substrate for COMT, converting 2-hydroxyestradiol into 2-methoxyestradiol, which cannot undergo further oxidation [22].

4.5   Acetylation

Acetylation is a reaction in which an acetyl group is transferred from a cofactor (acetyl coenzyme A) to a heteroatom in a substrate. Groups that can be acetylated are amines, hydroxyls, and thiols, although the most common acetylations are those on nitrogen-containing substrates: aliphatic and aromatic amines, hydrazides, hydrazines, sulfonamides, and hydroxylamines. Enzymes that catalyze these conjugations are N-acetyl transferases (NAT). Similarly to methylation, acetylation products are lipophilic which goes against the adage that all drug metabolism makes more polar products.

The acetyl group is activated in two step process. In the first step, the acetyl is activated by binding to a phosphate group of ATP. Acetyladenylate reacts with coenzyme A in the second step, liberating AMP and acetyl coenzyme A. Both steps are catalyzed by acetyl coenzyme A synthase:

$$CH_3COOH + ATP \xrightarrow{\text{AcCoA synthase}} CH_3COO - AMP + PP_i$$

$$CH_3COO - AMP + CoASH \xrightarrow{\text{AcCoA synthase}} CH_3CO - S - CoA + AMP$$

Acetylation is unique in a sense that the transfer of acetyl group does not go directly from coenzyme to substrate, as the acetyl group binds first to enzyme and then is transferred to substrate:

$$CoA - S - COCH_3 \xrightarrow[\begin{subarray}{c} NAT - SH \\ -CoA - SH \end{subarray}]{} NAT - S - COCH_3 \xrightarrow[\begin{subarray}{c} +RNH_2 \\ -NAT - SH \end{subarray}]{} RNHCOCH_3$$

NAT2 is a polymorphic enzyme that is associated with the toxic effect of the tuberculostatic drug isoniazid. Patients who are slow acetylators develop peripheral neuropathy, due to accumulation of isoniazid and its potential to inhibit the pyridoxine phosphokinase enzyme that converts pyridoxine to pyridoxal $5'$-phosphate, a prosthetic group in numerous biochemical reactions. This is manifested as pyridoxine deficiency, which manifests itself as a peripheral neuropathy. Consequently, slow acetylators should use vitamin B6 concomitantly with isoniazid [23].

Sulfonamides were extensively used as antibacterial drugs before penicillins emerged. Amino group of sulfonamides is susceptible to acetylation. Due to the poor solubility of acetylated metabolites, sulfonamides can precipitate in urine and cause nephrotoxicity. This, combined with the common allergic reactions to sulfonamides, has reduced the number of sulfonamides used to a handful.

4.6   Conjugation with Amino Acids

Conjugations with amino acids are not as common reactions as other conjugations due to low concentrations of free amino acids. The most common conjugating acid is glycine and, to a lesser extent, glutamine, serine, asparagine, and taurine. Substrates are aliphatic, aromatic, or heteroaromatic derivatives of carboxylic acids. The products are small, more polar molecules that are excreted in urine. Enzymes that catalyze these reactions are termed N-acyltransferases, e.g., in case of conjugation with glycine N-glycyltransferase.

Most conjugation reactions require activation of coenzyme. However, in conjugations with amino acids, it is the substrate that is activated. This process is similar to the generation of acetyl coenzyme A (see Sect. 4.5) and is catalyzed by acyl coenzyme A synthetase. An activated thioester form of substrate is then conjugated with the amino group of an amino acid. This step is catalyzed by an N-acyltransferase, and coenzyme A is product of the reaction.

Benzoic acid represents an oxidative metabolite of numerous xenobiotics such as amphetamine, toluene, cinnamic acid, and quinic acid (oxidation of quinic acid requires aromatization, which is catalyzed by gut microflora). The major metabolic product of benzoic acid is a conjugate with glycine named hippuric acid (first discovered in horse urine).

Salicylic acid is eliminated in the form of a glycine conjugate named salicyluric acid. Salicyluric acid represents the major metabolic pathway in the biotransformation of aspirin (~70%, Fig. 2) [24].

4.7   Conjugation with Glutathione

Glutathione (GSH) is the tripeptide γ-glutamyl-cysteinyl-glycine, which has numerous physiological functions, e.g., it participates in oxidoreductions and is one of the major cellular antioxidants. While the role of glutathione is mostly beneficial, glutathione has been linked to toxic effects of xenobiotics such as some halogenated hydrocarbons.

Conjugations with glutathione are catalyzed by glutathione transferase (GST) in the liver. Further sequential degradation of conjugate occurs in kidneys: γ-glutamyltransferase liberates glutamate, and cysteinyl-glycinyl dipeptidase then liberates the glycine residue. In the last step, an N-acetyltransferase acetylates the amino group of cysteine residue. The resulting conjugates are called mercapturic acids:

$$R_3C - X + GluCysGly \xrightarrow{GST} R_3C - GluCysGly + HX$$

$$R_3C - GluCysGly + H_2O \xrightarrow{\gamma\text{-glutamyltransferase}} R_3C - CysGly + Glu$$

$$R_3C - CysGly + H_2O \xrightarrow{cysteinyl-glycinyl\ dipeptidase} R_3C - Cys + Gly$$

$$R_3C - Cys + AcCoA \xrightarrow{NAT} R_3C - Cys - Ac + CoA$$

Substrates are reactive species that contain an electrophilic carbon atom or heteroatoms (N, O, S) that can directly bind to GSH (nonenzymatically) or enzymatically (with GST). These include oxidation products of aflatoxins, benzo[a]pyrene, pesticides, herbicides, and cytostatics. Conjugation with glutathione is relevant for many of the drugs whose metabolism results in reactive species. Acetaminophen is metabolized to NAPQI, which is detoxicated by conjugation with GST (Fig. 1). Similar detoxication and elimination are also observed in diclofenac metabolism. Profile of mercapturic acids obtained by biotransformation of drugs can help rationalize some idiosyncratic reactions and adverse effects observed with some medications, e.g., nevirapine is bioactivated to an arene oxide and quinone methide intermediates that cause fatal skin rash in some patients. Although not directly detected, mercapturic acid metabolites prove their existence [25].

5   Metabolic Reactions in Therapeutic Drug Monitoring

Therapeutic drug monitoring (TDM) is a clinical practice of ensuring that the dosing regime produces an optimal pharmacotherapeutic effect. This approach is especially important for drugs with narrow therapeutic range, i.e., small differences between sub-therapeutic and toxic levels. Successful therapy can be achieved by monitoring parent drug or metabolite concentration in serum or makers of biological activity, and TDM is especially useful in patients with renal or hepatic impairment. The absence of parent drug or metabolite can, among others, indicate patient non-compliance. Most commonly high-performance liquid chromatography (HPLC) coupled with appropriate detection (UV, fluorescence and mass spectrometry) is employed as analytical technique for monitoring concentrations of drugs and metabolites in serum. For some medications, other techniques can be more appropriate, e.g., immunoassays (digoxin, aminoglycosides, and monoclonal antibodies), prothrombin time (warfarin).

Interpretation of the results obtained can often be complex and requires a complete understanding of patient's medical record. In principle, recommendation for sub-therapeutic concentrations will require frequency adjustment (e.g., bid to tid) or dose reductions in case of supratherapeutic concentrations.

Some examples of TDM reliance upon metabolite measurement include oxcarbazepine (11-hydroxyoxcarbazepine), diazepam (nordiazepam, temazepam, and oxazepam) or antipsychotics such as risperidone in which case sum of both active compounds (drug + metabolite) is used for TDM (consult other chapters for specific drugs of interest).

References

1. Rendic S. Biotransformation of xenobiotics and endobiotics - for beginners. https://www.researchgate.net/publication/331286664_BIOTRANSFORMATION_OF_XENOBIOTICS_AND_ENDOBIOTICS-_for_the_beginners. Accessed 30 Sep 2021
2. Josephy PD, Guengerich FP, Miners JO. Phase I and Phase II" drug metabolism: terminology that we should phase out? Drug Metab Rev. 2005;37(4):575–80. https://doi.org/10.1080/036 02530500251220.
3. Flockhart DA. Drug Interactions Flockhart Table. Indiana University. https://drug-interactions.medicine.iu.edu/MainTable.aspx. Accessed 30 Sep 2021
4. Zanger UM, Schwab M. Cytochrome P450 enzymes in drug metabolism: regulation of gene expression, enzyme activities, and impact of genetic variation. Pharmacol Therap. 2013;138(1):103–41. https://doi.org/10.1016/j.pharmthera.2012.12.007.
5. Rendic SP, Guengerich FP. Human Family 1–4 cytochrome P450 enzymes involved in the metabolic activation of xenobiotic and physiological chemicals: an update. Arch Toxicol. 2021;95(2):395–472. https://doi.org/10.1007/s00204-020-02971-4.
6. Estabrook RW. A passion for P450s (rememberances of the early history of research on cytochrome P450). Drug Metab Dispos. 2003;31(12):1461–73. https://doi.org/10.1124/dmd.31.12.1461.
7. Nelson DR. Cytochrome P450 homepage. https://drnelson.uthsc.edu/. Accessed 30 Sep 2021

8. Sofi F, Giusti B, Marcucci R, Gori AM, Abbate R, Gensini GF. Cytochrome P450 2C19*2 polymorphism and cardiovascular recurrences in patients taking clopidogrel: a meta-analysis. Pharmacogenomics J. 2011;11(3):199–206. https://doi.org/10.1038/tpj.2010.21.
9. Dean L. Warfarin therapy and VKORC1 and CYP genotype. In: Pratt VM, Scott SA, Pirmohamed M, et al., editors. Medical Genetics Summaries. Bethesda (MD): National Center for Biotechnology Information (US). https://www.ncbi.nlm.nih.gov/books/NBK84174/. Accessed 30 Sep 2021
10. Alonzo MM, Lewis TV, Miller JL. Disulfiram-like reaction with metronidazole: an unsuspected culprit. J Pediatr Pharmacol Ther. 2019;24(5):445–9. https://doi.org/10.5863/1551-6776-24.5.445.
11. Berry CE, Hare JM. Xanthine oxidoreductase and cardiovascular disease: molecular mechanisms and pathophysiological implications. J Physiol. 2004;555:589–606. https://doi.org/10.1113/jphysiol.2003.055913.
12. Treacy EP, Akerman BR, Chow LM, Youil R, Bibeau C, Lin J, et al. Mutations of the flavin-containing monooxygenase gene (FMO3) cause trimethylaminuria, a defect in detoxication. Hum Mol Genet. 1998;7(5):839–45. https://doi.org/10.1093/hmg/7.5.839.
13. Bartlett D. Drug-induced serotonin syndrome. Crit Care Nurse. 2017;37(1):49–54. https://doi.org/10.4037/ccn2017169.
14. Bartsch G, Rittmaster RS, Klocker H. Dihydrotestosterone and the concept of 5α-reductase inhibition in human benign prostatic hyperplasia. World J Urol. 2002;19(6):413–25. https://doi.org/10.1007/s00345-002-0248-5.
15. Ye B, van Langenberg DR. Mesalazine preparations for the treatment of ulcerative colitis: are all created equal? World J Gastrointest Pharmacol Ther. 2015;6(4):137–44. https://doi.org/10.4292/wjgpt.v6.i4.137.
16. Šulc M, Indra R, Moserová M, Schmeiser HH, Frei E, Arlt VM, Stiborová M. The impact of individual cytochrome P450 enzymes on oxidative metabolism of benzo[a]pyrene in human livers. Environ Mol Mutagen. 2016;57(3):229–35. https://doi.org/10.1002/em.22001.
17. Comiran E, Kessler FH, Fröehlich PE, Limberger RP. Lisdexamfetamine: a pharmacokinetic review. Eur J Pharm Sci. 2016;89:172–9. https://doi.org/10.1016/j.ejps.2016.04.026.
18. Meech R, Hu DG, McKinnon RA, Mubarokah SN, Haines AZ, Nair PC, et al. The UDP-Glycosyltransferase (UGT) superfamily: new members, new functions, and novel paradigms. Physiol Rev. 2019;99(2):1153–222. https://doi.org/10.1152/physrev.00058.2017.
19. Smith HS. Opioid metabolism. Mayo Clin Proc. 2009;84(7):613–24. https://doi.org/10.1016/S0025-6196(11)60750-7.
20. Stein A, Voigt W, Jordan K. Chemotherapy-induced diarrhea: pathophysiology, frequency and guideline-based management. Ther Adv Med Oncol. 2010;2(1):51–63. https://doi.org/10.1177/1758834009355164.
21. Mazaleuskaya LL, Sangkuhl K, Thorn CF, FitzGerald GA, Altman RB, Klein TE. PharmGKB summary: pathways of acetaminophen metabolism at the therapeutic versus toxic doses. Pharmacogenet Genomics. 2015;25(8):416–26. https://doi.org/10.1097/FPC.0000000000000150.
22. Zhao YN, Zhang W, Chen YC, Fang F, Liu XQ. Relative imbalances in the expression of catechol O-methyltransferase and cytochrome P450 in breast cancer tissue and their association with breast carcinoma. Maturitas. 2012;72(2):139–45. https://doi.org/10.1016/j.maturitas.2012.03.003.
23. Wang P, Shehu AI, Lu J, Joshi RH, Venkataramanan R, Sugamori KS, et al. Deficiency of N-acetyltransferase increases the interactions of isoniazid with endobiotics in mouse liver. Biochem Pharmacol. 2017;145:218–25. https://doi.org/10.1016/j.bcp.2017.09.001.
24. Bojić M, Sedgeman CA, Nagy LD, Guengerich FP. Aromatic hydroxylation of salicylic acid and aspirin by human cytochromes P450. Eur J Pharm Sci. 2015;73:49–56. https://doi.org/10.1016/j.ejps.2015.03.015.
25. Dekker SJ, Zhang Y, Vos JC, Vermeulen NP, Commandeur JN. Different reactive metabolites of nevirapine require distinct glutathione S-transferase isoforms for bioinactivation. Chem Res Toxicol. 2016;29(12):2136–44. https://doi.org/10.1021/acs.chemrestox.6b00250.

Pharmacogenomics of Drug-Metabolizing Enzymes

Elizabeta Topić, Mario Štefanović, Dragan Primorac, Lidija Bach-Rojecky, and Wolfgang Höppner

Abstract

The pharmacogenetics of drug-metabolizing enzymes studies the relationship between an individual's genetic predisposition and ability to metabolize a drug or a foreign compound, and helps to understand why some people respond to drugs and others do not, or why some people need higher or lower doses. It also detects patients who will not respond to therapy and may experience toxic side effects. Unlike pharmacogenetics, which most often deals with the influence of individual polymorphisms on interindividual variations in response to drugs, the broader term pharmacogenomics includes levels of multi-gene (or whole genome) interaction. Today, there is a wealth of data on advances in pharmacogenetics and pharmacogenomics testing in gene-drug relationships. Still, there is also a large disparity in applying these data in everyday clinical practice. In order to reliably and systematically connect known gene variations with clinical

E. Topić
Croatian Society of Medical Biochemistry and Laboratory Medicine, Zagreb, Croatia

Croatian Academy of Medical Sciences, Zagreb, Croatia

M. Štefanović
Clinical Institute of Chemistry, University Hospital Sestre Milosrdnice, Zagreb, Croatia

D. Primorac (✉)
St. Catherine Specialty Hospital, Zagreb, Croatia
e-mail: dragan.primorac@svkatarina.hr; draganprimorac2@gmail.com

University of Split School of Medicine, Split, Croatia

University of Osijek Faculty of Medicine, Osijek, Croatia

University of Rijeka School of Medicine, Rijeka, Croatia

Josip Juraj Strossmayer University of Osijek Faculty of Dental Medicine and Health, Osijek, Croatia

Eberly College of Science, 517 Thomas St, State College, Penn State University, University Park, PA 16803, USA indicators of treatment efficacy, the Clinical Pharmacogenetics Implementation Consortium (CIPC) provides guidance to help physicians select and optimize the treatment of each individual patient, i.e., to personalize the treatment based on individual genotype and phenotype (https://cpicpgx.org/guidelines/).

Keywords

Drug metabolizing enzymes • Gene polymorphisms • Pharmacogenetics • Drug-gene interaction • CPIC

1   Introduction

Enzymes involved in drug or xenobiotic metabolism are classified as phase I or phase II enzymes. Phase I enzymes through oxygenation, oxidation, reduction and hydrolysis reactions of drug molecules create functional groups that in the next phase serve as a site for conjugation with glucuronic acid, sulfuric acid or glutathione, which are catalyzed by phase II enzymes. Through different biotransformation reactions, those enzymes increase the solubility of the drug in water by chemical modification to facilitate its excretion from the body. Most of them are in the liver, but they are also present in the intestines, skin, central nervous system (CNS) and almost all other tissues.

Each enzyme involved in drug metabolism is encoded by a specific gene that is expressed in the final protein of certain functional characteristics and enzymatic activity. Genes are inherited in allele pairs, one of several forms of DNA sequence that encodes a particular gene. The combination of allele pairs makes up the genotype (e.g., in the *CYP2C9* gene: the *1* allele (inherited from the mother) and the *2* allele (inherited from the father) form the heterozygote genotype *1/*2). The most common allele in the population is allele *1 (wild-type allele), while other alleles (*2, *3, etc.) are alleles with polymorphisms in their nucleotide sequence resulting in gene product with most often altered functional activity (reduced, enhanced, normal or even without activity). Combinations of

The Henry C. Lee College of Criminal Justice and Forensic Sciences, University of New Haven, West Haven, CT, USA

National Forensic Science University, Gandhinagar, Gujarat, India

College of Medicine and Forensics, Xi'an Jiaotong University, Xi'an, China

Medical School REGIOMED, 96450 Coburg, Germany

International Center For Applied Biological Sciences, Zagreb, Croatia

L. Bach-Rojecky
University of Zagreb Faculty of Pharmacy and Biochemistry, Zagreb, Croatia

W. Höppner
Bioglobe GmbH, 22529 Hamburg, Germany

inherited alleles can be homozygous or heterozygous (e.g., *1/*1 represents wild-type homozygote, *1/*2 heterozygote, *2/*2 mutated homozygote or *2/*3 mixed heterozygotes). Blocks of whole or parts of alleles that are inherited together are called haplotypes. Measurable, visible or presumed clinical manifestation arising from a genotype is called a phenotype.

The aim of pharmacogenetic testing is, by determining the genotype, to predict the phenotype and determine the risk of adverse effects and/or determine the need to change the dose or replace the drug with another drug that is metabolized by another metabolic pathway. Based on pharmacogenetic results, it is possible to assess in advance the risk of side effects when giving a particular drug, or to determine whether to give a higher or lower dose of the drug. In case the patient cannot use a drug due to his/her genetic profile or it is too dangerous for him/her, the drug should be replaced by another, with similar effect—but which is not a substrate of a polymorphic enzyme of a variant gene [1–4].

From the knowledge of the efficiency (functional activity) of individual polymorphic alleles in relation to the wild type, it is possible to estimate the total metabolic phenotype (metabolic ability, functional activity) based on the sum of presumed allele activities. Functional activity can be assessed by the ratio of phenotype activity to normal EM phenotype: values 0–0.5 correspond to poor metabolizer (PM) phenotype, 0.5–1 to intermediate (IM) phenotype, 1–2 to extensive (EM) phenotype, and values > 1.5 or 2.0 to fast or ultrafast metabolizer phenotype (UM) [5].

2   Enzymes Involved in Phase I Drug Metabolism

The most important phase I enzymes involved in drug biotransformation are cytochrome P450 (CYP) superfamily enzymes [1]. Sequencing of the human genome revealed 115 CYP genes, of which 57 are functional and encode individual enzymes, while the rest in the genome are present as pseudogenes without functional activity (but as a disruption in polymorphism detection methods). Of the greatest clinical importance are the isoenzymes CYP2D6, CYP2C19, CYP2C9, CYP3A4/CYP3A5, CYP1A2 and CYP2B6. Evaluation of the metabolic pathways of a large number of different drugs showed that about 50% of them are metabolized by CYP3A4/CYP3A5, 25% by CYP2D6, 15% by CYP2C9 and CYP2C19, and the rest by CYP1A2, CYP2A6, CYP2B6 and other enzymes [1, 2].

Although many of these enzymes exhibit gene polymorphism, not all variations are equally important for drug response. The most common change is the replacement of one base with another, i.e., a single nucleotide polymorphism (SNP), but there are also changes such as deletions, insertions or multiplication of parts or whole genes [1].

2.1 CYP2D6

The CYP2D6 enzyme, primarily expressed in the liver and central nervous system (CNS), is responsible for the metabolism of a number of antidepressants, neuroleptics, antiarrhythmics and β-adrenergic receptor blockers, and participates in the metabolism of endogenous substrates (serotonin, neurosteroides and dopamine precursors). The *CYP2D6* gene polymorphism is associated with four phenotypes that differ in their ability to metabolize the substrates: Extensive (EM), Poor (PM), Intermediate (IM) and Ultrarapid (UM) metabolizers, resulting in a therapeutically normal, high or low concentration of the drug (or its metabolite). There is also a difference in the safety of treatment, i.e., the manifestation of side effects [3, 6, 7].

In a person taking a drug that is a CYP2D6 substrate, the phenotypes given in Table 2 can be presented through the following clinical functional outcomes (Fig. 1).

Numerous polymorphisms of the *CYP2D6* gene are the result of point mutations, insertions or deletions and major rearrangements that include deletion of the entire gene, duplication or multiplication of genes, as well as creation of hybrid genes by recombination with neighboring pseudogene CYP2D7P. To date, more than 147 *CYP2D6* alleles are known, and the most common alleles are given in Table 1. The main alleles associated with the PM phenotype, leading to a complete lack of functional protein (null alleles), are: *3, *4, *5, *6, *7, *8, *9, *10A,

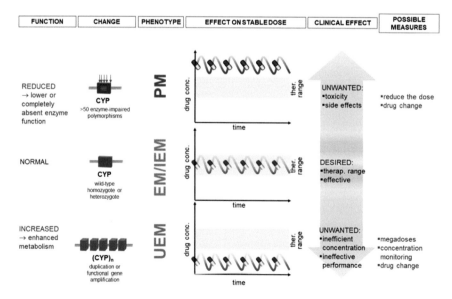

Fig. 1 Functional outcomes of *CYP2D6* polymorphism on CYP2D6 substrate drugs (with inactive metabolites), their clinical effect and possible therapeutic interventions. Modified according to Steimer W, Potter JM. Pharmacogenetic screening and therapeutic drugs. Clinica Chimica Acta 2002; 334: 137–55. https://doi.org/10.1016/s0009-8981(01)00713-6

Table 1 Most common *CYP2D6* alleles in different ethnic groups, their activity and phenotype characteristics

CYP2D6 allele	Ratio of functional activity	Activity	Predicted phenotype of homozygotes	Allele frequencies in ethnic groups					
				European (%)	African American (%)	East Asian (%)	American (%)	Latin American (%)
*1	1.0	Normal	EM	19.0	20.1	24.2	51.1	36.5
*1×2	2.0	Increased	MIND	0.8	0.8	0.3	2.9	1.5
*2	1.0	Normal	EM	27.7	15.6	12.1	22.1	22.7
*2×2	2.0	Increased	UM	0.8	1.9	0.5	0.6	1.2
*3	0	No	PM	1.6	0.3	0.0	0.0	0.7
*4	0	No	PM	18.5	4.8	0.5	10.2	12.1
*4≥2	0	No	PM	0.7	2.7	0.0	0.1	0.4
*5	0	No	PM	3.0	5.4	4.9	1.6	2.9
*6	0	No	PM	1.1	0.3	0.0	0.2	0.5
*9	0.5	Reduced	IM	2.8	0.4	0.2	0.4	1.6 lePara>
*10	0.25	Reduced	PM	1.6	3.8	43.6	1.4	2.6
*33	1.0	Normal	EM	1.9		0.0	0.2	
*34	1.0	Normal	EM	1.9		1.0		0.1
*35	1.0	Normal	EM	5.5	0.9	0.1	1.0	2.7
*39	1.0	Normal	EM	1.6	2.7	0.6		0.8
*41	0.5	Reduced	IM	9.2	3.7	2.3	2.3	5.1

Alleles and phenotype data are updated from https://cpicpgx.org/genes-drugs/ (January 2022)

Table 2 Frequency, functional activity, phenotype characteristics and allele combinations in CYP2D6

Phenotype	Frequency in the population (%)	Functional activity	Features	Example of a diplotype
UM	3.1	>2.0	Alleles (genes) in duplicate or multiple copies	*1/*1×N *1/*2×N *2/*2×N
EM	82	1.0–2.0	Two functional alleles, or two alleles of reduced function or one normal and the other allele of reduced function or a combination of multiple alleles with an activity ratio between 1.0 and 2.0	*1/*1, *1/*2, *1/*4, *1/*5, *1/*9, *1/*41, *2/*2, *41/*41
IM	7.1	0.25–1.0	One functional and the other non-functional allele (no-activity allele)	*4/*10, *4/*41, *5/*9
PM	7.3	<0.25	Without functional alleles	*3/*4, *4/*4, *5/*5, *5/*6

Alleles and phenotype data are updated from https://cpicpgx.org/genes-drugs/ (January 2022)

*17, *41, and two variants with reduced catalytic activity, alleles *17 and *41. Among PM phenotypes, the most common allele is *4 (70%), followed by allele *5 (26%), and allele *3 (3%), while alleles *17 and *41 are usually associated with the IM phenotype. The UM phenotype is the result of an amplified *CYP2D6 *1* or *CYP2D6 *2* allele, resulting in over-expression of the enzyme, and the product has functionally the same but catalytically multiple activity [1, 2].

The EM phenotype makes up the vast majority of the population (82%) and a person with two normal, active *CYP2D6* alleles will have a normal metabolic response to the drug substrate. Heterozygous individuals with one active and one altered allele (IM phenotype) exhibit a phenotype that will not be clearly distinguished from metabolism in individuals of the EM phenotype. The PM phenotype is made up of individuals who inherited two inactive alleles homozygously or heterozygously, in which a lack of CYP2D6 activity in CYP2D6 substrate metabolism is observed. The UM phenotype has been identified only in hetcrozygous amplified gene carriers and results in over-expression with a strong effect on CYP2D6 substrate metabolism and elimination. Such individuals may require larger doses of drugs that are metabolized to inactive ingredients, while for prodrugs, the higher rate of active metabolite production may result with increased risk of adverse effects. Characteristics of the phenotype, frequency and combination of alleles that make up the genotype (diplotype) of CYP2D6 and their ratio of functional activity to EM phenotype are given in Table 2. This ratio may range between 0 and 0.5 (PM phenotype, no activity or reduced and dose adjustment or drug change required). If the functional activity ratio is between 0.5 and 1.0 (EM or IM phenotype, normal or reduced activity that does not usually require a change in dosage) or it may be greater than 1.0 (UM phenotype, the activity is increased and requires a change dose or replacement of the drug) [5, 6].

Pharmacogenetic profile of CYP2D6
Based on most studies, in patients on CYP2D6 substrate therapy, screening for the UM phenotype (*CYP2D6*2×2*) and for the PM phenotype (especially for the *3, *4, *5, *6, *10* and *41* alleles) are recommended.

There are CPIC guidelines with strong recommendations for pharmacogenetics testing of some CYP2D6 drug substrates (e.g., atomoxetine, codeine, tamoxifen), in assessment of dose and effect of therapy (https://cpicpgx.org/genes-drugs/) [7–9].

2.2   CYP2C19

The enzyme CYP2C19 is responsible for the metabolism of a number of drugs from the groups of anticonvulsants, proton pump inhibitor, antidepressants, antiplatelet drug clopidogrel, etc. [10–12]. To date, more than 36 *CYP2C19* alleles are known, and the most common allele is given in Table 3.

The EM phenotype consists of carriers of alleles of normal or slightly impaired function in homozygous and heterozygous genotypes (e.g., *1/*1* and *1/*13*), which are inherited autosomally recessively. Specific mutations in genes result with alleles of significantly impaired function (*CYP2C19* alleles *2, *3, *4, *5, *6* and *8*) and lead to the PM phenotype. The fast and ultrafast metabolic phenotype consists of combinations of enhanced activity alleles (*CYP2C19 *17*) in homozygous or heterozygous form, which may, e.g., increase the risk of bleeding in clopidogrel-treated patients. Characteristics of the phenotype, frequency and combination of alleles that make up the genotype (diplotype) of the CYP2C19 enzyme are given in Table 4.

Homozygotes and heterozygotes of the PM and IM phenotypes may be at increased risk for adverse or uncommon reactions to certain drugs, and according to CPIC guidelines, testing is recommended with the use of drugs: amitriptyline, citalopram, escitalopram, clopidogrel, clomipramine, omeprazole, pantoprazole, sertraline, voriconazole and others.

Pharmacogenetic profile of CYP2C19
The PM phenotype detection strategy for CYP2C19 substrate drugs includes genotyping for the most common alleles, *2, *3, *4 and *8*. Testing for the *CYP2C19*17* allele is important to do in patients on clopidogrel, as the effect of prodrug clopidogrel may be increased (risk of bleeding) in these patients. According to CPIC

Table 3 Most common *CYP2C19* alleles in different ethnic groups, their activity and associated phenotype

CYP2C19 allele	Activity	Predicted phenotype	Allele frequencies in ethnic groups				
			European (%)	African American (%)	East Asian (%)	American (%)	Latin American (%)
*1	Normal	EM	62.5	54.7	59.6	79.2	71.7
*2	No	PM	14.7	18.2	28.4	12.1	10.4
*3	No	PM	0.2	0.3	7.3	0.0	0.1
*4	No	PM	0.2	0.0	0.0	0.0	0.1
*5	No	PM	0.0	0.0	0.3	0.0	0.0
*6	No	PM	0.0	0.0	0.1		0.0
*8	No	PM	0.3	0.1	0.0	0.0	0.1
*9	Reduced	IM	0.1	1.4	0.0		0.1
*13	Normal	EM	0.2	1.2	0.0		0.4
*15	Normal	EM	0.2	1.4	0.1		0.4
*17	Increased	RM, UM	21.6	20.7	2.1	8.6	16.7

Legend PM—poor metabolizer; EM—extensive metabolizer, RM—rapid metabolizer, UM—ultra-fast metabolizer, IM—intermediate metabolizer
Alleles and phenotype data are updated from https://cpicpgx.org/genes-drugs/ (January 2022)

Table 4 Frequency, phenotype characteristics and allele combinations in *CYP2C19*

Phenotype	Frequency in the population (%)	Genotype	Example of a diplotypes
UM	4.7	Two functional alleles of enhanced activity	*17/*17
RM	27.2	One functional allele of enhanced activity and one allele of normal activity	*1/*17, *3/*17
EM	39.6	Both functional alleles of normal activity	*1/*1, *1/*13
IM	26.0	One functional and the other non-functional allele (no-activity allele)	*1/*2, *1/*3, *1/*4
PM	2.4	Without functional alleles	*2/*2, *2/*4, *2/*3

UM—ultrafast metabolizer, RM—rapid (fast) metabolizer, EM—extensive (normal) metabolizer, IM—medium metabolizer, PM—poor (slow) metabolizer
Alleles and phenotype data are updated from https://cpicpgx.org/genes-drugs/ (January 2022)

Table 5 CPIC recommendations for amitriptyline dosing according to the combination of CYP2D6 and CYP2C19 phenotypes

Phenotype	CYP2D6 UM	CYP2D6 EM	CYP2D6 IM	CYP2D6 PM
CYP2C19 UM	Avoid	Replace medication	Replace medication	Avoid
CYP2C19 EM	Avoid or titrate to a higher dose	Standard dosing	Reduce the dose by 25%	Avoid or reduce the dose by 50%
CYP2C19 IM	Avoid	Standard dosing	Reduce the dose by 25%	Avoid or reduce the dose by 50%
CYP2C19 PM	Avoid	Avoid or reduce the dose by 50%	Avoid	Avoid

Alleles and phenotype data are updated from https://cpicpgx.org/genes-drugs/ (January 2022)

guidelines and the level of strong clinical evidence, a change in medication is recommended in patients treated with clopidogrel with the UM (increased risk of bleeding) and PM (reduced antiplatelet effect) phenotype [11].

In patients taking proton pump inhibitors, antidepressants citalopram, escitalopram, sertraline or tertiary amines such as amitriptyline, the recommendation for PM phenotype is to reduce the starting dose by 50% or even change the drug, while in UM phenotype, ineffective doses may be expected and should be considered drug replacement [12]. When taking amitriptyline, care should be taken to ensure that this drug is significantly metabolized by CYP2D6 in addition to CYP2C19, and both phenotypes should be considered in pharmacogenetic testing and treatment decisions [13] (Table 5).

2.3 CYP2C9

The CYP2C9 enzyme is involved in the metabolism of anticonvulsants, antidiabetics, anticoagulants, antiepileptics, non-steroidal anti-inflammatory drugs (NSAIDs) and some antimicrobials. In the assessment and selection of treatment, and based on CPIC guidelines, for some drugs (warfarin, acenocoumarol, piroxicam, tenoxicam, meloxicam, celecoxib, flurbiprofen, ibuprofen, lornoxicam, phenytoin), there are clinic evidence of benefit from pharmacogenetics CYP2C9 testing [14].

So far, 61 polymorphic *CYP2C9* alleles have been identified and all are due to point mutations. In addition to the wild-type allele (*CYP2C9 *1*), the two most important variants are *2 and *3, which encode PM phenotype enzyme with very low or without activity (Table 6).

The most common variants in the PM phenotype are the *2 and *3 alleles. To date, no gene rearrangements have been described that would lead to complete deletion or duplication of the *CYP2C9* gene (or UM phenotype). Characteristics of phenotype, functional activity, frequency and combination of alleles that make up the genotype (diplotype) of the CYP2C9 enzyme are given in Table 7.

Table 6 Most common *CYP2C9* alleles in different ethnic groups, their activity and phenotype characteristics

CYP2C9 allele	Activity (functional activity)	Phenotype	Allele frequencies in ethnic groups				
			European (%)	African American (%)	East Asian (%)	American (%)	Latin American (%)
*1	Normal (1)	EM	79.3	87.1	95.6	91.2	86.4
*2	No (0.5)	PM	12.7	2.2	0.2	3.3	7.6
*3	No (0)	PM	7.6	1.4	3.8	3.0	4.0
*8	Reduced (0.5)	IM	0.2	5.9	0.4	2.0	0.7
*11	Reduced (0.5)	IM	0.2	1.4	0.0	0.3	0.3

Alleles and phenotype data are updated from https://cpicpgx.org/genes-drugs/ (January 2022)

Table 7 Frequency, functional activity, phenotype characteristics and allele combinations in *CYP2C9*

Phenotype	Frequency in the population (%)	Functional activity	Features	Example of a diplotype
EM	62.9	2	Both functional alleles of normal activity	*1/*1, *1/*9
IM	34.5	1–1.5	One functional and the other non-functional allele (reduced activity or no)	*1/*2, *1/*3, *1/*8, *2/*2
PM	2.6	0–0.5	Without functional alleles or with one allele reduced and the other without function	*2/*3, *3/*3, *3/*8

Alleles and phenotype data are updated from https://cpicpgx.org/genes-drugs/ (January 2022)

Pharmacogenetic profile of CYP2C9

Since the *2 and *3 alleles were identified in 8–19% of whites and 6–7.4% of the black population, both alleles should be included in the pharmacogenetic profile when analyzing white and black pharmacogenetic polymorphisms, but only the allele *3 in Asians. The phenotype of poor metabolism is shown by heterozygous and homozygous carriers of variant alleles. *CYP2C9* polymorphism can significantly affect the toxicity of drugs with a narrow therapeutic range such as warfarin or phenytoin, which show interindividual variability [15]. The antiepileptic pheny-toin has a very small therapeutic range, so determining the appropriate (effective and safe) dose is time-consuming and expensive (due to therapeutic drug mon-itoring requirements), and testing for *CYP2C9* polymorphisms is recommended before starting therapy [16]. For individuals with an IM phenotype, a reduction in the starting dose of 25% is recommended, and in slow metabolizers (PM), it is rec-ommended that the starting dose of phenytoin be reduced by 50% compared to the standard dose. Since the effect of phenytoin is also affected by the *HLA-B* 15:02* genotype, if it is positive, it is indicated to avoid phenytoin therapy regardless of the CYP2C9 phenotype [17].

In anticoagulant therapy with warfarin, interindividual variability may be due in part to genetic polymorphisms of the *CYP2C9* gene and the *VKORC1* and *CYP4F2* genes involved in the metabolic cycle of vitamin K. For carriers of the combina-tion of or for those who have only one polymorphism of above three genes, there is a strong recommendation for pharmacogenetics testing [18, 19]. Genotyping of polymorphic alleles *CYP2C9* and *VKORC1* is now available in many laboratories. Based on test results, dosing tables, with support of calculating dose estimators available on the Internet (e.g., http://warfarindosing.org [20]), it is possible to estimate the required dose of the drug for each patient.

CYP2C9 testing is also recommended when using NSAIDs, and the CPIC has issued guidelines regarding drugs for which *CYP2C9* testing is recommended [21].

2.4   CYP3A4/A5

Enzymes of the CYP3A4 and CYP3A5 families are dominant CYP genes, expressed in the liver and involved in the oxidative metabolism of many drugs (50–60% of all drugs) from different groups. They have overlapping substrate speci-ficities, but CYP3A4 is predominant in Caucasian, while CYP3A5 is predominant in Blacks.

Although these genes have a number of polymorphic alleles, *CYP3A4 (*1–*35)* and *CYP3A5 (*1–*9)*, it has not been clearly shown that most of them show a significant effect on expression or enzyme activity. Non-functional *CYP3A5* alleles have been confirmed in different populations (Tables 8 and 9), but in *CYP3A4* (PM phenotype), they are rare (the most important non-functional allele is *CYP3A4 *22*, present in about 5% of Caucasians).

Pharmacogenetic profile of CYP3A4/A5

In pharmacogenetic testing, it is recommended to determine the presence of non-functional alleles for *CYP3A4 *22* and *CYP3A5 *3*, and less often the *CYP3A5 *6* and *CYP3A5 *7*, while other variants *2, *8* and *9* are of unknown func-tional significance. Testing according to available guidelines of high level evidence is indicated when administering the immunosuppressant tacrolimus to transplant recipients, which in patients with EM and IM phenotype should be given in 1.5–2

Table 8 Most common *CYP3A5* alleles in different ethnic groups and their activity

CYP3A5 alleles	Activity	Allele frequencies in ethnic groups			
		European (%)	African American (%)	East Asian (%)	American (%)
*1	EM	7.4	45.3	25.4	17.3
*2	Unknown				
*3	No activity	92.4	31.6	74.6	76.5
*4	Unknown				
*5	Unknown				
*6	No activity	0.2	11.1	0.1	3.7
*7	No activity	0.0	12.0	0.0	2.5
*8	Unknown				
*9	Unknown				

Alleles and phenotype data are updated from https://cpicpgx.org/genes-drugs/ (January 2022)

Table 9 Frequency, phenotype characteristics and allele combinations in CYP3A5

CYP3A5 phenotype	Allele frequencies in ethnic groups				Features	Example of a diplotype
	European (%)	African American (%)	East Asian (%)	American (%)		
EM	0.5	20.5	6.4	3.0	A person has both functional alleles of normal activity	*1/*1
IM	13.7	49.6	37.9	28.6	A person has one functional allele and the other a non-functional allele (non-activity allele)	*1/*3, *1/*6, *1/*7
PM	85.7	29.9	55.7	68.4	A person without functional alleles	*3/*3, *6/*6, *7/*7, *3/*6, *3/*7, *6/*7

Alleles and phenotype data are updated from https://cpicpgx.org/genes-drugs/ (January 2022)

times increased dose, while standard dose drug is given to people of PM phenotype [22].

2.5   Other Isoforms of Cytochrome CYP P450 Enzyme System (CYP1A2, 2A6, 2B6, 4F2)

CYP1A2 is highest in the liver, where it makes up approximately 13% of CYP protein, but is also found in the lungs, pancreas, gastrointestinal tract and brain. CYP1A2 can be induced by smoking, barbecue meat polyamine hydrocarbons, omeprazole and other proton pump inhibitors, while oral contraceptives, fluvoxamine, and fluoroquinolone antibiotics reduce its expression. More than 100 CYP1A2 substrates are known, including many clinically important drugs (e.g., clozapine, olanzapine, tacrine, fluvoxamine, haloperidol, theophylline), procarcinogens (e.g., benzopyrene, aromatic/heterocyclic amines, aflatoxin B1), endogenous substrates (steroids, arachidonic acid, melatonin, bilirubin, estrogen) and caffeine. Compared to other CYP enzymes, CYP1A2 is a metabolic enzyme of only about 9% of commonly used drugs and for many drugs, CYP1A2 is not the only metabolic enzyme that would limit their metabolic rate. Given the dominant role of CYP1A2 in the activation of toxic xenobiotics compared to drug metabolism, its role in procarcinogen metabolism and cancer risk is examined [1, 2].

To date, more than 60 polymorphic *CYP1A2* alleles are known. The most common wild-type allele is *CYP1A2 *1A* whose activity is normal. The most important alleles with reduced activity are *1C, *1K, *3, *4, *7*, and the allele *6* is without activity. The *1F* allele with increased activity is a feature of the UM phenotype, and is associated with a reduced risk of hypertension in non-smokers who consume more caffeine [23].

CYP2A6 is responsible for the metabolism of some xenobiotics (nicotine, caffeine) and about 3% of drugs (e.g., coumarin, tegafur, letrozole and efavirenz). The gene is highly polymorphic with variations resulting in altered enzyme activity. CYP2A6 represents approximately 4% of the CYP protein content in the liver, and more than 80 *CYP2A6* alleles are known. The normal allele activity is *CYP2A6 *1A*, while the *1X2A* and *1X2B* alleles have enhanced activity (those present in duplicate express the UM phenotype). Alleles *2* and *4A–*4H* are without, and alleles *9A, *10, *11* and *17* have decreased activity. CYP2A6 phenotypic traits (as with other CYP enzymes) are described as PM (slow metabolizers without, or with both reduced activity functional alleles), IM (heterozygotes) and UM phenotypes (with multiple copies of alleles). The metabolic activity of CYP2A6 varies by substrate. For example, the activity of the *CYP2A6 *18* allele against nicotine is similar to that of the wild-type enzyme, but is reduced when it metabolizes coumarin and tegafur. On the other hand, the activity of *CYP2A6 *17* is similar to the wild type when metabolizing coumarin, but significantly reduced toward nicotine. People with *CYP2A6 *12* are slow metabolizers of letrozole but intermediate of nicotine. Nicotine dependence is closely related to the pharmacokinetics of nicotine. For example, slow metabolizers (alleles *CYP2A6 *2, *4, *9* and *12*) are less likely to be smokers and have a lower level of dependence compared to normal metabolizers [24]. CYP2A6 also plays a role in caffeine metabolism and is a major enzyme in the biotransformation of tegafur (to 5-fluorouracil), with the *4C and *11 alleles responsible for poor metabolism of drug. CYP2A6 is also important in the degradation of letrozole and efavirenz (e.g., PM phenotype decreases efavirenz clearance) [25].

CYP2B6 accounts for approximately 2–10% of total liver CYP. It is responsible for the metabolism of 4% of most common drugs. 38 *CYP2B6* alleles are known (*1–*38), and the most common (> 1%) are: *1, *6, *5, *2, *4, *7, *9* and *22. *CYP2B6* alleles can be normal (e.g., *1, *2, *5), enhanced (e.g., *4, *22) and decreased activity (e.g., *6, *7, *9). Large interindividual variations in CYP2B6 expression (20–250-fold) are attributed to differences in transcriptional regulation and genetic variation. Many CYP2B6 substrates (cyclophosphamide, phenobarbitol, rifampicin, phenytoin, artimesin, carbamazepine, efavirenz and nevirapine) can induce its expression. CYP2B6 is the major enzyme involved in the metabolism of bupropion, efavirenz and nevirapine [26–28], and the pharmacogenomics testing of this enzyme are important in the treatment of AIDS. Efavirenz has a narrow therapeutic window with severe side effects on the central nervous system when present in high concentrations, with treatment failure at low concentrations. *CYP2B6 *4* and *CYP2B6 *6* variants are associated with adverse effects of efavirenz treatment, and based on high level of clinical evidence, CPIC recommends dosing adjustment to the *CYP2B* genotype [24]. The clinical significance of *CYP2B6* variants is also associated with ineffective cyclophosphamide therapy and may affect the effect of bupropion when administered as a smoking cessation drug [26–29].

CYP4F2 is an enzyme predominantly expressed in the liver and kidneys and it is responsible for the metabolism of fatty acids and eicosanoids. It regulates the bioavailability of vitamin E and vitamin K (which it metabolizes and thus suppresses the effects of the enzyme VKORC1). As CYP4F2 enzyme polymorphisms have a significant effect on the dosing of vitamin K antagonists (drugs such as warfarin or acenocoumarol), it is sometimes in pharmacogenetics assessments determined in combination (*CYP2C9, VKORC1* and *CYP4F2*), but its contribution is relatively small, up to 5%. Three alleles are known (*1, *2, *3), the *CYP4F2 *1* allele has normal activity (about 70% of the white population), while the second most common and most important allele is *3* (about 30%), associated with changes in amino acid metabolism, high blood pressure and decreased metabolism of vitamins E and K [18].

3   Enzymes Involved in Phase II Drug Metabolism

3.1   Thiopurine Methyltransferase—TPMT

The TPMT enzyme catalyzes the S-methylation of aromatic and heterocyclic sulfhydryl drugs, which have cytotoxic and immunosuppressive properties, such as azathioprine and 6-mercaptopurine (6-MP), and are used in the treatment of acute lymphoblastic leukemia, rheumatoid arthritis, organ transplantation, autoimmune and inflammatory diseases. S-methylation of these drugs is a major pathway in their biotransformation, which reduces cytotoxicity in hematopoietic tissues. Patients with TPMT deficiency (PM phenotype) produce more active thioguanine nucleotides, which accumulate and lead to potentially lethal hematopoietic toxicity with standard doses of drugs, while patients with moderate TPMT activity (IM phenotype) accumulate approximately 50% more thioguanine nucleotides and thus also have an increased risk [30].

Multiple non-functional *TPMT* alleles have been associated with inheritance of low enzyme activity (Table 10). 43 alleles *(*1–*43)* are known, and the most common variants are the alleles *3A and *3C, *3B and *2, which encode proteins with almost immeasurable activity.

Pharmacogenetic profile of TPMT
Due to the hematotoxicity of thiopurine caused by decreased TPMT activity, pharmacogenetic testing of the *TPMT *2, *3A, *3B, *3C* and *4 alleles is recommended, achieving 95% sensitivity of PM phenotype recognition. According to the guidelines of the CPIC and PharmGKB clinical pharmacogenetics consortium, azathioprine-treated patients who are heterozygous with at-risk variants of the

Table 10 Most common *TPMT* alleles in different ethnic groups, their activity and phenotype characteristics

TPMT allele	Activity	Predicted phenotype of homozygotes	Allele frequencies in ethnic groups			
			European (%)	African American (%)	East Asian (%)	Latin American (%)
*1	Normal	EM	95.3	92.3	98.0	94.3
*2	No	PM	0.2	0.5	0.0	0.3
*3A	No	PM	3.4	0.8	0.0	4.2
*3B	No	PM	0.3	0.0	0.0	0.2
*3C	No	PM	0.5	2.4	1.6	0.6
*4	No	PM	0.0	0.0	0.0	0.0
*16	Unclear	?	0.1	0.0	0.0	0.0

Alleles and phenotype data are updated from https://cpicpgx.org/genes-drugs/ (January 2022)

TPMT gene (and/or *NUDT15*, see later), the starting dose should be 30–80% of the normal dose. In the PM phenotype for TPMT, drug change or drastically reduced dose (tenfold reduction, up to 3 days/week only) is recommended [31]. The same recommendation applies to patients scheduled for treatment with 6-mercaptopurine or 6-thioguanine. If, in addition to the non-functional TPMT phenotype, the non-functional NUDT15 phenotype is further identified (see later), drug doses should be further reduced [32].

3.2   N-acetyltransferase 2-NAT2

The enzyme NAT2 is involved in the transfer of acetyl groups with coenzyme A to hydrophobic primary amine and hydrazine substrates thus increasing their solubility in water. 88 polymorphic variants of this enzyme are known in humans, and unlike the nomenclature of other drug metabolism enzymes, the wild-type allele is considered to be *NAT2 *4,* instead of **1* (Table 11). Variability in acetylation of NAT2 substrate distinguishes slow (slow acetylator—SA, with two slow alleles), medium fast (with one slow and one fast allele) and fast acetylation phenotypes (rapid acetylator—RA, with 2 fast alleles), resulting from SNP mutations. Rapid acetylation is encoded by wild-type *NAT2 *4* alleles (30–50% of the population), while the remaining are carriers of several mutated alleles. The SA phenotype is associated with the side effects of many drugs, and its frequency varies significantly in different populations: it is present in 90% of Arabs, 40%–60% of whites and 5%–25% of yellow race. It is assumed that the difference in the distribution of SA alleles among races was due to the relaxation of the evolutionary pressure of exposure to xenobiotics during the change of diet (transition from hunting and collecting to agricultural breeding). The three main variants of NAT2 that contribute to the slow acetylation phenotype are *NAT2 *5, NAT2 *6* and *NAT2 *14.*

Pharmacogenetic profile of NAT2

Table 11 Most common *NAT2* alleles, their activity and phenotype characteristics

Alleles	Activity	Associated phenotype	Allele frequency (%)
NAT2 *4	Normal	EM (RA)	23.0
NAT2 *5 (*5A–*5Z)	Reduced	PM (SA)	46.0[#]
NAT2 *6 (*6A–*6 V)	Reduced	PM (SA)	28.0
NAT2 *7 (*7A–*7G)	Reduced	PM (SA)	
NAT2 *10	Reduced	PM (SA)	
NAT2 *11	Normal	EM (RA)	
NAT2 *14 *(*14A–*14L)	Reduced	PM (SA)	0.1

RA—Rapid acetylator, SA—Slow acetylator, [#]—the highest frequency among blacks; Alleles and phenotype data are updated from https://cpicpgx.org/genes-drugs/ (January 2022)

By genotyping the alleles *5, *6, *14A and *14B, more than 97% of slow acetylators can be identified. Pharmacologically important NAT2 substrates include: aminoglutethimide, amonafid, amrinone, cisplatin, dapson, ethambutol, hydralazine, isoniazid, caffeine, clonazepam, nitrazepam, pyrazinamide, procainamide, rifampin, sulfamethyzole, sulfalazine and tamoxifen, but only for some of them (hydralazine and amifampridine), the guidelines based on pharmacogenetics results recommend drug dosing adjustment and precaution [32].

3.3   Glutathione S-transferase—GSTM1, GSTT1, GSTP1

Gutathione S-transferases (GST) are a multifunctional superfamily of enzymes that catalyze reactions, in which xenobiotics are conjugated to the glutathione. They are involved in the metabolism of drugs used to treat cancer, such as alkylating agents, anthracyclines, topoisomerase II inhibitors and corticosteroids. The group of soluble glutathione-S-transferases is divided into 7 genetically different classes of enzymes: A (alpha α), M (mi μ), P (pi π), T (theta θ), K (kappa k), O (omega ω) and Z (zeta ζ). Each class of GST enzymes is encoded by one or more highly polymorphic genes, the most important of which are GSTM1 (μ class), GSTT1 (θ class), GSTP1 (π class) and GSTA1 (α class). Deletions in the *GST* genes lead to non-functional alleles *GSTM1 *0* and *GSTT1 *0*, resulting in non-functional enzymes GSTM1 and GSTT1 [33, 34].

The frequency of occurrence of non-functional alleles in the *GST* gene varies significantly in different ethnic groups. The data indicate that the *GSTM1* gene is not found in 42–58% of whites and 27–41% of Africans due to deletion of both copies of the gene. The frequency of non-functional alleles of the *GSTT1* gene is present in 2–42% of whites, 50–60% of Asians, 15–20% of African Americans and less than 10% of Hispanics. Polymorphisms in the *GSTP1* gene occur in 40% of whites and 54% of Africans while in the GSTA1 gene in 40% of whites and 41% of Africans [35–37].

There are reports in which patients with allelic variants of *GSTM1 *0* or *GSTT1 *0* treated with platinum-based chemotherapy have a poorer response and reduced overall survival. Shortened survival in patients with reduced GST activity could be associated with severe toxicity, as indicated by a higher incidence of severe neutropenia in homozygous *GSTM1 *0* carriers treated with platinum-based chemotherapy. Due to inconsistent and insufficient evidence from published studies, there are currently no recommendations for prescribing these drugs.

Two polymorphisms of the *GSTP1* gene have been described: rs94 7894 (c.A1404G) and rs1799811 (c.C2294T). Point mutations in the *GSTA1* gene promoter (*GSTA1 *B*) results in lower promoter activity and consequently reduced gene expression.

3.4   UDP Glucuronyl Transferase—UGT1A1

The UGT family consists of 117 members within 4 families of *UGT1, UGT2, UGT3* and *UGT8* genes. UGT1 is the most important group of enzymes of phase II drug metabolism, catalyzing glucuronidation reactions, and the best studied isoform is UGT1A1 with 113 known allelic variants. UGT1A1 is responsible for the metabolism and detoxification of drugs and many endogenous substances such as bilirubin, steroid hormones, fat-soluble vitamins and biogenic amines. It is mostly present in the liver but also in other tissues such as the intestines, stomach and breast. UGT1A1 is the major enzyme responsible for conjugating bilirubin to glucuronic acid. Variants of alleles (many of which are in the promoter region) that lead to decreased enzyme activity (*6, *27, *28, *37) result in unconjugated hyperbilirubinemias (Crigler-Najjar disease and Gilbert's syndrome) [38], while other variants increase enzyme activity (*36) (Table 12). Mutations that lead to complete loss of activity are associated with severe Crigler-Najjar type 1 hyperbilirubinemia, and milder lack of activity phenotypes result in milder forms of Crigler-Najjar type 2 hyperbilirubinemia.

The mildest form of decreased UGT1A1 activity (benign unconjugated hyperbilirubinemia, Gilbert's syndrome) is associated with the *UGT1A1 *28* variant (which has 7 TA nucleotide repeats in the TATA promoter region versus wild-type *UGT1A1 *1* repeat, with 6T). Alleles containing a different number of TA repeats are *UGT1A1 *36* (5 repeats, increased activity relative to allele *1) and *UGT1A1 *37* (8 repeats, further decreased activity relative to allele *28). Gilbert's syndrome affects about 6% of the population and is important for differential diagnostics to distinguish from other much more serious icteric conditions. In the Asian population, Gilbert's syndrome and neonatal hyperbilirubinemia are more commonly caused by the *UGT1A1 *6* allele (the enzymatic activity of the PM phenotype is only 32% of normal). Some studies have shown that carriers of the *28 and *6 alleles have an increased risk of carcinogenicity mediated by exposure to aromatic

Table 12 Most common *UGT1A1* alleles in different ethnic groups and their activity

UGT1A1 allele	Activity	Allele frequencies in ethnic groups			
		European (%)	African American (%)	East Asian (%)	Latin American (%)
*1	Normal	36.1	3.1	70.6	20.6
*6	Reduced	0.8	0.4	14.6	1.2
*27	Reduced				
*28	Reduced	31.6	37.3	14.8	40.0
*36	Reinforced	0.0	8.4	0.0	0.0
*37	Reduced	0.1	5.7	0.0	0.0
*80	Unknown	31.4	45.0		38.3

Alleles and phenotype data are updated from https://cpicpgx.org/genes-drugs/ (January 2022)

Table 13 Frequency, functional activity, phenotype characteristics and allele combinations in *UGT1A1*

Phenotype	Activity	Frequencies in ethnic groups				Example of a diplotype
		European (%)	African American (%)	East Asian (%)	Latin American (%)	
EM	Normal	13.0	1.3	49.8	4.2	*1/*1, *1/*36, *1/*36,
IM	Medium	46.1	20.4	41.5	32.7	*1/*28, *1/*37, *36/*28, *36/*37
PM	Reduced	40.9	78.3	8.7	63.1	*28/*28, *28/*37, *37/*37, *80/*80, *6/*6

Alleles and phenotype data are updated from https://cpicpgx.org/genes-drugs/ (January 2022)

hydrocarbons (from food, cigarette smoke, etc.), while the effect of the *1 allele is protective. Due to the antioxidant effect of bilirubin, research also mentions the protective effect of allele *28 in the risk of cardiovascular disease [39].

Pharmacogenetic profile of UGT1A1

UGT1A1 is the major enzyme in the detoxification of SN38, the active metabolite of the cytostatic irinotecan. In the treatment with irinotecan and some other drugs (sacituzumab, govitecan, belinostat and atazanavir), determination of homozygous carriers of *UGT1A1* *28 polymorphism (10% of them in the white population; PM phenotype, Table 13) can help assess the risk of toxic side effects (leukopenia, diarrhea), which has been shown to be financially justified because there are as many as 7% of patients with such side effects. There are CPIC and PharmGKB recommendations based on highest level of clinical evidence for pharmacogenetic testing in patients scheduled for treatment with atazanavir [40].

3.5   Sulfotransferase—SULT

Sulfotransferases (SULT) are a superfamily of cytosolic enzymes that catalyze sulfoconjugation reactions. Sulfoconjugations are an important metabolic pathway for detoxification and elimination of key endogenous compounds including steroids, thyroid hormones, catechols, various drugs and other xenobiotics.

The enzymes SULT1A1, SULT1A3, SULT1B1, SULT1C4, SULT1E1 and SULT2A1 are the most important for drug metabolism. Of the three isoforms of the SULT1A enzyme, the SULT1A1 isoform plays a key role in the sulfonation of phenolic xenobiotics, including polyphenols and a number of drug metabolites. Typical substrates for SULT1A1 are p-nitrophenol, naphthol, acetaminophen (paracetamol) and minoxidil. The enzyme SULT1A3 is involved in the sulfonation of monoamines and structurally related compounds (e.g., dopamine, serotonin and isoproterenol). SULT1B1 is the only member of the subfamily SULT1B, whose main function is sulfonation of thyroid hormones. SULT1C expression is most pronounced in fetal tissues and it is thought that SULT1C4 enzymes may play a role in the metabolism of xenobiotics and thyroid hormones during fetal development. SULT isoform 1A1 is commonly associated with an increased risk of cancer as well as a response to various therapeutic agents [40, 41].

Eighteen *SULT* genes encoding sulfotransferases were identified and classified into gene families: *SULT1*, *SULT2*, *SULT3*, *SULT4* and *SULT6* and five pseudogenes without protein product. Point polymorphisms (SNPs) in sulfotransferase genes mainly lead to functional consequences on the protein product and they are ethnically differently distributed [42].

The *SULT1E1* gene is the only member of the *SULT1E* subfamily and is thought to have a major physiological function in estrogen sulfonation, including estrone (E1) and 17-β estradiol (E2), but also the xenobiotic 17-β ethinyl estradiol (EE2). The enzyme SULT2A1 is involved in the metabolism of androgens and bile acids, and its substrates are the steroids budesonide and tibolone. No significant sulfonation activity of enzymes from the SULT4 and SULT6 gene families was detected.

4   Vitamin K Epoxy Reductase—VKORC1

The *VKORC1* gene encodes a key enzyme in the vitamin K cycle (Vitamin K epoxy reductase), which is responsible for converting the inactive form of vitamin K epoxide into a biologically active reduced form that then further catalyzes the activation of coagulation factors II, VII, IX and X (Fig. 2). More than 30 variants of the *VKORC1* allele have been linked to vitamin K-dependent coagulation factors in a way that increases resistance or sensitivity to drugs—oral anticoagulants such as coumarins and warfarin, which inhibit VKORC1 function. *VKORC1* gene polymorphisms significantly contribute to the variability of therapeutic response, and the most important *VKORC1* polymorphisms are *G1639A (rs9923231)* and *C1173T (rs9934438)* [43].

The *G1639* allele is present in the *VKORC1 *1, *3* and *4* haplotypes and is associated with the standard dose of warfarin. The *1639A* allele is present in the *VKORC1 *2* haplotype and makes it more sensitive to warfarin, and the need for a lower dose of the drug. Other common polymorphisms in VKORC1 do not significantly affect warfarin dose prediction and are rarely determined.

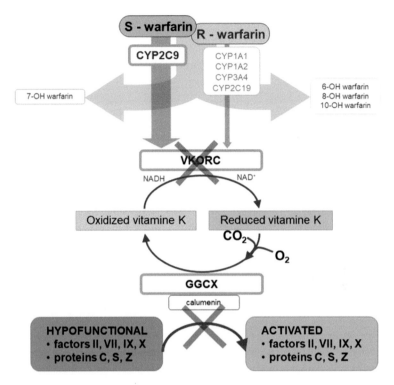

Fig. 2 Vitamin K cycle and the pharmacokinetic and pharmacodynamic pathways of warfarin. Warfarin is given as a racemic mixture of R- and S-enantiomers. The more potent, S-enantiomer, is mainly metabolized by CYP2C9, and the pharmacological effect of warfarin is mediated by inhibition of vitamin K epoxy reductase, complex 1 (VKORC1). This leads to a decrease in coagulation factor activity (II, VII, IX and X) and results in therapeutic anticoagulation (according to: www.medscape.com; 2008 Pharmacotherapy Publications). *Legend OH-hydroxy; NAD$^+$-oxidized form of nicotinamide adenine nucleotide; NADH-reduced form of NAD; GGCX-gamma glutamyl carboxylase*

---

5   Pharmacogenetic profile of CYP2C9 and VKORC1 in anticoagulant therapy

In anticoagulant therapy with warfarin, interindividual variability among patients can be largely explained by genetic polymorphisms *CYP2C9* (~ 10% variability) and *VKORC1* (~ 25% variability), while other, non-genetic factors, including age, BMI, sex, weight and INR, together contribute with about 20% of the total variability of the therapeutic response. Combinations of *CYP2C9* polymorphisms (polymorphisms *2 and *3) and *VKORC1* (polymorphisms *G1639A* and *C1173T*) carry an increased risk of a pronounced anticoagulant effect of coumarin drugs compared to individuals carrying at least one or both normal alleles. Heterozygous carriers of *VKORC1* polymorphisms in combination with *CYP2C9* polymorphism

Table 14 Example of predicted warfarin doses using the Sconce algorithm in individuals (height 182 cm and age 65 years) [43]

CYP2C9	Calculation of the daily dose (mg) of warfarin by genotype and the percentage difference of the usual dose		
	VKORC1 GG	VKORC1 AG	VKORC1 AA
*1/*1	6.8 mg/d	5.6 (−18%)	4.5 (−34%)
*1/*2	5.6 (−18%)	4.5 (−34%)	3.6 (−47%)
*1/*3	5.0 (−26%)	4.0 (−41%)	3.1 (−54%)
*2/*2	4.5 (−34%)	3.6 (−47%)	2.7 (−60%)
*2/*3	4.0 (−41%)	3.0 (−56%)	2.3 (−66%)
*3/*3	3.5 (−49%)	2.6 (−62%)	1.9 (−72%)

Table 15 CPIC and PharmGKB recommendations for treatment with coumarin anticoagulants (warfarin, phenprocoumon)

VKORC1/CYP2C9 genotype	Recommended therapy
VKORC1 wt/wt and CYP2C9 wt/wt	Therapy according to the instructions on the drug
VKORC1 wt/wt or risk variant heterozygous and CYP2C9 risk variant hetero or homozygote	Reducing the starting dose by 27–34%, frequent INR controls are required
VKORC1 risk variant homozygous and CYP2C9 wt/wt	To reduce the starting dose by 50%, frequent INR controls are required
VKORC1 risk variant homozygous and CYP2C9 risk variant hetero or homozygous	Reducing the starting dose by 55–61%, frequent INR controls are required

may have an enhanced and prolonged effect of coumarin drugs. Homozygous carriers of the VKORC1 polymorphism metabolize coumarin drugs slowly, thereby enhancing and prolonging the effect of the drug. The enhanced effect was particularly pronounced in combination with co-found polymorphism and in the CYP2C9 gene [43].

From the data of pharmacogenetic testing of CYP2C9 and VKORC1 (and some other involved genes, such as CYP4F2 and with the help of various available algorithms, it is possible to estimate the required dose of warfarin for each patient [42]. One of the simpler assessment algorithms based on pharmacogenetic testing CYP2C9 and VKORC1 shows Tables 14 and 15, and with the help of more complex online algorithms that include additional data, such as age, sex, INR, BMI and other genes (e.g., http://warfarindosing.org), the dose can be determined even more precisely [43–45].

6 Conclusion

The scientific literature cited in this review, as well as many other papers not cited here, show tremendous advances in understanding the drug-metabolizing enzymes concerning their functional properties, population variability of gene polymorphisms, genotype-phenotype correlation, and their impact on inter- and intra-individual variability in drug effects.

The clinical relevance of gene variants depends on the frequency of alleles and the magnitude of the effect of the clinical outcome parameters. Furthermore, it depends on the therapeutic range of the drug, the predictability of the drug response as well as the duration until the onset of therapeutic effect. The importance of genotyping can be in adjusting the dose according to the genotype, choosing the right therapeutic strategy, or even choosing a new drug. Dose adjustment based on pharmacogenetics is one of the tools to individualize drug treatment according to genetic factors to achieve optimal drug effect in each individual [46].

To link known gene variations for drug-metabolizing enzymes with clinical indicators of treatment efficacy reliably and systematically, the Clinical Pharmacogenetics Implementation Consortium (CIPC) provides guidelines to help physicians select, optimize, and personalize therapy to each patient, based on individual genotype and associated phenotype (https://cpicpgx.org/guidelines/).

References

1. Zanger UM. Schwab M. Cytochrome P450 enzymes in drug metabolism: regulation of gene expression, enzyme activities, and impact of genetic variation. Pharmacol Ther. 2013;138:103–41. https://doi.org/10.1016/j.pharmthera.2012.12.007.
2. Daly AK. Pharmacogenetics: a general review on progress to date. Br Med Bull. 2017;124(1):65–79. https://doi.org/10.1093/bmb/ldx035.
3. Steimer W, Potter JM. Pharmacogenetic screening and therapeutic drugs. Clin Chim Acta. 2002;315:137–55. https://doi.org/10.1016/s0009-8981(01)00713-6.
4. Sim S, Kacevska M, Ingelman-Sundberg M. Pharmacogenomics of drug-metabolizing enzymes: a recent update on clinical implications and endogenous effects. Pharm J. 2013;13:1–11. https://doi.org/10.1038/tpj.2012.45.
5. Gaedigk A, Dinh JC, Jeong H, Prasad B, Leeder JS. Ten years' experience with the CYP2D6 activity score: a perspective on future investigations to improve clinical predictions for precision therapeutics. J Pers Med. 2018;8:E15. https://doi.org/10.3390/jpm8020015].
6. Zanger UM, Raimundo S, Eichelbaum M. Cytochrome P450 2D6: overview and update on pharmacology, genetics, biochemistry. Naunyn Schmiedebergs Arch Pharmacol. 2004;369:23–37. https://doi.org/10.1007/s00210-003-0832-2.
7. Caudle KE, Klein TE, Hoffman JM, Muller DJ, Whirl-Carrillo M, Gong L, et al. Incorporation of pharmacogenomics into routine clinical practice: the Clinical Pharmacogenetics Implementation Consortium (CPIC) guideline development process. Curr Drug Metab. 2014;15(2):209–17. https://doi.org/10.2174/1389200215666140130124910.
8. Goetz MP, Kamal A, Ames MM. Tamoxifen pharmacogenomics: the role of CYP2D6 as a predictor of drug response. Clin Pharmacol Ther. 2008;83(1):160–6. https://doi.org/10.1038/sj.clpt.6100367.
9. Brown JT, Bishop JR, Sangkuhl K, Nurmi EL, Mueller DJ, Dinh JC, et al. Clinical Pharmacogenetics Implementation Consortium guideline for cytochrome P450 (CYP) 2D6 genotype

and atomoxetine therapy. Clin Pharmacol Ther. 2019;106(1):94–102. https://doi.org/10.1002/cpt.1409.

10. Desta Z, Zhao X, Shin J-G, Flockhart DA. Clinical significance of the cytochrome P450 2C19 genetic polymorphism. Clin Pharmacokinet Clin Pharmacol Ther. 2002;41(12):913–58. https://doi.org/10.2165/00003088-200241120-00002.

11. Scott SA, Sangkuhl K, Stein CM, Hulot JS, Mega JL, Roden DM, et al. Clinical Pharmacogenetics Implementation Consortium guidelines for CYP2C19 genotype and clopidogrel therapy: 2013 update. Clin Pharmacol Ther. 2013;94(3):317–23. https://doi.org/10.1038/clpt.2013.105.

12. Sim SC, Risinger C, Dahl ML, Aklillu E, Christensen M, Bertilsson L, Magnus Ingelman-Sundberg. A common novel CYP2C19 gene variant causes ultrarapid drug metabolism relevant for the drug response to proton pump inhibitors and antidepressants. Clin Pharmacol Ther. 2006;79(1):103–13. https://doi.org/10.1016/j.clpt.2005.10.002

13. Hicks JK, Sangkuhl K, Swen JJ, Ellingrod VL, Muller DJ, Shimoda K, et al. Clinical Pharmacogenetics Implementation Consortium guideline (CPIC) for CYP2D6 and CYP2C19 genotypes and dosing of tricyclic antidepressants: 2016 update. Clin Pharmacol Ther. 2017;102(1):37–44. https://doi.org/10.1002/cpt.597.

14. Miners JO, Birkett DJ. Cytochrome P4502C9: an enzyme of major importance in human drug metabolism. Br J Clin Pharmacol. 1998;45:525–38. https://doi.org/10.1046/j.1365-2125.1998.00721.x.

15. Aithal GP, Day CD, Kesteven JLP, Daly AK. Association of polymorphisms in the cytochrome P450 CYP2C9 with warfarin dose requirement and risk of bleeding complications. The Lancet. 1999;353(9154):717–9. https://doi.org/10.1016/S0140-6736(98)04474-2.

16. van der Weide J, Steijns LSW, van Weelden MJM, de Haan K. The effect of genetic polymorphism of cytochrome P450 CYP2C9 on phenytoin dose requirement. Pharmacogenetics. 2001;11(4):287–91. https://doi.org/10.1097/00008571-200106000-00002.

17. Karnes JH, Rettie AE, Somogyi AA, Huddart R, Fohner AE, Formea CM, et al. Clinical Pharmacogenetics Implementation Consortium (CPIC) guideline for CYP2C9 and HLA-B genotypes and phenytoin dosing: 2020 update. Clin Pharmacol Ther. 2021;109(2):302–9. https://doi.org/10.1002/cpt.2008.

18. Johnson JA, Caudle KE, Gong L, Whirl-Carrillo M, Stein CM, Scott CA, et al. Clinical Pharmacogenetics Implementation Consortium (CPIC) guideline for pharmacogenetics-guided warfarin dosing: 2017 update. Clin Pharmacol Ther. 2017;102(3):397–404. https://doi.org/10.1002/cpt.668.

19. Dean L. Warfarin therapy and the genotypes CYP2C9 and VKORC1. Created March 2012; Last update: June 11, 2018. Medical Genetics Summaries Internet. Available at: https://www.ncbi.nlm.nih.gov/books/NBK84174/. Accessed 26 June 2021.

20. IWPC Pharmacogenetic Dosing Algorithm—CPIC. Available at: https://cpicpgx.org › IWPC_dose_calculatorI

21. Theken KN, Craig R, Lee CR, Gong L, Caudle KE, Formea CM, et al. Clinical Pharmacogenetics Implementation Consortium guideline (CPIC) for CYP2C9 and nonsteroidal anti-inflammatory drugs. Clin Pharmacol Ther. 2020;108(2):191–200. https://doi.org/10.1002/cpt.1830

22. Birdwell KA, Decker B, Barbarino JM, Peterson JF, Stein CM, Sadee W, et al. Clinical Pharmacogenetics Implementation Consortium (CPIC) guidelines for CYP3A5 genotype and tacrolimus dosing. Clin Pharmacol Ther. 2015;98(1):19–24. https://doi.org/10.1002/cpt.113.

23. Koonrungsesomboon N, Khatsri R, Wongchompoo P, Teekachunhatean S. The impact of genetic polymorphisms on CYP1A2 activity in humans: a systematic review and meta-analysis. Pharmacogenomics J. 2018/12;18(6):760–8. https://doi.org/10.1038/s41397-017-0011-3

24. Nakajima M, Kwon JT, Tanaka N, Zenta T, Yamamoto Y, Yamamoto H, et al. Relationship between interindividual differences in nicotine metabolism and CYP2A6 genetic polymorphism in humans. Clin Pharmacol Ther. 2001;69(1):72–8. https://doi.org/10.1067/mcp.2001.112688.

25. Tanner J-A, Tyndale RF. Variation in CYP2A6 activity and personalized medicine. J Person Med. 2017;18(7):1–27. https://doi.org/10.3390/jpm7040018.
26. Zhang H, Sridar C, Kenaan C, Amunugama H, Ballou DP, Hollenberg PF. Polymorphic variants of cytochrome P450 2B6 (CYP2B6.4–CYP2B6.9) exhibit altered rates of metabolism for bupropion and efavirenz: a charge-reversal mutation in the K139E variant (CYP2B6.8) impairs formation of a functional cytochrome P450-reductase complex. J Pharmacol Exp Ther. 2011;338(3):803–9. https://doi.org/10.1124/jpet.111.183111
27. Desta Z, Gammal RS, Gong L, Whirl-Carrillo M, Gaur AH, Sukasem C, et al. Clinical Pharmacogenetics Implementation Consortium (CPIC) guideline for CYP2B6 and efavirenz-containing antiretroviral therapy. Clin Pharmacol Ther. 2019;106(4):726–33. https://doi.org/10.1002/cpt.1477.
28. Yoon HY, Cho YA, Yee J, Gwak HS. Effects of CYP2B6 polymorphisms on plasma nevirapine concentrations: a systematic review and meta-analysis. Nat Res Sci Rep. 2020;10:1–7. https://doi.org/10.1038/s41598-020-74506-x.
29. El-Serafi I, Afsharian P, Moshfegh A, Hassan M, Terelius Y. Cytochrome P450 oxidoreductase influences CYP2B6 activity in cyclophosphamide bioactivation. PLoS ONE. 2015;10(11): e0141979. https://doi.org/10.1371/journal.pone.0141979.
30. Wang L, Weinshilboum R. Thiopurine S-methyltransferase pharmacogenetics: insights, challenges and future directions. Oncogene. 2006;25:1629–38. https://doi.org/10.1038/sj.onc.1209372.
31. Relling MV, Schwab M, Whirl-Carrillo M, Suarez-Kurtz G, Ching-Hon Pui C-H, Stein CM, et al. Clinical Pharmacogenetics Implementation Consortium guideline for thiopurine dosing based on TPMT and NUDT15 genotypes: 2018 update. Clin Pharmacol Ther. 2019;105(5):1095–105. https://doi.org/10.1002/cpt.1304.
32. Sim E, Abuhammad A, Ryan A. Arylamine N-acetyltransferases: from drug metabolism and pharmacogenetics to drug discovery. Br J Pharmacol. 2014;171:2705–25. https://doi.org/10.1111/bph.12598.
33. Hayes JD, Strange RC. Glutathione S-transferase polymorphisms and their biological consequences. Pharmacology. 2000;61(3):154–66. https://doi.org/10.1159/000028396.
34. Cui JJ, Li Q, Yin J, Li L, Tan Y, Wei H, et al. GSTP1 and cancer: expression, methylation, polymorphisms and signaling (Review). Int J Oncol. 2020;56(4):867–78. https://doi.org/10.3892/ijo.2020.4979
35. Ding F, Li JP, Zhang Y, Qi GH, Song ZC, Yu YH. Comprehensive analysis of the association between the rs1138272 polymorphism of the GSTP1 gene and cancer susceptibility. Front Physiol. 2019;9:1897. https://doi.org/10.3389/fphys.2018.01897.
36. Gajecka M, Rydzanicz M, Jaskula-Sztul R, Kujawski M, Szyfter W, Szyfter K. CYP1A1, CYP2D6, CYP2E1, NAT2, GSTM1 and GSTT1 polymorphisms or their combinations are associated with the increased risk of the laryngeal squamous cell carcinoma. Mutat Res. 2005;574(1–2):112–23. https://doi.org/10.1016/j.mrfmmm.2005.01.027.
37. Aydin-Sayitoglu M, Hatirnaz O, Erensoy N, Ozbek U. Role of CYP2D6, CYP1A1, CYP2E1, GSTT1, and GSTM1 genes in the susceptibility to acute leukemias. Am J Hematol. 2006;81(3):162–70. https://doi.org/10.1002/ajh.20434.
38. Miners JO, McKinnon RA, Mackenzie PI. Genetic polymorphisms of UDP-glucuronosyltransferases and their functional significance. Toxicology. 2002;181–182:453–6. https://doi.org/10.1016/s0300-483x(02)00449-3.
39. Zulus B, Grünbacher G, Kleber ME, März W, Renner W. The UGT1A1*28 gene variant predicts long-term mortality in patients undergoing coronary angiography. Clin Chem Lab Med. 2018;56(4):560–4. https://doi.org/10.1515/cclm-2017-0692.
40. Gammal RS, Court MH, Haidar CE, Iwuchukwu OF, Gaur AH, Alvarellos M, et al. Clinical pharmacogenetics implementation consortium. Clinical Pharmacogenetics Implementation Consortium (CPIC) guideline for UGT1A1 and atazanavir prescribing. Clin Pharmacol Ther. 2016;99(4):363–9. https://doi.org/10.1002/cpt.269

41. Pachouri SS, Sobti RC, Kaur P, Singh J, Gupta SK. Impact of polymorphism in sulfotransferase gene on the risk of lung cancer. Cancer Genet Cytogenet. 2006;171(1):39–43. https://doi.org/10.1016/j.cancergencyto.2006.06.017.

42. Rasool MI, Bairam AF, Gohal SA, El Daibani AA, Alherz FA, Abunnaja MS, et al. Effects of the human SULT1A1 polymorphisms on the sulfation of acetaminophen, O-desmethylnaproxen, and tapentadol. Pharmacol Rep. 2019;71(2):257–65. https://doi.org/10.1016/j.pharep.2018.12.001.

43. Sconce EA, Khan TI, Wynne HA, Avery P, Monkhouse L, King BP, et al. The impact of CYP2C9 and VKORC1 genetic polymorphism and patient characteristics upon warfarin dose requirements: proposal for a new dosing regimen. Blood. 2005;106(7):2329–33. https://doi.org/10.1182/blood-2005-03-1108.

44. Obeng A, Kaszemacher T, Abul-Husn NS, Gottesman O, Vega A, Waite E, et al. Implementing algorithm-guided warfarin dosing in an ethnically diverse patient population using electronic health records and preemptive CYP2C9 and VKORC1 genetic testing. Clin Pharmacol Ther. 2016;100(5):427–30. https://doi.org/10.1002/cpt.425.

45. Johnson JA, Caudle KE, Gong L, Whirl-Carrillo M, Stein CM, Scott SA, et al. Clinical Pharmacogenetics Implementation Consortium (CPIC) guideline for pharmacogenetics-guided warfarin dosing: 2017 update. Clin Pharmacol Ther. 2017;102(3):397–404. https://doi.org/10.1002/cpt.668.

46. Primorac D, Höppner W, editors. Pharmacogenetics in clinical practice: experience with 55 commonly used drugs. Zagreb, Ham-burg, Philadelphia: St. Catherine Specialty Hospital, Bioglobe GmbH, ISABS; 2022. Available from: https://www.stcatherine.com/centre-of-excellence/10/individualized-and-preventive-medicine/pharmacogenomics/69

Role of Membrane Transporters in Pharmacogenomics

Lidija Bach-Rojecky, Dragan Primorac, Elizabeta Topić,
Mario Štefanović, and Wolfgang Höppner

Abstract

Protein membrane transporters are involved in various physiological processes, like the regulation of cell integrity, metabolism, and homeostasis. They transport multiple endogenous and exogenous substrates through cells. Most of the genes coding for these transporters are polymorphic with consequent modulated protein function by affecting either the activity of the transporter or expression level. Some transporters play a role in the disposition of many drugs, increasing or decreasing their intracellular and extracellular levels. Polymorphisms in

L. Bach-Rojecky
University of Zagreb Faculty of Pharmacy and Biochemistry, 10000 Zagreb, Croatia

D. Primorac (✉)
St. Catherine Specialty Hospital, 10000 Zagreb, Croatia
e-mail: dragan.primorac@svkatarina.hr; draganprimorac2@gmail.com

University of Split School of Medicine, 21000 Split, Croatia

Josip Juraj Strossmayer University of Osijek Faculty of Medicine, 31000 Osijek, Croatia

University of Rijeka School of Medicine, 51000 Rijeka, Croatia

Josip Juraj Strossmayer University of Osijek Faculty of Dental Medicine and Health, 31000 Osijek, Croatia

Eberly College of Science, State College, Penn State University, 517 Thomas St, State College, PA 16803, USA

The Henry C. Lee College of Criminal Justice and Forensic Sciences, University of New Haven, West Haven, CT, USA

Medical School REGIOMED, 96450 Coburg, Germany

National Forensic Science University, Gandhinagar, Gujarat, India

College of Medicine and Forensics, Xi'an Jiaotong University, Xi'an, China

International Center For Applied Biological Sciences, 10000, Zagreb, Croatia

© The Author(s), under exclusive license to Springer Nature Switzerland AG 2023   61
D. Primorac et al. (eds.), *Pharmacogenomics in Clinical Practice*,
https://doi.org/10.1007/978-3-031-45903-0_4

these transporters might be, among other factors, determinants of interindividual differences in the responses to many drugs.

Keywords

Transporter proteins • Gene variations • Pharmacogenetics • Pharmacokinetics • Efficacy • Adverse effects

1   Introduction

Membrane transport proteins play a crucial role in the absorption, distribution, metabolism, and excretion of many endogenous substances, such as glucose, bilirubin, and creatinine, as well as various xenobiotics, including drugs. They are expressed on the membranes of intestinal epithelial cells, hepatocytes, proximal renal tubule cells, brain capillary endothelial cells [1]. Changes in transporters' function due to various diseases or gene polymorphisms can change physiological processes. Also, they may affect the pharmacokinetics, efficacy, and toxicity of drugs, such as statins, calcium channel blockers, antidepressants, protease inhibitors, many anti-cancer drugs. Furthermore, changes in transporter function can significantly contribute to drug resistance, which is a major clinical problem, especially in oncology. A mechanism for cancer chemo-resistance might be a consequence of decreased expression and/or activity of influx transporters, or increased expression and/or activity of efflux transporters [2].

Transport proteins are the third most common class of pharmacological targets, corresponding to 15% of all human drug targets [3].

Membrane transport proteins are divided into two major superfamilies: ATP Binding Cassette Family (ABC) and Solute Carrier (SLC)-type membrane proteins [1].

With over 40% of genes among more than 900 transporter-encoding genes, the SLC superfamily encodes the largest group of membrane transporters in humans.

Genome-wide and candidate gene association studies show the significance for variants in breast cancer resistance protein (BCRP, encoded by *ABCG2* gene) and organic anion-transporting polypeptide 1B1 (OATP1B1, encoded by *SLCO1B1* gene*)* as major determinants of interindividual variation in drug absorption, disposition, and response. Therefore, according to the International Transporter

E. Topić
Croatian Society of Medical Biochemists, 10000 Zagreb, Croatia

Croatian Academy of Medical Sciences, 10000 Zagreb, Croatia

M. Štefanović
Clinical Institute of Chemistry, University Hospital Sestre Milosrdnice, 10000 Zagreb, Croatia

W. Höppner
Bioglobe GmbH, 22529 Hamburg, Germany

Consortium (ITC) and supported by the growing clinical data, common polymorphisms in BCRP *(ABCG2)*, OATP1B1 *(SLCO1B1)*, but also organic cation transporter (OCT1, encoded by *SLC22A1* gene), P-glycoprotein (P-pg encoded by *ABCB1* gene), OATP1B3 (encoded by *SLCO1B3* gene), OAT 1, 2 and 3 (encoded by *SLC22A6, SLC22A2 SLC22A8* genes, respectively), and multidrug and toxin extrusion protein (encoded by *SLC47A1* gene) should be considered during the relevant drug development program [4].

Although many polymorphic drug transporter variants may affect treatment outcomes, for the majority, there is insufficient evidence to introduce genotyping as a way to predict the efficacy and safety of the therapy. Because of inconsistent and often contradictory data, the Clinical Pharmacogenetics Implementation Consortium (CPIC) published guidelines just for several gene variant-drug combinations with the highest level of clinical importance [5].

This chapter gives brief overview of the clinically most important transporters and their relevance for pharmacogenomics.

2 ABC Superfamily

Within this group, 48 membrane transport proteins are known in humans, which are further distributed into seven subfamilies (ABCA, ABCB, ABCC, ABCD, ABCE/ABCF, and ABCG). They are involved in the regulation of cellular metabolism and homeostasis. Having four core domains, two transmembrane and two cytosolic domains, they utilize the energy of ATP binding and hydrolysis to serve as carriers for many endogenous substrates across biological membranes, like amino acids, sugars, nucleosides, vitamins, lipids, bile acids, eicosanoids, uric acid, antioxidants, and some natural toxins. In addition, they export many drug substrates to the extracellular space and contribute to drug resistance [6].

Previous clinical studies implicated genetic polymorphisms in at least 12 genes coding for ABC proteins connected with the risk of adverse drug reactions or altered therapeutic efficacy.

Up to now, 14 of ABC-transporter genes with clinical annotations related to drug response or adverse events have been included in The Pharmacogenomics Knowledge Base (PharmGKB): *CFTR, ABCA1, ABCB5, ABCB1, ABCC4, ABCC5, ABCC1, ABCC1, ABCC2, ABCC3, ABCC6, ABCC10, ABCG2,* and *ABCG1*. Only four have level 1 or 2 evidence of clinical annotations (according to PharmGKB classification, level 1 corresponds to high evidence and level 2 to moderate evidence). However, except for *CFTR* [7], no specific clinical recommendations are available due to a lack of more robust clinical evidence [8].

2.1   ABCB1 (P-gp, from P-Glycoprotein; MDR1, from Multidrug Resistance Protein)

P-gp is expressed in the plasma membrane of cells in a barrier and elimination organs. In the adrenal cortex, it is possibly involved in hormone transport, homeostasis, and glucocorticoid resistance. It mediates various cellular processes and is important for the exertion of hundreds of drugs from the cell, their passage through physiological barriers (blood–brain barrier, blood-placental barrier), and elimination from the body. It has a significant role in the first-pass elimination of drugs, limiting their bioavailability. P-gp also eliminates substrates from the systemic circulation via kidney and biliary excretion [9]. Numerous variants of the *ABCB1* gene are known that may be associated with altered protein expression and function. Gene polymorphisms that lead to increased expression and transporter function may explain resistance to cytostatic therapy since many cancer cells overexpress this transporter on their membranes [10]. Polymorphic transporters may also contribute to decreased efficacy of drugs with activity in the central nervous system (e.g., antiepileptics) due to their increased efflux to the periphery.

Three *ABCB1* polymorphisms have been most extensively studied: 1236C >T (rs1128503), 3435C > T (rs1045642), and 2677G > T/A (rs2032582). These polymorphisms are in linkage disequilibrium and define haplotype *ABCB1*2*, which is related to transporter increased activity. Polymorphic transporters might be associated with interindividual variability in treatment response to drug substrates, such as digoxin, nevirapine, simvastatin, methotrexate, and some opioids (Table 1) [8].

Additionally, these gene variants are associated with the risk of adverse reactions during therapy with cytostatics, like fluoropyrimidine, taxanes, and anthracyclines.

Variation rs1045642 is related to resistance to antiseizure drugs, like carbamazepine and valproate, although the results of studies are in discordance. The missense variants rs2229109 and rs9282564 found most frequently in Europeans (minor allele frequency = 4.3% and 10.8%) are possibly associated with paclitaxel toxicity [6].

According to a significant influence of P-gp on drugs' concentration in the cells and their clearance from the organism, currently clinical considerations are related to its role in multidrug resistance and drug-drug interactions. Although *ABCB1* gene polymorphisms might influence the efficacy and safety of different substrate drugs, further assessment and confirmation of their relevance for clinical practice are needed.

Table 1 Examples of gene variants-drug interaction (according to https://cpicpgx.org and https://www.pharmgkb.org/)

Gene	Variant	Drug	Clinical association/effect
ABCB1 (MDR1)	1236C > T (rs1128503)	Idarubicin plus cytarabine	Toxicity of induction chemotherapy in acute myeloid leukemia
		Geftinib	Toxicity
		Digoxin	Genotype AA is associated with increased likelihood of sudden cardiac death as compared to genotypes AG + GG
		Modafinil	Genotype AG is associated with increased response to modafinil in people with narcolepsy as compared to genotypes AA + GG
	3435C > T (rs1045642)	Methotrexate (level 2A)	Increased exposure and toxicity in acute lymphoblastic leukemia or non-Hodgkin lymphoma patients
		Nevirapine (level 2A)	Allele A is associated with decreased risk of toxic liver disease in people with HIV infections
		Digoxin (level 2A)	T allele carriers have higher bioavailability and plasma concentration and lower renal clearance
		Opioids	Patients with the AG genotype may have an increased risk of opioid dependence as compared to the AA or GG genotypes

(continued)

Table 1 (continued)

Gene	Variant	Drug	Clinical association/ effect
	2677G > T/A (rs2032582	Taxanes and platinum compounds	Toxicity in ovarian cancer patients
		Simvastatin (level 2A)	Genotype AA is associated with increased reduction in total cholesterol as compared to genotype CC
		Modafinil	Decreased response in narcolepsy patients
ABCC4	rs1751034	Tenofovir (level 2b)	TT genotype is associated with weaker effect because of lower intracelular drug concentration
ABCG2	rs2231142	Allopurinol (level 2B) Rosuvastatin (level 2A)	T allele carriers have reduced drug effect Genotypes GT + TT are associated with increased concentrations as compared to genotype GG
CFTR	rs75527207 rs397508537 rs11971167, etc	Ivacaftor[a] (level 1A)	Used in patients with at least one copy of a list of 33 CFTR genetic variants
SLCO1B1	rs4149056	Simvastatin[a] and atorvastatin[a] (level 1A)	CC + CT carriers may have an increased risk of myopathy as compared to the TT genotype.
SLC6A4	rs4795541	SSRI	*SLC6A4* HTTLPR long form (L allele) is associated with increased response as compared to*SLC6A4* HTTLPR short form (S allele)

(continued)

Table 1 (continued)

Gene	Variant	Drug	Clinical association/ effect
SLC1A	rs3087879	SSRI	Allele C is associated with increased severity of pharmacological resistance as compared to allele G

Legend SSRI—Selective serotonin reuptake inhibitors; [a] The highest level of clinical significance with CPIC guidelines; Level 1 clinical annotations describe variant-drug combinations that have variant-specific prescribing guidance available in a current clinical guideline annotation or an FDA-approved drug label annotation; Level 2A and 2B—These clinical annotations describe variant-drug combinations with a moderate level of evidence supporting the association. The association may be found in multiple cohorts, but there may be a minority of studies that do not support the majority assertion

2.2 ABCG2 (BCRP, from the Breast Cancer Resistance Protein, also Known as MXR or MCF-7)

ABC subfamily G, isoform 2 (*ABCG2*), is a gene encoding another efflux transporter with a broad substrate profile, like endogenous and naturally occurring polar molecules, flavonoids, antivirals, antibiotics, antivirals, and chemotherapeutics [11]. Increased activity and overexpression of the BCRP protein due to genetic variations are associated with resistance to different anti-cancer drugs, including tyrosine kinase inhibitors [12].

The BCRP protects tissues from xenobiotics and harmful metabolites and mediates their absorption, distribution, and elimination. It is distributed through the body, with the highest expression in brain tissue, the cervix, the small intestine, and the uterus. Additionally, its high expression in the kidney and liver mediates the elimination of substrates from the blood, while at the blood–brain barrier limits the entrance of substrates into the brain [11].

Many cancer cells, like stomach, colon, and esophageal cancer, can overexpress BCRP through gene amplification and chromosomal translocation. This can be associated with worse therapeutic outcomes since many chemotherapeutics (like imatinib, nilotinib, and dasatinib) are BCRP substrates [12].

Among many single nucleotide polymorphisms, the two most common and extensively studied variants are c.34G > A, which results in a V12M replacement, and rs2231142 c.421C > A, which results in a Q141K substitution. Both variants are most prevalent in East Asians and Latin Americans (22–32%), whereas their frequencies are lower in all other populations (4–10% in Europeans) [6].

While the rs2231137 variant does not affect the expression, localization, and function of BCRP or influence the pharmacokinetics of drug substrates, the rs2231142 variant decreases the expression of BCRP and is more important for the pharmacogenetics. For example, in individuals with the rs2231142 GG geno-type, a more pronounced therapeutic effect of allopurinol is achieved than in T allele carriers [13]. Also, carriers of the T allele who use rosuvastatin to treat hypercholesterolemia are exposed to higher drug plasma concentrations, as shown by most studies on the East Asian population [14]. Compared with Caucasian patients, Asian patients have a twofold increase in drug exposure, resulting in an increased risk for myopathy because of higher drug concentrations.

A strong association (at genome-wide level significance) of the C genotype with improved low-density lipoprotein cholesterol response to rosuvastatin was found in a genome-wide association study among near 7000 patients of European ancestry [15]. Additionally, *ABCG2* C421A variant A allele was significantly associated with a higher overall response to imatinib therapy, especially in Asian patients [16].

Undoubtedly, variation in BCRP activity affects the pharmacokinetics of many drugs and has been associated with their toxicity and efficacy. For now, the results of studies on the East Asian population strongly suggest the clinical implication of the rs2231142 gene variant. The significance of other variants needs further evaluation.

2.3   ABCC (MRP, from Multidrug Resistance Proteins)

Nine *ABCC* genes code for cellular plasma membrane transporters that function as efflux pumps. They have a broad specificity for the transport of endogenous and exogenous anionic substances, like glutathione conjugates (MRP1, MRP2, MRP4), bilirubin glucuronides (MRP2 and MRP3), cyclic AMP, and cyclic GMP (MRP4, MRP5, and MRP8). They are expressed on the liver and the kidney, exerting drugs from cells into bile and urine [17]. Many drugs and conjugated metabolites are substrates of these transporters, including methotrexate, etoposide, and the inactive metaboliteirinotecan glucuronide.

For example, *ABCC1* rs246240 G and *SLC22A11* rs11231809 T carriers are associated with an increased risk of non-response to methotrexate in the treatment of rheumatoid arthritis [18]. Rs45511401 allele T is associated with an increased risk of cardiotoxicity in patients treated with doxorubicin as compared to allele G carriers [19].

Moreover, multiple *ABCC* variants have been associated with irinotecan (rs3740066 in *ABCC2*, rs4148405 in *ABCC3* as well as rs3749438 and rs10937158 in *ABCC5*) or taxane drugs (rs12762549 in *ABCC2* as well as rs2238472 and rs2125739 in *ABCC6*) toxicity or response across populations. The *ABCC2* c.-24C >T polymorphism (rs717620), which causes reduced protein expression, has been the most studied, especially concerning cytostatics efficacy and safety [17]. As indicated by several studies, *ABCC2 c. −24C > T* TT or CT + TT genotypes can also contribute to antiseizure drug resistance in patients with generalized epilepsy [20].

2.4   CFTR (from, Cystic Fibrosis Transmembrane Conductance Regulator)

CFTR (or ABCC7), encoded by the *CFTR* gene, is an anion channel that transports chloride and bicarbonate ions and is expressed predominantly in epithelial tissues but is also found in other cell types such as smooth muscle, cardiac myocytes, macrophages, and erythrocytes. Therefore, defective CFTR results in widespread cellular homeostasis dysfunction. More than 2000 pathogenic *CFTR* gene variants associated with loss of channel function, grouped into six classes depending on the effect, have been reported to be associated with cystic fibrosis, an autosomal recessive disease. For example, two variants that cause severe disease phenotype are the most frequent *CFTR* variant F508del (c.1521_1523delCTT, rs199826652 or rs113993960), which results in an immature protein that is consequently mostly degraded, while second variant G551D (c.1652G > A, rs75527207) results in proteins which have defective channel gating when present in the plasma membrane [21]. Ivacaftor is a drug that potentiates CFTR gating function in patients having *CFTR* variant G551D (rs75527207). Ivacaftor is limited to patients with respective pathogenic gene variants (38 according to the US Food and Drug Administration) [7, 22].

2.5   ABCC8

ABCC8 (SUR1, sulfonylurea receptor) regulates ATP-sensitive K^+ channels and insulin secretion from pancreatic cells. Of clinical importance might be Ala1369Ser (rs757110) variant because some studies found that A/C carriers exhibited a higher response to sulfonylurea drugs compared to homozygous (A/A) and homozygous wild-type genotypes (C/C) [23]. However, because of inconsistent results regarding the association between the rs757110 variant and response to sulfonylureas, further evidence is needed.

3   SLC Superfamily

The large superfamily of SLC membrane transporters consists of more than 420 proteins organized into 65 families [24]. They are a heterogeneous group of broadly expressed membrane proteins with different substrate specificity. Many SLC members transport their substrates through secondary active transport or facilitative transport mechanisms. While some families, such as SLC2 and SLC27, carry glucose and long-chain fatty acids, others have a range of substrates (SLC22 transports different organic cations, anions, and zwitterions). The SLC superfamily also includes transporters of biogenic amines that participate in the regulation of signal transduction at the synapses of the peripheral and central nervous systems [25].

So far, numerous polymorphic variants of genes that change the expression and function of the transporter have been discovered, which possibly contribute to diseases, such as obesity, diabetes, central nervous system diseases, cancer. For example, genetic variations in the neurotransmitter transporters are associated with a range of neurological disorders to attention-deficit hyperactivity disorder, schizophrenia, and autism, while upregulation of the alanine serine cysteine transporter 2 (SLC1A5) is connected with poor prognosis in non-small cell lung cancer [25].

Given their abundance and role in the transport of essential organic and inorganic substances, they are investigated as potential sites of drug action. Even though the SLC family is generally druggable using small-molecule compounds, only 12 drug classes are approved by the Food and Drug Administration, whose primary mode of action is mediated selectively through one SLC or non-selectively through at least two. Some examples are drugs from the antidepressant, antidiabetic and diuretic classes. An example of recent successful blockbusters is a novel class of antidiabetics. These drugs inhibit sodium-glucose transporter type 2, encoded by the *SLC5A2* gene. They were developed based on associations between *SLC5A2* mutations and familial renal glucosuria. Other targeted proteins are the SLC6, SLC12, SLC18, SLC22, SLC25, and SLC29 families [26].

Several transporter families play a significant role in drug absorption, distribution, and elimination (e.g., SLC22 family, expressed in the kidney, liver, and blood–brain-barrier to regulate drug pharmacokinetics). Members of the SLC15 transporters represent another group of transporters that mediate the uptake of a broad range of peptides and peptide-like drugs. Most SLC transporters use an electrochemical and concentration gradient to transfer the substrate into the cell. Gene polymorphisms can therefore significantly affect the pharmacological profile of substrate drugs [25].

3.1   SLCO1B1 (formerly known as Organic Anion Transporter Protein, OAT1B1)

The solute carrier organic anion transporter family member 1B1 (*SLCO1B1*) gene encodes for a membrane-bound sodium-independent organic anion transporter protein (OATP1B1). Located predominantly on the basolateral membrane of hepatocytes, it actively transports many endogenous and xenobiotic anionic compounds into the cells. *SLCO1B1* is an important pharmacogene because OATP1B1 mediates the intrahepatic transport of many pharmaceutical agents [27]. The most studied is its influence on pharmacological characteristics of statins, widely used hypolipemic drugs for cardiovascular disease risk reduction. The liver is the site of action for statins, as well as for their metabolism before biliary elimination [28].

Hydrophilic drug pravastatin particularly relies on OATP1B1 transport since it cannot enter into hepatocytes through passive transport. Additionally, OATP1B1-dependent transport is important for the active form of simvastatin (acid), as well for other drugs, like the most used atorvastatin and rosuvastatin. Two common non-synonymous *SLCO1B1* variants rs2306283 (492A > G) rs2306283 (SLCO1B1: 492A > G) and rs4149056 (625T > C, or T521C) are in partial linkage disequilibrium. The minor allele of *SLCO1B1* T521C (the C allele is assigned a decreased function allele) is present in *5, *15, *16, *17 haplotypes and has been associated with elevated circulating concentrations of statins due to reduced protein function [29, 30].

Lower intrahepatic statins concentration can result in reduced hypolipemic effects, while elevated systemic concentrations are connected with extrahepatic side-effects, like muscle toxicity. It is estimated that the risk of myalgia and rhabdomyolysis is increased by 3–5 times in patients with reduced transporter function. Statin-induced myotoxicity (prevalence rate 7–30%) along with hepatotoxicity (prevalence rate 2–5%) are common dose-dependent drugs' adverse effects [28]. Patients with genotypes CC (up to 6% of patients) and CT (11–36% of patients) may have an increased risk of myopathy when treated with statins as compared to the TT genotype [29]. Statin dosing adjustments are suggested by CPIC, based on the *SLCO1B1* polymorphisms. It was found that even for the 40-mg simvastatin dose, the relative risk of myopathy is 2.6 per copy of the C allele at rs4149056. The risk is higher for the 80-mg simvastatin dose (myopathy odds ratio 4.5 for the TC genotype, ~20.0 for the CC genotype) [30].

3.2   SLC22A1

SLC22A1 gene encodes Organic Cationic Transporter 1 (OCT1), predominantly expressed in the liver, that mediates the uptake of a variety of endogenous ligands (dopamine, serotonin, choline) as well as cationic drugs, such as metformin, imatinib, oxaliplatin, morphine, and tramadol from the blood into cells thus impacting their pharmacokinetics and pharmacodynamics. Four nonsynonymous *SLC22A1* variants that have been most extensively studied are rs12208357, rs34130495, OCT1 420 deletion, and rs34059508. Carriers of loss-of-function *OCT1* polymorphisms had a 56% higher mean AUC of morphine compared to non-carriers, as well as significantly higher plasma concentrations of tramadol active metabolite of O-demethyltramadol [31]. However, because of the lack of data replication by multiple independent studies, the clinical applicability of these variants should be interpreted with caution.

3.3   SLC6A4 (5-HTTLPR)

Serotonin transporter (5-HTT, SERT) is a high-affinity protein for sodium and chloride ion-dependent serotonin (5-hydroxytryptamine, 5-HT) uptake into the cells. It is in the membranes of presynaptic neurons and participates in the reuptake of 5-HT. Due to its role in the regulation of serotonergic transmission, this protein is the primary target of selective serotonin reuptake inhibitors (SSRIs) such as fluoxetine, citalopram, fluvoxamine, sertraline, and paroxetine [32].

Of clinical importance are two *5-HTTLPR* polymorphisms. (1) VNTR polymorphism (L/S polymorphism) is a variable number of consecutive nucleotide repeats (from the Variable Number of Tandem Repeats). VNTR polymorphism is located outside the coding region of the exon and affects the change in the level of gene expression. Four polymorphic alleles are important: with nine (STin2.9), ten (STin2.10), eleven (STin2.11), or twelve (STin2.12) copies of the repetitive element. The most common STin2.12 is referred to as the 'L' allele, and the others are referred to as the 'S' allele. Several studies suggested that the STin2.12 allele of the STin2 VNTR polymorphism is likely a risk factor for schizophrenia susceptibility [33]. (2) Insertion / deletion polymorphism (rs4795541) within the gene promoter consists of 4 alleles with 14, 16, 18, or 20 repeating units of about 22pb in length. The common *5-HTTLPR* alleles are the long (L; 16 repeats) and short (S; 14 repeats) haplotypes, which are defined by a 43 bp insertion/deletion polymorphism. The 'L' allele is associated with enhanced transcription and biological activity of the transporter protein. The *5-HTTLPR* has been associated with antidepressant response in mood disorder patients, but findings are not consistent across studies [34]. Some studies found that *HTTLPR* S allele/L allele and S allele/S allele are associated with reduced response to antidepressants, as compared to L allele/L allele [35].

Considering other gene variants which significantly influence antidepressants' therapy efficacy and safety (e.g., gene variants for CYP enzymes), clinical implementation of *HTTLPR L/S* polymorphisms determination might also provide useful information when identifying patients who will not respond to antidepressant treatment.

3.4   SLC6A3 (DAT1)

SLC6A3 gene encodes a protein transporter that regulates the synaptic level of the neurotransmitter dopamine (DAT1, dopamine transporter). To date, polymorphic dopamine transporter alleles have been associated with an altered response to various drugs, like clozapine, disulfiram, and ethanol, as well as to methylphenidate in the treatment of attention-deficit hyperactivity disorder (ADHD). In the *SLC6A3* gene, the rs28363170 polymorphism of the VNTR region (2 to 11 repeats of part of the gene) is clinically relevant. The homozygous 10-repeat genotype of the 40 bp VNTR in the *SLC6A3* gene was associated with significantly reduced efficacy of methylphenidate in the treatment of ADHD [36], however there is no clinical guideline suggesting its determination in patients receiving the drug treatment.

3.5 SLC19A1 (Folate Transporter)

SLC19A1 encodes a high-capacity, bi-directional transporter of 5-methyl-tetrahydrofolate and thiamine monophosphate. It also actively transports methotrexate (MTX) into cells. MTX is used as an antifolate chemotherapeutic agent and as an immunomodulator in the therapy of inflammatory bowel diseases and rheumatoid arthritis. Human *SLC19A1* is highly polymorphic. The most extensively studied is a non-synonymous polymorphism Arg27His (80G > A; rs1051266), which has a total minor allele frequency of 44% and is found across all ethnic groups [37]. Several studies found an association between the probability of methotrexate-induced remission of rheumatoid arthritis symptoms in carriers of AA genotype as compared with patients with GG genotype, thus implicating that evaluation of *SLC19A1* 80G>A polymorphism may be a useful tool to optimize methotrexate therapy [38].

4 Conclusion

Despite the growing number of investigations of the influence of different transporter genotypes on drugs pharmacokinetics and pharmacological response, the majority of studies showed only weak associations and needed more proof before implementation in clinical practice [39].

Only a few of a large number of membrane transporters significantly affect the pharmacokinetics and pharmacodynamics of substrate drugs, where changes in their expression and function may alter the efficacy and safety of the therapy. Gene polymorphisms are the subject of intensive research, and only a few drugs have clinical guidelines suggesting pharmacogenomics testing of the respective transporter gene based on consistent and robust clinical evidence.

References

1. Yee SW, Brackman DJ, Ennis EA, Sugiyama Y, Kamdem LK, Blanchard R, et al. Influence of transporter polymorphisms on drug disposition and response: a perspective from the international transporter consortium. Clin Pharmacol Ther. 2018;104(5):803–17. https://doi.org/10.1002/cpt.1098.
2. Robey RW, Pluchino KM, Hall MD, Fojo AT, Bates SE, Gottesman MM. Revisiting the role of ABC transporters in multidrug-resistant cancer. Nat Rev Cancer. 2018;18:452–64. https://doi.org/10.1038/s41568-018-0005-8
3. Rask-Andersen M, Almén MS, Schiöth HB. Trends in the exploitation of novel drug targets. Nat Rev Drug Discov. 2011;10(8):579–90. https://doi.org/10.1038/nrd3478.
4. Giacomini KM, Galetin A, Huang SM. The International transporter consortium: summarizing advances in the role of transporters in drug development. Clin Pharmacol Ther. 2018;104(5):766–71. https://doi.org/10.1002/cpt.122410.1002/cpt.1098.
5. Clinical Pharmacogenetics Implementation Consortium (CPIC®). Available at: https://cpicpgx.org/guidelines/ Accessed: 29 Dec 2021.

6. Xiao Q, Zhou Y, Lauschke VM. Ethnogeographic and inter-individual variability of human ABC transporters. Hum Genet. 2020;139(5):623–46. https://doi.org/10.1007/s00439-020-021 50-6.
7. Primorac D, Höppner W, editors. Pharmacogenetics in clinical practice: Experience with 55 commonly used drugs. Zagreb, Hamburg, Philadelphia: St. Catherine Specialty Hospital, Bioglobe GmbH, ISABS; 2022. Available from: https://www.stcatherine.com/centre-of-excell ence/10/individualized-and-preventive-medicine/pharmacogenomics/69
8. López-Fernández LA. ATP-binding cassette transporters in the clinical implementation of pharmacogenetics. J Pers Med. 2018;8(4):40. https://doi.org/10.3390/jpm8040040.
9. Hodges LM, Markova SM, Chinn LW, Gow JM, Kroetz DL, Klein TE, Altman RB. Very important pharmacogene summary: ABCB1 (MDR1, P-glycoprotein). Pharmacogenet Genomics. 2011;21(3):152–61. https://doi.org/10.1097/FPC.0b013e3283385a1c.
10. Gottesman M, Fojo T, Bates S. Multidrug resistance in cancer: role of ATP–dependent transporters. Nat Rev Cancer. 2002;2:48–58. https://doi.org/10.1038/nrc706.
11. Fohner AE, Brackman DJ, Giacomini KM, Altman RB, Klein TE. PharmGKB summary: very important pharmacogene information for ABCG2. Pharmacogenet Genomics. 2017;27(11):420–7. https://doi.org/10.1097/FPC.0000000000000305.
12. Kukal, S., Guin, D., Rawat, C. et al. Multidrug efflux transporter ABCG2: expression and regulation. Cell Mol Life Sci. 2021;78:6887–939.
13. Brackman DJ, Yee SW, Enogieru OJ, Shaffer C, Ranatunga D, Denny JC, et al. Genome-wide association and functional studies reveal novel pharmacological mechanisms for allopurinol. Clin Pharmacol Ther. 2019;106(3):623–31. https://doi.org/10.1002/cpt.1439.
14. Zhang D, Ding Y, Wang X, Xin W, Du W, Chen W, et al. Effects of ABCG2 and SLCO1B1 gene variants on inflammation markers in patients with hypercholesterolemia and diabetes mellitus treated with rosuvastatin. Eur J Clin Pharmacol. 2020;76(7):939–46. https://doi.org/10.1007/s00228-020-02882-4.
15. Chasman DI, Giulianini F, MacFadyen J, Barratt BJ, Nyberg F, Ridker PM. Genetic determinants of statin-induced low-density lipoprotein cholesterol reduction: the justification for the use of statins in prevention: an intervention trial evaluating Rosuvastatin (JUPITER) trial. Circ Cardiovasc Genet. 2012;5(2):257–64. https://doi.org/10.1161/CIRCGENETICS.111.961144.
16. Jiang Z-P, Zhao X-L, Takahashi N, Angelini S, Dubashi B, Sun L, Xu P. Trough concentration and ABCG2 polymorphism are better to predict imatinib response in chronic myeloid leukemia: a meta-analysis. Pharmacogenomics. 2017;18(1):35–56. https://doi.org/10.2217/pgs-2016-0103.
17. Keppler D. Multidrug resistance proteins (MRPs, ABCCs): importance for pathophysiology and drug therapy. Handb Exp Pharmacol. 2011;201:299–323. https://doi.org/10.1007/978-3-642-14541-4_8.
18. Lima A, Bernardes M, Azevedo R, Medeiros R, Seabra V. Pharmacogenomics of methotrexate membrane transport pathway: can clinical response to methotrexate in rheumatoid arthritis be predicted? Int J Mol Sci. 2015;16(6):13760–80. https://doi.org/10.3390/ijms160613760.
19. Wojnowski L, Kulle B, Schirmer M, Schlüter G, Schmidt A, Rosenberger A, et al. NAD(P)H oxidase and multidrug resistance protein genetic polymorphisms are associated with doxorubicin-induced cardiotoxicity. Circulation. 2005;112(24):3754–62. https://doi.org/10.1161/CIRCULATIONAHA.105.576850.
20. Iannaccone T, Sellitto C, Manzo V, Colucci F, Giudice V, Stefanelli B, et al. Pharmacogenetics of carbamazepine and valproate: focus on polymorphisms of drug metabolizing enzymes and transporters. Pharmaceuticals (Basel). 2021;14(3):204. https://doi.org/10.3390/ph14030204.
21. McDonagh EM, Clancy JP, Altman RB, Klein TE. PharmGKB summary: very important pharmacogene information for CFTR. Pharmacogenet Genomics. 2015;25(3):149–56. https://doi.org/10.1097/FPC.0000000000000112.
22. CPIC® guideline for Ivacaftor and CFTR. Available at: https://cpicpgx.org/guidelines/guidel ine-for-ivacaftor-and-cftr/. Accessed: 29 Dec 2021
23. Sanchez-Ibarra HE, Reyes-Cortes LM, Jiang XL, Luna-Aguirre CM, Aguirre-Trevino D, Morales-Alvarado IA, et al. Genotypic and phenotypic factors influencing drug response in

Mexican patients with type 2 diabetes Mellitus. Front Pharmacol. 2018;9:320. https://doi.org/10.3389/fphar.2018.00320.

24. Bioparadigms. SLC tables. Available at: http://slc.bioparadigms.org; Accessed: 28 Dec 2021.
25. Garibsingh RA, Schlessinger A. Advances and challenges in rational drug design for SLCs. Trends Pharmacol Sci. 2019;40(10):790–800. https://doi.org/10.1016/j.tips.2019.08.006.
26. Schumann T, König J, Henke C, Willmes DM, Bornstein SR, Jordan J, et al. Solute carrier transporters as potential targets for the treatment of metabolic disease. Pharmacol Rev. 2020;72(1):343–79. https://doi.org/10.1124/pr.118.015735.
27. Oshiro C, Mangravite L, Klein T, Altman R. PharmGKB very important pharmacogene: SLCO1B1. Pharmacogenet Genomics. 2010;20(3):211–6.
28. Kee PS, Chin PKL, Kennedy MA, Maggo SDS. Pharmacogenetics of Statin-Induced Myotoxicity. Front Genet. 2020;11: 575678. https://doi.org/10.3389/fgene.2020.575678.
29. Turner RM, Fontana V, Zhang JE, Carr D, Yin P, FitzGerald R, et al. A genome-wide association study of circulating levels of atorvastatin and its major metabolites. Clin Pharmacol Ther. 2020;108(2):287–97. https://doi.org/10.1002/cpt.1820.
30. Ramsey LB, Johnson SG, Caudle KE, Haidar CE, Voora D, Wilke RA, et al. The clinical pharmacogenetics implementation consortium guideline for SLCO1B1 and simvastatin-induced myopathy: 2014 update. Clin Pharmacol Ther. 2014;96(4):423–8. https://doi.org/10.1038/clpt.2014.125.
31. Goswami S, Gong L, Giacomini K, Altman RB, Klein TE. PharmGKB summary: very important pharmacogene information for SLC22A1. Pharmacogenet Genomics. 2014;24(6):324–8. https://doi.org/10.1097/FPC.0000000000000048.
32. Nutt DJ, Forshall S, Bell C, Rich A, Sandford J, Nash J, Argyropoulos S. Mechanisms of action of selective serotonin reuptake inhibitors in the treatment of psychiatric disorders. Eur Neuropsychopharmacol. 1999;9(Suppl 3):S81–6. https://doi.org/10.1016/s0924-977x(99)000 30-9.
33. Fan J, Sklar P. Meta-analysis reveals an association between serotonin transporter gene STin2 VNTR polymorphism and schizophrenia. Mol Psychiatry. 2005;10:928–38. https://doi.org/10.1038/sj.mp.4001690.
34. Botton MR, Yang Y, Scott ER, Desnick RJ, Scott SA. Phased haplotype resolution of the SLC6A4 promoter using long-read single molecule real-time (SMRT) sequencing. Genes (Basel). 2020;11(11):1333. https://doi.org/10.3390/genes11111333.
35. Serretti A, Kato M, De Ronchi D, Kinoshita T. Meta-analysis of serotonin transporter gene promoter polymorphism (5-HTTLPR) association with selective serotonin reuptake inhibitor efficacy in depressed patients. Mol Psychiatry. 2007;12(3):247–57. https://doi.org/10.1038/sj.mp.4001926.
36. Myer NM, Boland JR, Faraone SV. Pharmacogenetics predictors of methylphenidate efficacy in childhood ADHD. Mol Psychiatry. 2018;23(9):1929–36. https://doi.org/10.1038/mp.2017.234.
37. Yee SW, Gong L, Badagnani I, Giacomini KM, Klein TE, Altman RB. SLC19A1 pharmacogenomics summary. Pharmacogenet Genomics. 2010;20(11):708–15. https://doi.org/10.1097/FPC.0b013e32833eca92.
38. Drozdzik M, Rudas T, Pawlik A, Gornik W, Kurzawski M, Herczynska M. Reduced folate carrier-1 80G>A polymorphism affects methotrexate treatment outcome in rheumatoid arthritis. Pharmacogenomics J. 2007;7(6):404–7. https://doi.org/10.1038/sj.tpj.6500438.
39. Bruckmueller H, Cascorbi I. ABCB1, ABCG2, ABCC1, ABCC2, and ABCC3 drug transporter polymorphisms and their impact on drug bioavailability: what is our current understanding? Expert Opin Drug Metab Toxicol. 2021;17(4):369–96. https://doi.org/10.1080/17425255.2021.1876661.

Role of Drug Receptors in Pharmacogenomics

Lidija Bach-Rojecky, Dragan Primorac, Elizabeta Topić, Mario Štefanović, and Wolfgang Höppner

Abstract

Membrane and intracellular receptors for various endogenous ligands differ in tissue/cell localization, structure, signaling mechanisms, cell-mediated effects, and their role in different pathophysiological conditions. The G-protein-coupled receptors, ion channels, enzymes, protein kinases, and nuclear hormone receptors represent targets for various drugs. Mutations in genes encoding receptors can change the drugs' pharmacodynamic properties, but more robust data are needed to develop evidence-based guidelines for clinical practice. Aberrantly activated receptor tyrosine kinase in cancers are of special interest because

L. Bach-Rojecky
University of Zagreb Faculty of Pharmacy and Biochemistry, 10000 Zagreb, Croatia

D. Primorac (✉)
St. Catherine Specialty Hospital, 10000 Zagreb, Croatia
e-mail: dragan.primorac@svkatarina.hr; dragaprimorac2@gmail.com

University of Split School of Medicine, 21000 Split, Croatia

Josip Juraj Strossmayer Faculty of Medicine, 31000 Osijek, Croatia

University of Rijeka School of Medicine, 51000 Rijeka, Croatia

University of Osijek Faculty of Dental Medicine and Health, 31000 Osijek, Croatia

Eberly College of Science, Penn State University, 517 Thomas St, State College, State College, PA 16803, USA

The Henry C. Lee College of Criminal Justice and Forensic Sciences, University of New Haven, West Haven, CT, USA

Medical School REGIOMED, 96450 Coburg, Germany

National Forensic Science University, Gandhinagar, Gujarat, India

College of Medicine and Forensics, Xi'an Jiaotong University, Xi'an, China

International Center for Applied Biological Sciences, 10000 Zagreb, Croatia

© The Author(s), under exclusive license to Springer Nature Switzerland AG 2023
D. Primorac et al. (eds.), *Pharmacogenomics in Clinical Practice*,
https://doi.org/10.1007/978-3-031-45903-0_5

they can influence the more precise diagnosis of the disease, ease the selection of therapies according to cancer genotype, and guide the development of new generations of targeted anti-cancer drugs.

Keywords

Receptors • Drug targets • Gene variations • Pharmacogenomics • Efficacy • Adverse effects

1   Introduction

Membrane and intracellular macromolecules (receptors) for various endogenous ligands are sites of action of many drugs. They differ in tissue/cell localization, structure, signaling mechanisms, cell-mediated effects, and the role they play in different pathophysiological conditions. Rhodopsin-like G-protein-coupled receptors (GPCRs, also known as 7TM), ion channels, protein kinases, and nuclear hormone receptors alone account for around 44% of all human protein targets and are "druggable" targets for 70% of small-molecule drugs [1].

At least 108 GPCRs are sites of action for over 475 drugs used to treat a wide range of diseases (about 34% of total drugs, according to the US Food and Drug Administration).

Mutations in genes encoding different receptors can result in a pathological variant of the protein that, among other factors, contributes to the development of a particular disease and can change the response to the exogenous ligands, i.e., drugs.

However, the impact of gene variations on the physiological function of receptors and the action of drugs has not been sufficiently investigated to develop evidence-based guidelines for clinical practice. In contrast to polymorphisms of genes involved in drug metabolism, disposition and fate in the organism, those connected to drug targets are less studied. A possible reason for this might be the extensive molecular diversity of drug targets, and the so-called multimodality in drug action or multiple drug targets affected by one drug [2, 3].

Numerous studies have shown the important role of tyrosine kinase receptor (RTK) gene mutations (whose intracellular domain has tyrosine kinase activity), such as EGFR, HER2/ErbB2, MET, VGFR in tumor formation. Four principal

E. Topić
Croatian Society of Medical Biochemists, 10000 Zagreb, Croatia

Croatian Academy of Medical Sciences, 10000 Zagreb, Croatia

M. Štefanović
Clinical Institute of Chemistry, University Hospital Sestre Milosrdnice, 10000 Zagreb, Croatia

W. Höppner
Bioglobe GmbH, 22529 Hamburg, Germany

mechanisms lead to constitutive RTK activation in human cancers: gain-of-function mutations, genomic amplification, chromosomal rearrangements, and autocrine activation. Understanding the mechanisms of aberrantly activated RTK in human cancers can significantly influence the more precise diagnosis of the disease, selection of anti-cancer therapies according to cancer genotype, and the development of new generations of targeted anti-cancer drugs [4].

Here, we briefly overview pharmacogenetics of some of the many receptors and their possible impact on disease prognosis and therapeutic outcomes.

2   Beta-Adrenoceptors

Beta2-adrenoreceptors are encoded by the *ADRB2* gene, which is abundantly expressed in bronchial smooth muscle cells, cardiac myocytes, and vascular smooth muscle cells. They play an important role in the regulation of the function of the heart, blood vessels, lungs, and metabolism in general. Drugs acting through this receptor are valuable therapeutic options for respiratory diseases (asthma and chronic obstructive respiratory disease), hypertension, ischemic heart disease, and heart failure. Studies have shown large variations in response after receptor stimulation with agonists, such as an increase in heart rate and strength, improved bronchial smooth muscle relaxation, and increased lipolysis in the subcutaneous adipose tissue [5].

The *ADRB2* gene has more than 80 polymorphisms. Two of more than 45 identified SNPs code for amino acid changes at positions 16 (Arg16Gly, rs1042713) and 27 (Glu27Gln, rs1042714). They are common, with minor allele frequencies between 40 and 50%, and have been well characterized in asthma pharmacogenetics. Polymorphism rs1042714 is an important genetic protective factor in decreasing asthma development risk, especially in children. The rs1042713 polymorphism may be involved in the risk of asthma in the Arab and Hispanic-Latino populations and a protective factor in the Indian population [6].

Polymorphisms of the *ADRB2* gene can affect the therapeutic response of drugs, acting either as agonists or antagonists at receptors. The Arg16Gly SNP (rs1042713) possibly affects respiratory disease treatment outcomes, as homozygotes for Arg (genotype AA) show poorer response to beta2-adrenoceptor agonists (salbutamol and salmeterol) in contrast to G allele carriers [7]. The second Gln27Glu polymorphism (rs1042714) is represented by about 43% in the population and is associated with reduced efficacy and duration of action of beta2-adrenergic agonists. It was observed that the G allele (Glu variant) increases electrostatic interactions (producing stronger bonding) between ligand drugs and the receptor-binding site, which can explain the variable therapeutic response to adrenergic agonists [8].

Thr164Ile polymorphism (loss of function) is less common (5%), and its role was investigated in relation to severe asthma, as well as heart failure. Namely, patients with severe asthma, carriers of the Ile164 allele, are more than twice as likely as Thr164 homozygotes to have uncontrolled, persistent symptoms and achieve poorer therapeutic responses after administration of long-acting beta2-adrenergic agonists (LABA) [9]. In patients with heart failure, Thr164Ile polymorphism seems to relate to reduced exercise tolerance and higher mortality, since the presence of the Ile164 variant is associated with attenuated contractile response to beta2-adrenergic-mediated stimulation that may contribute to the negative clinical outcome [10].

Although more than 80 polymorphisms have been detected in the *ADRB2* gene, studies have failed to justify the clinical significance of their routine pharmacogenetic testing.

Studies analyzing the possible link between variations in the *ADRB1* gene and response in patients with heart failure treated with beta-blockers have shown that there may be a differential drug dose requirement based on the *ADRβ1 389Arg/ Gly* polymorphism. Namely, patients who are Arg homozygotes might require a higher dose of beta-blocker to achieve a mortality risk reduction like that of Gly carriers [11].

3   Dopamine Receptors

Dopamine regulates numerous functions, from cognition, emotions, motor skills, hormone secretion, gastrointestinal tract motility, heart to kidney function, mediated through five subtypes of dopamine receptors (D1 - D5) distributed in the periphery and the central nervous system. Drugs acting via dopamine receptors, primarily D2, are used in the treatment of schizophrenia (receptor antagonists), Parkinson's disease (receptor agonists), addiction, and hyperprolactinemia [12]. *DRD2* and D2-like receptor genes, like *DRD3* and *DRD4*, have been investigated concerning antipsychotic treatment responses. The *DRD2* gene has more than 200 identified polymorphisms. The important *DRD2* variants are −141C Ins/Del (rs1799732), Taq1A (rs1800497), 957C > T (rs6277), and Ser311Cys (rs1801028). The −141C Ins/Del polymorphism in the *DRD2* promoter region (present in about 9% of Caucasians) has been associated as a risk factor with the development of schizophrenia and addiction and with the response to antipsychotics [13]. Classical antipsychotics act by blocking D2 receptors in the mesolimbic and striatal regions of the brain. Based on seven studies that investigated the association between polymorphisms of the *DRD2* gene and response to antipsychotics, three polymorphisms of *DRD2* (rs180498, rs2514218, and rs1079597) were significantly associated with treatment response [14]. The Taq1A polymorphism of the *DRD2* gene (present in about 22% of Caucasians) has been associated with the risk of nicotine and alcohol dependence and response to treatment [12]. Also, *DRD2* rs1076560, involved in regulating splicing of the gene that alters the ratio of DRD2 isoforms located pre- and postsynaptically, might be associated with cocaine and opioid abuse and dependence [15]. Several studies reported a significant correlation between the rs1800497 SNP and the frequency of motor fluctuations and dyskinesia in levodopa-treated patients. Furthermore, the *DRD2* Ins/Ins and *DRD3* Ser/Ser genotypes are associated with a higher risk of gastrointestinal side effects caused by levodopa in the treatment of Parkinson's disease [16].

Undoubtedly, dopamine receptors polymorphisms might, among other nongenetic risk factors, affect personal risk for the development of certain disorders, like schizophrenia or addiction, as well as therapeutic efficacy and safety of drugs acting through these widely distributed receptors. Despite the number of studies conducted on the association of particular polymorphisms of dopamine receptor genes with the therapeutic response to drugs, the results are often inconsistent and make it difficult to draw conclusions and specific recommendations.

4   Serotonergic Receptors

Serotonin (5-hydroxitryptamine, 5-HT), through 14 subtypes of 5-HT receptors categorized into 7 families, mediates numerous effects on the periphery and the central nervous system. 5-HT receptors are part of the G-protein-coupled receptor (GPCR) superfamily, except for the 5-HT3 receptor, a ligand-gated ion channel [17].

The most extensively studied 5-HT receptors are 5-HT2A, 2C, and 1A subtypes, which are targets for different antipsychotic and antidepressant drugs, mediating their therapeutic and adverse effects [18]. Polymorphisms in the *HTR1A* gene (e.g., rs6295) could explain individual differences in response to antidepressant treatment (some antidepressants act as partial agonists of the 5-HT1A receptor). However, the results of the studies are inconclusive. HTR2A is a postsynaptic receptor involved in enhancing excitatory signals to other neurons in brain tissue. The 5-HT2A is highly enriched in neocortex and regulates the function of prefrontal-subcortical circuits implicated in the pathophysiology of depression. Many antipsychotics, as well as some antidepressants, act as antagonists of this receptor. Studies of *HTR2A* gene polymorphisms have shown an association of 1438 A/G rs6311 and rs7997012 G/A with a better antidepressant response and a higher degree of remission, while 102 T/C rs6313 was associated with a lower risk of drug side effects [19]. The polymorphism 102 T/C rs6313 has also been associated with the action of the antipsychotic drugs olanzapine and risperidone, where T allele carriers are more likely to respond to therapy [18]. Blockade of HTR2C receptor is associated with increased appetite. Drugs, like atypical antipsychotics clozapine, olanzapine, and risperidone, exert high affinity for 5-HT2C receptors. It was shown that the polymorphism in *HTR2C* rs3813929 C > T (−759 C/T) increases the risk of weight gain [20].

Although implicated in the pathophysiology of different diseases and serving as targets for various drugs commonly used to treat mood and behavioral disorders, the role of genetic polymorphisms of 5-HT receptors as a predictive factor for therapeutic outcomes is still inconclusive due to inconsistent results coming from clinical studies.

5   Opioid Receptors

Opioid analgesics such as morphine, fentanyl, and oxycodone exert their analgesic effect by stimulating MOR opioid receptors. The efficacy of analgesia might be influenced by polymorphisms in the *OPRM1* gene encoding for the MOR-1, with more than 100 allelic variants identified so far. One of the most studied is the SNP. In vitro studies have shown that this SNP leads to: increased β-endorphin affinity, changes in post-receptor signalization, activation of G-protein-coupled inwardly rectifying potassium channels, inhibition of Cav2.2 voltage-gated calcium channels, and Gi/o activity, with additional decreased levels of MOR mRNA [21].

Its frequency in the population varies between 10 and 48%, and GG homozygotes need significantly higher doses of opioids for analgesic effect. Some clinical studies provided evidence in favor of this functional polymorphism, where GG genotype was related to a reduced analgesic effect and requirements for higher doses of morphine to achieve effective pain control in the postoperative setting [22, 23]. This polymorphism is also associated with the efficacy of opioid antagonist naltrexone in treating alcoholism and with opiate addiction development [24].

6   Estrogen Receptor

The estrogen receptor (ER) is an intracellular receptor for estrogens and has at least two isoforms, i.e., ERα and ERβ encoded by two distinct genes, highly polymorphic *ESR1* and *ESR2*. ERα has a higher level of expression in the breast tissue and is frequently implicated in the breast cancer development. ER-α, also known as NR3A1 (from nuclear receptor subfamily 3, group A, member 1), encodes the *ESR1* gene. More than 60% of breast tumors express ER, with many *ESR1* polymorphisms identified, such as rs9340799, rs3020364, rs9322335, rs2234693, rs1801132, rs2046210, rs3020314, rs1514348, rs3020314, rs1514348, rs1514348, and rs3020314, with different results obtained concerning cancer susceptibility to treatment and clinical outcome [25]. The more important polymorphisms associated with treatment success might be rs2207396 and rs9340799 (A allele carriers have an increased risk of aromatase inhibitor side effects, as well as a reduced response to conjugated estrogen administration on bone mineral density), rs2234693 (C allele carriers exibited a higher risk of musculoskeletal side effects due to the use of aromatase inhibitors) [26].

7   Oncopharmacogenetic Receptors

Understanding receptor tyrosine kinases (RTKs) signaling has provided fundamental insight into their functions in physiological, but also pathological conditions. Since RTKs play crucial roles in cancer development, targeting oncogenic driver mutations of RTKs has dramatically changed the treatment of cancer patients. The expanding spectrum of both established and candidate oncogenic driver mutations identified in different cancers (e.g., non-small-cell lung cancer, colorectal cancer, and breast cancer), associated with the signal transduction pathway inhibitors targeting these driver mutations, offers a tremendous opportunity to enhance cancer therapeutic outcomes.

Additionally, molecular classification of cancers has emerged, leading to new biological insights and targeted therapies directed toward specific molecular abnormalities not only in RTKs, but in their post-receptor signaling targets, as well. Some of them are mutations in *KRAS* (v-Ki-ras2-Kirsten rat sarcoma viral oncogene homolog), epidermal growth factor receptor (*EGFR*) and *HER2*, B-Raf proto-oncogene (*BRAF*) genes, translocations in anaplastic lymphoma kinase (*ALK*), Ret proto-oncogene (RET), or C-Ros-1 proto-oncogene (*ROS1*) gene [27].

8   KRAS (From v-Ki-ras2-Kirsten Rat Sarcoma Viral Oncogene Homolog)

KRAS is one of three proteins from the Ras family with GTPase activity and is essential in signaling intracellular processes. Rat sarcoma (RAS) is the most frequently mutated oncogene in human cancer, with KRAS as the most commonly mutated RAS isoform in lung adenocarcinoma (31–35%), mucosal adenoma, pancreatic duct carcinoma (88%), and colorectal cancer (45–50%). Dysregulation in KRAS can stimulate tumor growth by controlling interactions between cancer cells and the microenvironment, which finally affects therapeutic response. The most common variants are G12C (rs121913530), which accounted for 39% of *KRAS* mutations, followed by the mutations G12V (rs121913529), which accounts for 21%, and G12D (rs121913529), which accounts for 17% of *KRAS* mutations. Until about five years ago, direct targeting of KRAS was seen as highly challenging, but several small-molecule inhibitors of mutated KRAS in the advanced phase of development [28].

Contradictory results have been found about the prognostic and predictive values of *KRAS* mutations regarding therapy response and therapeutic outcome in different cancer types. For example, patients with metastatic colorectal cancer of the CC genotype have a poor response to therapy because of resistance to panitumumab and cetuximab, which act as antagonists of an epidermal growth factor receptor (EGFR). The primary tumor or metastases that carry activating mutations in the *KRAS* gene are responsible for possible lack of response and poorer prognosis in 30–50% of patients [29]. Current recommendations require testing for codon 12, and anti-EGFR drugs are not recommended for colorectal cancer patients with these variants.

8.1   EGFR

Mutations in different epidermal growth factor receptor (EGFR) domains have been found to influence tumor cells growth and proliferation. The tyrosine kinase domain (TKD) mutations hyperactivate the kinase and its downstream oncogenic signaling. As shown in large clinical trials, these TKD mutations are sensitive to the treatment with EGFR tyrosine kinase inhibitors (small molecules, like erlotinib and gefitinib). Approximately 90% of these mutations are small in-frame deletions within exon 19 or L858R point mutation within exon 21. Accumulating data shows that exon 19 deletions and L858R can both serve in terms of better prognosis and treatment outcomes in patients with non-small-cell lung cancers. In patients with advanced or metastatic non-small-cell lung cancer with mutations in the gene *EGFR*, which are sensitive to tyrosine kinase inhibitors (exon 19 deletions or L858R point mutations), guidelines recommend treatment with an EGFR-TKI [30].

8.2   BRAF

BRAF (serine/threonine-protein kinase B-Raf) is a protooncogenic protein, a part of the RAS-RAF-MEK-ERK pathway, involved in cellular signaling and cell growth regulation. Mutations in the *BRAF* gene have been found in many malignancies (non-Hodgkin's lymphoma, colorectal cancer, melanoma, thyroid cancer, lung cancer, and adenocarcinoma). *BRAF V600D/E/K/R* mutations are referred to as class I mutants, a group that results in strong activation of BRAF's kinase activity and constitutive activation of the MAPK pathway, thus causing cell proliferation even when no growth factors are bound to the respective receptor [31]. *BRAF* mutations in advanced colorectal cancers are observed in 8–12% of patients. T1799A transversion in exon 15, which results in a valine amino acid substitution, is the most frequent alteration. *BRAF* is considered a negative prognostic biomarker, and patients harboring mutations have limited chemotherapy response [32]. Almost half of all melanoma carry *BRAF* mutations. Accordingly, the success of melanoma treatment might depend on the pharmacogenetic determination of *BRAF* mutations and the application of BRAF-targeted therapy, like vemurafenib and dabrafenib (selective inhibitors of mutant BRAF protein) [33].

Based on positive experience with the current success of BRAF inhibitors in treating melanoma and colorectal cancers, further research is needed to understand the significance of other classes of *BRAF* mutations in tumorigenesis. Acquired knowledge could impact strategies to better diagnose and guide future targeted drug development.

8.3 HER2/ERBB2

HER2/ErbB2/NeuHER2 is a receptor with tyrosine kinase activity from the epidermal growth factor receptor family (EGFR and HER2-4/ErbB1-4) that are key regulators of replication and cell growth. *HER2* overexpression and activation, the most common abnormalities, have been associated with cell transformation and oncogenesis. Additionally, various mutations in the *HER2* gene are associated with the development of many solid tumors (lung, prostate, breast, head and neck, ovaries, colon, etc.), and overexpression in tumor cells is associated with disease progression, metastasis, and poorer prognosis. Despite their low frequency, activating *HER2* mutations has recently emerged as novel therapeutic targets for several human tumors [34].

The great value of pharmacogenetic testing for overexpression and amplification of the *HER2* gene is predicting responses to therapy with trastuzumab and pertuzumab and small inhibitors of the intracellular HER2 receptor domain. *HER2* gene amplification is an independent factor associated with a sensitivity to HER2-directed drugs and poor disease prognosis (shorter disease-free survival) [35]. Besides monoclonal antibodies, current HER2-targeted therapies include antibody–drug conjugates (trastuzumab-emtansine) and several small-molecule tyrosine kinase inhibitors: lapatinib (reversible inhibitor), afatinib, neratinib, and dacomitinib (irreversible inhibitors). Patients positive for mutated *HER2* have a better response to therapy, and *HER2* gene amplification testing has become part of the optimal therapeutic approach in breast cancer [36].

8.4 KIT (c-Kit, CD117, SCFR)

The *KIT (CD117)* gene encodes the protooncogenic receptor protein SCFR (Mast/Stem Cell Growth Factor Receptor). CD117 is also important surface marker that identifies some progenitor lineages of hematopoietic cells. Mutation activation and overexpression have been associated with gastrointestinal stromal tumors (mutations can occur in up to 85% cases), seminomas, melanoma, and leukemias [37]. Pharmacogenetic testing of *CD117* polymorphisms has been associated with the treatment efficacy with imatinib, a CD117 inhibitor. Imatinib is less effective in the presence of the activating mutations in the CD117 kinase domains, in contrast to activating mutations in the juxtamembrane domain encoded in exon 11. The S628N substitution in exon 13 is identified as a gain-of-function mutation, and tumors carrying this mutation demonstrate susceptibility to imatinib treatment. However, mutations in D816V and V560G conferred acquired resistance via activating mutations [38].

9 Conclusion

The field of pharmacogenomics related to drug receptors is still evolving. Mutations in genes encoding different receptors can result in pathological variants of the proteins that contribute to the development of a particular disease and can change the therapeutic response to the ligand drugs. Most research investigated the tyrosine kinase receptors and their role in cancer pathogenesis. The significant impact of the pathogenic gene variants on tumor cell progression influenced novel anti-cancer drug design and improved therapeutic outcomes for the patients. Still, more data are needed for other drug receptors associated with the common chronic diseases.

References

1. Santos R, Ursu O, Gaulton A, Bento AP, Donadi RS, Bologa CG, et al. A comprehensive map of molecular drug targets. Nat Rev Drug Discov. 2017;16:19–34. https://doi.org/10.1038/nrd. 2016.230).
2. Zhou Y, Arribas GH, Turku A, Jürgenson T, Mkrtchian S, Krebs K, et al. Rare genetic variability in human drug target genes modulates drug response and can guide precision medicine. Sci Adv. 2021;7(36):eabi6856. https://doi.org/10.1126/sciadv.abi6856.
3. Primorac D, Höppner W, editors. Pharmacogenetics in clinical practice: Experience with 55 commonly used drugs. Zagreb, Ham-burg, Philadelphia: St. Catherine Specialty Hospital, Bioglobe GmbH, ISABS; 2022. Available from: https://www.stcatherine.com/centre-of-exc ellence/10/individualized-and-preventive-medicine/pharmacogenomics/69. Accessed: 2 May 2022
4. Saraon P, Pathmanathan S, Snide J, et al. Receptor tyrosine kinases and cancer: oncogenic mechanisms and therapeutic approaches. Oncogene. 2021;40:4079–93. https://doi.org/ 10.1038/s41388-021-01841-2.
5. Litonjua AA, Gong L, Duan QL, Shin J, Moore MJ, Weiss ST, et al. Very important pharmacogene summary ADRB2. Pharmacogenet Genomics. 2010;20(1):64–9. https://doi.org/10.1097/ FPC.0b013e328333dae6.
6. Zhao S, Zhang W, Nie X. Association of β2-adrenergic receptor gene polymorphisms (rs1042713, rs1042714, rs1042711) with asthma risk: a systematic review and updated meta-analysis. BMC Pulm Med. 2019;19:202. https://doi.org/10.1186/s12890-019-0962-z.
7. Figueiredo RG, Costa RS, Figueiredo CA, Cruz AA. Genetic determinants of poor response to treatment in Severe Asthma. Int J Mol Sci. 2021;22(8):4251. https://doi.org/10.3390/ijms22 084251.
8. Bhosale S, Nikte SV, Sengupta D, Joshi M. Differential dynamics underlying the Gln27Glu population variant of the β2-adrenergic receptor. J Membr Biol. 2019;252(4–5):499–507. https://doi.org/10.1007/s00232-019-00093-2.
9. Ortega VE, Hawkins GA, Moore WC, Hastie AT, Ampleford EJ, Busse WW, et al. Effect of rare variants in ADRB2 on risk of severe exacerbations and symptom control during longacting β agonist treatment in a multiethnic asthma population: a genetic study. Lancet Respir Med. 2014;2(3):204–13. https://doi.org/10.1016/S2213-2600(13)70289-3.
10. Barbato E, Penicka M, Delrue L, Van Durme F, De Bruyne B, Goethals M, et al. Thr164Ile polymorphism of beta2-adrenergic receptor negatively modulates cardiac contractility: implications for prognosis in patients with idiopathic dilated cardiomyopathy. Heart. 2007;93(7):856–61. https://doi.org/10.1136/hrt.2006.091959.

11. Fiuzat M, Neely ML, Starr AZ, Kraus WE, Felker GM, Donahue M, et al. Association between adrenergic receptor genotypes and beta-blocker dose in heart failure patients: analysis from the HF-ACTION DNA substudy. Eur J Heart Fail. 2013;15(3):258–66. https://doi.org/10.1093/eur jhf/hfs175.
12. Mi H, Thomas PD, Ring HZ, Jiang R, Sangkuhl K, Klein TE, et al. PharmGKB summary: dopamine receptor D2. Pharmacogenet Genomics. 2011;21(6):350–6. https://doi.org/10.1097/ FPC.0b013e32833ee605.
13. Zhang JP, Lencz T, Malhotra AK. D2 receptor genetic variation and clinical response to antipsychotic drug treatment: a meta-analysis. Am J Psychiatry. 2010;167(7):763–72. https:// doi.org/10.1176/appi.ajp.2009.09040598.
14. Yoshida K, Müller DJ. Pharmacogenetics of Antipsychotic Drug Treatment: Update and Clinical Implications. Mol Neuropsychiatry. 2020;5(Suppl 1):1-26. https://doi.org/10.1159/000 492332
15. Clarke TK, Weiss AR, Ferarro TN, Kampman KM, Dackis CA, Pettinati HM, et al. The dopamine receptor D2 (DRD2) SNP rs1076560 is associated with opioid addiction. Ann Hum Genet. 2014;78(1):33–9. https://doi.org/10.1111/ahg.12046.
16. Politi C, Ciccacci C, Novelli G, Borgiani P. Genetics and treatment response in Parkinson's disease: an update on pharmacogenetic studies. Neuromolecular Med. 2018;20(1):1–17. https:// doi.org/10.1007/s12017-017-8473-7.
17. Berger M, Gray JA, Roth BL. The expanded biology of serotonin. Annu Rev Med. 2009;60:355–66. https://doi.org/10.1146/annurev.med.60.042307.110802.
18. Reynolds GP, McGowan OO, Dalton CF. Pharmacogenomics in psychiatry: the relevance of receptor and transporter polymorphisms. Br J Clin Pharmacol. 2014;77(4):654–72. https://doi. org/10.1111/bcp.12312.
19. Wan YS, Zhai XJ, Tan HA, Ai YS, Zhao LB. Associations between the 1438A/G, 102T/C, and rs7997012G/A polymorphisms of HTR2A and the safety and efficacy of antidepressants in depression: a meta-analysis. Pharmacogenomics J. 2021;21(2):200–15. https://doi.org/10. 1038/s41397-020-00197-2.
20. Hill MJ, Reynolds GP. Functional consequences of two HTR2C polymorphisms associated with antipsychotic-induced weight gain. Pharmacogenomics. 2011;12(5):727–34. 10.2217/ pgs.11.16ž.
21. Kumar S, Kundra P, Ramsamy K, Surendiran A. Pharmacogenetics of opioids: a narrative review. Anaesthesia. 2019;74(11):1456–70. https://doi.org/10.1111/anae.14813.
22. Trescot AM. Genetics and implications in perioperative analgesia. Best Pract Res Clin Anaesthesiol. 2014;28(2):153–66. https://doi.org/10.1016/j.bpa.2014.03.004.
23. Bach-Rojecky L, Čutura T, Lozić M, Husedžinović Kliškinjić, Matišić V, Primorac D. Personalized anesthetic pharmacology. In: Personalized medicine in Anesthesia. Pain and perioperative medicine. Cham: Springer Nature Switzerland, Switzerland; 2020. p. 65–92.
24. Haerian BS, Haerian MS. OPRM1 rs1799971 polymorphism and opioid dependence: evidence from a meta-analysis. Pharmacogenomics. 2013;14(7):813–24. https://doi.org/10.2217/ pgs.13.57.
25. Tan SC, Low TY, Mohamad Hanif EA, Sharzehan MAK, Kord-Varkaneh H, Islam MA. The rs9340799 polymorphism of the estrogen receptor alpha (ESR1) gene and its association with breast cancer susceptibility. Sci Rep. 2021;11:18619. https://doi.org/10.1038/s41598-021-979 35-8.
26. Wang J, Lu K, Song Y, Xie L, Zhao S, Wang Y, et al. Indications of clinical and genetic predictors for aromatase inhibitors related musculoskeletal adverse events in Chinese Han women with breast cancer. PLoS ONE. 2013;8(7): e68798. https://doi.org/10.1371/journal.pone.006 8798.
27. Du Z, Lovly CM. Mechanisms of receptor tyrosine kinase activation in cancer. Mol Cancer. 2018;17:58. https://doi.org/10.1186/s12943-018-0782-4.
28. Reck M, Carbone DP, Garassino M, Barlesi F. Targeting KRAS in non-small-cell lung cancer: recent progress and new approaches. Ann Oncol. 2021;32(9):1101–10. https://doi.org/10. 1016/j.annonc.2021.06.001.

29. Misale S, Yaeger R, Hobor S, Scala E, Janakiraman M, Liska D, et al. Emergence of KRAS mutations and acquired resistance to anti-EGFR therapy in colorectal cancer. Nature. 2012;486:532–6. https://doi.org/10.1038/nature11156.
30. Jiang H, Zhu M, Li Y, Li Q. Association between EGFR exon 19 or exon 21 mutations and survival rates after first-line EGFR-TKI treatment in patients with non-small cell lung cancer. Mol Clin Oncol. 2019;11(3):301–8. https://doi.org/10.3892/mco.2019.1881.
31. Dankner M, Rose AAN, Rajkumar S, et al. Classifying BRAF alterations in cancer: new rational therapeutic strategies for actionable mutations. Oncogene. 2018;37:3183–99. https://doi.org/10.1038/s41388-018-0171-x.
32. Takeda H, Sunakawa Y. Management of BRAF gene alterations in metastatic colorectal cancer: from current therapeutic strategies to future perspectives. Front Oncol. 2021;11: 602194. https://doi.org/10.3389/fonc.2021.602194.
33. Luke JJ, Flaherty KT, Ribas A, Long GV. Targeted agents and immunotherapies: optimizing outcomes in melanoma. Nat Rev Clin Oncol. 2017;14:463–82.
34. Cocco E, Lopez S, Santin AD, Scaltriti M. Prevalence and role of HER2 mutations in cancer. Pharmacol Ther. 2019;199:188–96. https://doi.org/10.1016/j.pharmthera.2019.03.010.
35. Connell CM, Doherty GJ. Activating HER2 mutations as emerging targets in multiple solid cancers. ESMO Open. 2017;2(5):e000279. https://doi.org/10.1136/esmoopen-2017-000279
36. Schlam I, Swain SM. HER2-positive breast cancer and tyrosine kinase inhibitors: the time is now. NPJ Breast Cancer. 2021;7(1):56. https://doi.org/10.1038/s41523-021-00265-1.
37. Ashman LK, Griffith R. Therapeutic targeting of c-KIT in cancer. Expert Opin Investig Drugs. 2013;22(1):103–15. https://doi.org/10.1517/13543784.2013.740010.
38. Patel M, Eckburg A, Gantiwala S, Hart Z, Dein J, Lam K, Puri N. Resistance to molecularly targeted therapies in Melanoma. Cancers (Basel). 2021;13(5):1115. https://doi.org/10.3390/cancers13051115.

Role of Drug Targets and Other Proteins Important in Pharmacogenomics

Lidija Bach-Rojecky, Dragan Primorac, Elizabeta Topić, Mario Štefanović, and Wolfgang Höppner

Abstract

Various physiological molecules, like enzymes, intracellular and membrane proteins, or soluble molecules, are important for drugs' pharmacological profile. While some mediate drug pharmacodynamic actions, others interfere with its biotransformation and clearance. Therefore, variations in genes encoding these proteins can influence the efficacy and safety of various drugs. Determination of specific genotypes might implicate drug dosage modification, or drug change, to avoid therapy failure and potentially fatal outcomes due to severe adverse effects. Based on the highest level of evidence, recommendations for therapy

L. Bach-Rojecky
University of Zagreb Faculty of Pharmacy and Biochemistry, 10000 Zagreb, Croatia

D. Primorac (✉)
St. Catherine Specialty Hospital, 10000 Zagreb, Croatia
e-mail: dragan.primorac@svkatarina.hr; draganprimorac2@gmail.com

University of Split School of Medicine, 21000 Split, Croatia

Josip Juraj Strossmayer University of Osijek Faculty of Medicine, 31000 Osijek, Croatia

University of Rijeka School of Medicine, 51000 Rijeka, Croatia

Josip Juraj Strossmayer University of Osijek Faculty of Dental Medicine and Health, 31000 Osijek, Croatia

Eberly College of Science, Penn State University, 517 Thomas St, State College, PA 16803, USA

The Henry C. Lee College of Criminal Justice and Forensic Sciences, University of New Haven, West Haven, CT, USA

Medical School REGIOMED, 96450 Coburg, Germany

National Forensic Science University, Gandhinagar, Gujarat, India

College of Medicine and Forensics, Xi'an Jiaotong University, Xi'an, China

International Center For Applied Biological Sciences, 10000, Zagreb, Croatia

D. Primorac et al. (eds.), *Pharmacogenomics in Clinical Practice*,
https://doi.org/10.1007/978-3-031-45903-0_6

adjustment according to specific genotype are already available for some drugs. But, for others, genotype-drug interactions need more robust data before clinical implementation.

Keywords

Gene variants • Drug safety • Adverse drug reactions • Therapy adjustment • Pharmacogenetics testing

1   Introduction

The pharmacological action of the drugs depends, among others, on their affinity for the target molecules, which might locate into the cells, or on the cell surface. Targets for drugs are chosen based on a high level of research detecting their physiological roles and function in specific pathophysiological processes.

In contrast to the previous approaches in drug design based on one drug-one target principle, novel drugs commonly have multiple targets, which mediate their pharmacological action. While some contribute to the drug therapeutic action, others mediate adverse effects.

Variations in genes encoding specific proteins with resultant functional changes have been demonstrated for some diseases. For example, some polymorphisms in the *CFTR* gene cause defective CFTR channel function and cystic fibrosis. Drugs specifically designed to modulate the pathogenic protein have revolutionized the therapy of this severe disease.

On the other side are polymorphisms in genes for drug targets that negatively influence drug binding and desired modulation of protein function. For example, evidence shows that polymorphisms in the gene encoding vitamin K epoxy reductase, an enzyme inhibited by warfarin, might influence anticoagulation.

Proteins not directly involved in drug action nor influencing its pharmacokinetics are also of interest because they can mediate some adverse effects that can be severe in presentation and fatal.

Human Leukocyte Antigens (HLA) are cell membrane proteins that regulate the immune system and are encoded by a complex of highly polymorphic genes. Specific *HLA* genotypes are associated with hypersensitivity and the risk of severe and potentially fatal cutaneous adverse reactions to some drugs, like anticonvulsants phenytoin and carbamazepine and anti-gout drug allopurinol.

E. Topić
Croatian Society of Medical Biochemistry and Laboratory Medicine, 10000 Zagreb, Croatia

Croatian Academy of Medical Sciences, 10000 Zagreb, Croatia

M. Štefanović
Clinical Institute of Chemistry, University Hospital Sestre Milosrdnice, 10000 Zagreb, Croatia

W. Höppner
Bioglobe GmbH, 22529 Hamburg, Germany

Additionally, gene variations for enzymes involved in the degradation of drugs can influence their elimination from the body. For example, dihydropyrimidine dehydrogenase degrades uracil and thymidine (pyrimidines) analogs used to treat various cancers. Mutations in the *DPYD* gene interfere with the breakdown of pyrimidine drugs. Consequently, drugs accumulate in the blood, urine, and cerebrospinal fluid, contributing to their increased toxicity.

It is more than clear that pharmacogenetic testing performed before introducing a drug to the therapy can optimize the drug dosing regime, predict the adverse effects, and individualize the treatment for each patient [1].

In this chapter, we describe some gene variations that can influence the pharmacological effects of different drugs. Based on collected data of the highest level of evidence, for some pathogenic gene variants there are clinical guidelines recommending therapy adjustments according to the results of pharmacogenetic testing to avoid drug failure and improve its safety [1].

2 Enzymes that Mediate Drugs Pharmacological Effects

2.1 Vitamin K Epoxy Reductase—VKORC1

The *VKORC1* gene encodes the vitamin K epoxide reductase (VKORC1), a crucial enzyme in the vitamin K cycle. Reduced vitamin K serves as a cofactor in the activation process of coagulation factors II, VII, IX, X. Warfarin, a widely used anticoagulant drug, is an inhibitor of vitamin K epoxide reductase complex, thus interfering with the coagulation process. Warfarin has a narrow therapeutic index and large inter-patient variability in the dose required to achieve targeted anticoagulation. One of the causative factors for this is polymorphisms in the *VKORC1* gene since it accounts for 15–30% of the variability in warfarin response [1]. Several polymorphisms and haplotypes have been detected in the *VKORC1* gene. The G3673A variant has been genotyped in different populations, with a high prevalence in the Asian population (around 90%), and around 40% in Caucasians. This variant results in fewer functional copies of the mature VKORC1 protein. Carriers of the A allele respond to a lower initial warfarin dose than do carriers of the G allele [2].

A common variant c.−1639G>A rs9923231 is significantly associated with warfarin sensitivity, where patients with one or two −1639A require progressively lower warfarin doses than −1639G/G homozygotes. The c.−1639G>A allele frequency largely explains the differences in average dose requirements between Whites, Blacks, and Asians. Several rare nonsynonymous *VKORC1* variants, like G9041A, or 3730 G>A, explain high dose requirements to achieve anticoagulation [2].

2.2   Angiotensin-Converting Enzyme

Angiotensin-converting enzyme (ACE) indirectly raises blood pressure by converting angiotensin I to a potent vasoconstrictor angiotensin II. So far, 78 variants and 13 haplotypes of the *ACE* gene have been identified, the most well-known variant being the insertion deletion polymorphism (I/D, rs1799752) in intron 16, showing different allele frequencies among racial groups (D allele is less common in Asians). The I/D genetic polymorphism of this enzyme is also considered to be one of the risk factors for cardiovascular diseases including hypertension, heart attack, and stroke [3].

Drugs ACE inhibitors (like lizinopril, ramipril, etc.) exert their effect by blocking the conversion of angiotensin I to angiotensin II, and polymorphisms in the *ACE* gene may affect their effectiveness, making *ACE* a potentially interesting gene for pharmacogenetic testing. Many studies have linked variant D to stronger (homozygous) or moderately increased (heterozygous) plasma ACE activity, leading to a reduced response to ACE inhibitor therapy. On the other hand, some studies with the D/D genotype have linked an enhanced effect of drugs from the β-blocker group. However, most research on *ACE* gene polymorphism to date has focused on their impact on disease and clinical outcomes rather than drug response and has not been strong enough to detect complex interactions, focusing almost exclusively on I/D polymorphisms [3, 4].

2.3   Catechol-O-Methyltransferase

COMT gene encode enzyme Catechol-*O*-Methyltransferases (COMT), whose substrates are catechols (dopamine, adrenaline, noradrenaline, and some other endogenous substrates), which are inactivated by methylation. *COMT* gene variants have been associated with psychiatric disorders, including schizophrenia, perception of opioid receptor-mediated pain, and breast cancer. In neuropsychiatric diseases, *COMT* polymorphisms are associated with catecholamine neurotransmitter metabolism, while the role of *COMT* in breast cancer is associated with catecholestrogens methylation. COMT is able to metabolize some drugs (e.g. levodopa, methyldopa, entacapone, methadone, oxycodone, tramadol), but so far no solid evidence has been found to establish its pharmacogenetic significance.

The most well-known polymorphism is the Val158Met (rs4680), Met allele, which reduces COMT activity, and some studies have linked this allele to personality disorders and risks of schizophrenia [5].

2.4   Glucose-6-Phosphate Dehydrogenase

Glucose-6-Phosphate Dehydrogenase (G6PD) mediates the production of NADPH and ribose-5-phosphate in the pentose phosphate pathway of glucose metabolism. The G6PD enzyme reduces cellular NADP in the oxidation of glucose-6-phosphate by providing an energy source to keep cellular glutathione in reduced form. In the absence of reduced glutathione, drugs oxidatively damage erythrocytes and hemolysis occurs.

G6PD enzyme deficiency is a sex-linked disorder that affects about 300 million people worldwide, and which, given the number of people affected, can be considered the most important disorder of its kind. Although the enzyme is present in all tissues, its deficiency is most pronounced in erythrocytes. Increased oxidative load of erythrocytes may cause hemolysis due to insufficient amounts of NADPH in individuals with the deficiency of G6PD enzyme activity. The most common clinical manifestations of G6PD deficiency are acute acquired hemolytic anemia, chronic congenital hemolytic anemia, and favism [6]. The population frequency of G6PD deficiency varies depending on gender and ethnicity. The disorder is more common in hemizygous men, and very rarely in women, and is more common in individuals of African, Asian, and Mediterranean descent (*G6PD* 563T/1311T haplotype). The *G6PD* gene is extremely polymorphic. So far, about 400 polymorphic variants are known, mostly caused by point mutation, deletion polymorphisms, and less often de-novo mutations. *G6PD* variants were classified into five categories according to the severity of the clinical manifestation resulting from the genotype. In-frame deletions are usually associated with the most severe clinical manifestations of class I (such as the *G6PD* Tondel variant, identified in a heterozygous woman with chronic hemolytic anemia) [7]. Class II and III are the most common type of polymorphic variants of G6PD deficiency associated with the phenotype of acute hemolytic anemia.

The *G6PD* gene is one of the first genes found to be associated with a variable drug response. People with G6PD deficiency may be at increased risk of side effects from a number of medications including primaquine, chloroquine, dapsone, rasburicase, rosiglitazone, metformin/glibenclamide combination, for which the FDA (U.S. Food and Drug Administration) has issued warnings and precautions. Aspirin, vitamin C and chloroquine should be used with caution, especially in combination with other drugs or in high doses [8]. The prevalence of G6PD deficiency in endemic regions (where malaria drugs are needed) is an important public health problem, as malaria can provoke a hemolytic phenotype, making it difficult to identify drug effects. There is the CPIC guideline with strong recommendation for pharmacogenetics testing of *G6PD* before rasburicase therapy starts [9].

2.5   Dihydropyrimidine Dehydrogenase

Dihydropyrimidine dehydrogenase (DPYD) is involved in the breakdown of uracil and thymidine (pyrimidines) and their elimination from the body. Mutations in the *DPYD* gene interfere with the breakdown of pyrimidines, resulting in their accumulation in blood, urine, and cerebrospinal fluid. Excess uracil and thymidine have also been linked to neurological problems in some people with congenital DPYD deficiency [10].

Table 1 Functional activity and phenotype characteristics in DPYD and relevance for fluoropy-rimidine drugs (5-fluorouracil, capecitabine and tegafur) dosing

DPYD phenotype	Functional activity	Features
EM	2	Standard dosing
IM	1–1.5	Possible side effects and dose adjustment is recommended
PM	0–0.5	Possible side effects and dose adjustment or drug replacement is recommended

Alleles and phenotype data are updated from https://cpicpgx.org/genes-drugs/ (January 2022)

DPYD plays a major role in the hepatic degradation of the anticancer drugs 5-fluorouracil, capecitabine and tegafur (fluoropyrimidine drugs). Deficiency of this enzyme is present in about 3–5% of the population, and complete deficiency in about 0.2%. Due to the size of the genes and the low frequency of variants in *DPYD*, it is not possible to establish a single nomenclature of haplotypes. Therefore, mutations are marked individually, and only a small number of alleles are marked with an asterisk system (*). Many mutations have been found in the *DPYD* gene, and the most important mutated alleles of candidates for pharmacogenetic testing (present in about 7% of the European population) are: c.1905+1G>A (*2A), c.1679T>G (*13), c.1129-5923C>G, c.1236G>A (HapB3) and c.2846A>T.

Homozygotes (PM phenotype, with a functional activity ratio of 0–0.5) have an increased risk of severe toxicity at the standard dose of fluoropyrimidine drug, and in these patients, the starting dose should be reduced by more than 50%, or even drug replacement initiated (Table 1). In heterozygotes (IM phenotype, with a functional activity ratio of 1–1.5) the current CPIC guidelines recommend a 50% reduction in fluoropyrimidine drug dose, titratation the dose and monitoring the drug concentration [10].

2.6 Methylenetetrahydrofolate Reductase

Methylenetetrahydrofolate reductase (MTHFR) is an enzyme important in folate metabolism, where it participates in the conversion of homocysteine to methionine, and is involved in the pharmacodynamics of several drugs. There are several documented variants of *MTHFR* gene, which differentiate allele frequencies between different racial and ethnic groups, and research highlights the importance of the two most common *MTHFR* polymorphisms: C667T (rs1801133) and A1298C (rs1801131) [11]. Point mutation in the *MTHFR* gene (C667T, T-allele) is present in about 10–15% of Whites and causes a 50% decrease in enzyme activity, resulting in an accumulation of serum homocysteine (so-called hyperhomocysteinemia), which is associated with increased risk according to the defect of intrauterine neural tube development, pregnancy complications, and the risk of cardiovascular diseases. In heterozygous carriers of C677T polymorphism, MTHFR activity is moderate, and in homozygous carriers significantly reduced [11, 12].

MTHFR is also involved in the metabolism of several chemotherapeutic antineoplastic, and antirheumatic drugs, such as methotrexate, carboplatin, and 5-fluorouracil, which is why some studies report an association of T allele homozygotes with increased toxicity of these drugs. The A1298C polymorphism has been shown to increase the risk of methotrexate toxicity in Caucasians if they are carriers of the C allele [13].

So far, there have been attempts to establish recommendations for genetic testing of *MTHFR*, but the clinical benefit of polymorphism testing has never been proven and it is not recommended. Some authorities consider testing justified in patients with depression, coronary heart disease, acute myocardial infarction, peripheral vascular artery disease, stroke, and venous thromboembolism (if they have elevated homocysteine levels, > 13 μmol/L, or abnormal methionine loading test) [14].

2.7 Nucleoside Diphosphatase

Nucleoside Diphosphate Linked Moiety X-type motif 15, Nudix, is an enzyme associated with thiopurine metabolism and is important for their use in the treatment of inflammatory diseases and cancer. *NUDT15* gene belongs to the nucleoside diphosphatase gene family (also known as *MTH2*—MutT homolog 2) and is involved in preventing DNA mutations by removing bases damaged by residual peroxides and superoxides that are not detoxified by glutathione. Through its metabolic activity, it participates in the elimination of thiopurine drugs (azathioprine, mercaptopurine, and thioguanine) and is therefore important in pharmacogenetic testing. Twenty alleles of *NUDT15* are known, and the most common 9 shows Table 2.

Table 2 The most common *NUDT15* alleles in different ethnic groups, their activity and phenotype characteristics

NUDT15 allele	Activity	Allele frequencies in ethnic groups (%)		
		European	East Asian	Latin American
*1	Normal	99.3	87.9	93.6
*2	No	0.0	3.5	3.7
*3	No	0.2	6.1	0.8
*4	Unclear	0.0	0.1	1.8
*5	Unclear	0.0	1.1	0.0
*6	Unclear	0.3	1.3	0.2
*7	Unclear	0.0	0.1	0.0
*8	Unclear	-	-	-
*9	No	0.002	0.0	0.0

Alleles and phenotype data are updated from https://cpicpgx.org/genes-drugs/ (January 2022)

Thiopurines are used in the treatment of malignant and nonmalignant conditions, so the approach to dose adjustment and initiation of therapy based on *NUDT15* status is similar to that of *TPMT* and depends on the clinical indication. In the treatment of many malignancies, normal starting doses of thiopurine analogs are high because about 90% of the wild-type population for *TPMT* and *NUDT15* receive the maximum tolerated doses. For normal *NUDT15* metabolizers (*NUDT15*1/*1*), no initial dose adjustment is required. For the IM phenotype (e.g., *NUDT15*1/*3*), a reduction in the starting dose should be considered to reduce toxicity. For the PM phenotype NUDT15 (e.g., *NUDT15*3/*3*), a significant dose reduction is required and the concentration and side effects should be monitored or drug replaced [15, 16].

2.8   Thymidylate Synthase

Thymidylate synthase (TYMS, TS) is an enzyme very important for DNA synthesis and cell cycle, and catalyzes the conversion of deoxyuridine monophosphate (dUMP) to deoxythymidine monophosphate (dTMP). This process is important for the formation of thymine, a nucleotide required for DNA synthesis and repair. Inhibition of TS leads to deoxynucleotide imbalance and an increase in dUMP levels, causing DNA damage. Because of its key role in DNA replication, TS is the target of antitumor drugs such as capecitabine, 5-fluorouracil (5-FU), and methotrexate. 5-FU acts as an inhibitor of TS and prevents the methylation reaction of dUMP to dTMP. The expression of this gene encoding TS and the antisense transcript of a member of the superfamily 1 mitochondrial enolase (GeneID: 55556) varies inversely as cell growth progresses from the late log phase to the plateau phase. The sensitivity of TS to its inhibitors is a key part of its effect in the treatment of colon, pancreatic, ovarian, and gastric and breast cancers. Polymorphisms in this gene may be associated with the etiology of the neoplasm as well as the response to 5-FU-based chemotherapy (17).

The *TYMS* promoter region in humans contains a polymorphic enhancer with two (*2R*) or three (*3R*) 28-bp consecutive repeats that affect TS mRNA expression and results in genotypes with two tandem repeats (*2R/2R*), three tandem repeats (*3R/3R*) or heterozygous genotype (*2R/3R*). Tandem repeats can contain up to nine copies of a repeated 28 bp sequence. The *TSER*2(2R)* variant has low enzyme expression, while *TSER*3 (3R)* has approximately 2.6× higher expression than *TSER*2*. In addition, the point polymorphism (SNP) *G>C* within the second repeat of *TSER*3* is associated with altered TS transcription. Overexpression of TS has been associated with increased resistance to 5-FU, while SNPs has been associated with increased toxicity of 5-FU in different populations [17]. There is currently no protocol for cancer patients at risk of 5-FU resistance that may affect drug dosing or replacement according to TS gene variants.

3   Channels that Mediate Drugs Pharmacological Effects

3.1   Calcium Channels—Ryanodine Receptors (RYR) and Dihidropyrimidine Receptors

Ryanodine receptors (RYR) are intracellular calcium channels located at the membranes of sarcoplasmic reticulum and endoplasmic reticulum. Three isoforms of RYR differ according to their localization: RYR1 is primarily localized in skeletal muscle, RYR2 is expressed in cardiac muscle, while expression of more widely localized RYR3 dominates in the brain. They mediate the efflux of the calcium ions into the cytosol of cells. In skeletal muscle, activation of ryanodine receptors occurs via a coupling to the voltage-dependent L-type calcium channel (dihidropyrimidine receptors) on plasma membranes [18].

Mutations in the *RYR1* gene are strongly associated with malignant hyperthermia susceptibility. Even 48 *RYR1* nucleotide polymorphisms and one deletion, together with two mutations in the gene for the L-type calcium channel (dihidropyrimidine receptor), are connected with the increased risk of malignant hyperthermia (MH). MH is a hypermetabolic reaction with symptoms, such as muscle rigidity, high body temperature, tachycardia, rhabdomyolysis, and hyperkalemia [18]. Administration of halogenated volatile anesthetics (e.g., halothane, isoflurane, desflurane, sevoflurane) and the depolarizing neuromuscular blocker succinylcholine can induce MH in susceptible persons. Based on available evidence, clinical guidelines recommend a genetic test before starting these drugs to determine the susceptibility to MH [18–20].

3.2   Anion (Chloride) Channel

The cystic fibrosis transmembrane conductance regulator (CFTR, ATP-binding cassette sub-family C, and member 7, ABCC7) is expressed predominantly in epithelial tissues, where it serves as an anion channel that transports chloride (Cl^-) and bicarbonate. More than 2100 variants in the *CFTR* gene have been reported. Cystic Fibrosis (CF) is an autosomal recessive disease resulting from a defect-causing variant on each *CFTR* allele. Even 360 variants based on the clinical and functional criteria were defined as CF-causing and classified in 6 classes (classes I to III cause more severe disease). However, one single mutation—the deletion of a phenylalanine at position 508 (F508del) is found in at least one allele of 80% of individuals with CF worldwide [21].

Drugs developed to correct specific defects of the CFTR protein represent novel therapies for CF. They act either as correctors of defective CFTR protein to increase its expression at the cell surface or as potentiators that enhance the transmembrane channel opening of the defective protein. Ivacaftor, the first approved potentiator drug was indicated in CF patients with at least one G551D variant (rs75527207 genotype AA or GA), but the indication was later extended to 33 different *CFTR* variants. G551D variant is SNP at position c.1652G>A that causes a Gly to Asp change resulting in a protein expressed at the plasma membrane but defective in ATP hydrolysis and channel gating. Ivacaftor targets the gating defect of to enhance channel activity. The most common pathogenic mutation is a deletion mutant F508del (with deletion of phenylalanine at site 508 caused by genomic deletion of three nucleotides). Because this mutation results in minimal cell surface protein expression, to increase treatment efficacy, ivacaftor is combined with corrector drugs lumacaftor and tezacaftor [22].

4   Immune Response Gene Polymorphism—Human Leukocyte Antigens (HLA)

Human Leukocyte Antigens—HLA (also known as the human form of the Major Histocompatibility Complex—MHC) are cell-surface proteins that present intracellular antigens to the immune cells (T cells) to initiate their antigen-specific responses. They are encoded by a large cluster of *MHC* genes which contains class I, II, and III subgroups. The *HLA-A, HLA-B,* and *HLA-C* genes are part of the class I complex and are among the most highly polymorphic genes in the human genome. For example, more than 7000 *HLA-B* alleles and more than 3000 *HLA-A* alleles have been identified in populations worldwide and deposited to the World Health Organization Nomenclature Committee for Factors of the HLA System [23].

The HLA genes are highly relevant for pharmacogenetics research since allelic variants have been associated with susceptibility and resistance to numerous diseases, as well as adverse reactions to a wide range of pharmaceuticals (Table 3). For example, *HLA-B*53* is connected with resistance to malaria, *HLA-B*51* with susceptibility to the Beçhet's disease, and *HLA-B*46* with increased risk of Graves' disease. Strong associations are also found for *HLA-B*57* and HIV long-term non-progression, and *HLA-B*27* and ankylosing spondylitis [24].

The most important HLA genes for pharmacogenetics, with a significant effect on therapeutic outcomes, are *HLA-A*31:01 and HLA-A*33:03,* as well as *HLA-B*15:02, HLA-B*57:01, HLA-B*58:01.* The frequency of *HLA-A*31:01* and *HLA-B*15:02* alleles in Caucasians is less than 0.1%, while they are more common in Asians. About 6% of the population has the *HLA-B*57:01* allele, and about 1–5% has the *HLA-B*58:01* allele. These genotypes increase the risk of adverse effects to abacavir, allopurinol, phenytoin, carbamazepine, and oxcarbazepine. Based on the highest level of evidence, available clinical guidelines suggest *HLA* genotype screening in all drug-naive individuals before initiation of the therapy [24, 25].

Abacavir is an antiviral drug used to treat HIV-infected patients. In approximately half of the patients with the *HLA-B*57:01* allele, it causes severe immune system-mediated hypersensitivity reactions after repeated dosing, which can be fatal. Hypersensitivity reactions may include fever, rash, nausea, vomiting, abdominal pain, fatigue, cough, and dyspnea. The *HLA-B*57:01* allele frequency varies—it is the lowest in African and Asian populations and is absent in the Japanese. In the European population frequency is 6–7%, and the highest (up

Table 3 Drugs and recommendations for therapy based on *HLA* genotype (according to https://cpicpgx.org)

HLA risk allele	Drug/indication	Associated phenotype	Recommendation/CPIC guideline
HLA-B*57:01	Abacavir/HIV treatment	Hypersensitivity reaction	In individuals with the *HLA-B*57:01* variant allele ("*HLA-B*57:01*-positive"), abacavir is not recommended and should be considered only under exceptional circumstances*
HLA-B*57:01:01	Flucloxacillin/ antibacterial drug	Patients with one or two copies have an increased risk of drug-induced liver injury	Monitor for liver function and select an alternative drug instead of flucloxacillin if liver enzymes or bilirubin is elevated (Dutch Pharmacogenetics Working Group Guidelines, August 2019)
HLA-B*58:01	Allopurinol/drug for hyperuricemia	Patients with one or two copies of the *HLA-B*58:01* allele may have an increased risk of severe cutaneous adverse reactions, such as SJS, TEN and MPE	Drug is contraindicated in individuals with the *HLA-B*58:01* variant allele ("*HLA-B*58:01*-positive")*
HLA-B*15:02	Phenytoin and phosphophenytoine/ epilepsia treatment	Patients with one or two copies of the *HLA-B*15:02:01* allele may have an increased risk of severe cutaneous adverse reactions such as SJS/TEN	Drugs are contraindicated in individuals with the *HLA-B*15:02* variant allele ("*HLA-B*15:02*-positive")*
HLA-B*15:02 *HLA-A*31:01*	Carbamazepine and oxcarbazepine/ epilepsia treatment	Patients carrying at least one copy of either *HLA-B*15:02* or *HLA-A*31:01* have an increased risk of SJS/ TEN *HLA-A*31:01* is associated with an increased risk of drug reaction with eosinophilia and systemic symptoms and MPE	An alternative drug for carbamazepine-naive patients carrying at least one copy of either *HLA-B*15:02* or *HLA-A*31:01* is recommended*

SJS Stevens-Johnson syndrome, *TEN* toxic epidermal necrolysis, *MPE* maculopapular erythem; *Clinical Pharmacogenetics Implementation Consortium (CPIC) issued clinical guidelines to 20%) is estimated in the Southwest Asian population. Abacavir use is not recommended in abacavir-naive individuals who are *HLA-B*57:01* positive [26].

Allopuriol, a xanthine oxidase inhibitor, is used to treat hyperuricemia and gout. It can cause severe hypersensitivity reactions with an estimated 0.1–0.4% risk. These may include cutaneous reactions, such as toxic epidermal necrolysis and Stevens-Johnson syndrome, or drug reaction with systemic symptoms that may include fever, leukocytosis, eosinophilia, hepatitis, and acute renal failure. Strong evidence associates the *HLA-B*57:01* allele and the risk of these potentially fatal adverse effects. Because of its high predictive value in some populations (Han-Chinese, Taiwan, and Japanese), clinical guidelines recommend avoiding allopurinol usage in *HLA-B*57:01* positive individuals [27].

Antiseizure drug *phenytoin* and its prodrug *fosphenytoin* should be avoided in patients with the *HLA-B*15:02* allele because of the increased risk of SJS and TEN. *HLA-B*15:02* is most prevalent in East Asian and Central/South Asian populations (allele frequency ranging from 1% to over 20%) and is less frequent in the European population (0–1%). Because of substantial evidence linking this genotype with the risk of potentially fatal cutaneous adverse reactions, guidelines recommend avoiding phenytoin use in the *HLA-B*15:02* positive individuals [24].

The same risk is detected for other antiseizure drugs *carbamazepine* and *oxcarbazepine,* where substantial evidence associates *HLA-B*15:02* genotype and cutaneous adverse reactions [28].

Additionally, evidence suggests the association of the *HLA-A*31:01* genotype with carbamazepine-induced hypersensitivity syndrome. This is characterized by skin rash, plus two of fever, lymphadenopathy, and hematologic abnormalities, with the involvement of at least one internal organ (there is no evidence for oxcarbazepine). The frequency of the *HLA-A*31:01* allele is higher than the *HLA-B*15:02* allele in Caucasians (3%) and Hispanic/South Americans (6%), and is also highly expressed in Japanese (8%) and South Koreans (5%). Based on the highest level of evidence, in carriers of *HLA-B*15:02* and *HLA-A*31: 01* alleles, carbamazepine therapy is not recommended [28].

5 Other Genes of Interest for Specific Drugs

5.1 Mitochondrially Encoded 12s rRNA—*MT-RNR1*

MT-RNR1 is one of the 37 mitochondrial genes which encode the 12s rRNA subunit and is the mitochondrial homolog of the bacterial 16s rRNA. Commonly used aminoglycoside antibiotics (like amikacin, gentamicin, streptomycin, etc.) bind to the 16s rRNA subunit of the bacterial 30S ribosome, with consequent inhibition of bacterial protein synthesis. These drugs can cause sensorineural hearing loss (cochleototoxicity) and vestibulotoxicity, dose-dependent adverse effects when applied for a protracted period [29].

Variants in *MT-RNR1 m.1095T>C* (rs267606618); *m.1494C>T* (rs267606619); *m.1555A>G* (rs267606617) cause the 12s rRNA subunit to closely resemble the procaryotic 16s rRNA subunit. These allow aminoglycosides to bind more readily to the eukaryotic 12s rRNA subunit. Sensory cells (or hair cells) in the inner ear are rich in mitochondria because of the high energy demand. Hearing loss is a common symptom across many mitochondrial conditions and is also a consequence of aminoglycosides-induced sensory cells injury [30].

Although the frequency of the pathogenic alleles within the different populations is low, there is consistent evidence of strong and moderate levels that associate m.1555A>G, m.1494C>T, and the m.1095T>C variants with aminoglycoside drugs-induced hearing loss. Therefore, clinical guidelines suggest avoiding aminoglycosides in individuals with pathogenic *MT-RNR1* variants unless the increased risk of permanent hearing loss is outweighed by the risk of infection and in the absence of effective alternative therapies [30].

5.2   Interferon-λ 3 (IFN-λ 3)

Interferon-λ 3 (IFN-λ 3), encoded by *IFNL3* (also known as *IL28B*), is a member of the type 3 IFN-λ family, with antiviral, antiproliferative, and immune-modulatory activities. Variations in *IFNL3* gene have the strongest predictive value of treatment response following pegylated interferon-α (PEG-IFN-α) and ribavirin (RBV) therapy for previously untreated patients with hepatitis C virus (HCV) genotype 1 [31].

Until a decade ago, the treatment for chronic HCV infection relied on PEG-IFN-α and RBV combination therapy lasting 24 weeks for HCV genotypes 2 and 3, while for other HCV genotypes, the treatment continued for 48 weeks. Except for long duration and low to modest therapy outcomes (measured as a sustained virologic response, SVR), this treatment regime is expensive and associated with many side effects. Also, it is unpredictable, with SVR varying significantly among different races and ethnicities, thus implicating genetic variabilities, among other factors, as important factors that influence treatment outcomes.

The two most tested single variants are rs12979860 and rs8099917. Rs12979860 allele frequency varies among different ethnic groups (C allele is most frequently present in East Asians, followed by Caucasians and Hispanics, and is the least common among individuals of African origin; allele frequencies of 0.9, 0.63, 0.55, and 0.39, respectively). Genotypes CC for rs12979860 and TT for rs8099917 are associated with favorable therapeutic response, with an approximately two-fold increase in SVR for HCV genotype 1 patients. However, rs8099917 is better in predicting response to PEG-IFN-α and RBV therapy in Japanese patients as compared with rs12979860. Also, the duration of treatment can be shorter (especially with a concomitant protease inhibitor in combination) in individuals with favorable genotypes [32].

Based on the highest level of evidence, CPIC guidelines recommend the use of PEG-IFN-α–containing regimens based on *IFNL3* genotype, and a shorter therapy duration when protease inhibitor is in combination (24–28 versus 48 weeks) [32].

6   Conclusion

Different genes encoding intracellular or membrane proteins might influence a drug's efficacy and safety. Some genes are highly polymorphic, where pathogenic variants might increase the risk for serious adverse effects, with potentially fatal outcomes. For some pathogenic genotypes, substantial evidence of the highest level and prognostic value resulted in clinical guidelines for therapy adjustments to avoid therapy failure and improve its safety.

References

1. Primorac D, Bach-Rojecky L, Vađunec D, Juginović A, Žunić K, Matišić V, et al. Pharmacogenomics at the center of precision medicine: challenges and perspective in an era of Big Data. Pharmacogenomics. 2020;21(2):141–56. https://doi.org/10.2217/pgs-2019-0134.
2. Owen RP, Gong L, Sagreiya H, Klein TE, Altman RB. VKORC1 pharmacogenomics summary. Pharmacogenet Genomics. 2010;20(10):642–4. https://doi.org/10.1097/FPC.0b013e328 33433b6.
3. Liu M, Yi J, Tang W. Association between angiotensin converting enzyme gene polymorphism and essential hypertension: a systematic review and meta-analysis. J Renin Angiotensin Aldosterone Syst. 2021;22(1):1470320321995074. https://doi.org/10.1177/1470320321995074.
4. Heidari F, Vasudevan R, Mohd Ali SZ, Ismail P, Arkani M. RAS Genetic variants in interaction with ace inhibitors drugs influences essential hypertension control. Arch Med Res. 2017;48(1):88–95. https://doi.org/10.1016/j.arcmed.2017.03.003.
5. Stein MB, Fallin MD, Schork NJ, Gelernter J. COMT polymorphisms and anxiety-related personality traits. Neuropsychopharmacology. 2005;30(11):2092–102. https://doi.org/10.1038/sj. npp.1300787.
6. Belfield KD, Tichy EM. Review and drug therapy implications of glucose-6-phosphate dehydrogenase deficiency. Am J Health Syst Pharm. 2018;75(3):97–104. https://doi.org/10.2146/ ajhp160961.
7. Cappellini MD, Fiorelli G. Glucose-6-phosphate dehydrogenase deficiency. Lancet. 2008;2008371(9606):64–74. https://doi.org/10.1016/S0140-6736(08)60073-2.
8. McDonagh EM, Thorn CF, Bautista JM, Youngster I, Russ B, Altman RB, Klein TE. PharmGKB summary: very important pharmacogene information for G6PD. Pharmacogenet Genomics. 2012;22(3):219–28. https://doi.org/10.1097/FPC.0b013e32834eb313.
9. Relling MV, McDonagh EM, Chang T, Caudle KE, McLeod HL, Haidar CE, et al. Clinical Pharmacogenetics Implementation Consortium (CPIC) guidelines for rasburicase therapy in the context of G6PD deficiency genotype. Clin Pharmacol Ther. 2014;96(2):169–74. https:// doi.org/10.1038/clpt.2014.97.
10. Amstutz U, Henricks LM, Offer SM, Barbarino J, Schellens JHM, Swen JJ, et al. Clinical pharmacogenetics implementation consortium (CPIC) guideline for dihydropyrimidine dehydrogenase genotype and fluoropyrimidine dosing: 2017 update. Clin Pharmacol Ther. 2018;103(2):210–6. https://doi.org/10.1002/cpt.911.
11. Sahasranaman S, Howard D, Roy S. Clinical pharmacology and pharmacogenetics of thiopurines. Eur J Clin Pharmacol. 2008;64(8):753–67. https://doi.org/10.1007/s00228-008-0478-6.
12. Ueland PM, Hustad S, Schneede J, Refsum H, Vollset SE. Biological and clinical implications of the MTHFR C677T polymorphism. Trends Pharmacol Sci. 2001;22(4):195–201. https://doi. org/10.1016/s0165-6147(00)01675-8.
13. Su Y, Yan H, Guo L, Lu T, Zhang D, Yue W. Association of MTHFR C677T polymorphism with antipsychotic-induced change of weight and metabolism index. Front Psychiatry. 2021;12:673715. https://doi.org/10.3389/fpsyt.2021.673715.

14. Fisher MC, Cronstein BC. Metaanalysis of methylenetetrahydrofolate reductase (MTHFR) polymorphisms affecting methotrexate toxicity. J Rheumatol. 2009;36(3):539–45. https://doi.org/10.3899/jrheum.080576.

15. Yang JJ, Whirl-Carrillo M, Scott SA, Turner AJ, Schwab M, Tanaka Y, et al. Pharmacogene Variation Consortium Gene Introduction: NUDT15. Clin Pharmacol Ther. 2019;105(5):1091–4. https://doi.org/10.1002/cpt.1268.

16. Relling MV, Schwab M, Whirl-Carrillo M, Suarez-Kurtz G, Pui CH, Stein CM, et al. Clinical pharmacogenetics implementation consortium guideline for thiopurine dosing based on TPMT and NUDT15 genotypes: 2018 update. Clin Pharmacol Ther. 2019;105(5):1095–105. https://doi.org/10.1002/cpt.1304.

17. Rose MG, Farrell MP, Schmitz JC. Thymidylate synthase: a critical target for cancer chemotherapy. Clin Colorectal Cancer. 2002;1(4):220–9. https://doi.org/10.3816/CCC.2002.n.003.

18. Riazi S, Kraeva N, Hopkins PM. Malignant hyperthermia in the post-genomics era: new perspectives on an old concept. Anesthesiology. 2018;128(1):168–80. https://doi.org/10.1097/ALN.0000000000001878.

19. Gonsalves SG, Dirksen RT, Sangkuhl K, Pulk R, Alvarellos M, Vo T, et al. Clinical pharmacogenetics implementation consortium (CPIC) guideline for the use of potent volatile anesthetic agents and succinylcholine in the context of RYR1 or CACNA1S genotypes. Clin Pharmacol Ther. 2019;105(6):1338–44. https://doi.org/10.1002/cpt.1319.Erratum.In:ClinPharmacolTher. 2019;106(6):1408.

20. Bach-Rojecky L, Čutura T, Lozić M, Husedžinović Kliškinjić, Matišić V, Primorac D. Personalized anesthetic pharmacology. in personalized medicine in anesthesia. In: Dabbagh A, editors. Pain and Perioperative Medicine. Cham: Springer Nature Switzerland, Switzerland; 2020. p. 65–92.

21. Pranke I, Golec A, Hinzpeter A, Edelman A, Sermet-Gaudelus I. Emerging therapeutic approaches for cystic fibrosis: from gene editing to personalized medicine. Front Pharmacol. 2019;10:121. https://doi.org/10.3389/fphar.2019.00121.

22. Elborn JS, Ramsey BW, Boyle MP, Konstan MW, Huang X, Marigowda G, et al. Efficacy and safety of lumacaftor/ivacaftor combination therapy in patients with cystic fibrosis homozygous for Phe508del CFTR by pulmonary function subgroup: a pooled analysis. Lancet Respir Med. 2016;4(8):617–26. https://doi.org/10.1016/S2213-2600(16)30121-7.

23. Nomenclature for Factors of the HLA System. http://hla.alleles.org/. Accessed 13 Feb 2022

24. Barbarino JM, Kroetz DL, Klein TE, Altman RB. PharmGKB summary: very important pharmacogene information for human leukocyte antigen B. Pharmacogenet Genomics. 2015;25(4):205–21. https://doi.org/10.1097/FPC.0000000000000118.

25. Primorac D, Höppner W, editors. Pharmacogenetics in clinical practice: Experience with 55 commonly used drugs. Zagreb, Ham-burg, Philadelphia: St. Catherine Specialty Hospital, Bioglobe GmbH, ISABS; 2022. https://www.stcatherine.com/centre-of-excellence/10/individualized-and-preventive-medicine/pharmacogenomics/69. Accessed 2 March 2022.

26. Martin MA, Klein TE, Dong BJ, Pirmohamed M, Haas DW, Kroetz DL. Clinical Pharmacogenetics Implementation Consortium. Clinical pharmacogenetics implementation consortium guidelines for HLA-B genotype and abacavir dosing. Clin Pharmacol Ther. 2012;91(4):734–8. https://doi.org/10.1038/clpt.2011.355.

27. Hershfield MS, Callaghan JT, Tassaneeyakul W, Mushiroda T, Thorn CF, Klein TE, Lee MT. Clinical Pharmacogenetics Implementation Consortium guidelines for human leukocyte antigen-B genotype and allopurinol dosing. Clin Pharmacol Ther. 2013;93(2):153–8. https://doi.org/10.1038/clpt.2012.209.

28. Phillips EJ, Sukasem C, Whirl-Carrillo M, Müller DJ, Dunnenberger HM, Chantratita W, et al. Clinical pharmacogenetics implementation consortium guideline for HLA genotype and use of carbamazepine and oxcarbazepine: 2017 update. Clin Pharmacol Ther. 2018;103(4):574–81. https://doi.org/10.1002/cpt.1004.

29. Barbarino JM, McGregor TL, Altman RB, Klein TE. PharmGKB summary: very important pharmacogene information for MT-RNR1. Pharmacogenet Genomics. 2016;26(12):558–67. https://doi.org/10.1097/FPC.0000000000000247.
30. McDermott JH, Wolf J, Hoshitsuki K, Huddart R, Caudle KE, Whirl-Carrillo M, et al. Clinical pharmacogenetics implementation consortium guideline for the use of aminoglycosides based on MT-RNR1 genotype. Clin Pharmacol Ther. 2022;111(2):366–72. https://doi.org/10.1002/cpt.2309.
31. Suppiah V, Moldovan M, Ahlenstiel G, Berg T, Weltman M, Abate ML, et al. IL28B is associated with response to chronic hepatitis C interferon-alpha and ribavirin therapy. Nat Genet. 2009;41(10):1100–4. https://doi.org/10.1038/ng.447.
32. Muir AJ, Gong L, Johnson SG, Lee MT, Williams MS, Klein TE, et al. Clinical Pharmacogenetics Implementation Consortium (CPIC). Clinical Pharmaco-genetics Implementation Consortium (CPIC) guidelines for IFNL3 (IL28B) geno-type and PEG interferon-α-based regimens. Clin Pharmacol Ther. 2014;95(2):141–6. https://doi.org/10.1038/clpt.2013.203.

Pharmacogenetic Algorithms

Bernard Esquivel, Cristina Verzosa, Hagit Katzov-Eckert, and Marysol Garcia-Patino

Abstract

Pharmacogenetic clinical algorithms represented by logistic steps in the decision-making process are designed to shift pharmacogenetics from research to clinical practice. Algorithms have been developed to guide treatment recommendations based on studies and clinical trials. The availability of guidelines and databases provide evidence for the use of validated pharmacogenetic algorithms and demonstrate a benefit when implemented compared to standard treatment. This chapter focuses on conditions that have validated pharmacogenetic algorithms or established clinically actionable drug-gene associations. Clinical algorithms in cardiovascular disease, neurology and mental health, pain, rheumatology, oncology, and anti-viral treatments will be described as well as the evidence and studies supporting these algorithms. In many cases, clinical guidelines do not recommend routine genotyping before start of treatment; however, if genotypes are known, there is no harm in considering pharmacogenetic algorithms for personalized treatment. While pharmacogenetic considerations may guide medication selection and clinical treatment plans, a holistic approach should be considered in the context of the patient.

B. Esquivel (✉) · C. Verzosa · H. Katzov-Eckert · M. Garcia-Patino
GenXys Health Care Systems Inc., Vancouver, BC, Canada
e-mail: ber.doc@gmail.com

C. Verzosa
e-mail: cristina.verzosa@genxys.com

H. Katzov-Eckert
e-mail: hagit.ke@genxys.com

M. Garcia-Patino
e-mail: marysol.garcia@genxys.com

© The Author(s), under exclusive license to Springer Nature Switzerland AG 2023   105
D. Primorac et al. (eds.), *Pharmacogenomics in Clinical Practice*,
https://doi.org/10.1007/978-3-031-45903-0_7

Keywords

Pharmacogenetics • Clinical algorithms • Guidelines • CPIC • DPWG • Implementation

1 Introduction—Clinical Algorithms

Clinical algorithms represent the steps involved in clinical decision making. Algorithms guide the user to specific treatment recommendations based on a series of questions or differentiators. They are commonly presented as diagrams or flow charts for ease of use, although often specific details of clinical application are given in text. Algorithms consolidate multiple treatment considerations into a single guide.

Validated algorithms have clinical outcomes trial data that demonstrate a benefit when implemented compared to standard treatment.

The implementation of clinical algorithms has changed over time. In the past, clinical algorithms were available only in hard copy formats and clinicians needed to access reference texts at point of care, or have the algorithm memorized. Online tools have allowed clinicians to access algorithms in a more accessible and flexible manner. Recently, advances in clinical decision support software allow for real time integration of patient data into a programmed algorithm to produce an instantaneous result.

2 Pharmacogenetic Guidelines

Guidelines are systematically developed statements and recommendations to improve and enhance best clinical practices. Clinical guidelines typically use GRADE as a standardized system of level of evidence.

A pharmacogenetic guideline specifically addresses gene-drug and gene–disease associations and standardizes genotypic and phenotypic interpretations for these associations in an evidence-based approach. These guidelines can then be used to implement pharmacogenetics into clinical care.

Resources are needed to evaluate literature and provide clinical guidance for the increasing amount of pharmacogenomic information. Several public, online pharmacogenetics databases are available to assist with clinical decision-making. In addition to the multiple, public databases there are pharmacogenetic databases available via subscription. Educational opportunities are needed to increase awareness and understanding. This need is growing to educate patients and providers, as personalized medicine and specifically pharmacogenomics is frequently mentioned. The online databases not only include regulatory databases but also pharmacogenomic referential databases. As pharmacogenomic resources are developed and more readily available, clinicians are more likely to integrate pharmacogenomics into clinical practice with accessible information. The integration of pharmacogenomics into clinical practice will enhance patient care and patient outcomes when personalizing a patient's medication therapy, increasing efficacy, and decreasing the risk of adverse effects.

The Clinical Pharmacogenetics Implementation Consortium (CPIC) [1, 2], the Dutch Pharmacogenetics Working Group (DPWG) [3–5], the Canadian Pharmacogenomics Network for Drug Safety (CPNDS), French National Network of Pharmacogenetics (RNPGx) [6], and other societies are working on standardization efforts for genotype translations, phenotype terms, and reporting of PGx recommendations. Variants influencing drug metabolizing genes may have changing functional assignments or new clinical implications as new evidence is discovered. As new evidence becomes available the guidelines change or new guidelines are established. This requires continuous updates to the interpretation of drug-gene interactions.

3 Differentiating Between Pharmacokinetic and Clinical Significance

Pharmacokinetics and pharmacodynamics are closely linked together. Pharmacokinetics analyzes the Absorption, Distribution, Metabolism, and Excretion (ADME) of a drug, while pharmacodynamics evaluates drug effects and their relationship to plasma concentration. Genetic variations in enzymes, transporters or receptors that participate in these mechanisms introduce differences in drug pharmacokinetics and action (therapeutic and unwanted). However, these differences are not always translated into the clinical setting. This is relevant in the decision-making of clinical algorithms using pharmacogenetics information. Depending on the scope of the algorithm, a pharmacokinetic effect might not have the same value as a gene-drug interaction with a proven clinical effect. This section discusses the effects of pharmacogenetic variability and its clinical significance.

CYP enzymes play an important role in drug metabolism. At least 57 functional CYP genes have been detected [7], but only a portion of them is responsible for metabolizing 70–80% of all drugs used in the clinic [8]. Their metabolizing activity is affected by several factors, such as genetic variability and the presence of specific xenobiotics. The high degree of genetic variability in *CYP* genes leads to different functional status. Depending on the presence of specific single-nucleotide polymorphisms (SNPs) and the number of copies detected, a patient can be categorized as an ultrarapid, normal, intermediate or poor metabolizer.

Different CYP metabolizer status will lead to different pharmacokinetic profiles. For instance, if a drug is metabolized by a CYP enzyme to less active compounds, poor metabolizers will have higher plasma concentrations of the active compound compared to normal metabolizers. In many cases, this scenario can lead to a higher probability of side effects in poor metabolizers; however, this is not always the case.

CYP2D6 alone is responsible for the metabolism of 25% of drugs used in clinical care [7]. It is involved in the metabolism of drugs used to treat mental health conditions, chronic pain, and heart disease, among others. However, some of the CYP2D6 gene–drug interactions that have effects on the plasma concentration do not have an influence on drug response. An example of this is oxycodone, an opioid medication used for pain management.

Oxycodone is metabolized into oxymorphone by CYP2D6, a metabolite 14 times more active than its parent drug [9]. In healthy individuals, it has been shown that CYP2D6 metabolizer status has an effect on oxycodone plasma concentrations. CYP2D6 poor metabolizers (PMs) have a significantly lower plasma concentration of oxymorphone compared to normal and ultrarapid metabolizers [10, 11]. However, there is conflicting data on whether CYP2D6 variants have a clinical effect on drug response or oxycodone-induced adverse reactions [12]. Several studies have found no significant differences in pain control between CYP2D6 genotypes [13–15]. The CPIC guideline [12] does not provide therapeutic recommendations for the use of this drug due to the lack of evidence supporting a clinical effect dependent on CYP2D6 genotype.

In some cases, a pharmacodynamic effect might be present, but therapeutic modifications may not be recommended due to the nature of the condition. For instance, gefitinib, a drug used to treat nonsmall cell lung cancer, is metabolized into ortho-desmethyl-gefitinib by CYP2D6. Ortho-desmethyl-gefitinib is a less active form of gefitinib, and it has been shown that CYP2D6 PMs have no detectable levels of this metabolite [16].

It has been shown that gefitinib can be tolerated by CYP2D6 PMs and that drug toxicity is not associated with CYP2D6 genotype [17, 18]. However, there are reports that indicate that other factors, such as the concomitant use of CYP3A4 inhibitors, can increase the probability of gefitinib-induced hepatotoxicity in patients carrying CYP2D6 variants [19]. The US Food and Drug Administration (FDA) provides drug monograph that does not include dose adjustment recommendations based on CYP2D6 metabolizer status, since higher plasma levels of gefitinib is clinically important for the treatment of non-small cell lung cancer. Closely monitoring CYP2D6 PMs is suggested.

CYP2C9 has been associated with the clearance of nonsteroidal anti-inflammatory drugs (NSAIDs), a group of drugs commonly used as analgesics. More than 60 CYP2C9 alleles have been identified so far [20], but the decreased and no function alleles CYP2C9*2 and CYP2C9*3 are the most prevalent CYP2C9 variants. Patients carrying decreased and no function CYP2C9 alleles have a higher risk of NSAID exposure, which is associated with an increased risk of gastrointestinal bleeding [21].

The CPIC guideline for CYP2C9 and the use of NSAIDs includes recommendations for celecoxib, flurbiprofen, lornoxicam, ibuprofen meloxicam, piroxicam and tenoxicam [22]. However, the pharmacokinetic differences caused by CYP2C9 variants are much smaller for other drugs in this group, reducing the probability of a clinical effect. For instance, CYP2C9 is responsible for less than 20% of the clearance of other NSAIDs such as diclofenac [23], and CYP2C9 metabolizer status has not been associated to a higher risk of diclofenac-induced toxicity [24].

Sulfonylureas, a group of drugs used to treat type 2 diabetes, are also metabolized by CYP2C9. The metabolites formed by CYP2C9 are less effective or inactive compared to the parent drugs. Subjects carrying genetic variants such as *CYP2C9*2* or *CYP2C9*3*, have higher sulfonylurea plasma levels than those detected in wild-type subjects (*CYP2C9*1*) [25–28]. However, the clinical effect of *CYP2C9* genetic variation is not clear.

Some studies have shown that subjects carrying *CYP2C9* variants may have better clinical outcomes. For instance, Zeng et al. [29] reported that in diabetic patients treated with gliclazide, *CYP2C9*3* (**1/*3* and **3/*3*) was associated with lower fasting plasma glucose. Similarly, Suzuki et al. [28] analyzed hemoglobin A1C (HbA1c) levels in diabetic patients treated with glimepiride and reported that patients carrying *CYP2C9*3* had a significant decrease HbA1c levels after 6 months of treatment. Nonetheless, the presence of *CYP2C9* genetic variants has also been associated with hypoglycemic adverse events in diabetic patients taking sulfonylureas [30–32], although this tendency has not been observed in all studies [33]. Because of the complexity of type 2 diabetes, recommendations based on *CYP2C9* genetic variants for the use of sulfonylureas is not supported.

4 Pharmacogenetics in Selected Disease States

This chapter focuses on disease states that utilize pharmacogenetic algorithms or are treated with drugs that have evidence for clinically actionable gene-drug associations. The therapeutic areas included are cardiovascular disease, neurology and mental health, pain, rheumatology, oncology, and anti-viral treatments.

4.1 Cardiovascular Diseases

Warfarin is a highly prescribed medication for the treatment of oral anticoagulation. Warfarin is challenging to manage due to variability in response and has a high rate of serious adverse drug reactions leading to hospitalization [34].

Warfarin is dosed to achieve an International Normalized Ratio (INR) of 2 to 3 for most conditions. Inappropriate dosing increases the risk for warfarin-related adverse events. There is increased risk of cardiovascular events during the initial months of warfarin therapy [35, 36]. Patients of African descent have a high rate of cardiovascular events and a high risk of major bleeding from warfarin [37]. Factors such as race, age, sex, body surface area, smoking, concomitant medication, liver and kidney function, absorption, or elimination of vitamin K account for only 15% to 20% of interpatient variability in warfarin dose requirements, and therefore, genetics may play a role in accurately predicting therapeutic dose [38].

Genetic studies have shown that genotype contributes to interpatient variability in warfarin dose requirements. The main genes implicated are *CYP2C9* and *VKORC1* [39–42]. Other genes involved to a lesser extent in warfarin dose requirement is *CYP4F2*, which encodes a vitamin K oxidase and *GGCX* which encodes gamma-glutamyl carboxylase which uses reduced vitamin K to activate clotting factors.

In 2010, the FDA changed warfarin label to note that if *CYP2C9* and *VKORC1* genotypes are known then these genetic factors should be considered in dose selection and follow-up [43]. Dosing algorithms that predict maintenance warfarin dose requirements based on a combination of demographic, clinical and genetic factors have been developed and there are several retrospective studies and clinical trials that have tested these algorithms. These studies have validated four pharmacogenetic warfarin algorithms. First, the International Warfarin Dose Refinement Collaboration algorithm for warfarin dosage adjustment may be used for the first warfarin adjustment on day 4 or 5 of treatment, after the first INR reading [44]. Second, the International Warfarin Pharmacogenetics Consortium (IWPC) algorithm a well validated algorithm which was shown to explain 46% interindividual variability in warfarin response [45]. Other well validated warfarin clinical algorithms include the IWPC modified algorithm by Anderson et al. [46] which is an algorithm for warfarin initiation. The algorithm includes important demographics and genetics into the calculation of the weekly dose. Finally, the Gage algorithm [47] has a "mini loading dose" for CYP2C9 IMs, CYP2C9 PMs and does not include CYP2C9 variants for first two doses.

The CPIC guideline recommends the use of warfarin validated pharmacogenetic dosing algorithms. Even though, these may not be applicable to non-Caucasians or for patients with INR targets outside the 2–3 range [48]. The CPIC guideline includes *CYP2C9*5, CYP2C9*6, CYP2C9*8, CYP2C9*11*, and *CYP2C* rs12777823 which are variants more frequent in individuals with African ancestry. CPIC guideline recommends only using pharmacogenetics in African ancestry if testing for *CYP2C9*5, CYP2C9*6, CYP2C9*8, CYP2C9*11* and *CYP2C* rs12777823 variants. For pediatric patients, CPIC guideline recommends using a validated pharmacogenetics algorithm if *VKORC1* −1639G>A, *CYP2C9*2* and *CYP2C9*3* genotypes are available.

In conclusion, warfarin dose recommendations that incorporate genotype and clinical information can be generated for individual patients. It is important to note that there are other factors such as diet, concomitant medications, poor compliance, and dosing errors that affect patient response to warfarin. Thus, the use of pharmacogenetic dosing should not be considered a substitute for clinical and INR monitoring.

Clopidogrel is a highly prescribed thienopyridine antiplatelet drug used to prevent cardiovascular events after an Acute Coronary Syndrome (ACS) or Percutaneous Coronary Intervention (PCI). Clopidogrel is a prodrug metabolized by CYP2C19. The implications of individuals taking clopidogrel and carriers of *CYP2C19* no function alleles are reduced metabolism of clopidogrel to the active compound, less antiplatelet effect, and higher risk of bleeding and atherothrombotic events [49].

There are several prospective studies and clinical trials examining *CYP2C19* genotype-guided antiplatelet therapy on clinical outcomes. The studies demonstrated that a genotype-guided strategy, whereby alternative medications to clopidogrel are prescribed in CYP2C19 IMs and PMs, may lower the risk for platelet reactivity and adverse cardiovascular events without increasing bleeding risk [50–56].

In the litigation case of Hawaii vs. Bristol Myers Squibb Co. and Sanofi-Aventis U.S. in 2021 it was ruled that the companies violated Hawaii's consumer protection laws by not disclosing that Plavix (trade name for clopidogrel) would be ineffective for as many as 30% of patients over a 12-year period from 1998 to 2010 [57].

The FDA includes a black box warning against the use of clopidogrel in CYP2C19 PMs and recommends the use of alternative antiplatelet therapy such as ticagrelor. The CPIC guideline recommends that CYP2C19 IMs avoid standard clopidogrel dose if possible and PMs receive alternative antiplatelet [58].

The CPIC guideline recommendations applies to ACS patients undergoing PCI while the DPWG as well as CPIC provides recommendations for acute stroke and transient ischemic attack patients (TIA): CYP2C19 PMs: avoid clopidogrel if possible.

The American College of Cardiology Foundation, American Heart Association, and the Society for Cardiovascular Angiography and Interventions (ACCF/AHA/ SCAI) PCI guideline recommends CYP2C19 genetic testing, with use of prasugrel or ticagrelor in CYP2C19 IMs and PMs, may be considered in patients undergoing PCI who are at high risk of poor outcome due to inadequate platelet inhibition [59].

The benefit of having a CYP2C19 metabolizer status available may be most beneficial for patients post myocardial infarction standard discharge with clopidogrel and may provide useful prognostic data about cardiovascular risk in patients undergoing PCI for ACS.

Statins are highly prescribed lipid-lowering therapies for the treatment and prevention of cardiovascular disease. Statins have been associated with myopathy which can range from mild to severe [60]. The gene *SLCO1B1* was identified in a genome wide association study to influence simvastatin induced myopathy [61]. The *SLCO1B1**5 (rs4149056, Val174Ala) loss of function allele was associated with reduced activity of the hepatic OATP1B1 (organic anion-transporting polypeptide) transporter and increased plasma concentrations of simvastatin. The effect of *SLCO1B1* rs4149056 drug clearance is statin specific with largest effect on simvastatin, followed by pitavastatin, atorvastatin, pravastatin, and rosuvastatin, and no effect observed for fluvastatin [62]. Other genes that are involved in statin clearance and metabolism include *CYP2C9* and fluvastatin and *ABCG2* and rosuvastatin.

The FDA includes *SLCO1B1* rs4149056 simvastatin in its list of Table of Pharmacogenetic associations and individuals carrying *SLCO1B1* rs4149056 loss of function alleles may have increased risk of myopathy [63].

CPIC guideline includes myopathy risk implications and prescribing recommendations or *SLCO1B1* decreased and poor function alleles for simvastatin, atorvastatin, lovastatin, pitavastatin, and pravastatin [64]. For fluvastatin the guideline provides an algorithm for both *CYP2C9* and *SLCO1B1* and for rasuvastatin the guideline provides an algorithm for both *ABCG2* and *SLCO1B1*.

There is growing evidence for utility of pharmacogenetic guided treatment algorithms however, clinical guidelines recommendations do not advise on routine genotyping for *CYP2C9, VKORC1* warfarin, *CYP2C19* clopidogrel, or *SLCO1B1* statins and call for prospective trials. With availability of direct-to-consumer genetic tests there is a potential to include genotype guided strategies in treatment selection.

Metoprolol is a racemate cardioselective β1-adrenoreceptor blocking agent used for hypertension, heart failure, angina pectoris, arrhythmias, and migraine prophylaxis (3. Metoprolol is predominantly metabolized by CYP2D6 to its inactive metabolites. Retrospective and prospective studies have shown that carriers of *CYP2D6* loss of function alleles may have a higher systemic exposure to metoprolol, which may indicate a greater reduction in heart rate and blood pressure. There is inconclusive data showing increased risk of bradycardia for CYP2D6 PMs [65]. The DPWG guideline for metoprolol in CYP2D6 PM and IM patients recommends a dose reduction (to 25% and 50% of the standard dose, respectively) where a gradual reduction in heart rate is required (for example, in chronic heart failure) or symptomatic bradycardia occurs and to consider other beta-blocker such as atenolol or bisoprolol which are not predominantly metabolized by CYP2D6 [3].

4.2   Neurology and Mental Health

Pharmacogenetics has demonstrated to be of great value for the treatment of neurological and mental health conditions. Its clinical implementation is taking off throughout the world; however, pharmacogenetic testing is still not part of standard protocols. The FDA drug monographs, as well as the CPIC and DPWG guidelines, provide therapeutic recommendations for the use of drugs for the treatment of neurological and mental health conditions. The integration of these recommendations into electronic health record (EHR) systems optimizes drug selection and ensures a more widespread use of pharmacogenetic information [66].

Gene–drug interactions integrated in neurology and mental health decision support systems

Selective serotonin reuptake inhibitors (SSRIs) are widely used for the treatment of depression and anxiety disorders. They are commonly prescribed as a first-line treatment due to their tolerability and safety profile. However, about half of the patients treated with a SSRI, will fail initial therapy [67]. The use of pharmacogenetic information has the potential to improve clinical outcomes.

SSRIs prevent the reuptake of serotonin and increase serotonergic activity. CYP2D6 and CYP2C19 play an important role in the metabolism of SSRIs. Paroxetine and fluvoxamine are extensively metabolized by CYP2D6, while CYP2C19 is responsible for the metabolism of citalopram, escitalopram, and sertraline [68]. The pharmacogenetic recommendations and indications provided by clinical guidelines for the use of SSRIs are discussed in this section.

Paroxetine is a highly potent and specific SSRI [69]. It has been shown that CYP2D6 ultrarapid metabolizers have significantly lower plasma concentrations of paroxetine compared to CYP2D6 normal metabolizers [70]. Both the CPIC [68] and DPWG guidelines [3] support the contraindication of paroxetine in patients that are CYP2D6 ultrarapid metabolizers since low plasma concentrations of paroxetine may increase the risk of therapeutic failure. Alternatively, CYP2D6 poor metabolizers have a higher plasma concentration of paroxetine. The CPIC guideline recommends a 25–50% dose reduction due to risk of adverse drug events, while the DPWG does not provide a therapeutic recommendation.

Fluvoxamine has a similar profile to paroxetine. CYP2D6 poor metabolizers may require dosage adjustments to avoid the risk of side effects, due to a higher plasma concentration of fluvoxamine. The most current version of the CPIC guideline recommends reducing fluvoxamine dose by 25–50% for patients that are CYP2D6 poor metabolizers. Unlike paroxetine, there is insufficient data to provide recommendations to CYP2D6 ultrarapid metabolizers [68]. The FDA Table of Pharmacogenetic Associations categorizes both fluvoxamine and paroxetine as pharmacogenetic associations for which data demonstrate a potential impact on pharmacokinetic properties only [63].

Citalopram and escitalopram. CYP2C19 plays an important role in the metabolism of citalopram and escitalopram. Citalopram is a racemic mixture, whereas escitalopram is the (S)-stereoisomer of citalopram. Compared to patients that are CYP2C19 normal metabolizers (NMs), CYP2C19 PMs have a significantly higher exposure to both citalopram and escitalopram, while CYP2C19 UMs have significantly lower plasma levels of these two drugs [71]. Due to their similarity, the CPIC has the same therapeutic recommendations for citalopram and escitalopram. The CPIC guideline recommends selecting an alternative drug for CYP2C19 UMs to reduce the probability of therapeutic failure, and a 50% dose reduction for CYP2C19 PMs to avoid adverse events [68]. The DPWG guideline recommends that both CYP2C19 IMs and PMs are given a lower dose of citalopram and escitalopram, while the use of escitalopram but not citalopram is contraindicated in CYP2C19 ultrarapid metabolizers [3]. The FDA states that CYP2C19 PMs have higher systemic concentrations of citalopram and an increased risk of adverse drug reactions such as QT prolongation [63].

Sertraline The effect of CYP2C19 genotype on the plasma concentration of sertraline is supported by evidence [72]. CYP2C19 PMs have significantly higher serum concentrations of this drug, although only a minor increase in the metabolism of sertraline was detected in CYP2C19 UMs. Based on this evidence, both the DPWG and CPIC guidelines recommend reducing sertraline dose for CYP2C19 PMs [3, 68].

Anti-epileptics. The use of pharmacogenetic information is a valuable tool in the treatment of epilepsy. Patients with the presence of specific genetic variants taking anti-epileptic drugs are highly susceptible to potentially severe cutaneous adverse reactions. The CPIC and DPWG guidelines have provide recommendations for the therapeutic use of phenytoin and fosphenytoin, as well as carbamazepine and oxcarbazepine. This section provides an overview of the pharmacogenetic recommendations that can be integrated in decision supports systems used by clinicians.

Phenytoin and fosphenytoin are commonly used for the treatment of status epilepticus. Fosphenytoin is a prodrug of phenytoin, and it produces the same therapeutic effect. Unlike phenytoin, fosphenytoin does not cause the same cardiac rhythm complications that phenytoin produces when given intravenously [73]. Phenytoin is primarily metabolized by CYP2C9, and polymorphisms on this gene can affect the plasma levels of this drug [74]. Additionally, human leukocyte antigen (HLA) genes have been associated to severe cutaneous adverse drug reactions. HLA-B is a highly polymorphic gene, and carriers of the HLA-B*15:02 have a high incidence of developing phenytoin-induced Stevens-Johnson syndrome (SJS) and toxic epidermal necrolysis (TEN). SJS and TEN affect 10% and 30% of the body surface area, TEN being the more severe of these two conditions, with mortality rates as high as 30% mostly due to sepsis [75].

The CPIC guideline has developed an algorithm with therapeutic recommendations based on the presence of HLA-B*15:02 and CYP2C9 phenotype [76]. In this algorithm, the presence of HLA-B*15:02 contraindicates the use of phenytoin and fosphenytoin in patients that have not used these drugs before. If a patient is not a carrier of HLA-B*15:02, the genotype of CYP2C9 is evaluated. Patients carrying two normal function CYP2C9 alleles (normal metabolizers) or one normal function allele plus one decreased function allele (intermediate metabolizers with an activity score of 1.5) do not require dosing adjustments based on pharmacogenetic information. Patients carrying a normal function allele and a no function allele or two decreased function alleles (intermediate metabolizers with an activity score of 1.0) may initiate phenytoin or fosphenytoin with the standard dose, but a dose reduction of 25% is recommended for the following doses. Finally, patients carrying two no function alleles or one no function allele and a decreased function allele can initiate with the standard dose of phenytoin or fosphenytoin, but a dose reduction of 50% is recommended for subsequent doses. In all cases, doses require to be adjusted based on drug monitoring and response.

The DPWG guidelines include similar recommendations based on a patient's CYP2C9 genotype; however, therapeutic annotations based on HLA-B*15*02 status are not available [3]. The FDA drug monographs of phenytoin and fosphenytoin highlight the relevance of pharmacogenetic information and recommend avoiding the use of these drugs in HLA-B*15:02 and CYP2C9*3 carriers.

Carbamazepine and oxcarbazepine are anti-convulsant drugs used to treat patients with epilepsy. Oxcarbazepine is an analog of carbamazepine, and although the former is better tolerated, both drugs have similar efficacy and adverse effects [3]. The CPIC guidelines provide therapeutic recommendations for the use of these drugs in epileptic patients based on the presence of HLA-B*15:02 and HLA-A*31:01.

The presence of *HLA-B*15:02* is strongly correlated with carbamazepine- and oxcarbazepine-induced SJS/TEN; however, the severity and incidence of these adverse events are lower in patients taking oxcarbazepine [77, 78]. The CPIC guideline recommends avoiding the use of carbamazepine and oxcarbazepine and patients that have not been treated with these drugs due to the high risk of SJS/TEN [79]. The FDA drug monographs for carbamazepine and oxcarbazepine contraindicate the use of these drugs in *HLA-B*15:02* carriers and recommend that patients with ancestry of populations where *HLA-B*15:02* incidence is higher (Hong Kong, Thailand, Malaysia, Philippines) are tested for *HLA-B*15:02* presence.

The *HLA-A*31:01* allele has been associated with carbamazepine-induced SJS/TEN and other cutaneous adverse drug reactions such as maculopapular exanthema (MPE) and drug reaction with eosinophilia and systemic symptoms (DRESS). DRESS is a potentially life-threatening condition characterized by eruptions of long durations, while MPE involves a diffuse cutaneous erythema. In populations where *HLA-B*15:02* is less common, the presence of *HLA-A*31:01* represents a higher risk for the development of severe carbamazepine-induced cutaneous adverse reactions. The CPIC guideline recommends avoiding the use of carbamazepine in drug-naïve patients due to the greater risk of developing SJS/TEN, MPE and DRESS [79]. The FDA drug monograph of carbamazepine recommends avoiding the use of this drug in patients known to be *HLA-A*31:01* positive, but unlike *HLA-B*15:02*, it does not recommend testing for the presence of this allele in high-risk populations.

Antipsychotics are mainly prescribed for the treatment of schizophrenia, although their use for in conditions such as major depressive disorder, anxiety, insomnia, and anxiety disorder has increased over the past years. There are two main classes of antipsychotics, typical or first-generation antipsychotics and atypical or second-generation antipsychotics. Typical antipsychotics are effective, but patients taking this type of drugs have a higher probability of developing motor side effects such as dystonia and tardive dyskinesia. The probability of developing motor side effects while using atypical antipsychotics is lower; however, they are associated with other adverse events such as weight gain and the development of metabolic syndrome [80].

First- and second-generation antipsychotics are largely metabolized by CYP enzymes such as CYP1A2, CYP2C9, and CYP3A4/5. However, it has been shown that CYP2D6 and CYP2C19 play a more important role in the variation of drug metabolism [81]. Although CPIC guidelines are not yet available for the optimization of antipsychotic therapy, the DPWG and FDA have included recommendations and dosage adjustments based on pharmacogenetic information.

Aripiprazole and brexpiprazole are second-generation antipsychotics approved by the FDA for the treatment of schizophrenia. Both act as dopamine D2 partial agonists. Brexpiprazole has a similar structure and efficacy to aripiprazole [82], and both drugs are metabolized by CYP2D6 to their inactive metabolites. It has been shown that compared to CYP2D6 NMs and PMs have a higher exposure to aripiprazole and that patients with *CYP2D6* polymorphisms accumulate higher levels of brexpiprazole [83, 84]. The DPWG guideline and the FDA monographs of aripiprazole and brexpiprazole recommend a dose reduction for patients that are known CYP2D6 PMs. For brexpiprazole, both the DPWG and the FDA drug monograph recommend using half the dose in CYP2D6 PMs. For aripiprazole, the DPWG guideline recommends using no more than 10 mg/day [3], while the FDA drug monograph establishes that half a dose should be used in this group of patients [85]. In practice, this recommendation is easier to follow considering that this drug is used for the treatment of several conditions other than schizophrenia with different recommended doses.

Iloperidone is a second-generation antipsychotic that acts as a dopamine D2 and serotonin 2A receptor antagonist. Iloperidone is metabolized via hydroxylation by CYP2D6, and it has been shown that CYP2D6 PMs and patients carrying decreased function alleles have higher plasma concentrations of the active metabolite compared to normal metabolizers [86, 87]. The DPWG guideline does not include iloperidone, but the FDA drug monograph recommends reducing iloperidone dose by half in CYP2D6 PMs due to their higher risk of developing QT prolongation [3, 87].

Clozapine is the first second-generation antipsychotic that was used for the treatment of schizophrenia. Unlike first-generation antipsychotics, it did not show a strong blockage of the dopamine D2 receptor, reducing the risk of motor side effects [88]. Clozapine is also metabolized by CYP2D6, and the FDA drug monograph states that CYP2D6 poor metabolizers have a higher risk of high plasma levels compared to normal metabolizers [89]. The FDA drug monograph also states that CYP2D6 metabolizers may need a lower dose of clozapine. The DPWG guideline acknowledges that CYP2D6 phenotype influences clozapine plasma levels; however, it does not recommend making dosing modifications. This decision is based on the conflicting evidence linking CYP2D6 phenotype and clozapine-induced side effects [3].

Risperidone is second-generation antipsychotic commonly prescribed for the treatment of schizophrenia, bipolar disorder and autism. Risperidone is metabolized by CYP2D6 to its metabolite 9-hydroxyrisperidone (9-OHR). Compared to CYP2D6 normal metabolizers, poor metabolizers have lower 9-OHR and higher risperidone plasma concentrations [90]. Since the activity of 9-OHR and risperidone is similar, the pharmacokinetic differences detected due to CYP2D6 gene variability do not translate into dose adjustments. The FDA drug monograph of risperidone states that therapeutic changes based on CYP2D6 genotype are not required [91]. The most recent version of the DPWG guideline argues that although the activity of 9-OHR and risperidone is the same, risperidone is able cross the blood–brain barrier more easily than 9-OHR [3]. Therefore, compared to CYP2D6 NMs, PMs have a higher brain concentration of the active moiety, while ultra-rapid metabolizers have a lower one. This is supported by a study that found that, compared to CYP2D6 NMs, treatment failure was higher in poor and ultrarapid metabolizers treated with risperidone [92]. The DPWG guideline recommends choosing an alternative treatment for CYP2D6 UMs and a dose reduction for PMs [3].

Algorithms that integrate pharmacogenetics for mental health treatment.

Pharmacogenetic testing allows clinicians to enhance the predictive value of clinical algorithms used to treat neurological and mental health conditions. However, few clinical algorithms have integrated this information as part of their input. Shelton et al. [93] analyzed the ability of CYP2C19, CYP2D6 and CYP3A4 to predict citalopram and escitalopram levels in patients treated for major depressive disorder as individual genes or in combination. A weighted algorithm that considered all three genotypes was able to better predict the variability in citalopram and escitalopram blood concentrations, compared to a single-gene approach [93].

This algorithm included both pharmacokinetic and pharmacodynamic gene-drug interactions to predict the outcomes of patients treated for major depressive disorder. The algorithm was clinically validated through a secondary analysis of the Genomics Used to Improve Depression Decisions (GUIDED) trial. Compared to CPIC guidelines that provide recommendations based on CYP2D6 and CYP2C19 genotypes, the combinatorial algorithm was able to better predict clinical outcomes [94].

Another approach that has been explored is the use of machine learning-based algorithms that integrate pharmacogenetic data. For instance, Athreya et al. [95] validated an algorithm that used genome-wide association biomarkers associated to SSRI response. The SNPs included in the algorithm were in or near the *TSPAN5*, *ERICH3*, *DEFB1* and *AHR*. The machine learning model was trained using depression scores at baseline and after 8 weeks of treatment and was able to separate patients in different severity-based clusters.

Although pharmacogenetic information plays an important role in treatment prediction, it is only a piece of the puzzle. The integration of other relevant clinical factors will improve the performance of these algorithms and bring precision prescribing into routine clinical care.

4.3 Oncology

Fluoropyrimidines are antimetabolite drugs widely used to treat cancer, including colorectal and breast cancer and cancers of the aerodigestive tract.

5-fluorouracil (5-FU) is commonly given intravenously, where more than 80% of it is metabolized in the liver [96]. Capecitabine is an oral prodrug of 5-FU that passes unaltered through the gut wall and is converted into 5'dFCR then 5'-deoxy-5-fluorouridine (5'dFUR) in the liver by carboxylesterase and cytidine deaminase, respectively. 5'dFUR is then converted to 5-FU via thymidine phosphorylase or uridine phosphorylase [97]. Tegafur is another prodrug of 5-FU that CYP2A6 converts to an unstable intermediate, 5-hydroxytegafur, which spontaneously breaks down to form 5-FU [98].

There are several routes for metabolism of 5-FU, some of which lead to activation and pharmacodynamic actions of the drug. The rate-limiting step of 5-FU catabolism is DihydroPyrimidine Dehydrogenase (DPYD) conversion of

5-FU to dihydrofluorouracil (DHFU). DHFU is then converted to fluoro-beta-ureidopropionate (FUPA) and subsequently to Fluoro-Beta-Alanine (FBAL) by dihydropyrimidinease (DPYS) and beta-ureidopropionase (UPB1), respectively [98]. Deficiency in enzymes in this pathway can result in severe and even fatal 5-FU toxicity. Several variants in *DPYD* have been associated with toxicity including (see the *DPYD* VIP and curated annotations for more details). Variants in *DPYS* have also been shown to influence 5-FU toxicity [99, 100]. A rare variant *DPYS:833G>A* (*DPYS:Gly278Asp*) in exon 5 was shown to be the determining variant of severe toxicity in a Dutch patient receiving 5-FU [101]. Variants *DPYS:1635delC* and *DPYS:Leu7Val* were shown in vitro to have reduced activity [102]. To modulate the activity of fluoropyrimidines, inhibitors of DPYD such as uracil and eniluracil can be coadministered. This slows the degradation of 5-FU and can improve response rate.

The main mechanism of 5-FU activation is conversion to fluorodeoxyuridine monophosphate (FdUMP) which inhibits the enzyme thymidylate synthase (TYMS), an important part of the folate-homocysteine cycle and purine and pyrimidine synthesis The conversion of 5-FU to FdUMP can occur via thymidylate phosphorylase (TYMP) to fluorodeoxyuridine (FUDR) and then by the action of thymidine kinase to FdUMP or indirectly via fluorouridine monophosphate (FUMP) or fluroridine (FUR) to fluorouridine diphosphate (FUDP) and then ribonucleotide reductase action to FdUDP and FdUMP. FUDP and FdUDP can also be converted to FUTP and FdUTP and incorporated into RNA and DNA, respectively, contributing to fluoropyrimidines' pharmacodynamic actions [98].

An essential consideration in the use of 5-FU and related drugs is the development of drug resistance by the tumor. Some mechanisms of resistance involve expression changes in pharmacodynamic gene candidates (*TYMS* and *P53*). Drug resistance can also involve changes in drug transport. There is conflicting data about the transporters involved in the pharmacokinetics of 5-FU. *SLC29A1* expression was not associated with survival in one study of pancreatic tumors but resistance/sensitivity was associated with its expression in another study of pancreatic tumor cell lines [103, 104]. Transport of 5-FU has been reported in an in vitro expression system of SLC22A7 [105]. Several transporters have been implicated in 5-FU resistance, including ABCG2, ABCC3, ABCC4 and ABCC5 [98, 106].

4.4   Pain

Clinical algorithms used in pharmacologic pain treatment typically focus on tiering drug class options based on risk-benefit analysis, but rarely include patient specific considerations such as pharmacogenetics that may impact appropriate drug choice.

Most pain treatment algorithms recommend non-opioids except in severe acute pain that cannot be managed by other means [107–109]. Opioids are then used only when non-opioid therapy fails. Depending on origin and severity, chronic pain may be treated with a variety of drug classes, including acetaminophen (paracetamol), NSAIDs, antidepressants, anticonvulsants, gabapentinoids, and opioids.

Within each of these broad categories, there are several individual drugs that have pharmacogenetic associations.

It is important to note that databases of pharmacogenetic associations may include gene-drug interactions that have high level evidence of pharmacokinetic differences between phenotypes that might not necessarily translate to clinically actionable dose changes. This may be due to compensatory metabolic pathways, or other unknown mechanisms.

The drugs listed in the following section have FDA or CPIC clinical recommendations for pharmacogenetic associations.

NSAIDs are commonly used in both acute and chronic pain. They are considered effective, inexpensive, and non-addictive. However, they carry the risk of serious adverse effects such as gastrointestinal bleeds, renal toxicity, and cardiovascular events. CYP2C9 poor and intermediate metabolizers are at higher risk of adverse effects due to reduced clearance and consequent higher plasma levels of the drug. In general, the longer the half-life of the drug, the more pronounced this effect will be. The 2020 CPIC Guideline for CYP2C9 and Nonsteroidal Anti-inflammatory Drugs [22] lists therapeutic recommendations for celecoxib, flurbiprofen, ibuprofen, lornoxicam, meloxicam, and piroxicam. Generally, a lower starting dose or alternate drug is recommended for poor metabolizers, and a lower starting dose or increased monitoring is recommended for intermediate metabolizers.

Tricyclic antidepressants (TCAs) are frequently used as a first-line treatment in chronic neuropathic pain and fibromyalgia, as well as treating comorbid depression and pain. Commonly used TCAs include amitriptyline, desipramine, imipramine, and nortriptyline. All of these are influenced by CYP2D6 phenotype, with poor and intermediate metabolizers at higher risk of adverse events and ultra-rapid metabolizers at risk of reduced response [110]. Additionally, amitriptyline and imipramine are also influenced by CYP2C19 phenotype, again with poor and intermediate metabolizers at higher risk of adverse events and ultra-rapid metabolizers at risk of reduced response. Generally, lower starting doses or an alternate drug is recommended for poor metabolizers, and an alternate drug should be considered for ultra-rapid metabolizers. Additional caution should be used in patients who are poor, intermediate, or ultra-rapid metabolizers for both CYP2D6 and CYP2C19, and are considering treatment with amitriptyline or imipramine. It should be noted that TCAs have a large dosing range depending on the condition treated, and specific dosing recommendations due to pharmacogenetics may be based on evidence taken from studies observing patient populations with a specific condition and dose range.

Serotonin-norepinephrine reuptake inhibitors. Venlafaxine is a commonly used antidepressant used in chronic neuropathic pain and comorbid depression and pain. CYP2D6 poor metabolizers have reduced metabolism to less active compounds and are at higher risk of adverse effects [68]. The FDA Table of pharmacogenetic associations recommends considering dose reductions in patients who are poor metabolizers for CYP2D6 [63].

Opioids. While current prescribing guidelines recommend opioids only in cases where pain cannot be managed with other treatments, they remain commonly used in all areas of pain management. The 2020 Clinical Pharmacogenetics Implementation Consortium Guideline for CYP2D6, OPRM1, and COMT Genotypes and Select Opioid Therapy [12] notes:

"Excluding morphine, tapentadol, and levorphanol, which are largely glucuronidated, multiple CYP pathways, predominantly CYP3A, CYP2B6, and CYP2D6, metabolize opioid agonists. CYP3A is a major inactivating enzyme for some, such as N-dealkylation of synthetic phenylpiperidines (e.g., fentanyl and alfentanil) and semisynthetic morphinan (e.g., hydrocodone and oxycodone) opioids. The opioids codeine and tramadol are O-demethylated by CYP2D6 to the more active metabolites morphine and O-desmethyltramadol, respectively. CYP2D6 converts hydrocodone and oxycodone into the active metabolites hydromorphone and oxymorphone, respectively, but both hydrocodone and oxycodone have clinical opioid activity. The main biotransformation of methadone is N-demethylation and this is predominantly by CYP2B6. Active metabolites can mediate none, little, or as much as all of the pharmacologic effect of an administered opioid, depending on metabolite concentration, relative efficacy, and potency compared with that of the parent drug. Other genes that have been studied for their association with opioid clinical effect or adverse events include OPRM1 and COMT".

While multiple genes have been studied for their association with opioid effectiveness or safety, this section focuses on drugs mediated by CYP2D6 pathways. Codeine, tramadol, hydrocodone, and to a lesser extent oxycodone, are either prodrugs (codeine), or have more potent active metabolites after conversion of the parent drug via CYP2D6 pathways. It is important to note that unlike in the drugs listed in previous sections, it is ultra-rapid metabolizers who are at risk of toxicity and adverse events, and poor metabolizers who are at risk of reduced response.

Codeine and tramadol. FDA labeling for codeine and tramadol include warnings that CYP2D6 ultra-rapid metabolizers are at risk of respiratory depression or death due to higher active metabolite concentrations. CPIC 2020 recommendations for codeine and tramadol include avoiding use in CYP2D6 ultra-rapid metabolizers due to risk of severe toxicity and using alternate agents in CYP2D6 poor metabolizers due to lack of effect [12].

Hydrocodone. While hydrocodone is also converted to active metabolites via CYP2D6 pathways, CPIC 2020 guidelines note that there is insufficient evidence to guide clinical practice at this time, and only recommends considering alternate agents in CYP2D6 poor or intermediate metabolizers if no response is observed with standard label dosing [12].

Oxycodone is partially metabolized to a more potent metabolite by CYP2D6. However, the association between CYP2D6 phenotype and oxycodone safety or effectiveness has not been consistently demonstrated in clinical trials [12]. CPIC 2020 guidelines do not make any clinical recommendations for oxycodone use based on CYP2D6 metabolizer status.

Anticonvulsants. Carbamazepine, oxcarbazepine, and lamotrigine are recommended treatments for trigeminal neuralgia [111]. All three of these drugs are associated with cutaneous reactions, which can be serious and potentially fatal. *HLA-B*1502* positive status is associated with increased risk of cutaneous reactions in carbamazepine, oxcarbazepine, and lamotrigine [112]. *HLA-A*3101* positive status is associated with increased risk in carbamazepine and oxcarbazepine, and *HLA-B*5801* positive status is associated with increased risk in lamotrigine only.

4.5   Rheumatology

Allopurinol is the preferred urate-lowering therapy for treating chronic gout, with multiple guidelines citing its efficacy, tolerability, safety, and low cost. However, its use is associated with potentially fatal severe cutaneous adverse drug reactions, including SJS and TENS. The presence of *HLA-B*5801* is associated with a significantly increased risk of allopurinol induced severe cutaneous reactions and is contraindicated in those who are positive for *HLA-B*5801* [113]. The American College of Rheumatology recommends testing for the *HLA-B*5801* allele in patients of Southeast Asian descent (e.g., Han Chinese, Korean, Thai) or African American descent, due to the higher prevalence of this allele in these populations.

4.6   Anti Virals and Aminoglycosides

Abacavir. Certain medications can induce inappropriate hypersensitivity/immune response ranging from milder forms, such as urticarial and MPE, to more severe clinical presentations such as acute generalized exanthematous pustulosis (AGEP), SJS, TEN, and Drug Rash with Eosinophilia and Systemic Symptoms (DRESS). All these conditions are classified as Ssevere Cutaneous Adverse drug Reactions (SCAR). The immune mechanism of SCAR is classified as type-IV hypersensitivity reaction characterized by the activation of lymphocytes such as CD4+ and CD8+ T cells. Type-IV hypersensitivity is also called delayed-type hypersensitivity and often develops a few days or weeks after drug exposure [114].

Abacavir is a nucleoside reverse-transcriptase inhibitor with activity against the human immunodeficiency virus (HIV), available for once-daily use in combination with other antiretroviral agents, that has shown efficacy, few drug interactions, and a favourable long-term toxicity profile. The most significant adverse effect of abacavir that limits its use in therapy and mandates a high degree of clinical vigilance is an immunologically mediated hypersensitivity reaction affecting 5 to 8% of patients during the first six weeks of treatment [115]. Since 2002, an association between a diagnosis of hypersensitivity reaction to abacavir and carriage of the major histocompatibility complex class I allele *HLA-B*5701* was reported independently by two research groups and was subsequently corroborated by several independent studies.

Excerpt from the CPIC abacavir dosing guidelines [114]:

> We agree with others* that *HLA-B*57:01* screening should be performed in all abacavir-naive individuals before initiation of abacavir-containing therapy; this is consistent with the recommendations of the FDA, the US Department of Health and Human Services, and the European Medicines Agency. In abacavir-naive individuals who are *HLA-B*57:01*-positive, abacavir is not recommended and should be considered only under exceptional circumstances when the potential benefit, based on resistance patterns and treatment history, outweighs the risk.

Nowadays, the correlation between hypersensibility and *HLA-B*5701*, in fact, several global regulatory agencies (FDA, EMA, Swiss Agency of Therapeutic Products, Health Canada) state that *HLA-B*5701* testing prior to prescribing abacavir is required.

Aminoglycosides. The death of hair cells causes aminoglycoside-induced hearing loss (AIHL) in the inner ear following exposure to aminoglycosides. Aminoglycosides cross the blood-labyrinth barrier in the inner ear and enter the endolymph. They then selectively enter sensory hair cells through mechanoelectrical transduction (MET) channels in a calcium-dependent manner. The exact composition of the MET channel has not been ascertained but is known to contain the TMC1 protein le. This pathway displays the MET channel components

Tip-link protein chains consisting of cadherin 23 and protocadherin 15 (PCDH15) regulate MET channel gating [116]. Gentamicin uptake and subsequent cell death was found to be prevented in hair cells derived from *CDH23* knockout mice [117].

The Clinical Pharmacogenetics Implementation Consortium (CPIC) guidelines recognized the risk of developing aminoglycoside-induced hearing loss (AIHL) when specific *MT-RNR1* variants are present. CPIC 2021 guideline provides recommendations for both adult and pediatric patients. Excerpts from the guideline [118]:

– "The critical pharmacogenetics recommendation for a person with an *MT-RNR1* variant which predisposes to AIHL is that aminoglycoside antibiotics are relatively contraindicated, meaning that aminoglycosides should be avoided unless the increased risk of hearing loss is outweighed by the severity of infection and lack of safe or effective alternative therapies."
– "There is insufficient evidence to suggest that the adverse drug reaction may be more profound with some members of the aminoglycoside class than others. As such, this guidance covers all aminoglycoside antibiotics irrespective of class. We provide a strong recommendation that carriers of *MT-RNR1* variants that predispose to AIHL should avoid aminoglycosides unless the risk of infection

outweighs the increased risk of permanent hearing loss without safe or effective alternative therapies."

– "If no effective alternative to an aminoglycoside is thought to be available, we advise use for the shortest possible time, consultation with an infectious disease expert for alternative approaches, therapeutic drug monitoring and frequent assessment for hearing loss, both during and after therapy, in consultation with an audiovestibular physician."

– "An individual with no detectable MT-RNR1 variant or carrying *MT-RNR1* variants not considered to be predisposing to AIHL (normal risk), including the *m.827A > G* variant, should still be considered at risk of AIHL."

5   Multi-Factor Considerations

While pharmacogenetic considerations can and should guide drug selection and clinical treatment plans, they must be considered in the context of the patient. For example, a drug that may be suitable from a pharmacogenetic standpoint may be inappropriate for a patient given their renal or hepatic status, or interactions with current medications.

When considering multiple factors in selecting an appropriate drug, the type of pharmacogenetic impact should be assessed—the given phenotype may affect pharmacokinetics (metabolism) or pharmacodynamics, or increase risk of an adverse event in a non-linear, non-dose-dependent way.

When pharmacokinetics is influenced by a genetic variant, it is important to look at other patient specific factors that influence pharmacokinetics and the specific drug involved. For example, amitriptyline clearance is affected by both genetics and hepatic function [110]. A CYP2D6 poor metabolizer with hepatic impairment has two factors that significantly affect drug clearance. The clinical decision should consider both of these. If only one of these factors were present, a clinician may decide to use a lower dose to account for lowered metabolism. Knowing that two factors are present, it may be more appropriate to select a different drug entirely, given that two clearance pathways are reduced.

Another way to incorporate specific patient factors is to consider multiple risk factors for a given adverse event. For warfarin, *VKORC1 −1639G>A* is associated with lower dose requirements [119]—the net effect is that a standard dose of warfarin will be more likely to cause over-anticoagulation (i.e. bleed risk) and lower doses should be used with patients carrying this allele. While *VKORC1* itself does not affect active drug clearance, any additional bleeding risk (e.g. *CYP2C9 *2* or *3* status, amiodarone use) needs to be taken into account when considering warfarin dose.

6   Conclusion

- Pharmacogenetic algorithms allow clinicians to integrate gene-drug interactions into existing clinical decision-making tools.
- Pharmacogenetic algorithms for warfarin prescribing are among the most well-validated, with a high number of clinical trials used in their development.
- Complex conditions such as mental health would benefit from well-validated pharmacogenetic algorithms, but more prospective trials are needed.
- Genetic variations in enzymes, transporters or receptors that participate in these mechanisms introduce differences in drug metabolism and action. However, these differences are not always translated into the clinical setting.
- Pharmacogenetic considerations can and should guide drug selection and clinical treatment plans, but they must be considered in the context of the patient as a whole.

References

1. Relling MV, Klein TE, Gammal RS, Whirl-Carrillo M, Hoffman JM, Caudle KE. The clinical pharmacogenetics implementation consortium: 10 years later. Clin Pharmacol Ther. 2020;107(1):171–5. https://doi.org/10.1002/cpt.1651.
2. CPIC the clinical pharmacogenetics implementation consortium https://cpicpgx.org/. Accessed Oct 2022.
3. DPWG: Dutch Pharmacogenetics Working Group https://www.pharmgkb.org/page/dpwg. Accessed Oct 2022.
4. Swen JJ, Wilting I, de Goede AL, Grandia L, Mulder H, Touw DJ, et al. Pharmacogenetics: from bench to byte. Clin Pharmacol Ther. 2008;83(5):781–7. https://doi.org/10.1038/sj.clpt. 6100507.
5. Swen JJ, Nijenhuis M, de Boer A, Grandia L, Maitland-van der Zee AH, Mulder H et al. Pharmacogenetics: from bench to byte--an update of guidelines. Clin Pharmacol Ther. 2011;89(5):662–673. https://doi.org/10.1038/clpt.2011.34.
6. Picard N, Boyer JC, Etienne-Grimaldi MC, Barin-Le Guellec C, Thomas F, Loriot MA, et al. Pharmacogenetics-based personalized therapy: levels of evidence and recommendations from the French Network of Pharmacogenetics (RNPGx). Therapie. 2017;72(2):185–92. https://doi.org/10.1016/j.therap.2016.09.014.
7. Tornio A, Backman JT. Cytochrome P450 in pharmacogenetics: an update. Adv Pharmacol. 2018;83:3–32. https://doi.org/10.1016/bs.apha.2018.04.007.
8. Zanger UM, Schwab M. Cytochrome P450 enzymes in drug metabolism: regulation of gene expression, enzyme activities, and impact of genetic variation. Pharmacol Ther. 2013;138(1):103–41. https://doi.org/10.1016/j.pharmthera.2012.12.007.
9. Samer CF, Daali Y, Wagner M, Hopfgartner G, Eap CB, Rebsamen MC, et al. Genetic polymorphisms and drug interactions modulating CYP2D6 and CYP3A activities have a major effect on oxycodone analgesic efficacy and safety. Br J Pharmacol. 2010;160(4):919–30. https://doi.org/10.1111/j.1476-5381.2010.00709.x.
10. Samer CF, Daali Y, Wagner M, Hopfgartner G, Eap CB, Rebsamen MC, et al. The effects of CYP2D6 and CYP3A activities on the pharmacokinetics of immediate release oxycodone. Br J Pharmacol. 2010;160(4):907–18. https://doi.org/10.1111/j.1476-5381.2010.00673.x.

11. Deodhar M, Turgeon J, Michaud V. Contribution of CYP2D6 functional activity to oxy-codone efficacy in pain management: genetic polymorphisms, phenoconversion, and tissue-selective metabolism. Pharmaceutics. 2021;13(9):1466. https://doi.org/10.3390/pharmaceu tics13091466.

12. Crews KR, Monte AA, Huddart R, Caudle KE, Kharasch ED, Gaedigk A, et al. Clinical pharmacogenetics implementation consortium guideline for CYP2D6, OPRM1, and COMT genotypes and select opioid therapy. Clin Pharmacol Ther. 2021;110(4):888–96. https://doi. org/10.1002/cpt.214.

13. Cajanus K, Neuvonen M, Koskela O, Kaunisto MA, Neuvonen PJ, Niemi M, et al. Analgesic plasma concentrations of oxycodone after surgery for breast cancer-which factors matter? Clin Pharmacol Ther. 2018;103(4):653–62. https://doi.org/10.1002/cpt.771.

14. Andreassen TN, Eftedal I, Klepstad P, Davies A, Bjordal K, Lundstrom S, et al. Do CYP2D6 genotypes reflect oxycodone requirements for cancer patients treated for cancer pain? A cross-sectional multicentre study. Eur J Clin Pharmacol. 2012;68(1):55–64. https://doi.org/ 10.1007/s00228-011-1093-5.

15. Zwisler ST, Enggaard TP, Mikkelsen S, Brosen K, Sindrup SH. Impact of the CYP2D6 genotype on post-operative intravenous oxycodone analgesia. Acta Anaesthesiol Scand. 2010;54(2):232–40. https://doi.org/10.1111/j.1399-6576.2009.02104.x.

16. Swaisland HC, Cantarini MV, Fuhr R, Holt A. Exploring the relationship between expres-sion of cytochrome P450 enzymes and gefitinib pharmacokinetics. Clin Pharmacokinet. 2006;45(6):633–44. https://doi.org/10.2165/00003088-200645060-00006.

17. Hirose T, Fujita K, Kusumoto S, Oki Y, Murata Y, Sugiyama T, et al. Association of pharma-cokinetics and pharmacogenomics with safety and efficacy of gefitinib in patients with EGFR mutation positive advanced non-small cell lung cancer. Lung Cancer. 2016;93:69–76. https:// doi.org/10.1016/j.lungcan.2016.01.005.

18. Kobayashi H, Sato K, Niioka T, Miura H, Ito H, Miura M. Relationship among gefitinib exposure, polymorphisms of its metabolizing enzymes and transporters, and side effects in Japanese patients with non-small-cell lung cancer. Clin Lung Cancer. 2015;16(4):274–81. https://doi.org/10.1016/j.cllc.2014.12.004.

19. Takimoto T, Kijima T, Otani Y, Nonen S, Namba Y, Mori M, et al. Polymorphisms of CYP2D6 gene and gefitinib-induced hepatotoxicity. Clin Lung Cancer. 2013;14(5):502–7. https://doi.org/10.1016/j.cllc.2013.03.003.

20. Gaedigk A, Sangkuhl K, Whirl-Carrillo M, Twist PG, Klein TE, Miller NA, et al. The evo-lution of pharmVar. Clin Pharmacol Ther. 2019;105(1):29–32. https://doi.org/10.1002/cpt. 1275.

21. Macias Y, Gomez Tabales J, Garcia-Martin E, Agundez JAG. An update on the pharmacoge-nomics of NSAID metabolism and the risk of gastrointestinal bleeding. Expert Opin Drug Metab Toxicol. 2020;16(4):319–32. https://doi.org/10.1080/17425255.2020.1744563.

22. Theken KN, Lee CR, Gong L, Caudle KE, Formea CM, Gaedigk A, et al. Clinical pharma-cogenetics implementation consortium guideline (CPIC) for CYP2C9 and nonsteroidal anti-inflammatory drugs. Clin Pharmacol Ther. 2020;108(2):191–200. https://doi.org/10.1002/cpt. 1830.

23. Rodrigues AD. Impact of CYP2C9 genotype on pharmacokinetics: are all cyclooxygenase inhibitors the same? Drug Metab Dispos. 2005;33(11):1567–75. https://doi.org/10.1124/dmd. 105.006452.

24. Aithal GP, Day CP, Leathart JB, Daly AK. Relationship of polymorphism in CYP2C9 to genetic susceptibility to diclofenac-induced hepatitis. Pharmacogenetics. 2000;10(6):511–8. https://doi.org/10.1097/00008571-200008000-00004.

25. Yin OQ, Tomlinson B, Chow MS. CYP2C9, but not CYP2C19, polymorphisms affect the pharmacokinetics and pharmacodynamics of glyburide in Chinese subjects. Clin Pharmacol Ther. 2005;78(4):370–7. https://doi.org/10.1016/j.clpt.2005.06.006.

26. Vormfelde SV, Brockmoller J, Bauer S, Herchenhein P, Kuon J, Meineke I, et al. Relative impact of genotype and enzyme induction on the metabolic capacity of CYP2C9 in healthy volunteers. Clin Pharmacol Ther. 2009;86(1):54–61. https://doi.org/10.1038/clpt.2009.40.

27. Chen K, Wang R, Wen SY, Li J, Wang SQ. Relationship of P450 2C9 genetic polymorphisms in Chinese and the pharmacokinetics of tolbutamide. J Clin Pharm Ther. 2005;30(3):241–9. https://doi.org/10.1111/j.1365-2710.2005.00639.x.

28. Suzuki K, Yanagawa T, Shibasaki T, Kaniwa N, Hasegawa R, Tohkin M. Effect of CYP2C9 genetic polymorphisms on the efficacy and pharmacokinetics of glimepiride in subjects with type 2 diabetes. Diab Res Clin Pract. 2006;72(2):148–54. https://doi.org/10.1016/j.diabres. 2005.09.019.

29. Zeng W, Guo Y, Chen P, Liu Z, Chen D, Han C. CYP2C93 variant is associated with antidiabetes efficacy of gliclazide in Chinese type 2 diabetes patients. J Diab Investig. 2016;7(5):764–8. https://doi.org/10.1111/jdi.12486.

30. Holstein A, Plaschke A, Ptak M, Egberts EH, El-Din J, Brockmoller J, et al. Association between CYP2C9 slow metabolizer genotypes and severe hypoglycaemia on medication with sulphonylurea hypoglycaemic agents. Br J Clin Pharmacol. 2005;60(1):103–6. https://doi. org/10.1111/j.1365-2125.2005.02379.x.

31. Gokalp O, Gunes A, Cam H, Cure E, Aydin O, Tamer MN, et al. Mild hypoglycaemic attacks induced by sulphonylureas related to CYP2C9, CYP2C19 and CYP2C8 polymorphisms in routine clinical setting. Eur J Clin Pharmacol. 2011;67(12):1223–9. https://doi.org/10.1007/ s00228-011-1078-4.

32. Ragia G, Petridis I, Tavridou A, Christakidis D, Manolopoulos VG. Presence of CYP2C9*3 allele increases risk for hypoglycemia in Type 2 diabetic patients treated with sulfonylureas. Pharmacogenomics. 2009;10(11):1781–7. https://doi.org/10.2217/pgs.09.96.

33. Surendiran A, Pradhan SC, Agrawal A, Subrahmanyam DK, Rajan S, Anichavezhi D, et al. Influence of CYP2C9 gene polymorphisms on response to glibenclamide in type 2 diabetes mellitus patients. Eur J Clin Pharmacol. 2011;67(8):797–801. https://doi.org/10.1007/ s00228-011-1013-8.

34. Budnitz DS, Lovegrove MC, Shehab N, Richards CL. Emergency hospitalizations for adverse drug events in older Americans. N Engl J Med. 2011;365(21):2002–12. https://doi.org/10. 1056/NEJMsa1103053.

35. Wadelius M, Chen LY, Lindh JD, Eriksson N, Ghori MJ, Bumpstead S, et al. The largest prospective warfarin-treated cohort supports genetic forecasting. Blood. 2009;113(4):784– 92. https://doi.org/10.1182/blood-2008-04-149070.

36. Hylek EM, Evans-Molina C, Shea C, Henault LE, Regan S. Major hemorrhage and tolerability of warfarin in the first year of therapy among elderly patients with atrial fibrillation. Circulation. 2007;115(21):2689–96. https://doi.org/10.1161/CIRCULATIONAHA.106. 653048.

37. Dang MT, Hambleton J, Kayser SR. The influence of ethnicity on warfarin dosage requirement. Ann Pharmacother. 2005;39(6):1008–12. https://doi.org/10.1345/aph.1E566.

38. Gage BF, Eby C, Johnson JA, Deych E, Rieder MJ, Ridker PM, et al. Use of pharmacogenetic and clinical factors to predict the therapeutic dose of warfarin. Clin Pharmacol Ther. 2008;84(3):326–31. https://doi.org/10.1038/clpt.2008.10.

39. Aithal GP, Day CP, Kesteven PJ, Daly AK. Association of polymorphisms in the cytochrome P450 CYP2C9 with warfarin dose requirement and risk of bleeding complications. Lancet. 1999;353(9154):717–9. https://doi.org/10.1016/S0140-6736(98)04474-2.

40. Rieder MJ, Reiner AP, Gage BF, Nickerson DA, Eby CS, McLeod HL, et al. Effect of VKORC1 haplotypes on transcriptional regulation and warfarin dose. N Engl J Med. 2005;352(22):2285–93. https://doi.org/10.1056/NEJMoa044503.

41. Aquilante CL, Langaee TY, Lopez LM, Yarandi HN, Tromberg JS, Mohuczy D, et al. Influence of coagulation factor, vitamin K epoxide reductase complex subunit 1, and cytochrome P450 2C9 gene polymorphisms on warfarin dose requirements. Clin Pharmacol Ther. 2006;79(4):291–302. https://doi.org/10.1016/j.clpt.2005.11.011.

42. Cooper GM, Johnson JA, Langaee TY, Feng H, Stanaway IB, Schwarz UI, et al. A genome-wide scan for common genetic variants with a large influence on warfarin maintenance dose. Blood. 2008;112(4):1022–7. https://doi.org/10.1182/blood-2008-01-134247.

43. Squibb B-M. Coumadin (warfarin sodium) package insert Princeton NJ. http://packagein serts.bms.com/pi/pi_coumadin.pdf. (2019).
44. Lenzini P, Wadelius M, Kimmel S, Anderson JL, Jorgensen AL, Pirmohamed M, et al. Integration of genetic, clinical, and INR data to refine warfarin dosing. Clin Pharmacol Ther. 2010;87(5):572–8. https://doi.org/10.1038/clpt.2010.13.
45. The International Warfarin Pharmacogenetics Consortium. Estimation of the warfarin dose with clinical and pharmacogenetic data. N Engl J Med. 2009;360(8):753–64. https://doi.org/10.1056/NEJMoa0809329.
46. Anderson JL, Horne BD, Stevens SM, Woller SC, Samueson KM, Mansfield JW, et al. A randomized and clinical effectiveness trial comparing two pharmacogenetic algorithms and standard care for individualizing warfarin dosing (CoumaGen-II). Circulation. 2012;125(16):1997–2005. https://doi.org/10.1161/CIRCULATIONAHA.111.070920.
47. Gage BF, Bass AR, Lin H, Woller SC, Stevens SM, Al-Hammadi N, et al. Effect of genotype-guided warfarin dosing on clinical events and anticoagulation control among patients undergoing hip or knee arthroplasty: the GIFT randomized clinical trial. JAMA. 2017;318(12):1115–24. https://doi.org/10.1001/jama.2017.11469.
48. Johnson JA, Caudle KE, Gong L, Whirl-Carrillo M, Stein CM, Scott SA, et al. Clinical pharmacogenetics implementation consortium (CPIC) guideline for pharmacogenetics-guided warfarin dosing: 2017 update. Clin Pharmacol Ther. 2017;102(3):397–404. https://doi.org/10.1002/cpt.668.
49. Mega JL, Close SL, Wiviott SD, Shen L, Hockett RD, Brandt JT, et al. Cytochrome p-450 polymorphisms and response to clopidogrel. N Engl J Med. 2009;360(4):354–62. https://doi.org/10.1056/NEJMoa0809171.
50. Collet JP, Hulot JS, Anzaha G, Pena A, Chastre T, Caron C, et al. High doses of clopidogrel to overcome genetic resistance: the randomized crossover CLOVIS-2 (clopidogrel and response variability investigation study 2). JACC Cardiovasc Interv. 2011;4(4):392–402. https://doi.org/10.1016/j.jcin.2011.03.002.
51. Price MJ, Murray SS, Angiolillo DJ, Lillie E, Smith EN, Tisch RL, et al. Influence of genetic polymorphisms on the effect of high- and standard-dose clopidogrel after percutaneous coronary intervention: the GIFT (Genotype Information and Functional Testing) study. J Am Coll Cardiol. 2012;59(22):1928–1937. https://doi.org/10.1016/j.jacc.2011.11.068.
52. Sibbing D, Gebhard D, Koch W, Braun S, Stegherr J, Morath T, et al. Isolated and interactive impact of common CYP2C19 genetic variants on the antiplatelet effect of chronic clopidogrel therapy. J Thromb Haemost. 2010;8(8):1685–93. https://doi.org/10.1111/j.1538-7836.2010.03921.x.
53. Claassens DMF, Vos GJA, Bergmeijer TO, Hermanides RS, van 't Hof AWJ, van der Harst P, et al. A genotype-guided strategy for oral P2Y12 inhibitors in primary PCI. N Engl J Med. 2019;381(17):1621–1631. https://doi.org/10.1056/NEJMoa1907096.
54. Pereira NL, Avram R, So DY, Iturriaga E, Byrne J, Lennon RJ, et al. Rationale and design of the TAILOR-PCI digital study: transitioning a randomized controlled trial to a digital registry. Am Heart J. 2021;232:84–93. https://doi.org/10.1016/j.ahj.2020.10.069.
55. Tuteja S, Glick H, Matthai W, Nachamkin I, Nathan A, Monono K, et al. Prospective CYP2C19 genotyping to guide antiplatelet therapy following percutaneous coronary intervention: a pragmatic randomized clinical trial. Circ Genom Precis Med. 2020;13(1): e002640. https://doi.org/10.1161/CIRCGEN.119.002640.
56. Pereira NL, Farkouh ME, So D, Lennon R, Geller N, Mathew V, et al. Effect of genotype-guided oral P2Y12 inhibitor selection vs conventional clopidogrel therapy on ischemic outcomes after percutaneous coronary intervention: the TAILOR-PCI randomized clinical trial. JAMA. 2020;324(8):761–71. https://doi.org/10.1001/jama.2020.12443.
57. Bellon T, Raymond N. Bristol-Myers, Sanofi Must Pay $834 Million Over Plavix: Bloomberg; https://www.reuters.com/article/us-bristol-myers-sanofi-plavix-idUSKBN2A F1YI (2021).
58. Scott SA, Sangkuhl K, Stein CM, Hulot JS, Mega JL, Roden DM, et al. Clinical pharmacogenetics implementation consortium guidelines for CYP2C19 genotype and clopidogrel

therapy: 2013 update. Clin Pharmacol Ther. 2013;94(3):317–23. https://doi.org/10.1038/clpt.
2013.105.

59. Musa T, Mgbemena O, Franchi F. De-escalation of P2Y12-inhibiting therapies to reduce the
risk of bleeding after PCI: American college of cardiology. Available from: https://www.acc.
org/latest-in-cardiology/articles/2021/10/06/17/50/de-escalation-of-p2y12-inhibiting-therap
ies-to-reduce-the-risk-of-bleeding-after-pci. Accessed: 11 Oct 2022

60. Sathasivam S. Statin induced myotoxicity. Eur J Intern Med. 2012;23(4):317–24. https://doi.
org/10.1016/j.ejim.2012.01.004.

61. Group SC, Link E, Parish S, Armitage J, Bowman L, Heath S, et al. SLCO1B1 variants and
statin-induced myopathy–a genomewide study. N Engl J Med. 2008;359(8):789–99. https://
doi.org/10.1056/NEJMoa0801936.

62. Vassy JL, Gaziano JM, Green RC, Ferguson RE, Advani S, Miller SJ, et al. Effect of pharmacogenetic testing for statin myopathy risk versus usual care on blood cholesterol: a randomized clinical trial. JAMA Netw Open. 2020;3(12): e2027092. https://doi.org/10.1001/jamane
tworkopen.2020.27092.

63. Table of Pharmacogenetic Associations: US Food and Drug Administration; https://www.fda.
gov/medical-devices/precision-medicine/table-pharmacogenetic-associations. Accessed Oct
2022.

64. Rhonda MCD, Mikko N, Laura BR, Jasmine AL, Katriina TE, Robert JS, et al. The
clinical pharmacogenetics implementation consortium (CPIC) guideline for SLCO1B1,
ABCG2, and CYP2C9 and statin-associated musculoskeletal symptoms. Clin Pharmacol
Ther 2022;111(5):1007–1021. https://doi.org/10.1002/cpt.2557.

65. Meloche M, Khazaka M, Kassem I, Barhdadi A, Dube MP, de Denus S. CYP2D6 polymorphism and its impact on the clinical response to metoprolol: a systematic review and
meta-analysis. Br J Clin Pharmacol. 2020;86(6):1015–33. https://doi.org/10.1111/bcp.14247.

66. Hicks JK, Dunnenberger HM, Gumpper KF, Haidar CE, Hoffman JM. Integrating pharmacogenomics into electronic health records with clinical decision support. Am J Health Syst
Pharm. 2016;73(23):1967–76. https://doi.org/10.2146/ajhp160030.

67. Barak Y, Swartz M, Baruch Y. Venlafaxine or a second SSRI: switching after treatment failure
with an SSRI among depressed inpatients: a retrospective analysis. Prog Neuropsychopharmacol Biol Psychiatry. 2011;35(7):1744–7. https://doi.org/10.1016/j.pnpbp.2011.06.007.

68. Hicks JK, Bishop JR, Sangkuhl K, Muller DJ, Ji Y, Leckband SG, et al. Clinical pharmacogenetics implementation consortium (CPIC) guideline for CYP2D6 and CYP2C19 genotypes
and dosing of selective serotonin reuptake inhibitors. Clin Pharmacol Ther. 2015;98(2):127–
34. https://doi.org/10.1002/cpt.147.

69. Mellerup ET, Plenge P. High affinity binding of 3H-paroxetine and 3H-imipramine to rat neuronal membranes. Psychopharmacology. 1986;89(4):436–9. https://doi.org/10.1007/BF0241
2117.

70. Charlier C, Broly F, Lhermitte M, Pinto E, Ansseau M, Plomteux G. Polymorphisms in the
CYP2D6 gene: association with plasma concentrations of fluoxetine and paroxetine. Ther
Drug Monit. 2003;25(6):738–42. https://doi.org/10.1007/s40262-014-0162-1.

71. Chang M, Tybring G, Dahl ML, Lindh JD. Impact of cytochrome P450 2C19 polymorphisms on citalopram/escitalopram exposure: a systematic review and meta-analysis. Clin
Pharmacokinet. 2014;53(9):801–11. https://doi.org/10.1007/s40262-014-0162-1.

72. Rudberg I, Hermann M, Refsum H, Molden E. Serum concentrations of sertraline and N-
desmethyl sertraline in relation to CYP2C19 genotype in psychiatric patients. Eur J Clin
Pharmacol. 2008;64(12):1181–8. https://doi.org/10.1007/s00228-008-0533-3.

73. DeToledo JC, Ramsay RE. Fosphenytoin and phenytoin in patients with status epilepticus:
improved tolerability versus increased costs. Drug Saf. 2000;22(6):459–66. https://doi.org/
10.2165/00002018-200022060-00004.

74. Chang WC, Hung SI, Carleton BC, Chung WH. An update on CYP2C9 polymorphisms and
phenytoin metabolism: implications for adverse effects. Expert Opin Drug Metab Toxicol.
2020;16(8):723–34. https://doi.org/10.1080/17425255.2020.1780209.

75. Duong TA, Valeyrie-Allanore L, Wolkenstein P, Chosidow O. Severe cutaneous adverse reactions to drugs. Lancet. 2017;390(10106):1996–2011. https://doi.org/10.1016/S0140-673 6(16)30378-6.
76. Karnes JH, Rettie AE, Somogyi AA, Huddart R, Fohner AE, Formea CM, et al. Clinical pharmacogenetics implementation consortium (CPIC) guideline for CYP2C9 and HLA-B genotypes and phenytoin dosing: 2020 update. Clin Pharmacol Ther. 2021;109(2):302–9. https://doi.org/10.1002/cpt.2008.
77. Tangamornsuksan W, Scholfield N, Lohitnavy M. Association between HLA genotypes and oxcarbazepine-induced cutaneous adverse drug reactions: a systematic review and meta-analysis. J Pharm Sci. 2018;21(1):1–18. https://doi.org/10.18433/J36S7D.
78. Chen CB, Hsiao YH, Wu T, Hsih MS, Tassaneeyakul W, Jorns TP, et al. Risk and association of HLA with oxcarbazepine-induced cutaneous adverse reactions in Asians. Neurology. 2017;88(1):78–86. https://doi.org/10.1212/WNL.0000000000003453.
79. Phillips EJ, Sukasem C, Whirl-Carrillo M, Muller DJ, Dunnenberger HM, Chantratita W, et al. Clinical pharmacogenetics implementation consortium guideline for HLA genotype and use of carbamazepine and oxcarbazepine: 2017 update. Clin Pharmacol Ther. 2018;103(4):574–81. https://doi.org/10.1002/cpt.1004.
80. Zhang JP, Malhotra AK. Pharmacogenetics and antipsychotics: therapeutic efficacy and side effects prediction. Expert Opin Drug Metab Toxicol. 2011;7(1):9–37. https://doi.org/10.1517/17425255.2011.532787.
81. van Westrhenen R, Aitchison KJ, Ingelman-Sundberg M, Jukic MM. Pharmacogenomics of antidepressant and antipsychotic treatment: how far have we got and where are we going? Front Psychiatry. 2020;11:94. https://doi.org/10.3389/fpsyt.2020.00094.
82. Kishi T, Ikuta T, Matsuda Y, Sakuma K, Iwata N. Aripiprazole versus brexpiprazole for acute schizophrenia: a systematic review and network meta-analysis. Psychopharmacology (Berl). 2020;237(5):1459–1470. https://doi.org/10.1007/s00213-020-05472-5.
83. Jukic MM, Smith RL, Haslemo T, Molden E, Ingelman-Sundberg M. Effect of CYP2D6 genotype on exposure and efficacy of risperidone and aripiprazole: a retrospective, cohort study. Lancet Psychiatry. 2019;6(5):418–26. https://doi.org/10.1016/S2215-0366(19)300 88-4.
84. Ishigooka J, Iwashita S, Higashi K, Liew EL, Tadori Y. Pharmacokinetics and safety of Brex-piprazole following multiple-dose administration to Japanese patients with Schizophrenia. J Clin Pharmacol. 2018;58(1):74–80. https://doi.org/10.1002/jcph.979.
85. Otsuka Pharmaceutical. ABILIFY® (aripiprazole) drug monograph. Rockville, MD. https://www.accessdata.fda.gov/drugsatfda_docs/label/2020/021436s044s045,021713s035s036,021 729s027s028,021866s029s030lbl.pdf. (2019).
86. Pei Q, Huang L, Huang J, Gu JK, Kuang Y, Zuo XC, et al. Influences of CYP2D6(*)10 polymorphisms on the pharmacokinetics of iloperidone and its metabolites in Chinese patients with schizophrenia: a population pharmacokinetic analysis. Acta Pharmacol Sin. 2016;37(11):1499–508. https://doi.org/10.1038/aps.2016.96.
87. Vanda Pharmaceuticals. FANAPT (iloperidone) drug monograph. Washington, DC. https://www.accessdata.fda.gov/drugsatfda_docs/label/2017/022192s018s021lbl.pdf. (2017).
88. Lesche D, Mostafa S, Everall I, Pantelis C, Bousman CA. Impact of CYP1A2, CYP2C19, and CYP2D6 genotype- and phenoconversion-predicted enzyme activity on clozapine exposure and symptom severity. Pharmacogenomics J. 2020;20(2):192–201. https://doi.org/10.1038/s41397-019-0108-y.
89. Therapeutics H. CLOZARIL (clozapine) drug monograph. Rosemont, PA. https://www.acc essdata.fda.gov/drugsatfda_docs/label/2021/019758s088lbl.pdf. (2020).
90. de Leon J, Schoretsanitis G. CYP2D6 pharmacogenetics and risperidone: reflections after 25 years of research. Pharmacogenomics. 2020;21(16):1139–44. https://doi.org/10.2217/pgs-2020-0115.
91. Limited IU. PERSERIS (risperidone) drug monograph: https://www.accessdata.fda.gov/dru gsatfda_docs/label/2018/210655s000lbl.pdf. North Chesterfield, VA. (2018).

92. de Leon J, Wynn G, Sandson NB. The pharmacokinetics of paliperidone versus risperidone. Psychosomatics. 2010;51(1):80–8. https://doi.org/10.1176/appi.psy.51.1.80.

93. Shelton RC, Parikh SV, Law RA, Rothschild AJ, Thase ME, Dunlop BW, et al. Combinatorial pharmacogenomic algorithm is predictive of citalopram and escitalopram metabolism in patients with major depressive disorder. Psychiatry Res. 2020;290: 113017. https://doi.org/10.1016/j.psychres.2020.113017.

94. Rothschild AJ, Parikh SV, Hain D, Law R, Thase ME, Dunlop BW, et al. Clinical validation of combinatorial pharmacogenomic testing and single-gene guidelines in predicting psychotropic medication blood levels and clinical outcomes in patients with depression. Psychiatry Res. 2021;296: 113649. https://doi.org/10.1016/j.psychres.2020.113017.

95. Athreya AP, Neavin D, Carrillo-Roa T, Skime M, Biernacka J, Frye MA, et al. Pharmacogenomics-driven prediction of antidepressant treatment outcomes: a machine-learning approach with multi-trial replication. Clin Pharmacol Ther. 2019;106(4):855–65. https://doi.org/10.1002/cpt.1482.

96. Diasio RB, Harris BE. Clinical pharmacology of 5-fluorouracil. Clin Pharmacokinet. 1989;16:215–37. https://doi.org/10.2165/00003088-198916040-00002.

97. Miwa M, Ura M, Nishida M, Sawada N, Ishikawa T, Mori K, et al. Design of a novel oral fluoropyrimidine carbamate, capecitabine, which generates 5-fluorouracil selectively in tumours by enzymes concentrated in human liver and cancer tissue. Eur J Cancer. 1998;34:1274–81. https://doi.org/10.1016/s0959-8049(98)00058-6.

98. Thorn CF, Marsh S, Carrillo MW, McLeod HL, Klein TE, Altman RB. PharmGKB summary: fluoropyrimidine pathways. Pharmacogenet Genomics. 2011;21(4):237–42. https://doi.org/10.1097/FPC.0b013e32833c6107.

99. Zhang H, Li YM, Jin X. *DPYD*5 gene mutation contributes to the reduced *DPYD* enzyme activity and chemotherapeutic toxicity of 5-FU: results from genotyping study on 75 gastric carcinoma and colon carcinoma patients. Med Oncol. 2007;24:251–8. https://doi.org/10.1007/BF02698048.

100. Gross E, Busse B, Riemenschneider M, Neubauer S, Seck K, Klein HG, et al. Strong association of a common dihydropyrimidine dehydrogenase gene polymorphism with fluoropyrimidine-related toxicity in cancer patients. PLoS ONE. 2008;3: e4003. https://doi.org/10.1371/journal.pone.0004003.

101. Van Kuilenburg AB, Meinsma R, Zonnenberg BA, Zoetekouw L, Baas F, Matsuda K, et al. Dihydropyrimidinase deficiency and severe 5-fluorouracil toxicity. Clin Cancer Res. 2003;9:4363–7.

102. Holly TR, Hany EH, Vincenzo G, Lori MK, Fridley, Brooke L. Genetic regulation of dihydropyrimidinase and its possible implication in altered uracil catabolism. Pharmacogenet Genomics. 2007;17(11):973–87. https://doi.org/10.1097/FPC.0b013e3282f01788.

103. Farrell JJ, Elsaleh H, Garcia M, Lai R, Ammar A, Regine WF, et al. Human equilibrative nucleoside transporter 1 levels predict response to gemcitabine in patients with pancreatic cancer. Gastroenterology. 2009;136:187–95. https://doi.org/10.1053/j.gastro.2008.09.067.

104. Tsujie M, Nakamori S, Nakahira S, Takahashi Y, Hayashi N, Okami J, et al. Human equilibrative nucleoside transporter 1, as a predictor of 5-fluorouracil resistance in human pancreatic cancer. Anticancer Res. 2007;27:2241–9.

105. Kobayashi Y, Ohshiro N, Sakai R, Ohbayashi M, Kohyama N, Yamamoto T. Transport mechanism and substrate specificity of human organic anion transporter 2 (hOat2 [SLC22A7]). J Pharm Pharmacol. 2005;57:573–8. https://doi.org/10.1211/0022357055966.

106. Hagmann W, Jesnowski R, Faissner R, Guo C, Lohr JM. ATP-binding cassette C transporters in human pancreatic carcinoma cell lines. Upregulation in 5-fluorouracil-resistant cells. Pancreatology. 2009;9:136–144. https://doi.org/10.1159/000178884.

107. Bates D, Schultheis BC, Hanes MC, Jolly SM, Chakravarthy KV, Deer TR, et al. A comprehensive algorithm for management of neuropathic pain. Pain Med. 2019;20(Suppl 1):S2–12. https://doi.org/10.1093/pm/pnz075.

108. Dowell D, Haegerich TM, Chou R. CDC guideline for prescribing opioids for chronic pain—United States, 2016. MMWR Recomm Rep. 2016;65(1):1–49. https://doi.org/10.15585/mmwr.rr6501e1.
109. Qaseem A, Wilt TJ, McLean RM, Forciea MA, Denberg TD, Barry MJ, et al. Noninvasive treatments for acute, subacute, and chronic low back pain: a clinical practice guideline from the American college of physicians. Ann Intern Med. 2017;166(7):514–30. https://doi.org/10.7326/M16-2367.
110. Hicks JK, Sangkuhl K, Swen JJ, Ellingrod VL, Muller DJ, Shimoda K, et al. Clinical pharmacogenetics implementation consortium guideline (CPIC) for CYP2D6 and CYP2C19 genotypes and dosing of tricyclic antidepressants: 2016 update. Clin Pharmacol Ther. 2017;102(1):37–44. https://doi.org/10.1002/cpt.597.
111. Bendtsen L, Zakrzewska JM, Abbott J, Braschinsky M, Di Stefano G, Donnet A, et al. European Academy of Neurology guideline on trigeminal neuralgia. Eur J Neurol. 2019;26(6):831–49. https://doi.org/10.1111/ene.13950.
112. Grover S, Kukreti R. HLA alleles and hypersensitivity to carbamazepine: an updated systematic review with meta-analysis. Pharmacogenet Genomics. 2014;24(2):94–112. https://doi.org/10.1097/FPC.0000000000000021.
113. Hershfield MS, Callaghan JT, Tassaneeyakul W, Mushiroda T, Thorn CF, Klein TE, et al. Clinical pharmacogenetics implementation consortium guidelines for human leukocyte antigen-B genotype and allopurinol dosing. Clin Pharmacol Ther. 2013;93(2):153–8. https://doi.org/10.1038/clpt.2012.209.
114. Martin MA, Klein TE, Dong BJ, Pirmohamed M, Haas DW, Kroetz DL, et al. Clinical pharmacogenetics implementation consortium. Clinical pharmacogenetics implementation consortium guidelines for HLA-B genotype and abacavir dosing. Clin Pharmacol Ther. 2012;91(4):734–738. https://doi.org/10.1038/clpt.2011.
115. Mallal S, Phillips E, Carosi G, et al. HLA-B*5701 screening for hypersensitivity to abacavir. N Engl J Med. 2008;358(6):568–79. https://doi.org/10.1056/NEJMoa0706135.
116. Alharazneh A, Luk L, Huth M, Monfared A, Steyger PS, Cheng AG. Functional hair cell mechanotransducer channels are required for aminoglycoside ototoxicity. PlosOne. 2011;6(7): e22347. https://doi.org/10.1371/journal.pone.0022347.
117. Vu1 AA, Nadaraja GS, Huth ME, Luk L, Kim J, Chai R. Integrity and regeneration of mechanotransduction machinery regulate aminoglycoside entry and sensory cell death. PlosOne 2013;8(1):e54794. https://doi.org/10.1371/journal.pone.0054794.
118. McDermott JH, Wolf J, Hoshitsuki K, et al. Clinical pharmacogenetics implementation consortium guideline for the use of aminoglycosides based on MT-RNR1 genotype. Clin Pharmacol Ther. 2022;111(2):366–72. https://doi.org/10.1002/cpt.2309.
119. Tang W, Shi QP, Ding F, Yu ML, Hua J, Wang YX. Impact of VKORC1 gene polymorphisms on warfarin maintenance dosage: a novel systematic review and meta-analysis of 53 studies. Int J Clin Pharmacol Ther. 2017;55(4):304–21. https://doi.org/10.5414/CP202833.
120. Lennard MS, Silas JH, Freestone S, Ramsay LE, Tucker GT, Woods HF. Oxidation phenotype–a major determinant of metoprolol metabolism and response. N Engl J Med. 1982;307(25):1558–60. https://doi.org/10.1056/NEJM198212163072505.

Pharmacogenomics in Pain Treatment

Dragan Primorac and Lidija Bach-Rojecky

Abstract

Chronic pain affects almost every fourth adult individual and is connected with suffering and reduced quality of life. The pain treatment relies on two drug classes: non-steroidal anti-inflammatory drugs (NSAIDs) and opioids. However, substances from different therapeutic classes, like antidepressants and anticonvulsants, can alleviate some chronic pain syndromes. Responses to classical analgesics can vary, where every second affected patient experiences inadequate

D. Primorac (✉)
St. Catherine Specialty Hospital, 10000 Zagreb, Croatia
e-mail: dragan.primorac@svkatarina.hr; draganprimorac2@gmail.com

University of Split School of Medicine, 21000 Split, Croatia

Josip Juraj Strossmayer University of Osijek Faculty of Medicine, 31000 Osijek, Croatia

University of Rijeka School of Medicine, 51000 Rijeka, Croatia

Josip Juraj Strossmayer University of Osijek Faculty of Dental Medicine and Health,
31000 Osijek, Croatia

Eberly College of Science, Penn State University, 517 Thomas Street, State College, PA 16803,
USA

The Henry C. Lee College of Criminal Justice and Forensic Sciences, University of New Haven,
West Haven, CT, USA

National Forensic Science University, Gandhinagar, Gujarat, India

College of Medicine and Forensics, Xi'an Jiaotong University, Xi'an, China

Medical School REGIOMED, 96450 Coburg, Germany

International Center For Applied Biological Sciences, 10000 Zagreb, Croatia

L. Bach-Rojecky
University of Zagreb Faculty of Pharmacy and Biochemistry, 10000 Zagreb, Croatia

© The Author(s), under exclusive license to Springer Nature Switzerland AG 2023
D. Primorac et al. (eds.), *Pharmacogenomics in Clinical Practice*,
https://doi.org/10.1007/978-3-031-45903-0_8

133

pain reduction and different side effects. NSAIDs have the risks of gastrotox-icity, cardiotoxicity, and renal failure. The use of opioid drugs is associated with tolerance, development of dependence, addiction, and risk of abuse. Adju-vant analgesics, because of differences in pharmacologic profile, cause diverse adverse reactions that influence their applicability in different chronic pain states. Nowadays, studies have identified several genes or gene clusters, which can influence drugs' mechanisms of action and pharmacokinetic profile, and consequently affect therapeutic outcomes. Therefore, genotype-guided therapy adjustment can increase drug efficacy, diminish adverse effects, and improve patients' quality of life.

Keywords

Pain • Non-steroidal anti-inflammatory drugs • Opioid analgesics • Adjuvant analgesics • Pharmacogenomics

1   Introduction

Chronic pain is a growing public health problem representing a leading cause of disability and disease burden worldwide. Among chronic pain conditions, low back pain and headache disorders are the most common. It is estimated that some 30–50% of the world's population and almost 20% of the Europeans suffer from chronic pain with a devastating cost for the health care systems, society, and economy [1].

Understanding pain genetic background (540 so-called pain genes have been documented) can predict the individual risk of developing chronic pain. In addition, variations in genes affecting drugs' pharmacological profile (pharma-codynamics and pharmacokinetics) can elucidate differences in the efficacy and safety of analgesic drugs noticed in clinical practice [2].

Acute and chronic pain conditions are commonly treated with two phar-macologically distinct groups of drugs—non-steroidal anti-inflammatory drugs (NSAIDs) and opioids. Other non-opioid analgesics, like paracetamol (also known as acetaminophen), are used alone or in combination with other drugs to obtain a synergistic analgesic effect. Additionally, drugs from different therapeutic classes, such as antidepressants and anticonvulsants, are applied as adjunct analgesics for some chronic pain conditions [3].

Despite a well-established pharmacological profile and clinical usefulness proven during several decades in combating various pain syndromes, analgesic drugs are still under the loop because of their ineffectiveness in a significant pro-portion of patients and the profile of adverse reactions. Therapy failure, partial or incomplete, and side effects negatively affect desired therapeutic outcomes and patients' adherence to the therapy [4].

Several distinct but important and interconnected factors can influence the chal-lenges in pain treatment. Patient characteristics such as age, sex, body weight, and medical conditions (such as depression, cancer, obesity, and diabetes) are some of them. Among patient-related factors, variants in genes encoding different proteins involved in the drug's pharmacological profile can significantly impact pain perception and treatment outcomes [1].

2   Non-steroidal Anti-inflammatory Drugs (NSAIDs)

NSAIDs are among the most frequently used drugs for the pain of low to medium intensity, often associated with inflammation, such as osteoarthritis, postoperative surgical conditions, menstrual cramps, and headaches. This class of drugs includes more than 40 chemically distinct compounds, available in different pharmaceutical forms and intended for application by different routes. They also have antipyretic and anti-inflammatory effects, although some other potential uses have been proposed. For example, NSAIDs are investigated for their antitumor actions, and as preventive therapy for neurodegenerative diseases, like Alzheimer's dementia [5]. Apart from chemical structure, NSAIDs differ in their pharmacological characteristics, which might govern the choice of one drug over the other in a specific patient [4].

The principal mechanism of NSAIDs action relies on the inhibition of various prostanoid productions. They primarily inhibit the enzyme cyclooxygenase (prostaglandin G/H synthases), which catalyzes production of the unstable prostaglandins G2/H2 from arachidonic acid. Two isoenzymes of cyclooxygenase (COX) have been recognized: COX-1 and COX-2. COX-1 is constitutively expressed in many tissues and plays a role in homeostasis by producing prostanoids with different physiological roles and thromboxane A2 in platelets. COX-2 is an inducible isoform in inflammatory cells that produce pro-inflammatory prostaglandins. However, COX-2 has a physiological role in maintaining the normal function of the cardiovascular system because of its distribution in the kidney and endothelial cells. All NSAIDs are reversible inhibitors of both COX-1 and COX-2 but differ in the affinity and selectivity for each isoform. Acetylsalicylic acid acts as the irreversible inhibitor of primarily COX-1. While older traditional NSAIDs act as non-selective inhibitors of both isoenzymes, several drugs of newer generation (coxibs) exert more COX-2 selective inhibition [6].

NSAIDs can cause numerous adverse effects: some are rare, while others are common or very common. Serious complications that may occur in particular patient populations include gastrointestinal bleeding, hypertension, myocardial infarction, heart failure, and renal impairment. Since the risks for the above-mentioned serious complications are dependent on the applied dose and the duration of treatment, the golden rule for NSAIDs use states that they should be taken in the "lowest effective doses and for the shortest period possible" [7].

Inhibition of COX-1 is associated with ulcerations and bleeding of the gastric mucosa and slows mucosal regeneration due to prolonged bleeding time. These gastro pathological changes are consequence of NSAIDs-reduced production of cytoprotective prostaglandins PGE2 and PGI2, with decreased secretion of mucus and bicarbonates. In addition, some acidic NSAIDs can produce a direct cytotoxic effect on gastric epithelial cells [4, 6].

On the other hand, drugs with higher-degree selectivity for the COX-2 enzyme can impair vasodilatation, increase activity of platelets, and change renal hemodynamics, thus leading to an increased risk of cardiovascular adverse events [4, 7].

Two types of kidney injury are connected with NSAIDs use: acute kidney injury after high doses of NSAIDs and chronic kidney disease developed with long-term drugs use. Existing heart failure, or usage of angiotensin-converting enzyme inhibitors, angiotensin receptor blockers, or diuretics increase the risk of nephrotoxicity [8].

NSAIDs differ in their pharmacokinetic properties, like bioavailability, biotransformation pathways, and plasma elimination half-life. Metabolic reactions of celecoxib, diclofenac, flurbiprofen, indomethacin, ibuprofen, lornoxicam, meloxicam, nabumetone, naproxen, piroxicam, and tenoxicam are associated with the CYP2C subfamily, including the highly variable CYP2C8, CYP2C9, and CYP2C19 isoforms. Polymorphisms in these genes may result in modified enzyme expression or functionality, thus influencing drugs' bioavailability, clearance, and half-life [4]. The *CYP2C9* gene which encodes enzyme involved in the metabolism of some NSAIDs (like celecoxib, piroxicam, and lornoxicam) has at least 61 variant alleles with multiple sub-alleles. Commonly reported alleles are classified as those with normal function (e.g., *CYP2C9*1*), decreased function (e.g., *CYP2C9*2, *5, *8, *11*), and no function (e.g., *CYP2C9*3, *6, *13*). Based on the highest level of clinical evidence, CPIC recommends NSAIDs therapy adjustment according to the patient's *CYP2C* genotype (Table 1) in order to decrease the risk of therapy failure and adverse drug reactions [9].

There are indices for peptic ulcer pathogenesis to be influenced by functional polymorphisms in the *COX*-encoding genes. Individuals carrying reduced function COX-enzymes may be potentially susceptible to NSAID-induced peptic ulceration, but there is insufficient evidence currently to determine whether the *COX* gene polymorphisms predispose to NSAID-induced peptic ulcer disease [10].

Allelic variants *UGT2B7*2* encoding UDP-glucuronosyltransferase-2B7 and *ABCC2 C-24T* encoding the transporter for the biliary excretion of drug metabolites may predispose to the formation and accumulation of reactive diclofenac metabolites. However, more evidence supporting those gene polymorphisms with hepatotoxicity risk after diclofenac use is needed [11].

3   Paracetamol (Acetaminophen)

Paracetamol is one of the most frequently used analgesic drugs worldwide. It is available in many over-the-counter formulations, either alone or in combination with other substances. Because of a well-established synergistic effect, it is also

Table 1 Recommendations for NSAIDs therapy according to the *CYP2C9* genotype (*modified according to Ref.* [9])

CYP2C9 genotype/phenotype	Recommendations for celecoxib, flurbiprofen, lornoxicam, ibuprofen, meloxican, piroxicam and tenoxicam
CYP2C9*1/*1/normal metabolizer *CYP2C9*1/*2*/intermediate metabolizer	**All drugs**
CYP2C9*1/*3, *2/*2/intermediate metabolizer	**Celecoxib, flurbiprofen, lornoxicam, and ibuprofen** Therapy should be initiated with the lowest recommended starting dose and titrated upward to clinical effect or maximum recommended dose with caution, especially in individuals with other factors affecting clearance, such as hepatic impairment or advanced age **Meloxicam** Therapy should be initiated with 50% of the lowest recommended starting dose and titrated upward to clinical effect or 50% of the maximum recommended dose with caution. Alternatively, the other drug not primarily metabolized by CYP2C9 can be considered **Piroxicam and tenoxicam** An alternative therapy not metabolized by CYP2C9 or not significantly impacted by *CYP2C9* genetic variants, or a drug metabolized by CYP2C9 but with a shorter half-life can be introduced
CYP2C9*2/*3, *3/*3/poor metabolizer	**Celecoxib, flurbiprofen, lornoxicam, and ibuprofen** Therapy should be initiated with 25–50% of the lowest recommended starting dose and titrated upward to clinical effect. Alternatively, the other drug not primarily metabolized by CYP2C9 can be considered **Meloxicam, piroxicam, and tenoxicam** An alternative therapy not metabolized by CYP2C9 or not significantly impacted by *CYP2C9* genetic variants, or an NSAID metabolized by CYP2C9 but with a shorter half-life can be considered

Content published by CPIC is available free of restriction under the CC0 1.0 Universal (CC0 1.0) Public Domain Dedication combined with mild opioids, like codeine and tramadol to treat the pain of moderate intensity. Paracetamol differs in pharmacological properties, as well as safety profile from COX-inhibitors, and is not considered an NSAID [4, 12].

Paracetamol inhibits the peroxidase activity of the COX-2 enzyme, thus reducing prostaglandin synthesis only in the presence of low levels of peroxide. This is the main reason of its negligible anti-inflammatory action. It readily enters the central nervous system (CNS), which is the primary site of its action. Besides inhibition of central COX-2 and prostaglandin production, paracetamol, through its active metabolite N-arachidonoylphenolamine (AM-404), modulates the endocannabinoid, opioid, and serotoninergic systems involved in pain processing [12].

Paracetamol is primarily metabolized in hepatocytes by glucuronidation and sulfation, while oxidation via CYP2E1 plays a minor role at therapeutic drug doses (<4 g/day). The reactive metabolite N-acetyl-p-benzoquinone imine (NAPQI) is produced via oxidation and is detoxified with glutathione (GSH), either spontaneously, or catalyzed by glutathione-S-transferase [13].

At supra-therapeutic doses of paracetamol (more than 4 g/day), the glucuronidation and oxidation increase, while the sulfation pathways become saturated. After a very high doses (>7 g), higher proportions of the drug get oxidized to NAPQI (>15%). This toxic metabolic product depletes GSH levels in the hepatocytes, leading to cell death after disturbing the function of mitochondrial proteins and ion channels [13].

Polymorphisms in genes encoding paracetamol metabolizing enzymes: UDP-glucuronosyl transferases (UGT1A1, UGT1A6, UGT1A9), sulfotransferases (SULT1A1 and SULT2A1), and CYP2E1 might be responsible for differences in drug's metabolism and toxicity observed in certain patients populations. However, further studies are necessary to determine to what extent gene polymorphisms account for the ethnic differences in paracetamol pharmacokinetics. The most studied polymorphisms with possible influence on paracetamol efficacy and toxicity are *UGT1A-3'UTR rs10929303*, rs1042640, and rs8330. One study suggested that rs8330 is associated with increased glucuronidation and decreased risk of paracetamol-induced acute liver failure [14].

Since other reactions play a role in paracetamol biotransformation, more studies are warranted to establish the relationship between polymorphisms in genes connected with paracetamol inactivation and detoxification of toxic metabolites. The obtained results could help to explain inter-individual variability in response to paracetamol.

4   Opioid Analgesics

Prescription opioids are used to treat acute and chronic non-malignant and malignant pain of moderate to severe intensity. However, their use is accompanied by some serious risks, such as misuse, opioid use disorder (addiction), and fatal overdoses. In the USA, nearly 218,000 deaths from prescription opioids overdose were detected in a period from 1999 to 2017 [15].

Opioid drugs overprescribing for chronic pain during the 1990s was just the beginning of the growing problem during the following decades which is even more complicated with illegal highly potent and toxic fentanyl-like compounds distributed on streets. Deaths from fentanyl and other synthetic opioids increased from around 3000 in 2010 to over 28,466 in 2017 [16]. These data urge the necessary steps to stop the opioid misuse-related problems and to save this valuable class of drugs from further social stigmatization.

Opioid analgesics differ in their origin (natural, semi-synthetic, synthetic), the intensity of the analgesic effect, duration of action, and risk of adverse effects, including the development of tolerance and addiction. Differences exist when it comes to their mechanism of action: drugs like morphine, codeine, oxycodone, methadone, fentanyl, tramadol, and tapentadol are full agonists of opioid receptors, primarily μ subtype (MOR), buprenorphine is a partial agonist of MOR with antagonistic activity on κ subtype (KOR), while oliceridine—the newest drug in the class acts as a biased agonist of MOR, thus preferentially activating particular intracellular pathways (related to G-protein) over β-arrestin [4, 17]. Additionally, opioid drugs differ in the postreceptor signaling pathways which they activate or inhibit upon binding on the opioid receptors. As a consequence, there are also differences in MOR desensitization, re-sensitization, endocytosis, and recycling. Interference with opioid pathways in the central nervous system and at the periphery results with variety of adverse effects, which include sedation, dizziness, nausea, constipation, pruritus, bradycardia, paradoxical hyperalgesia, and respiratory depression. Tolerance and development of dependence with a severe withdrawal syndrome upon drug discontinuation are also their negative characteristics [4].

Opioid analgesics have different pharmacokinetic properties like bioavailability, plasma half-life, biotransformation pathways, distribution, and elimination. The duration of the analgesic effect is dependent on the degree of the drug's biotransformation, activity of metabolites, and their half-lives [4].

CYP2D6 enzyme is important for metabolism of some drugs, like codeine, tramadol, hydrocodone, oxycodone, and methadone.

The enzyme CYP2D6 catalyzes the demethylation reaction of prodrug codeine to its active metabolite morphine. Therefore, CYP2D6 enzyme activity determines the codeine/morphine ratio and the strength of the opiate effect. For the *CYP2D6* gene, numerous activity-reducing variants, as well as activity-increasing gene duplications, are recognized. Specific gene duplications (denoted as *1/*1xN or *1/*2xN) correspond to the phenotype of ultrarapid metabolizer. The prevalence of this CYP2D6 phenotype has been estimated at 1–10% for European and

North Americans, 3–4% for African Americans, 1–2% for East Asians, and greater than 10% in certain racial/ethnic groups. Ultrarapid metabolizers convert codeine more rapidly and completely with a consequent higher than expected morphine levels. These may result in signs of overdose and respiratory depression, even at the therapeutic dosages [17].

The FDA-approved drug label for codeine warns that respiratory depression and death can occur in children who receive codeine following a tonsillectomy and/or adenoidectomy and are CYP2D6 ultrarapid metabolizers [18].

Tramadol is a weaker synthetic opioid agonist with additional effects on the monoaminergic system at the level of the dorsal horn of the spinal cord, where it interferes with pain signal processing. Tramadol is metabolized by O- and N-demethylation, followed by conjugation into final metabolites glucuronides and sulfates. After demethylation via CYP2D6, an active metabolite O-desmethyl tramadol binds to the MOR with 200 times higher affinity and is more potent than tramadol in producing analgesia [19].

Since CYP2D6 plays a significant role in tramadol biotransformation, variations in enzyme activity might be important for drugs efficacy and safety. A lot of evidence accumulated over time suggesting that specific CYP2D6 gene duplications contribute to the risk of toxicity with standard tramadol dosing. According to CPIC dosing recommendations (https://cpicpgx.org/guidelines/guideline-for-codeine-and-cyp2d6/) for an individual identified as CYP2D6 ultrarapid metabolizer, "a different analgesic should be used to avoid the risk of severe toxicity," but it is also suggested to avoid tramadol use, or to increase tramadol dose in individuals identified as CYP2D6 poor metabolizers (the no-function CYP2D6*4 and *5 alleles largely account for the poor metabolizer phenotype in Caucasian population) because of the possible reduced analgesic effect with the standard dosing [19].

Additionally, the FDA released a safety announcement recommending against the use of codeine and tramadol by mothers during lactation because an increased risk of adverse effects and respiratory depression in the infants. Also, they issued strongest warning because of safety concern that "codeine should not be used to treat pain or cough and tramadol should not be used to treat pain in children younger than 12 years" [18].

Other genes that have been studied for their association with opioids efficacy and safety include UGT2B (encoding glucuronosyltransferase), OPRM1 (encoding MOR), and COMT (encoding catechol-O-methyltransferase, which degrades catecholamines).

Polymorphisms in UGT2B7 were investigated in relation to morphine use. This gene encodes enzyme which catalyzes morphine glucuronidation, and could potentially change the drug efficacy, but studies showed contradictory and inconclusive results.

The OPRM1 SNP rs1799971 (118 A>G) is one of the most studied. The frequency of this polymorphism largely varies among individuals of Asian (35–50%), European (15.4%), Hispanic (14%), and African (4.7%) origin. Although studies suggested that the rs1799971 G allele in OPRM1 is associated with increased morphine dose requirements, the alteration in dose is minor and not clinically actionable [4, 20]. For now, there is insufficient evidence to provide any other recommendations for *OPRM1* variants [19]. Similarly, there was mixed evidence about the association between variants in *COMT* and clinical response to opioid drugs. Functional SNP of *COMT* rs4680 is also of clinical interest, because this polymorphism is associated with the lower enzyme activity. Despite several clinical studies that showed that AA carriers have an increased sensitivity to the analgesic effects of opioids (compared to G allele carriers), more evidence is needed before implementing this genotype in drugs dosing adjustments [19].

Updated CPIC guidelines recommend the use of *CYP2D6* genotype for prescribing codeine and tramadol and show the limited and/or weak evidence for other opioids partially metabolized by this enzyme, like hydrocodone, oxycodone, and methadone. Due to inconclusive data, CPIC does not recommend genetic testing for *OPRM1* and *COMT* in routine clinical settings until more comprehensive studies on larger patient populations will be available [19].

5   Adjunct Analgesics

Besides two major analgesic groups described in the previous text, for chronic pain treatment, drugs from other therapeutic classes can be used, like tricyclic antidepressants (TCA), anticonvulsants (gabapentinoids, carbamazepine, oxcarbazepine), musculoskeletal agents (baclofen, tizanidine), topical analgesics (capsaicin, lidocaine), and cannabinoids (dronabinol), among others. Each medication has its benefit/risk profile, as well as the more or less known mechanism of action on nociception pathways.

5.1   Antidepressants

Antidepressants (e.g., desipramine, nortriptyline, amitriptyline, duloxetine, and venlafaxine) are commonly used in various chronic pain conditions, including neuropathic pain, fibromyalgia, low back pain, and headaches. In comparison with doses and onset of antidepressant effects, their effect on pain occurs in lower doses and in shorter period. The main mechanism of analgesic action involves an increase in the noradrenergic and serotonergic neurotransmission in the synaptic cleft at supraspinal and spinal levels, thus reinforcing the descending inhibitory pain pathways. Additional mechanisms include inhibition of ion channels, blockade of glutamate NMDA receptors, and reduction of PGE2 production [20].

TCA has numerous adverse effects, including dry mouth, dizziness, sedation, memory impairment, orthostatic hypotension, urinary retention, and cardiac conduction abnormalities.

Since TCA clearance depends on the complex biotransformation pathways, understanding the differences in the metabolism of each drug is helpful in the prediction of their efficacy and safety. Most TCA are tertiary amines, and their metabolism is mediated by CYP2D6 and CYP2C19 enzymes. A drug that is a tertiary amine is first de-methylated by CYP2C19 to an active metabolite, which is then hydroxylated by CYP2D6 to inactive metabolites. Thus, the treatment failure or adverse effects might be predicted based on the *CYP2D6* genotype (e.g., SNPs *1XN, *2, *2XN, *3, *4, *5, *6, *9, *10, *41*) and the *CYP2C19* genotype (e.g., *2,*3,*17*), which influence drug clearance, and the ratio of parent drug to active metabolites, respectively [21].

CPIC recommends adjusting the dosage of individual TCA in patients according to their metabolizer status. While guidelines are referring to the doses used in the treatment of depression, for lower doses used to treat pain, no dose adjustment in intermediate or poor CYP2D6/CYP2C19 metabolizers is recommended, because it is less likely that those patients will experience adverse effects. However, individuals with ultrarapid CYP2D6 metabolizer status might experience drug failure because of lower than needed drug concentrations. In those patients, the use of an alternative drug is suggested [21].

Venlafaxine and duloxetine are the other two antidepressants drugs commonly used to treat pain. Since their biotransformation pathways also involve the before-mentioned enzymes, the determination of CYP2D6 and CYP2C19 genotypes might potentially explain inter-individual differences in treatment outcomes seen in the practice. However, more studies are necessary before recommendations for dosage adjustments according to the genotype can be suggested. As with TCA, most studies are performed on patients treated for depression with higher dosages of drugs [22].

5.2   Anticonvulsants

Anticonvulsants are used to treat various types of epilepsy, but some drugs from the class are useful in the treatments of chronic pain syndromes. They decrease neuronal excitability due to blocking different presynaptic and postsynaptic ion channels. Gabapentinoids pregabalin and gabapentin are the first-line agents for postherpetic neuralgia, painful diabetic peripheral neuropathy, fibromyalgia, and central neuropathic pain. Carbamazepine and oxcarbazepine are usually used to treat trigeminal neuralgia as drugs of first choice [23].

Gabapentinoids are distributed to the CNS using the L-type amino acid transporter 1 (*LAT1* or *SLC7A5*). Evaluation of the *LAT1 rs4240803* genetic polymorphism in Pakistani patients with neuropathic pain showed that maximum responders ($\geq$50%) were in the GG genotype group, while 72.5% of patients with GA genotype experienced drugs adverse effects. These results need further confirmation from studies on a larger cohort of patients treated for chronic pain [24].

Carbamazepine and its keto-analog oxcarbazepine share a pharmacological profile, as well as many therapeutic indications and adverse effects. The majority of adverse effects like dizziness, ataxia, and nystagmus are concentration-dependent.

However, serious adverse effects, such as aplastic anemia, hyponatremia, leukopenia, osteoporosis, liver injury, and hypersensitivity reactions (drug reaction with eosinophilia and systemic symptoms, maculopapular exanthema, Stevens-Johnson syndrome, and toxic epidermal necrolysis), does not show a clear linear dose–response relationship [25].

There is evidence linking the *HLA-B*15:02* and *HLA-A*31:01* genotypes with the risk of potentially fatal cutaneous hypersensitivity reactions, which usually occur in drug-naive patients and within the first month of the therapy. Based on strong evidence, CPIC recommends for a patient *HLA-B*15:02* and/or *HLA-A*31:01* positive "avoidance of carbamazepine/oxcarbazepine and use of an alternative drug," if possible.

Therefore, determination of *HLA-B*15:02* and *HLA-A*31:01* can predict the risk of serious, and potentially fatal cutaneous adverse reactions to carbamazepine and oxcarbazepine, thus improving treatment outcomes and patients safety [25, 26].

6   Conclusion

Successful pain management requires the delivery of analgesia with minimal risk of ADRs. Despite a plethora of drugs from pharmacologically well-characterized classes, almost half of all patients suffering from chronic pain experience inadequate analgesia and serious adverse effects. Among other factors, allelic variants in genes encoding for target proteins, transporters, and metabolizing enzymes might explain observed inter-individual variability in pain experience, as well as drug-induced analgesia and ADRs. Therefore, PGx could serve as a powerful tool for personalization of the pain treatment.

References

1. Mills SEE, Nicolson KP, Smith BH. Chronic pain: a review of its epidemiology and associated factors in population-based studies. Br J Anaesth. 2019;123(2):e273–83. https://doi.org/10.1016/j.bja.2019.03.023.
2. Kringel D, Malkusch S, Kalso E, Lötsch J. Computational functional genomics-based AmpliSeq™ panel for next-generation sequencing of key genes of pain. Int J Mol Sci. 2021;22(2):878. https://doi.org/10.3390/ijms22020878.
3. Nicol AL, Hurley RW, Benzon HT. Alternatives to opioids in the pharmacologic management of chronic pain syndromes: a narrative review of randomized, controlled, and blinded clinical trials. Anesth Analg. 2017;125(5):1682–703. https://doi.org/10.1213/ANE.0000000000002426.
4. Bach-Rojecky L, Vađunec D, Žunić K, Kurija J, Šipicki S, Gregg R, et al. Continuing war on pain: a personalized approach to the therapy with nonsteroidal anti-inflammatory drugs and opioids. Per Med. 2019;16(2):171–84. https://doi.org/10.2217/pme-2018-0116.
5. Kaduševičius E. Novel applications of NSAIDs: insight and future perspectives in cardiovascular, neurodegenerative, diabetes and cancer disease therapy. Int J Mol Sci. 2021;22(12):6637. https://doi.org/10.3390/ijms22126637.

6. Brune K, Patrignani P. New insights into the use of currently available non-steroidal anti-inflammatory drugs. J Pain Res. 2015;8:105–18. https://doi.org/10.2147/JPR.S75160.
7. Tacconelli S, Bruno A, Grande R, Ballerini P, Patrignani P. Non-steroidal anti-inflammatory drugs and cardiovascular safety—translating pharmacological data into clinical readouts. Expert Opin Drug Saf. 2017;16(7):791–807. https://doi.org/10.1080/14740338.2017.1338272.
8. Bindu S, Mazumder S, Bandyopadhyay U. Non-steroidal anti-inflammatory drugs (NSAIDs) and organ damage: a current perspective. Biochem Pharmacol. 2020;180: 114147. https://doi.org/10.1016/j.bcp.2020.114147.
9. Theken KN, Lee CR, Gong L, Caudle KE, Formea CM, Gaedigk A, et al. Clinical Pharmacogenetics Implementation Consortium Guideline (CPIC) for CYP2C9 and nonsteroidal anti-inflammatory drugs. Clin Pharmacol Ther. 2020;108(2):191–200. https://doi.org/10.1002/cpt.1830.
10. Agúndez JA, Blanca M, Cornejo-García JA, García-Martín E. Pharmacogenomics of cyclooxygenases. Pharmacogenomics. 2015;16(5):501–22. https://doi.org/10.2217/pgs.15.6.
11. Daly AK, Aithal GP, Leathart JB, Swainsbury RA, Dang TS, Day CP. Genetic susceptibility to diclofenac-induced hepatotoxicity: contribution of UGT2B7, CYP2C8, and ABCC2 genotypes. Gastroenterology. 2007;132(1):272–81. https://doi.org/10.1053/j.gastro.2006.11.023.
12. Graham GG, Davies MJ, Day RO, Mohamudally A, Scott KF. The modern pharmacology of paracetamol: therapeutic actions, mechanism of action, metabolism, toxicity and recent pharmacological findings. Inflammopharmacology. 2013;21:201–32. https://doi.org/10.1007/s10787-013-0172-x.
13. Mazaleuskaya LL, Sangkuhl K, Thorn CF, FitzGerald GA, Altman RB, Klein TE. PharmGKB summary: pathways of acetaminophen metabolism at the therapeutic versus toxic doses. Pharmacogenet Genomics. 2015;25(8):421–6. https://doi.org/10.1097/FPC.0000000000000150.
14. Court MH, Freytsis M, Wang X, Peter I, Guillemette C, Hazarika S, et al. The UDP-glucuronosyltransferase (UGT) 1A polymorphism c.2042C>G (rs8330) is associated with increased human liver acetaminophen glucuronidation, increased UGT1A exon 5a/5b splice variant mRNA ratio, and decreased risk of unintentional acetaminophen-induced acute liver failure. J Pharmacol Exp Ther. 2013;345(2):297–307. https://doi.org/10.1124/jpet.112.202010.
15. Centers for Disease Control. Opioid overdose. Prescription opioid data. Available at: https://www.cdc.gov/drugoverdose/deaths/prescription/index.html. Accessed 13 Aug 2021
16. Jones CM, Einstein EB, Compton WM. Changes in synthetic opioid involvement in drug overdose deaths in the United States, 2010–2016. JAMA. 2018;319(17):1819–21. https://doi.org/10.1001/jama.2018.2844.
17. Crews KR, Monte AA, Huddart R, Caudle KE, Kharasch ED, Gaedigk AD, et al. Clinical Pharmacogenetics Implementation Consortium Guideline for CYP2D6, OPRM1, and COMT genotypes and select opioid therapy. Clin Pharmacol Ther. 2021. https://doi.org/10.1002/cpt.2149.https://doi.org/10.1002/cpt.2149.
18. Annotation of FDA label for codeine and CYP2D. Available at: https://www.pharmgkb.org/labelAnnotation/PA166104916. Accessed 13 Aug 2021
19. Dean L, Kane M. Tramadol therapy and CYP2D6 genotype. 2015 Sep 10 [updated 2021 Jul 20]. In: Pratt VM, Scott SA, Pirmohamed M, Esquivel B, Kane MS, Kattman BL, Malheiro AJ, editors. Medical genetics summaries [Internet]. Bethesda (MD): National Center for Biotechnology Information (US); 2012.
20. Dharmshaktu P, Tayal V, Kalra BS. Efficacy of antidepressants as analgesics: a review. J Clin Pharmacol. 2012;52(1):6–17. https://doi.org/10.1177/0091270010394852.
21. Hicks JK, Sangkuhl K, Swen JJ, Ellingrod VL, Müller DJ, Shimoda K, et al. Clinical Pharmacogenetics Implementation Consortium Guideline (CPIC) for CYP2D6 and CYP2C19 genotypes and dosing of tricyclic antidepressants: 2016 update. Clin Pharmacol Ther. 2017;102(1):37–44. https://doi.org/10.1002/cpt.597.
22. Sangkuhl K, Stingl JC, Turpeinen M, Altman RB, Klein TE. PharmGKB summary: venlafaxine pathway. Pharmacogenet Genomics. 2014;24(1):62–72. https://doi.org/10.1097/FPC.0000000000000003.

23. Li CT, Watson JC. Anticonvulsants in the treatment of pain. In: Deer T, Pope J, Lamer T, Provenzano D (eds) Deer's treatment of pain. Cham: Springer; 2019. Available at: https://doi.org/10.1007/978-3-030-12281-2_19. Accessed 14 Aug 2021.

24. Shaheen A, Alam SM, Azam F, Khan M, Ahmad Saleem S, Liaquat A, Mumtaz S. Influence of single nucleotide polymorphism of LAT1 on therapeutic response to gabapentinoids in Pakistani patients with neuropathic pain. Basic Clin Pharmacol Toxicol. 2021;128(3):503–10. https://doi.org/10.1111/bcpt.13534.

25. Phillips EJ, Sukasem C, Whirl-Carrillo M, Müller DJ, Dunnenberger HM, Chantratita W, et al. Clinical Pharmacogenetics Implementation Consortium Guideline for HLA genotype and use of carbamazepine and oxcarbazepine: 2017 update. Clin Pharmacol Ther. 2018;103(4):574–81. https://doi.org/10.1002/cpt.1004.

26. Primorac D, Höppner W, editors. Pharmacogenetics in clinical practice: experience with 55 commonly used drugs. Zagreb, Hamburg, Philadelphia: St. Catherine Specialty Hospital, Bioglobe GmbH, ISABS; 2022. Available from: https://www.stcatherine.com/centre-of-excellence/10/individualized-and-preventive-medicine/pharmacogenomics/69. Accessed 13 Aug 2021.

Pharmacogenomics in Psychiatric Diseases

Adrijana Kekic

Abstract

Mental health disorders are prevalent, complex, and difficult to treat illnesses. Psychopharmacotherapy is the cornerstone of their treatment. Drug selection is still heuristic, due to the lack of reliable biological biomarkers to predict treatment response. Genetic variants of pharmacokinetics and pharmacodynamic genes contribute to a quarter of total drug response variability across the population. The promise of pharmacogenomics in psychiatry is a better prediction of psychotropic drug response. This chapter will focus on genetic variants with demonstrated clinical impact related to antidepressants, antipsychotics, mood stabilizers, and other psychotropics.

Keywords

Mental disorders · Psychiatry · Psychopharmacology · Pharmacogenetics · Pharmacogenomics

1 Introduction

Mental health disorders are prevalent, complex, and difficult to treat illnesses. Mental health disorders reduce life expectancy by 10.1 years and increase the risk of mortality compared to the general population. The Institute for Health Metrics and Evaluation estimates that globally 280 million people suffer from depression [1]. Major depression disorder (MDD), anxiety, alcohol use disorders, schizophrenia, bipolar disorder, and dysthymia (persistent mild depression) are leading causes of disability in the US, according to the US Burden of Disease Collaborators 2013

A. Kekic (✉)
Department of Pharmacy, Mayo Clinic, Phoenix, AZ, USA
e-mail: Kekic.adrijana@mayo.edu

[2]. Treatment of neuropsychiatric disorders can be costly and involve multiple drug trials. The U.S spent $187.8 billion on mental health disorders in 2013 and over $70 billion on depression treatment [3].

Psychopharmacotherapy is the cornerstone of treatment for most mental health disorders. Drug selection is primarily heuristic, due to the lack of reliable biological biomarkers to predict treatment response. In addition to trial-and-error prescribing, clinicians are tasked with maximizing benefits with existing and older drugs, since very few new ones enter the market. Therefore, the goal for clinicians is to personalize and optimize pharmacotherapy with available drugs. Unfortunately, response to pharmacotherapy varies widely among patients. A variety of intrinsic and extrinsic factors contribute to interindividual differences in drug response (efficacy and toxicity). Depending on a drug, genetic factors are estimated to account for 20–95% of the variability observed in drug disposition and effects [4] which means after accounting for all other intrinsic and extrinsic factors, genetics contributes to a quarter of total drug response variability across the population. After oncology drugs, psychotropics drugs have the greatest number of PGx markers in their drug labels ($n = 35$) [5].

The promise of pharmacogenomics in psychiatry is a better prediction of psychotropic drug response. This chapter will focus on genetic variants with demonstrated clinical impact related to antidepressants, antipsychotics, and other psychotropics. The chapter is divided into two main sections to allow for easier navigation based on the reader's interest: the first section covers genes that affect pharmacokinetics and pharmacodynamics of psychotropics medications, and the second section covers drug classes with evidence to support their clinical implementation. As the field of psycho-pharmacogenomics continues to evolve, so will guidelines and algorithms. Emerging technologies, reduced cost for testing, uptake in implementation efforts, integration of other "omics" biomarkers will continue to drive and guide more individualized drug selection and outcomes.

2   Pharmacogenes in Psychiatry

2.1   Pharmacokinetic Genes

Pharmacokinetics (what the body does to a drug) refers to proteins involved in drug absorption, distribution, metabolism, and elimination. Genetic variability influences the activity of these proteins and contributes to drug toxicity and treatment failure [6, 7]. Genes that encode for drug-metabolizing enzymes (DMEs) are associated with treatment response traits that follow a simple Mendelian pattern of inheritance [8]. Polymorphisms in several DME genes are clinically relevant, as reflected in prescribing recommendations from The Clinical Pharmacogenetics Implementation Consortium (CPIC), The Dutch Pharmacogenetics Working Group (DPWG), and US Food and Drug Administration (FDA) labels for several medications [4, 5, 9–13].

Drug metabolism is divided into three phases: phase I (oxidation, demethylation, reduction, and hydrolysis), phase II (conjugation), and phase III (modification and excretion) [14, 15]. Phase I enzymes make drugs more water soluble, enabling their elimination. Phase I enzymes involved in the transformation of psychotropics include the cytochrome P450 (CYP) family, epoxide hydrolases (EH), flavin-containing monooxygenases (FMOs), esterases, and microsomal epoxide hydrolases (mEH). The most studied are the CYP P450 superfamily of enzymes, named because they absorb 450 nm wavelength light when reduced and bound by carbon monoxide. This superfamily of heme-containing proteins is embedded within the endoplasmic reticulum of the liver, kidneys, brain, etc. Their primary role is the biotransformation of endogenous substances and xenobiotics, including drugs [16, 17]. Approximately forty isoforms have been identified. However, only six enzymes are responsible for the metabolism of almost 90% of all phase I drugs, including psychotropic drugs: CYP1A2, CYP2B6, CYP2C9, CYP2C19, CYP2D6, and CYP3A4 [18]. Overall, the human genome encodes 57 functional CYP genes and 58 pseudogenes [19]. Their expression is influenced by many patient-specific factors including genetic polymorphisms, sex, age, regulation by cytokines, hormones, disease states, as well as induction and inhibition by xenobiotics. Pharmacogenomics studies done in the early 1990s identified the first *CYP2D6* loss-of-function alleles [20–22]. Since, over a hundred mutations have been identified in *CYP*s involved in the metabolism of psychotropics and with differences in allelic frequency worldwide [23].

Mutations in *CYP*s can be considered in terms of genetics, such as loss or gain of function [24] and pharmacology or enzyme activity. Phenotype (enzyme activity) has been often simplified into four categories: poor metabolizer (no to little activity), intermediate metabolizer (reduced activity), extensive metabolizer (normal activity), and ultrarapid metabolizer (increased activity) [25]. For an active drug, loss-of-function alleles may reduce its clearance and increase the parent drug concentration (drug toxicity risk). For a prodrug, loss-of-function can do the opposite by reducing conversion to its active metabolite (lack of efficacy risk). Considering that almost 80% of drugs used in clinical practice, including psychotropics, are metabolized by CYPs, polymorphisms of human CYP450 have a substantial clinical impact [23, 26].

In addition to genetics, several non-genetic factors influence CYP450 enzyme expression and function. They include but are not limited to sex, age, presence of other drugs, disease states, and epigenetic influences. For example, one genome-wide gene expression profiling study found that sex affected mRNA expression of genes in the human liver. Out of 1249 sex-biased genes that were identified, 70% showed higher mRNA expression in females. Of 40 ADME-related genes identified in this study, *CYP1A2* and *CYP3A4* showed female bias [27], confirming earlier pharmacokinetics studies of hepatic CYP3A4 that found almost two-fold higher levels of proteins in females compared to males [28, 29]. Age is another important and well-established factor. This is of significant clinical relevance in neonates (immaturity of several CYP450 enzymes) and the elderly (diminished clearance) when prescribing medications with narrow therapeutic windows, such as antidepressants and antipsychotics [19, 30–33]. In the elderly, other factors of diminished clearance are drug interactions that are due to polypharmacy (more than five drugs), reduced hepatic blood flow, and reduced renal function [34].

CYP1A2

The *CYP1A2* is a member of the *CYP1A* subfamily and is located on chromosome 15q24.1 is expressed hepatically [35].

CYP1A2 (P450 family 1, subfamily A, polypeptide 2) mediates the rate-limiting steps of many clinically relevant drugs [36]. It is one of the major DMEs [37], and it accounts for 13–15% of hepatic cytochrome P450 [37–39]. Significant interindividual and intraindividual differences exist in the clearance of its substrates related to variability to the enzyme activity [37, 40]. Consequentially, the knowledge of CYP1A2 as an important contributor to drug interactions has increased over the past twenty years [41–43]. Variations in the enzyme activity are affected by genetics (up to 75%) and environmental factors such as smoking (induction) and oral birth control use (inhibition) [44].

Substrates of CYP1A2 subfamily include antipsychotics (chlorpromazine, trifluoperazine, clozapine, olanzapine, and haloperidol), tertiary amine tricyclics (amitriptyline, nortriptyline, and clomipramine), selective serotonin reuptake inhibitors (fluvoxamine), serotonin-norepinephrine reuptake inhibitors (duloxetine), and atypical antidepressant such as mirtazapine [45, 46]. CYP1A2 is inhibited by ciprofloxacin and fluvoxamine, both considered strong CYP1A2 inhibitors [47]. CYP1A2 enzyme is highly inducible by many substances, including drugs (carbamazepine, modafinil, omeprazole, phenobarbital, rifampin, etc.), dietary substances (caffeine, cruciferous vegetables, and meat cooked at high temperatures), and products of combustion such as cigarettes or cannabis smoke [48–50]. Smoking increases CYP1A2 enzyme activity and metabolism of CYP1A2 substrates [50–52], making it an important drug–substance interaction in a clinical setting. Studies show that a greater percentage of the variations is attributed to smoking, rather than genetic polymorphism of *CYP1A2 *1F* [53].

Caffeine is a common substrate and inducer of CYP1A2. It is often used as a probe for enzyme activity. *CYP1A2 *1F* was initially considered to be a relatively frequent variant, due to erroneous haplotype assignment. *CYP1A2 *1F* c.-163C>A SNP is associated with higher inducibility (increased enzyme activity) and increased metabolism of caffeine in Caucasian smokers [51]. *CYP1A2*1F/*1F* genotype might significantly influence olanzapine concentrations and treatment response [54].

Although evidence lacks for *CYP1A2* genotype-based guidance (drug-gene interactions), clinicians should consider the impact of inducers and inhibitors on concentration of CYP1A2 substrates (drug–drug and drug–exposome interactions).

CYP2B6

Historically, CYP2B6 (P450 family 2, subfamily B, polypeptide 6) has not attributed a significant role in drug metabolism. However, with the development of biologics, more drugs are metabolized through this pathway [55]. In addition, improvement in techniques to assess its expression and function revealed that CYP2B6 represents about 2–10% of total hepatic P450 content, responsible for the metabolism of about 10% of approved drugs [32, 40, 56, 57]. In all, it metabolizes about 90 substrates. However, there is wide variability in its enzyme expression with estimates of 20 to 250-fold in interindividual variations [56]. CYP2B6 metabolizes only a handful of psychiatry drugs including bupropion, clobazam, and ketamine [32, 56, 58]. The enzyme is inhibited by ticlopidine (strong), voriconazole (moderate), and induced by carbamazepine, phenobarbital, phenytoin, and some antivirals. In addition to being expressed in the liver, it is also found extra-hepatically in the brain, digestive tract, kidneys, and lungs [59].

CYP2B6 enzyme is encoded by *CYP2B6* (a functional gene) and *CYP2B7* (a nonfunctional gene or a pseudogene) with a wide variance in expression of up to 300-fold [39, 56, 57, 60, 61]. Both are located on chromosome 19 and within the CYP2ABFGST cluster [35]. Among 38 alleles and over 100 SNPs currently identified, several alleles are associated with changes in enzyme function. Pharmacokinetics studies of *CYP2B6* found that *4 allele carriers had 1.66-fold higher total bupropion clearance compared to *1 homozygous genotype ($p = 0.001$) and significantly higher Cmax of 4-hydroxybupropion compared to all other studied genotypes (*1, *2, *5, and *6) [62].

Evidence of intra and interethnic variabilities exist for *6 and *18 alleles. *CYP2B6* *6, a combination of *4 and *9 alleles, represents a decreased function allele frequently found in Africans. Individuals with *CYP2B6* *6/*6 genotype are at increased risk of side effects from some CYP2B6 substrates [32, 62–64]. An increased function allele, *4, reported as more frequent in Africans and Americans compared to other populations. Its average frequency is about 9% with the greatest prevalence found in African (up to 45%), Hispanic (27%), European (21%), and Asian (19%) populations [65].

CYP2C
The *CYP2C9* (P450 family 2, subfamily C, polypeptide 9) enzyme metabolizes about 15% to 20% of drugs that undergo phase I metabolism, including warfarin and phenytoin [66, 67]. It is encoded by *CYP2C9* as one of the several *CYP2C* clusters on chromosome 10q24. Four members of the *CYP2C* subfamily, *CYP2C8, CYP2C9, CYP2C18,* and *CYP2C19,* are found in a single gene locus on chromosome 10 [35, 68, 69]. Encoded enzymes are involved in the metabolism of approximately 20% of drugs, including psychotropics. Expressed primarily in the liver, CYP2C enzymes account for 20% of hepatic CYP content [37]. Quantitatively, CYP2C9 it is the second-highest among all hepatic CYP isoforms, right after CYP3A4 [70]. In psychiatry, substrates of CYP2C9 include amitriptyline, doxepin, fluoxetine, phenytoin, valproic acid, and venlafaxine. Substrates of CYP2C19 include diazepam, phenytoin, some selective serotonin reuptake inhibitors (SSRIs), and tricyclic antidepressants (TCAs) [9, 71–74].

CYP2C19. The CYP2C19 (P450 family 2, subfamily C, polypeptide 19) enzyme is expressed in various tissues, including the liver, gut, and brain [75]. It metabolizes 8% to 10% of prescription drugs, including many psychotropics [38, 76, 77]. Psychotropic substrates for CYP2C19 enzyme are SSRIs (esp. citalopram, escitalopram, and sertraline), TCAs (esp. amitriptyline, clomipramine, and imipramine), clozapine, diazepam, olanzapine, and others. The enzyme is inhibited in pregnancy and can be either inhibited or induced by several drugs. For example, fluoxetine is a moderate CYP2C19 inhibitor [78, 79].

The CYP2C19 enzyme is encoded by *CYP2C19*, spanning nine coding exons [80]. *CYP2C19* is a highly polymorphic gene with phenotypes ranging from poor to ultrarapid metabolizers. A splice mutation *2 (rs4244285) is the most common loss of function allele with the highest allelic frequency in Asians (30%), Africans (18%), and Caucasians (18%). The majority of PMs have *2 allele (86% in Caucasians and 69–87% in East Asians [23, 80, 81].

Another common loss-of-function allele is *3 (rs4986893), resulting from a premature stop codon. It is found more frequently in East Asians (7%) compared to other populations [79]. The most common increased function allele or gain-of-function is *17 (rs12248560), found in Caucasians and Africans at 23% frequency and virtually absent in East Asians [23].

Of psychotropics, the pharmacokinetics of several drugs from SSRIs and TCA classes of antidepressants are affected by *CYP2C19* polymorphisms. The clinically meaningful impact is documented with an altered concentration ratio of racemic citalopram, escitalopram, and sertraline [82, 83].

CYP2D6

CYP2D6 is one of the most studied and polymorphic pharmacogenes. Currently over 130 alleles have been identified [84]. It belongs in the *CYP2D* subfamily that also includes two pseudogenes, *CYP2D7* and *CYP2D8* [85]. Nine exons that encode for CYP2D6 (P450 family 2, subfamily C, polypeptide 19) enzyme are found on chromosome 22 (22q13.2). The enzyme is embedded in the phospholipid bilayer of the endoplasmic reticulum found in the brain, intestinal, liver, and lymphoid cells [13, 75, 84, 86, 87]. Although its hepatic content is only 1.5–4% [23, 26, 88], CYP2D6 is involved in the metabolism of 20–25% of commonly used drugs, including many antidepressants and antipsychotic drugs [89, 90]. CYP2D6 is largely non-inducible by other drugs. In vivo studies show that endo- and xenobiotics, along with cortisol rise in pregnancy, can induce the enzyme [91]. On the other hand, many drugs can inhibit it, including psychotropics such as bupropion, duloxetine, fluoxetine, haloperidol, paroxetine, etc. [92–94]. Among 70 drugs that have *CYP2D6* listed in their FDA-approved product label, 35 are psychiatry drugs. (Please refer to Table 1 with the FDA pharmacogenomic biomarkers in drug labeling, CPIC, and DPWG drug-gene pairs.)

Table 1 Worldwide distribution of common variants in the *CYP2C19* and *CYP2D6* genes and their allelic frequency [23]

Allele	Enzyme activity	Europeans	Africans	East Asian	South Asians	Americans
CYP2C19*2	Decreased	18.3	18.1	31.0	34.0	10.1
CYP2C19*3	Decreased	Rare	Rare	6.7	Rare	Rare
CYP2C19*17	Increased RM, UM	22.4	23.5	1.5	13.6	12.0
CYP2D6xN Amplification	Increased	2.3	9.3	2	1.5	1
CYP2D6 *3	Inactive	4.1	Rare	Rare	Rare	Rare
CYP2D6*4	Inactive	15.5	11.9	Rare	11.6	15.7
CYP2D5*5 Depletion	Inactive	3	4	6.5	2	3
CYP2D6*6	Inactive	2.2	Rare	Rare	Rare	Rare
CYP2D6*9	Decreased	1.6	Rare	Rare	Rare	1.3
CYP2D6*10	Decreased	Rare	3.2	58,7	6.5	Rare
CYP2D6*17	Decreased	Rare	19.7	Rare	Rare	1
CYP2D6*29	Decreased	Rare	9.2	Rare	Rare	Rare
CYP2D6*41	Decreased	3.0	3.0	3.0	13.5	3.5

CYP2D6 is the most studied DME gene [71, 90, 95–98]. Realizing that many drugs in psychiatry are CYP2D6 substrates and much intraindividual difference exist in the enzyme activity, commercially available pharmacogenomics clinical decision support tools typically include common alleles of *CYP2D6*. This means that many rare variants are often left unassessed. Although rare, these variants can contribute to changes in enzyme activity. Therefore, testing for only common alleles can lead to false-negative results defined as normal (wild) metabolizer phenotype or activity score 1.

Worldwide distribution and frequency of *CYP2D6* variants are excellently summarized by Zhou et al., based on their meta-analysis of population-scale DME genes sequenced [23]. There are three types of *CYP2D6* genetic variants: null allele (no functional enzyme), decrease transcription allele (reduced enzyme activity), and increased transcription allele (increased enzyme activity). For example, *4 allele (haplotype) accounts for the majority of poor metabolizer (PM) phenotype and is commonly found in Caucasians and Africans with an estimated frequency of 15.5 and 11.9, respectively. Another common PM is a complete deletion allele *5, found to be highest in East Asians (6.5%), then in Africans (4%) and European Caucasians and Americans (3%). Allele *10 is associated with reduced activity and is the highest in East Asians (58.7%) compared to South Asians (6.5%), while rare in Europeans and Americans. Similarly, *17 is a reduced function allele, found majorly in Africans (19.7%). Another reduced activity allele *41 is the most common intermediate metabolizer (IM) phenotype in South Asians (13.5%) and the most common in Europeans and Americans (3% and 3.5%). (Refer to the allelic frequency in Table 1, adapted from Zhou et al., 2017 study).

3   Pharmacodynamic Genes

Several genes encoding drug transporters and drug receptors have been investigated for their potential association with psychotropics drug response. The strongest association is with *HLA* and antiepileptic hypersensitivity reaction that led to the genotype-based guidelines. For antidepressants, *SLC64A*, *5HTR2A*, *5HTR1A*, and *GRIK4* were found with the most significant associations. For antipsychotics, *DRD2*, *DRD3*, *SL6A4*, and others were investigated for associations.

3.1   *HLA* genes

The human leukocyte antigens (HLA) are proteins that help recognize self from non-self and are associated with drug-induced hypersensitivity reactions. HLAs present non-self proteins, such as microbial peptides, to the immune system for the destruction of infected cells. They are encoded by HLA genes, which are some of the most polymorphic genes in humans [99]. Of many variants examined, *HLA-B*15:02* and *HLA-A*31:01* genotypes have the strongest evidence of prediction for drug-induced hypersensitivity reactions [100, 101].

*HLA-B*15:02* is associated with mood stabilizers-induced hypersensitivity reactions. The strongest association is with carbamazepine (OR = 80.7) and oxcarbazepine (OR = 26.1) [102, 103]. In patients taking carbamazepine, *HLA-A*31:01* is also predictive for severe drug reactions that can be life-threatening, such as, Stevens-Johnson syndrome, toxic epidermal necrolysis, and drug rash with eosinophilia and systemic symptoms (OR = 5.65) [102, 104, 105]. Carbamazepine has a black box warning against use in *HLA-B*15:02* positive patients, stating they "should not be treated unless the benefit clearly outweighs the risk." Caution is also advised in patients positive for *HLA-A*31:0*. Oxcarbazepine label cautions of "increased risk of SJS" but does not advise drug avoidance [106].

Drug-gene pairs of carbamazepine and *HLA-B*15:02*/HLA-A*31:01 have the highest level of evidence by CPIC (A) and PharmGKB (1A). For treatment naïve patients, the CPIC guidelines recommend avoiding carbamazepine use if positive for both variants and avoiding oxcarbazepine if positive for *HLA-B*15:02. If taken more than 3 months, SJS/TEN are unlikely to develop [107].

3.2   *SCL6A4*

Serotonin transporter, also known as a solute carrier family 6, member 4 (SLC6A4), transports serotonin from the synaptic cleft into pre-synaptic neurons. This protein, encoded by *SLC64A*, is a primary drug target of both SSRIs and

SNRIs. There are several polymorphisms of *SLC6A4* examined for their role in SSRI and SNRI response. Of these, two polymorphisms stand out [108, 109].

L or S alleles. The first is a functional polymorphism in the transporter-linked polymorphic region (5-HTTLPR or rs4795541). It results in the insertion/deletion of 44-base pair repeats represented by either the L allele (increased transcription) or S allele (decreased transcription). Studies have shown an association between homozygous S allele and inadequate or reduced response to SSRIs when compared to patients who were homozygous L allele [110, 111]. A 2006 meta-analysis by Serretti et al. of 1,433 SSRI-treated patients from 15 studies showed that the presence of the L allele in Caucasians was associated with increased remission and better response rates (OR = 2.21 and OR = 1.72) [112].

The lack of association in Asian patients was again found in another meta-analysis of 5408 patients from 28 studies [113, 114].

Ethnic differences exist in allelic frequencies, where the L allele is found most frequently in people of African and Caucasian European descent (83%, 60%) and less frequently in Japanese, Korean, and Chinese descent (20%, 23%, and 26%) [115–119]. On the other hand, the S allele was more common in the Japanese, Korean, and Chinese populations than the African or Caucasian populations (17%, 40%). Additionally, in Korean and Japanese patients, S allele was associated with a better therapeutic response compared to the L allele [110, 120, 121].

LA or LG alleles. The second is the SNP rs25531, found within the L allele of the promoter region (*5-HTTLPR*). There are two variations called L_G and L_A, depending on the presence of G or A. In L_G, the functional A>G variation reduces mRNA expression to the level of S allele ("lower function" phenotype), while L_A increased mRNA expression that results in a "higher function" phenotype.

There are no SLC6A4 genotype-based guidelines for any psychotropics. The CPIC comments on "increasing evidence" of these variants and drug response that may warrant future dosing recommendations [9, 72].

3.3   *HTR2A, HTR1A*

HTR2A encodes the postsynaptic serotonin 2A receptor, 5-HTR$_{2A}$. The receptor is a drug target of antidepressants and antipsychotics. These drugs downregulate and block it [122]. Several polymorphisms of *HTR2A* have been investigated for variation in drug response. These include: rs6311 (-1438G>A) promoter polymorphism and two coding region polymorphisms, rs6313 (102C>T), and rs6314 (135C>T). A 2020 meta-analysis of 16 studies did not find a significant difference in predicting an antidepressant response, citing more research needed [123].

The only other SNP, rs7997012 (IVS2 A>G), showed predictive value for citalopram in a Caucasian population from the STAR*D cohort. Homozygous A carriers had an 18% reduction in absolute risk of treatment failure compared to homozygous G carriers [124, 125]. Contradicting results were described by

[126]. They evaluated 637 German Caucasians with MDD treated with a variety of antidepressants. Those with the A allele did worse, compared to the G allele.

There are currently no *5HTR2A* genotype-based recommendations with level 1 evidence per PharmGKB. They annotate 2B level of evidence for citalopram and *HTR2A* while the rest of antidepressants have an even lower level of evidence.

HTR1A encodes serotonin receptor 1A (5-HT$_{1A}$) The receptor is downregulated by chronic SSRIs treatment and blocked by other antidepressants, resulting in increased serotonin transmission and levels [127–129]. Of several *HTR1A* polymorphisms, rs6295 is associated with increased receptor expression and antidepressant response with fluoxetine, nefazodone, or flibanserin with Homozygous G carriers that were more prevalent in those who responded. Opposite results were shown in other studies, including, where the G allele was associated with better treatment response in female patients [130]. Heterogeneity of major depressive disorder, ethnicity, and differences in allelic frequencies may have contributed to these conflicting findings. There are currently no HTR1A genotype-based guidelines for any psychotropics.

3.4   *GRIK4*

Glutamate receptors bind glutamate, an excitatory neurotransmitter in the brain. Increased levels of glutamate were seen in patients with MDD and other conditions such as autism spectrum disorders [131, 132]. Chronic use of SSRIs is associated with reduced glutamate activity. In a STAR*D genome-wide association study, an SNP rs1954787 had a significant association with antidepressant response. This SNP, found on the first intron of the glutamate receptor, ionotropic, and kainite 4 gene (*GRIK4*), was associated with a better response to citalopram in homozygous C allele carriers compared to T allele carriers [133]. There are currently no *GRIK4* genotype-based guidelines for antidepressants, including citalopram.

3.5   *DRD2, DRD3,* and *DRD4*

There are five types of dopamine receptors and of those, D2, D3, and D4 have an association with an antipsychotic response.

DRD2 encodes the D2 receptor, blocked by all antipsychotics, ith higher specificity by the first-generation such as haloperidol compared to the second-generation antipsychotics such as aripiprazole. Excessive blockade at D2 receptors is associated with extrapyramidal side effects (acute dystonic reactions, akathisia, rigidity, tremors, etc.) [135–138]. Of the several polymorphisms identified with DRD2, the −141-C Ins/Del polymorphism (rs1799732) in the promoter region is associated with altered D2 receptor density and antipsychotic response. Either no association or conflicting findings from several studies [133, 134, 139–141]. There are currently no DRD2 nor DRD3 genotype-based guidelines for antipsychotics.

DRD3 encodes the D3 receptor. Its Ser9Gly polymorphism is associated with an antipsychotic response. Gly allele is associated with less response seen in patients treated with chlorpromazine, clozapine, and risperidone [142–145].

DRD4 encodes the D4 receptor, the preferential binding site of clozapine (tenfold higher activity compared to D2 and D3 receptors). A common variable number of tandem repeat polymorphisms was investigated for clozapine response. Although an initial study showed a positive association, subsequent studies did not [146 148].

4   PGx of Psychotropic Drugs

4.1   Antidepressants

Antidepressants are the cornerstone pharmacotherapy for the treatment of mental health disorders. They are the first-line therapy for major depressive disorder (MDD) that affects more than 280 million people worldwide [149]. MDD is a highly heterogeneous and prevalent illness associated with significant disability, morbidity, and mortality [150]. Various factors likely contribute to adverse outcomes, including increased risk of suicide. pre-existing conditions pathophysiological changes that may lead to other chronic diseases, decreased treatment adherence, and unhealthy lifestyle [151–153]. Antidepressants regulate serotonin, norepinephrine, dopamine, and neurotransmitters hypothesized to be associated with mood and other psycho-neurological disorders [154]. There are several classes of antidepressants, based on their target site and effects on neurotransmitters: serotonergic only (SSRIs, SRAs), serotonergic/noradrenergic (SNRIs, TCAs, mirtazapine), dopaminergic/noradrenergic (bupropion), and drugs that mediate serotonin, epinephrine (noradrenaline), and dopamine (MAOIs). Their desired effects and side effects are closely tied to their mechanism of action.

Pharmacogenetics and Evidence

Despite several drug classes used in MDD treatment, many patients experience a lack of efficacy and adverse drug events [155]. The pivotal STAR*D trial (the sequenced treatment alternatives to relieve depression) found that 49% of first-episode patients responded to an antidepressant, 37% achieved remission after the first-line treatment, and only 13% after the fourth line treatment [156]. It is estimated that in the US about 25,000 patients per year seek emergency department services due to antidepressant-induced or related adverse events [157]. According to the National Institute of Mental Health, many contributing factors affect pharmacotherapy outcomes, both patients specific and environmental [158]. Genetics was assumed to play a role too, but it was not until 2013 that data showed how extensively. Tansey et al. were the first to demonstrate that genetics contributed significantly to an antidepressant response [159]. They performed genome-wide association studies of 2899 patients, including those from the STAR*D trial.

They found that genetic variants accounted for 42% of interindividual variations, suggesting a polygenic (more than one gene) trait of antidepressant response.

Numerous pharmacogenetics (a single gene-drug) and pharmacogenomics (many genes-drug) studies examined the effect of genetic variants on psychotropic drugs [139]. While many more are underway, the current evidence supports only four genes as "clinically actionable" [11]. "Clinically actionable" refers to the genotype-based guidelines from the CPIC and/or DPWG that gives prescribing information and guidance for psychotropics. These four genes are *CYP2D6, CYP2C19, HLA-A*31:01*, and *HLA-B*15:02*. The first two, *CYP2D6* and *CYP2C19,* are **pharmacokinetic genes of drug-metabolizing enzymes** associated with altered drug levels and drug response of several antidepressants and antipsychotics. *HLA* refers to human leukocyte complex genes that encode proteins that help the immune system distinguish self from non-self. To date, there are no HLA-antidepressant clinically actionable drug-gene pairs. CPIC and CPNDS guidelines warn of increased risk of hypersensitivity reactions with carbamazepine (for more, see Anti-epileptics).

In addition to drug-metabolizing enzyme genes, **drug transporters and drug targets** genes have been studied for their effects on the **pharmacodynamics** of antidepressants. The most significant evidence to date is for *SLC64A* and *HTR2A*. *SLC6A4*, the serotonin transporter gene, is associated with treatment outcomes in MDD and depression [160–164]. Pharmacogenetics of SLC6A4 short and long alleles are described in part 1 of this chapter. L allele seems to be associated with better response to antidepressants, with ethnic differences, but further studies are needed for conclusive clinical guidance.

The postsynaptic 5-HT$_{2A}$, (serotonin receptor type 2A) was observed to be overexpressed in the frontal cortex of patients with depression, especially suicide victims (Stanley 1983, 86). SSRIs block and downregulate 5-HT$_{2A}$, thought to account for their therapeutic effects. Studies that investigated polymorphism of **HTR2A**, encoding the receptor, have conflicting results. McMahon et al. study searched for genetic predictors of antidepressant treatment outcome among 1953 citalopram treated patients with MDD in the STAR*D study. Out of 768 SNPs, only IVS2 A>G (rs7997012) was associated with treatment outcome (*P* range $1 \times 10(-6)$ to $3.7 \times 10(-5)$ in the total sample), but with racial differences. Carriers of the A allele were predominantly white patients (six times more compared to black patients), and those who carried two copies of this variant (AA genotype) had an 18% reduction in absolute risk of treatment failure compared to the GG genotype [124].

A 2020 study by Kao et al. aimed to identify which genetic variants are related to both MDD susceptibility and antidepressant response. Their meta- and mega-analysis found the association between 5-HT$_{2A}$ variants and antidepressant response. A total of 14 polymorphisms were identified as potential markers for therapeutic response: 13 were related for remission and 1 for a response. However, they did not find an association with MDD susceptibility [165]. Lack of association was also found in a 2021 meta-analysis by Yan et al. between −1438

A>G variant with bulimia nervosa. However, Caucasian carriers of the A allele had a significantly higher risk of anorexia nervosa compared to Asian patients [166].

The most promising results related to antidepressant response were published in 2021. In a meta-analysis of forty-two studies, Wan et al. found significant associations of 5-HT$_{2A}$ polymorphisms (1438A/G, 102T/C, and rs7997012G/A) correlating with the safety and efficacy of antidepressants [167]. It remains to be seen how this and other emerging evidence may inform the genotype-guided prescribing based on this pharmacodynamic gene.

Drug Classes and Guidelines

Based on the existing evidence, SSRIs and TCAs have the highest level (1A) of guideline recommendations among antidepressants. Recently, Murphy et al., found that genotype-based guidelines for antidepressants and antipsychotics help implementation of pharmacogenomics into clinical practice [168]. Refer to Table 2 for a list of other drugs with PGx biomarkers found in their FDA labels and other professional guidelines.

Selective serotonin reuptake inhibitors (SSRI). Most SSRIs have genotype-based guideline recommendations. Substrates of CYP2C19 (citalopram, escitalopram, and sertraline) and CYP2D6 (fluvoxamine and paroxetine) have prescribing information by CPIC and DPWG and drug label annotations from several sources, including the FDA based on CYP2C19 and CYP2D6 genotypes. Currently, there is no clinical recommendation based on pharmacodynamic genes such as *SLC6A4* or *HTR2A*.

For CYP2C19 UMs, predicted to be at risk of therapy failure, the CPIC guideline for citalopram and escitalopram recommends an alternative not metabolized by CYP219. For CYP2C19 PMs, predicted to be at increased risk of side effects, the CPIC guideline for citalopram and escitalopram recommends a 50% dose reduction of the recommended starting dose. Additionally, they advise prescribers to titrate to response or to use an alternative not metabolized by CYP2C19 [9]. These drug-gene pairs have the highest level of evidence 1A by PharmGKB. The rest of the drug-gene pairs such as *ABCB1*, *GRIK4*, *HTR2A*, and *SLC6A4* has a lower level of evidence 3 or 4 [169].

The DPWG guidelines recommendations differ for citalopram and escitalopram compared to the CPIC guidelines. The DPWG recommends "no action needed" for CYP2C19 UMs. They also updated their guidelines in 2018 [11]. The updated guidelines recommend that IMs and PMs do not exceed recommended daily dose of citalopram based on age: 30 mg (tablet) or 22 mg (drops) in IMs up to 65 years and 15 mg (tablet) or 10 mg (drops) in PMs older than 65 years, due to increased risk of QT prolongation and torsades de pointes associated with increased plasma levels of citalopram. For CYP2C19 UMs, they recommend not to use escitalopram and instead use CYP2D6 substrates, such as fluvoxamine and paroxetine. Similar to citalopram, escitalopram's max dose is based on genotype and age: for IMs that dose should not exceed 75% of the standard max dose (if or older than 65 years, max dose is 7.5 mg), and for PMs dose should not exceed 50% of the standard

Table 2 Common psychotropic drugs with PGx biomarkers in FDA label and other professional guidelines

Drug	Class	FDA label	Drug label annotations	CPIC	DPWG
Amitriptyline	TCA	Precaution	FDA	CYP2C19 CYP2D6	CYP2D6 CYP2C19*
Amphetamine	Stimulant	Clinical pharmacology	FDA		
Aripiprazole, aripiprazole lauroxil	Antipsychotic (atypical)	Dosage and administration, use in specific populations, clinical pharmacology	EMA FDA HCSC Swissmedic		CYP2D6
Atomoxetine	Stimulant	Dosage and administration, warnings and precautions, adverse reactions, drug interactions, use in specific populations, clinical pharmacology	FDA HCSC PMDA Swissmedic	CYP2D6	CYP2D6
Brexpiprazole	Antipsychotic (atypical)	Dosage and administration, use in specific populations, clinical pharmacology	EMA FDA Swissmedic		CYP2D6
Bupropion	DNRI	Clinical pharmacology	FDA		
Cariprazine		Clinical pharmacology	FDA		
Citalopram	SSRI	CYP2D6 Clinical pharmacology	FDA HCSC Swissmedic	CYP2C19	CYP2C19 CYP2D6*
Citalopram	SSRI	CYP2C19 dosage and administration, warnings, clinical pharmacology			
Clomipramine	TCA	Precautions	FDA Swissmedic	CYP2C19 CYP2D6	CYP2C19 CYP2D6

(continued)

Table 2 (continued)

Drug	Class	FDA label	Drug label annotations	CPIC	DPWG
Clozapine	Antipsychotic (atypical)	Dosage and administration, use in specific populations, clinical pharmacology	FDA		CYP2D6*
Desipramine	TCA	Precautions	FDA	CYP2D6	
Desvenlafaxine	SNRI	Clinical pharmacology CYP2D6	FDA		
Doxepin	TCA	CYP2C19 Clinical pharmacology	FDA	CYP2C19 CYP2D6	CYP2C19* CYP2D6
Duloxetine	SNRI	Drug interactions	EMA FDA Swissmedic		CYP2D6*
Escitalopram	SSRI	CYP2C19 adverse reactions CYP2D6 drug interactions	FDA HCSC	CYP2C19	CYP2C19 CYP2D6*
Fluoxetine	SSRI	Precautions, clinical pharmacology	FDA Swissmedic		CYP2D6*
Fluvoxamine	SSRI	Drug interactions	FDA Swissmedic	CYP2D6	CYP2C19* CYP2D6*
Iloperidone	Antipsychotic (atypical)	Dosage and administration, warnings and precautions, drug interactions, clinical pharmacology	FDA		
Imipramine	TCA	Precautions	FDA	CYP2C19 CYP2D6	CYP2C19 CYP2D6
Modafinil	Stimulant	Clinical pharmacology	FDA		
Nefazodone	TCA	Precautions	FDA		
Nortriptyline	TCA	Precautions	FDA HCSC	CYP2D6	CYP2D6
Paliperidone	Antipsychotic (atypical)	Clinical pharmacology	FDA Swissmedic		

(continued)

Table 2 (continued)

Drug	Class	FDA label	Drug label annotations	CPIC	DPWG
Paroxetine	SSRI	Drug interactions, clinical pharmacology	FDA	CYP2D6	CYP2D6
Perphenazine	Antipsychotic (typical)	Precautions, clinical pharmacology	FDA PMDA		
Pimozide	Antipsychotic (typical)	Dosage and administration, precautions	FDA		CYP2D6
Protriptyline	TCA	Precautions	FDA		
Risperidone	Antipsychotic (atypical)	Clinical pharmacology	FDA HCSC Swissmedic		CYP2D6
Thioridazine	Antipsychotic (typical)	Contraindications, warnings, precautions	FDA		
Trimipramine	TCA	Precautions	FDA	CYP2C19 CYP2D6	
Venlafaxine	SNRI	Drug interactions, use in specific populations, clinical pharmacology	FDA Swissmedic		CYP2D6
Vortioxetine	SPARI	Dosage and administration, clinical pharmacology	EMA FDA HCSC Swissmedic		

dose (if or older than 65 years, max dose is 5 mg/day) due to increased risk of WT prolongation and torsades de pointes [10].

Both *CYP2B6* and *CYP2C19* genetic variants can affect sertraline metabolism in patients with MDD [170]. However, *CYP2C19* polymorphisms have a greater pharmacokinetic effect than other *CYP*s. Increased metabolism and reduced plasma levels of sertraline are seen in UMs, while reduced metabolism and increased plasma levels are seen in PMs [83, 171–173]. Currently, the CPIC guideline recommends that CYP2C19 PMs are initiated at 50% dose reduction and titrated to response or prescribed an alternative drug not metabolized by CYP2C19 [9]. In contrast, the DPWG recommends that in PMs maximum dose should not exceed 75 mg per day. They also recommend monitoring patients and guiding dose by the response, side effect, and/or sertraline plasma concentration [10]. For citalopram, escitalopram, and sertraline, *CYP2C19* is considered as "actionable PGx" by the FDA, HCSC, Swissmedic [169].

Of SSRIs metabolized by CYP2D6, only fluvoxamine and paroxetine have genotype-based guidelines. For fluvoxamine, CPIC recommends a 25–50% reduction of recommended starting dose for CYP2D6 PMs. Additionally, they recommend titrating to response or using an alternative drug not metabolized by CYP2D6 [9]. The DPWG does not have CYP2D6 genotype-based recommendations at this time [10]. For paroxetine, the CPIC recommends that UMs and PMs are prescribed an alternative drug not metabolized by CYP2D6. In case that paroxetine is strongly indicated in PMs, they advise initiating at 50% dose reduction of the recommended dose and titrate to response [9]. The DPWG only has recommendations for UMs currently. Like CPIC they also recommend an alternative to paroxetine for CYP2D6 UMs [10]. Drug label annotations for fluvoxamine as "actionable PGx" by the FDA and Swissmedic [11].

Serotonin partial agonist reuptake inhibitors (SPARI). *Vilazodone* is both an SSRI and $5HT_{1A}$ receptor partial agonist or serotonin partial agonist reuptake inhibitor (SPARI) approved for the treatment of MDD [174, 175]. Practically speaking, vilazodone is a crossover between SSRIs antidepressants and anxiolytic buspirone. At doses over 40 mg, it occupies about 50% of serotonin transporters and serotonin receptor type 1A [176]. It is primarily metabolized by CYP3A4, with minor metabolism by CYP2C19 and CYP2D6 [174]. Currently, there are no clinical or drug label annotations to guide prescribing.

Multimodal antidepressant. *Vortioxetine* has a unique mechanism of action, compared to other serotonin-modulating drugs. Like vilazodone, it has two pharmacodynamic targets: the serotonin transporter (it inhibits SERT) and serotonin receptors (it is an agonist at $5\text{-}HT_{1A}$ receptor). Unlike vilazodone, vortioxetine is also a $5\text{-}HT_3$, $5\text{-}HT_7$, and $5\text{-}HT_{1D}$ receptor antagonist, and $5\text{-}HT_{1B}$ receptor partial agonist [177]. Due to its complex neuromodulating activity in multiple systems beyond serotonin (norepinephrine, dopamine, acetylcholine, histamine, glutamate, and GABA), vortioxetine may affect the neuronal network involved in the mood and cognition changes seen in MDD [178–182]. It is firstly and primarily metabolized by hepatic CYP2D6, with smaller contributions from many other CYPs, to inactive metabolites, further metabolized by UGTs [183]. There are currently no genotype-based recommendations. The only clinical annotation is for CYP2D6 but with level 3 evidence (low level). It is based on a meta-analysis of vortioxetine in healthy individuals. They observed decreased clearance of vortioxetine and twice as high increased exposure in CYP2D6 PMs compared to NMs in healthy volunteers but did not report on the significance of such association [184]. Actionable PGx is considered by the EMA, FDA, HCSC, and Swissmedic.

Tricyclic antidepressants (TCA). Polymorphisms of *CYP2C19* and *CYP2D6* can significantly affect the pharmacokinetics of TCAs [173, 185, 186]. CYP2C19 metabolizes the tertiary amines (e.g., amitriptyline and imipramine) to their active metabolites, the secondary amines (nortriptyline and desipramine). CYP2D6 enzyme metabolizes both the tertiary and secondary amines into less active hydroxy metabolite [185]. Prescribing guidelines exist based on these two genes.

Recently, PGx experts recommended standardizing CYP2D6 genotype translation to metabolizer phenotypes for greater consistency in interpreting CYP2D6 genotype. This discord is due to a lack of standardization across clinical PGx laboratories and PGx guidelines (CPIC and DPWG) [25].

Amitriptyline is a tertiary amine with many label-approved uses (MDD, OCD, PTSD, bulimia, etc.) and many off-label uses (enuresis, fibromyalgia, irritable bowel syndrome migraine prevention, neuropathic pain, etc.). Amitriptyline is metabolized by CYP2C19 to its active metabolite nortriptyline, further metabolized by CYP2D6 to its less active metabolite, hydroxy- nortriptyline [185]. CYP2C19 PMs have greatly reduced metabolism of amitriptyline to nortriptyline, associated with an increased risk of side effects from amitriptyline compared to NMs. CYP2D6 UMs have significantly increased metabolism to the less active metabolite compared to NMs, associated with an increased risk of therapy failure [72, 187–189]. Both the CPIC and DPWG give prescribing guidance. The CPIC guidelines, from December 2016 update, are based on combinatory results of *CYP2C19* and *CYP2D6*. They recommend that an alternative drug be used for CYP2D6 UMs or PMs and CYP2C19 URs, RMs, and PMs. If amitriptyline is clinically necessary for phenotypes aforementioned, they recommend a 50% dose reduction in either PMs of CYP2C19 or CYP2D6 and a 25% dose reduction for CYP2D6 IMs [72]. Since the 2016 update, CPIC conducted a modified-Delphi project for a uniform system for translating CYP2D6 genotype to phenotype, using an activity score (AS). In the most recent CPIC update from October 2019, they incorporate their consensus terminology. Specifically, 25% dose reduction in IMs correlates to AS of 1, making it an "optional recommendation." They also downgraded the value of the *CYP2D6*10* allele from 0.5 to 0.25, which for homozygous *10*, changed their phenotype from 1 (NM) to 0.5 (IM). Currently, the authors of the original TCA guidelines are in the process of updating them [25, 72].

The DPWG does not have CYP219 genotype-based recommendations for amitriptyline. They do recommend a dose decrease for CYP2D6 IMs (75% of the standard dose) and PMs (70% of the standard dose) with monitoring for both efficacy and side effects. For Ums, they recommend dose increase for UMs (1.4 times the standard dose) or if to avoid amitriptyline if dose increase results in increased cardiotoxicity risk [10].

The FDA has an "actionable PGx" annotation stating that CYP2D6 PMs may have higher drug concentration and recommends drug monitoring with concomitant use of a CYP2D6 inhibitor. These discrepancies between regulatory bodies present a challenge to clinicians and implementors of PGx [11, 190].

Nortriptyline is an active metabolite of amitriptyline. It is further metabolized by CYP2D6 into a less active metabolite, 10-hydroxynortriptyline. The CPIC guideline recommends reducing the dose by 25% for CYP2D6 IMs, 50% for PMs (if use is warranted), and using an alternative for UMs or PMs [72]. The DPWG also recommend reducing dose for IMs or PMs and using an alternative for UMs. Additionally, for UMs, they advise using 1.7 times the standard dose and monitoring of nortriptyline and its metabolite for IMs, PMs, and UMs [10].

Imipramine is a tertiary amine metabolized by CYP2C19 into its active metabolite desipramine (secondary amine). Polymorphism of *CYP2C19* can affect pharmacokinetics and plasma concentration of imipramine, associated with drug response [185, 191]. The CPIC has specific recommendations for amitriptyline and nortriptyline, as prototypical representatives of the tertiary and secondary amines [72]. Therefore, considering their similar pharmacokinetic profiles within the class, the CPIC guidelines can be applied to other TCAs. For example, tertiary amines clomipramine and imipramine have the CPIC guidelines that reflect amitriptyline's prescribing recommendations based on a combinatory dosing algorithm of *CYP2C19* and *CYP2D6* genotypes.

Selective serotonin and norepinephrine reuptake inhibitors (SNRIs). *Venlafaxine* is metabolized by several CYPs enzymes. However, CYP2D6 is considered rate-limiting due to converting venlafaxine to its active metabolite, O-desmethylvenlafaxine. Currently, the only prescribing information is provided by the DPWG. For CYP2D6 UMs, they recommend increasing the dose or using an alternative drug to venlafaxine (lack of efficacy). Specifically, they advise being alert to a decrease in the plasma concentration of venlafaxine and its active metabolite (O-desmethylvenlafaxine) and to increasing the dose by 150% if clinically necessary. If a dose increase is not possible, they recommend a drug not metabolized by CYP2D6. For CYP2D6 IMs and PMs, they recommend prescribing an alternative drug (ex. Duloxetine, mirtazapine, citalopram, and sertraline) or reducing the dose for patients who are CYP2D6 PMs and IMs [10].

Desvenlafaxine is an active metabolite of venlafaxine and is marketed as a standalone drug. It is primarily metabolized by CYP3A4. There are currently no clinical annotations or prescribing information based on any drug-gene pairs. Interestingly, the FDA has an annotation for desvenlafaxine but as an "informative PGx" stating no difference in pharmacokinetics between CYP2D6 PMs and NMs [192].

Duloxetine is majorly metabolized by CYP1A2 and CYP2D6, while other CYPs contribute minorly. Several drug-gene pairs have been described, but all with level 3 evidence. Of these, gene *ANO2* anoctamin 2 (calcium-activated chloride channel) was found with several polymorphisms (rs61908409, rs61908410, rs61908410, etc.) associated with drug response (efficacy) to treatment with duloxetine in MDD [193]. Several other genes were also investigated, such as *DRD3* (dopamine receptor D3), *FCN2* (ficolin 2), *MIEF2* (mitochondrial elongation factor 2), *TEX10* (testis expressed 10), and others [193, 194].

Milnacipran is not metabolized by CYPs. Several variants, including adenoreceptor alpha 2A or *ADRA2A* (rs1800544), serotonin receptor 1A or *HTR1A* (rs6295, rs1364043, and rs10042486), and MAM domain-containing glycosylphosphatidylinositol anchor 2 or *MDGA2* (rs1160351), have been reported in respect to drug response, but with level 3 evidence [114, 195, 196]. There is currently no prescribing information based on *CYP2D6* or any other genotypes for desvenlafaxine, duloxetine, milnacipran, or levomilnacipran.

Norepinephrine and dopamine reuptake inhibitor (NDRI). *Bupropion* hydrochloride is a norepinephrine and dopamine reuptake inhibitor, available in three oral forms: immediate release or IR (dosed three times a day), sustained-release, or SR (dosed two times a day), and extended-release or XR (dosed once a day). It is approved as an antidepressant and non-nicotine smoking cessation treatment [197, 198]. Due to its unique mechanism of action and absence of sero-tonergic side effects (sexual dysfunction, weight gain, and somnolence), it is also used as an adjunct to other antidepressants in partial or non-responders [199, 200]. It is metabolized by hepatic CYPs to three major active metabolites [201]. The most active of the three is hydroxybupropion (HB), formed by CYP2B6. Although the parent drug and HB metabolite have similar half-lives (~20 h), C_{max} of hydroxybupropion is 4- to 7-fold higher, and the AUC is ~10-fold greater, compared with those of the parent drug [202].

Polymorphisms of CYP2B6 were associated with variations in the pharmacokinetics of bupropion [32, 62, 63]. In vitro studies showed that CYP2C19 is also involved in metabolism through alternative hydroxylation pathways and found to be concentration-dependent [203]. Supratherapeutic concentrations of bupropion and hydroxybupropion were described in a CYP2C19 RM (*1/*17 genotype), suggesting CYP2C19's role in the metabolism of the parent drug [204].

Although many more clinical annotations exist (*ANKK1, CHRNA5, COMT, DRD1, DRD2, SACM1L,* etc.), there are all level 3 evidence. Currently, there are no clinical annotations or prescribing guidance based on either *CYP2B6* or *CYP2C19* genotypes. Level 2A evidence is assigned for decreased function *CYP2B6* alleles (*6, and *18) in people with tobacco use disorder and decreased active metabo-lites when compared to NMs [205]. Adding bupropion into the patient's drug therapy should be taken with caution. Bupropion is a potent CYP2D6 inhibitor [202]. Annotation for the FDA drug label warns of its inhibitory effect and increased plasma concentration of antidepressants, antipsychotics, beta-blockers, and antiarrhythmics type 1C [206].

Tetracyclic amines. *Mirtazapine* is an atypical antidepressant, sometimes catego-rized as a noradrenergic and specific serotonergic antidepressant (NaSSA). The pharmacokinetics depend on age and sex: elderly and females have higher plasma concentrations compared to young and male adults. Mirtazapine, a racemic mixture of R and S enantiomers, is metabolized primarily by CYP2C6 and CYP3A4. Poly-morphisms of CYP2D6 were found to affect S-enantiomer with AUC 79% larger in PMs compared to NMs [207]. Although level 2A evidence exists for CYP2D6 in respect to mirtazapine clearance, there are currently no genotype-based guidelines by the CPIC, DPWG, or others [42].

Monoamine oxidase inhibitors (MAOIs). Monoamine oxidase inhibitors are unique among antidepressants due to their ability to increase levels of dopamine, epinephrine, and serotonin neurotransmitters. They inhibit the activity of the monoamine oxidase enzyme, a mitochondrial enzyme that breaks down these three neurotransmitters [208]. The consequent increase in the neurotransmitters is thought to be responsible for their therapeutic effects, especially in treatment-resistant MDD [209, 210].

There are two isoforms of MAO encoded by the *MAO-A* and *MAO-B* genes located on the X chromosome. Low MAO-A activity has been associated with a high risk of alcoholism, drug abuse, and impulsive behavior [211, 212]. The non-selective MAOIs cause irreversible inhibition and include isocarboxazid, phenelzine, and tranylcypromine. Selegiline is a selective inhibitor of MAO-B and is available in the US. Moclobemide is another reversible inhibitor, selective of MAO-A and available outside of the US [213]. A study by Becker et al. reported that the *SLC22A1* (rs622342) C allele was associated with an increased dose of selegiline in European patients with Parkinson's disease [214]. However, evidence is limited in respect to genetic variants and drug response. There are currently no genotype-based guidelines for any member of MAOIs drug class.

4.2   Antipsychotics

Antipsychotics are the first-line pharmacotherapy for the management of schizophrenia. They are also used for the treatment of other mental illnesses such as bipolar disorder. They are often prescribed for off-label uses, including management of agitations, anorexia nervosa, and chemotherapy-induced emesis [215, 216]. Considering their wide use, it should not be surprising that over 1% of the population uses antipsychotics [217]. A global 12-month lifetime psychosis prevalence is 0.7% while the prevalence of antipsychotic use in the US is estimated at 1.6% [218, 219]. Additionally, there is great variability in an antipsychotic response. An estimated 30–50% of patients have an inadequate response and significant, long-lasting side effects [220]. Several factors are thought to contribute including the age of symptom onset, adherence, comorbidities, diet, drug use, environment, gender, and genetics [220].

Pharmacogenetics and Evidence

Since the 1990s, many pharmacogenetics (a single gene-drug) and pharmacogenomics (many genes-drug) studies found associations between pharmacokinetic and/or pharmacodynamic genes and antipsychotic response [53, 173, 190, 221–226]. Candidate gene studies confirmed that variants in *CYP1A2, CYP2D6, CYP2C19. ABCB1, DRD2, DRD3, HTR2A, HTR2C, BDNF, COMT, and MC4R* were indeed associated with an antipsychotic response. Additionally, several genome-wide association studies discovered new associations between glutaminergic pathways and drug response [220, 227]. Despite such evidence, clinically actionable PGx markers of drug response are not fully solidified to guide prescribing. They are mostly confined to DME genes. Their genetic variants, especially of *CYP2D6*, have been implemented.

Antipsychotics undergo metabolism by several hepatic CYPs, including CYP1A2, CYP2C9, CYP2C19, CYP2D6, and CYP3A4 [227]. Of those, genetic variants in *CYP2D6* and *CYP1A2* have the most evidence of altered pharma-cokinetics and corresponding clinical outcomes. For example, patients who were CYP2D6 PMs or RMs were switched more frequently from risperidone to another antipsychotic. This was due to either increased risk of side effects in PMs or lack of efficacy in RMs [11]. Variants in the *CYP1A2* associated with increased plasma levels were behind a better response to olanzapine [8]. Concerning side effects, traditive dyskinesia (TD) is a common one. It causes repetitive, involuntary move-ments that are concerning to many patients. Several studies showed that a higher risk of traditive dyskinesia in patients with *CYP1A2* (*1D and *1F) and *CYP2D6* (*4) variants [228–230]. Pharmacogenomics studies also found that variants in genes encoding for serotonin (HTR$_{2A}$, HTR$_{2C}$) and dopamine receptors (DRD2, DRD3) were also associated with TD [231]. Like other pharmacodynamic studies of psychotropics, these potential biomarkers are of limited clinical value, likely due to the combinatory profile needed to predict antipsychotic response.

A recent assessment by Arranz et al. provides a comprehensive summary of pharmacogenomics studies done in the past five years with antipsychotics [220]. Citing the lack of guidelines by the CPIC and DPWG, they also included several publications containing recommendations on how to adjust a dose according to functional CYP polymorphisms [232, 233]. The DPWG comments on "reducing the maximum dose of aripiprazole for patients carrying poor metabolizer alleles of *CYP2D6*." For haloperidol, they recommend a dose reduction of 50% or an alter-native for CYP2D6 PMs. In patients who are CYP2D6 IMs needing pimozide, they recommend they "should be given no more than 80% of the standard max-imum dose" and that CYP2D6 PMs "should be given no more than 50% of the standard maximum dose" [10].

4.3   Mood Stabilizers

Mood stabilizers, such as carbamazepine, lamotrigine, oxcarbazepine, and val-proic acid, are used for the management of bipolar disorder. Bipolar disorder is a type of mood disorder that is characterized by episodes of depression and mania and is one of the leading causes of disability worldwide [234].

Carbamazepine (CBZ) and oxcarbazepine (OXC) are similar in structure but differ in their mechanism of action and metabolic pathways [235, 236]. They both strongly block sodium channels, but modulate different calcium channels. Both drugs are metabolized by CYP3A4. However, CBZ is a potent CYP inducer (many drug interactions), while OXC is a significantly weaker CYP inducer (fewer drug interactions) [237]. Genetic testing before their initiation and ongoing therapeutic monitoring are recommended.

Pharmacogenetics and Evidence

The CPIC guideline warns of *HLA-B* *15:02 genotype and risk of **carbamazepine- and oxcarbazepine**-induced Steven-Johnson syndrome (SJS) or toxic epidermal necrolysis (TEN), both potentially life-threatening hypersensitivity skin reactions

[238]. The *HLA-B*15:02* is associated with a greatly increased risk of CBZ-induced skin reactions. Its allelic frequency varies across the population at 7–16% found in Chinese, Malaysian, and Thai [239–241] and less than 1% found in Japanese and European populations [242]. The Canadian Pharmacogenomics Network for Drug Safety (CPDNS) guidelines also warns of the risk, recommend testing, and to use an alternative for CBZ-naïve patients with at least one *HLA-A*31:01* allele [11]. The DPWG recommends that CBZ be avoided and to select an alternative if positive for *HLA-B*15:02*, *HLA-A*31:01*, and *HLA-B*15:11* [106, 107]. For lamotrigine, the DPWG recommends weighting the risk versus benefits of the life-threatening cutaneous side effects such as Steven-Johnson syndrome/toxic epidermal necrolysis (SJS/TEN) that occurs more often in individuals with HLA*15:02. They recommend to select an alternative if available, other than CBZ [243]. For valproic acid, the FDA drug label indicates required testing for a mutation in mitochondrial DNA polymerase gamma (POLG) and suspected POLG-related disorder in children under 2 years old [5].

4.4   ADHD Medications

Atomoxetine and stimulants are used for symptom improvement and management of attention-deficit/hyperactivity disorder (ADHD). ADHD is a common neurodevelopment disorder in children and adolescents. It is considered a chronic disorder, and twin studies indicate a strong genetic component [244].

Atomoxetine (ATX) is a selective norepinephrine reuptake inhibitor that inhibits the norepinephrine transporter (SLC6A2). Of the pharmacokinetics studies done with *CYP2D6, CYP2C19, and SLC6A2* variations, the greatest impact was observed with CYP2D6 genetic variations, which was 10-fold higher in CYP2D6 PMs compared to non-PMs. Both the CPIC and DPWG have annotations for atomoxetine and CYP2D6. The CPIC has dosing recommendation based on CYP2D6 genotype for pediatric and adult patients. CYP2D6 PM status is associated with lower final dose requirements compared to non-PMs. In addition, greatly decreased metabolism of ATX may be associated with increased risk of side effects and greater improvement of symptoms [245]. Amphetamine, dextroamphetamine, lisdexamfetamine, methamphetamine, and methylphenidate lack genotype guided prescribing. The FDA drug label for amphetamine extended-release brand name has CYP2D6 as a PGx biomarker, acknowledging a possibility of variation in its metabolism due to *CYP2D6* polymorphisms [5].

4.5   Benzodiazepines

Benzodiazepines are some of the most frequently used drugs in a clinical practice, including psychiatry. They are used for many indications such as for management of anxiety disorders, sleep, and others. There are more than 20 drugs in the class and their primary receptor target is the GABA receptor. Many of them are metabolized by CYPs, such as CYP3A4/5 and CYP2C19 [246, 247]. However, evidence is limited related to *CYPs* polymorphism, drug concentration, and clinical impact. Clozapine's FDA indicates that reduced dose may be needed for CYP2D6 PMs [206]. They currently lack the CPIC, DPWG, or other genotype-based recommendations.

5 Conclusion

Despite numerous pharmacogenetics and pharmacogenomics studies, the current evidence supports only four genes as clinically actionable: *CYP2D6, CYP2C19, HLA-A*31:01*, and *HLA-B*15:02*. Consensus exists among professional organizations including the CPIC and DPWG that CYP2C19 and CYP2D6 be used to inform prescribing of several psychotropic drugs. While implementation efforts are rapidly growing, rare variants that are currently not assessed need to be taken into consideration. In addition to incorporating whole genomic sequencing for common and rare variants, clinicians will need to continue to assess other clinical factors, such as other drugs and substances, to help predict a drug response phenotype. Future algorithms will need to be built to help integrate genetics and clinical biomarkers to help clinicians in selecting the optimal pharmacotherapy for a patient.

References

1. Institute of Health Metrics and Evaluation. Global Health Data Exchange (GHDx). [Internet]. 2019. Available from: http://ghdx.healthdata.org/gbd-results-tool?params=gbd-api-2019-per malink/d780dffbe8a381b25e1416884959e88b. Accessed 13 Nov 2022.
2. Global Burden of Disease Studies. Implications for mental and substance use disorders. Health Aff. 2016;35(6):1114–20. https://doi.org/10.1377/hlthaff.2016.0082.
3. Dieleman JL, Baral R, Birger M, Bui AL, Bulchis A, Chapin A, et al. US spending on personal health care and public health, 1996–2013. JAMA. 2016;316(24):2627–46. https://doi.org/10.1001/jama.2016.16885.
4. Hiemke C, Bergemann N, Clement HW, Conca A, Deckert J, Domschke K, et al. Consensus guidelines for therapeutic drug monitoring in neuropsychopharmacology: update 2017. Pharmacopsychiatry. 2018;51(1–02):9–62. https://doi.org/10.1055/s-0037-1600991.
5. Kim JA, Ceccarelli R, Lu CY. Pharmacogenomic biomarkers in US FDA-approved drug labels (2000–2020). J Pers Med. 2021;11(3). https://doi.org/10.3390/jpm11030179.
6. Paugh SW, Stocco G, McCorkle JR, Diouf B, Crews KR, Evans WE. Cancer pharmacogenomics. Clin Pharmacol Ther. 2011;90(3):461–6. https://doi.org/10.1038/clpt.2011.126.
7. Coate L, Cuffe S, Horgan A, Hung RJ, Christiani D, Liu G. Germline genetic variation, cancer outcome, and pharmacogenetics. J Clin Oncol. 2010;28(26):4029–37. https://doi.org/10.1200/JCO.2009.27.2336.
8. Nebert DW, Zhang G, Vesell ES. From human genetics and genomics to pharmacogenetics and pharmacogenomics: past lessons, future directions. Drug Metab Rev. 2008;40(2):187–224. https://doi.org/10.1080/03602530801952864.
9. Hicks J, Bishop J, Sangkuhl K, Müller D, Ji Y, Leckband S, et al. Clinical Pharmacogenetics Implementation Consortium (CPIC) guideline for CYP2D6 and CYP2C19 genotypes and

dosing of selective serotonin reuptake inhibitors. Clin Pharmacol Ther. 2015;98(2):127–34. https://doi.org/10.1002/cpt.147.

10. DPWG. The Dutch Pharmacogenomic Working Group. Phamacogenomic recommendations, farmacogenetica-update 2020. Available at: https://www.pharmgkb.org/page/dpwg. Accessed 13 Nov 2022.

11. Abdullah-Koolmees H, van Keulen AM, Nijenhuis M, Deneer VHM. Pharmacogenetics guidelines: overview and comparison of the DPWG, CPIC, CPNDS, and RNPGx guidelines. Front Pharmacol. 2020;11: 595219. https://doi.org/10.3389/fphar.2020.595219.

12. Table of Pharmacogenetic Associations. Available at: https://www.fda.gov/medical-devices/precision medicine/table-pharmacogenetic-associations. Accessed 13 Nov 2022.

13. Carvalho Henriques B, Yang EH, Lapetina D, Carr MS, Yavorskyy V, Hague J, et al. How can drug metabolism and transporter genetics inform psychotropic prescribing? Front Genet. 2020;11(1277). https://doi.org/10.3389/fgene.2020.491895.

14. Ishikawa T. The ATP-dependent glutathione S-conjugate export pump. Trends Biochem Sci. 1992;17(11):463–8. https://doi.org/10.1016/0968-0004(92)90489-v.

15. Xu C, Li CY, Kong AN. Induction of phase I, II and III drug metabolism/transport by xenobiotics. Arch Pharm Res. 2005;28(3):249–68. https://doi.org/10.1007/BF02977789.

16. Kanamura S, Watanabe J. Cell biology of cytochrome P-450 in the liver. Int Rev Cytol. 2000;198:109–52. https://doi.org/10.1016/s0074-7696(00)98004-5.

17. Mansuy D. The great diversity of reactions catalyzed by cytochromes P450. Comp Biochem Physiol C Pharmacol Toxicol Endocrinol. 1998;121(1–3):5–14. https://doi.org/10.1016/s0742-8413(98)10026-9.

18. Sikka R, Magauran B, Ulrich A, Shannon M. Bench to bedside: pharmacogenomics, adverse drug interactions, and the cytochrome P450 system. Acad Emerg Med. 2005;12(12):1227–35. https://doi.org/10.1197/j.aem.2005.06.027.

19. Zanger UM, Schwab M. Cytochrome P450 enzymes in drug metabolism: regulation of gene expression, enzyme activities, and impact of genetic variation. Pharmacol Ther. 2013;138(1):103–41. https://doi.org/10.1016/j.pharmthera.2012.12.007.

20. Gough AC, Miles JS, Spurr NK, Moss JE, Gaedigk A, Eichelbaum M, et al. Identification of the primary gene defect at the cytochrome P450 CYP2D locus. Nature. 1990;347(6295):773–6. https://doi.org/10.1038/347773a0.

21. Hanioka N, Kimura S, Meyer UA, Gonzalez FJ. The human CYP2D locus associated with a common genetic defect in drug oxidation: a G1934—a base change in intron 3 of a mutant CYP2D6 allele results in an aberrant 3′ splice recognition site. Am J Hum Genet. 1990;47(6):994–1001.

22. Kagimoto M, Heim M, Kagimoto K, Zeugin T, Meyer UA. Multiple mutations of the human cytochrome P450IID6 gene (CYP2D6) in poor metabolizers of debrisoquine. Study of the functional significance of individual mutations by expression of chimeric genes. J Biol Chem. 1990;265(28):17209–14.

23. Zhou Y, Ingelman-Sundberg M, Lauschke VM. Worldwide distribution of cytochrome P450 alleles: a meta-analysis of population-scale sequencing projects. Clin Pharmacol Ther. 2017;102(4):688–700. https://doi.org/10.1002/cpt.690.

24. van der Weide J, Steijns LS. Cytochrome P450 enzyme system: genetic polymorphisms and impact on clinical pharmacology. Ann Clin Biochem. 1999;36(Pt 6):722–9. https://doi.org/10.1177/000456329903600604.

25. Caudle KE, Sangkuhl K, Whirl-Carrillo M, Swen JJ, Haidar CE, Klein TE, et al. Standardizing CYP2D6 genotype to phenotype translation: consensus recommendations from the Clinical Pharmacogenetics Implementation Consortium and Dutch Pharmacogenetics Working Group. Clin Transl Sci. 2020;13(1):116–24. https://doi.org/10.1111/cts.12692.

26. Zhou SF, Liu JP, Chowbay B. Polymorphism of human cytochrome P450 enzymes and its clinical impact. Drug Metab Rev. 2009;41(2):89–295. https://doi.org/10.1080/03602530902843483.

27. Zhang YKK, Sugathan A, Nassery N, Dombkowski A, Zanger UM, et al. Transcriptional profiling of human liver identifies sex-biased genes associated with polygenic dyslipidemia and

coronary artery disease. PLoS ONE. 2011;6(8):e23506. https://doi.org/10.1371/journal.pone. 0023506.

28. Lamba V, Panetta JC, Strom S, Schuetz EG. Genetic predictors of interindividual variability in hepatic CYP3A4 expression. J Pharmacol Exp Ther. 2010;332(3):1088–99. https://doi.org/ 10.1124/jpet.109.160804.

29. Yang X ZB, Molony C, Chudin E, Hao K, Zhu J, et al. Systematic genetic and genomic analysis of cytochrome P450 enzyme activities in human liver. Genome Res. 2010;20(8):1020–1036. https://doi.org/10.1101/gr.103341.109.

30. Lu H, Rosenbaum S. Developmental pharmacokinetics in pediatric populations. J Pediatr Pharmacol Ther. 2014;19(4):262–76. https://doi.org/10.5863/1551-6776-19.4.262.

31. Fernandez E, Perez R, Hernandez A, Tejada P, Arteta M, Ramos JT. Factors and mechanisms for pharmacokinetic differences between pediatric population and adults. Pharmaceutics. 2011;3(1):53–72. https://doi.org/10.3390/pharmaceutics3010053.

32. Zanger U, Klein K. Pharmacogenetics of cytochrome P450 2B6 (CYP2B6): advances on polymorphisms, mechanisms, and clinical relevance. Fron Genet. 2013;4(24). https://doi.org/ 10.3389/fgene.2013.00024.

33. Zanger UM, Raimundo S, Eichelbaum M. Cytochrome P450 2D6: overview and update on pharmacology, genetics, biochemistry. Naunyn Schmiedebergs Arch Pharmacol. 2004;369(1):23–37. https://doi.org/10.1007/s00210-003-0832-2.

34. Cotreau MM, von Moltke LL, Greenblatt DJ. The influence of age and sex on the clearance of cytochrome P450 3A substrates. Clin Pharmacokinet. 2005;44(1):33–60. https://doi.org/ 10.2165/00003088-200544010-00002.

35. Nelson DR, Zeldin DC, Hoffman SM, Maltais LJ, Wain HM, Nebert DW. Comparison of cytochrome P450 (CYP) genes from the mouse and human genomes, including nomenclature recommendations for genes, pseudogenes and alternative-splice variants. Pharmacogenetics. 2004;14(1):1–18. https://doi.org/10.1097/00008571-200401000-00001.

36. Zhou S-F, Wang B, Yang L-P, Liu J-P. Structure, function, regulation and polymorphism and the clinical significance of human cytochrome P450 1A2. Drug Metab Rev. 2010;42(2):268–354. https://doi.org/10.3109/03602530903286476.

37. Shimada T, Yamazaki H, Mimura M, Inui Y, Guengerich FP. Interindividual variations in human liver cytochrome P-450 enzymes involved in the oxidation of drugs, carcinogens and toxic chemicals: studies with liver microsomes of 30 Japanese and 30 Caucasians. J Pharmacol Exp Ther. 1994;270(1):414–23.

38. Kazui M, Nishiya Y, Ishizuka T, Hagihara K, Farid NA, Okazaki O, et al. Identification of the human cytochrome P450 enzymes involved in the two oxidative steps in the bioactivation of clopidogrel to its pharmacologically active metabolite. Drug Metab Dispos. 2010;38(1):92–9. https://doi.org/10.1124/dmd.109.029132.

39. Ohtsuki S, Schaefer O, Kawakami H, Inoue T, Liehner S, Saito A, et al. Simultaneous absolute protein quantification of transporters, cytochromes P450, and UDP-glucuronosyltransferases as a novel approach for the characterization of individual human liver: comparison with mRNA levels and activities. Drug Metab Dispos. 2012;40(1):83–92. https://doi.org/10.1124/dmd.111.042259.

40. Rendic S. Summary of information on human CYP enzymes: human P450 metabolism data. Drug Metab Rev. 2002;34(1–2):83–448. https://doi.org/10.1081/dmr-120001392.

41. Pragyan P, Kesharwani SS, Nandekar PP, Rathod V, Sangamwar AT. Predicting drug metabolism by CYP1A1, CYP1A2, and CYP1B1: insights from MetaSite, molecular docking and quantum chemical calculations. Mol Divers. 2014;18(4):865–78. https://doi.org/10. 1007/s11030-014-9534-6.

42. Lind AB, Reis M, Bengtsson F, Jonzier-Perey M, Powell Golay K, Ahlner J, et al. Steady-state concentrations of mirtazapine, N-desmethylmirtazapine, 8-hydroxymirtazapine and their enantiomers in relation to cytochrome P450 2D6 genotype, age and smoking behaviour. Clin Pharmacokinet. 2009;48(1):63–70. https://doi.org/10.2165/0003088-200948010-00005.

43. Kapelyukh Y, Henderson CJ, Scheer N, Rode A, Wolf CR. Defining the Contribution of CYP1A1 and CYP1A2 to drug metabolism using humanized CYP1A1/1A2 and Cyp1a1/

Cyp1a2 knockout mice. Drug Metab Dispos. 2019;47(8):907–18. https://doi.org/10.1124/dmd.119.087718.

44. Rasmussen BB, Brix TH, Kyvik KO, Brøsen K. The interindividual differences in the 3-demthylation of caffeine alias CYP1A2 is determined by both genetic and environmental factors. Pharmacogenetics. 2002;12(6):473–8. https://doi.org/10.1097/00008571-200208000-00008.

45. Faber MS, Jetter A, Fuhr U. Assessment of CYP1A2 activity in clinical practice: why, how, and when? Basic Clin Pharmacol Toxicol. 2005;97(3):125–34. https://doi.org/10.1111/j.1742-7843.2005.pto_973160.x.

46. Lobo ED, Bergstrom RF, Reddy S, Quinlan T, Chappell J, Hong Q, et al. In vitro and in vivo evaluations of cytochrome P450 1A2 interactions with duloxetine. Clin Pharmacokinet. 2008;47(3):191–202. https://doi.org/10.2165/00003088-200847030-00005.

47. Polasek TM, Lin FPY, Miners JO, Doogue MP. Perpetrators of pharmacokinetic drug–drug interactions arising from altered cytochrome P450 activity: a criteria-based assessment. Br J Clin Pharmacol. 2011;71(5):727–36. https://doi.org/10.1111/j.1365-2125.2011.03903.x.

48. Rost KL, Brösicke H, Heinemeyer G, Roots I. Specific and dose-dependent enzyme induction by omeprazole in human beings. Hepatology. 1994;20(5):1204–12.

49. Parker AC, Pritchard P, Preston T, Choonara I. Induction of CYP1A2 activity by carbamazepine in children using the caffeine breath test. Br J Clin Pharmacol. 1998;45(2):176–8. https://doi.org/10.1046/j.1365-2125.1998.00684.x.

50. Qian Y, Gurley BJ, Markowitz JS. The potential for pharmacokinetic interactions between cannabis products and conventional medications. J Clin Psychopharmacol. 2019;39(5):462–71. https://doi.org/10.1097/JCP.0000000000001089.

51. Ghotbi R, Christensen M, Roh H-K, Ingelman-Sundberg M, Aklillu E, Bertilsson L. Comparisons of CYP1A2 genetic polymorphisms, enzyme activity and the genotype-phenotype relationship in Swedes and Koreans. Eur J Clin Pharmacol. 2007;63(6):537–46. https://doi.org/10.1007/s00228-007-0288-2.

52. Dobrinas M, Cornuz J, Oneda B, Kohler Serra M, Puhl M, Eap C. Impact of smoking, smoking cessation, and genetic polymorphisms on CYP1A2 activity and inducibility. Clin Pharmacol Ther. 2011;90(1):117–25. https://doi.org/10.1038/clpt.2011.70.

53. Lesche D, Mostafa S, Everall I, Pantelis C, Bousman CA. Impact of CYP1A2, CYP2C19, and CYP2D6 genotype- and phenoconversion-predicted enzyme activity on clozapine exposure and symptom severity. Pharmacogenomics J. 2020;20(2):192–201. https://doi.org/10.1038/s41397-019-0108-y.

54. Laika B, Leucht S, Heres S, Schneider H, Steimer W. Pharmacogenetics and olanzapine treatment: CYP1A2*1F and serotonergic polymorphisms influence therapeutic outcome. Pharmacogenomics J. 2010;10(1):20–9. https://doi.org/10.1038/tpj.2009.32.

55. Li Y, Meng Q, Yang M, Liu D, Hou X, Tang L, et al. Current trends in drug metabolism and pharmacokinetics. Acta Pharm Sin B. 2019;9(6):1113–44. https://doi.org/10.1016/j.apsb.2019.10.001.

56. Wang H, Tompkins LM. CYP2B6: new insights into a historically overlooked cytochrome P450 isozyme. Curr Drug Metab. 2008;9(7):598–610. https://doi.org/10.2174/138920008785821710.

57. Lamba V, Lamba J, Yasuda K, Strom S, Davila J, Hancock ML, et al. Hepatic CYP2B6 expression: gender and ethnic differences and relationship to CYP2B6 genotype and CAR (constitutive androstane receptor) expression. J Pharmacol Exp Ther. 2003;307(3):906–22. https://doi.org/10.1124/jpet.103.054866.

58. Hedrich WD, Hassan HE, Wang H. Insights into CYP2B6-mediated drug–drug interactions. Acta Pharm Sin B. 2016;6(5):413–25. https://doi.org/10.1016/j.apsb.2016.07.016.

59. Lonsdale J, Thomas J, Salvatore M, Phillips R, Lo E, Shad S, et al. The Genotype-Tissue Expression (GTEx) project. Nature Genet. 2013;45(6):580–5. https://doi.org/10.1038/ng.2653.

60. Lang T, Klein K, Fischer J, Nüssler AK, Neuhaus P, Hofmann U, et al. Extensive genetic polymorphism in the human CYP2B6 gene with impact on expression and function in human

liver. Pharmacogenet Genomics. 2001;11(5). https://doi.org/10.1097/00008571-200107000-00004.

61. Desta Z, Saussele T, Ward B, Blievernicht J, Li L, Klein K, et al. Impact of CYP2B6 polymorphism on hepatic efavirenz metabolism in vitro. Pharmacogenomics. 2007;8(6):547–58. https://doi.org/10.2217/14622416.8.6.547.

62. Kirchheiner J, Klein C, Meineke I, Sasse J, Zanger UM, Mürdter TE, et al. Bupropion and 4-OH-bupropion pharmacokinetics in relation to genetic polymorphisms in CYP2B6. Pharmacogenet Genomics. 2003;13(10). https://doi.org/10.1097/00008571-200310000-00005.

63. Klein K, Lang T, Saussele T, Barbosa-Sicard E, Schunck WH, Eichelbaum M, et al. Genetic variability of CYP2B6 in populations of African and Asian origin: allele frequencies, novel functional variants, and possible implications for anti-HIV therapy with efavirenz. Pharmacogenet Genomics. 2005;15(12):861–73. https://doi.org/10.1097/01213011-200512000-00004.

64. Hofmann MH, Blievernicht JK, Klein K, Saussele T, Schaeffeler E, Schwab M, et al. Aberrant splicing caused by single nucleotide polymorphism c.516G>T [Q172H], a marker of CYP2B6*6, is responsible for decreased expression and activity of CYP2B6 in liver. J Pharmacol Exp Ther. 2008;325(1):284–92. https://doi.org/10.1124/jpet.107.133306.

65. Langmia IM, Just KS, Yamoune S, Brockmöller J, Masimirembwa C, Stingl JC. CYP2B6 functional variability in drug metabolism and exposure across populations—implication for drug safety, dosing, and individualized therapy. Front Genet. 2021;12(1205). https://doi.org/10.3389/fgene.2021.692234.

66. Ali ZK, Kim RJ, Ysla FM. CYP2C9 polymorphisms: considerations in NSAID therapy. Curr Opin Drug Discov Devel. 2009;12(1):108–14.

67. Lee CR, Goldstein JA, Pieper JA. Cytochrome P450 2C9 polymorphisms: a comprehensive review of the in-vitro and human data. Pharmacogenetics. 2002;12(3):251–63. https://doi.org/10.1097/00008571-200204000-00010.

68. Goldstein JA, de Morais SM. Biochemistry and molecular biology of the human CYP2C subfamily. Pharmacogenetics. 1994;4(6):285–99. https://doi.org/10.1097/00008571-199412000-00001.

69. Gelboin HV, Krausz K. Monoclonal antibodies and multifunctional cytochrome P450: drug metabolism as paradigm. J Clin Pharmacol. 2006;46(3):353–72. https://doi.org/10.1177/0091270005285200.

70. Rettie AE, Jones JP. Clinical and toxicological relevance of CYP2C9: drug–drug interactions and pharmacogenetics. Annu Rev Pharmacol Toxicol. 2005;45:477–94. https://doi.org/10.1146/annurev.pharmtox.45.120403.095821.

71. Bertilsson L. Geographical/interracial differences in polymorphic drug oxidation. Current state of knowledge of cytochromes P450 (CYP) 2D6 and 2C19. Clin Pharmacokinet. 1995;29(3):192–209. https://doi.org/10.2165/00003088-199529030-00005.

72. Hicks J, Sangkuhl K, Swen J, Ellingrod V, Müller D, Shimoda K, et al. Clinical Pharmacogenetics Implementation Consortium guideline (CPIC) for CYP2D6 and CYP2C19 genotypes and dosing of tricyclic antidepressants: 2016 update. Clin Pharmacol Ther. 2017;102(1):37–44. https://doi.org/10.1002/cpt.597.

73. Hicks JK, Bishop JR, Gammal RS, Sangkuhl K, Bousman CA, Leeder JS, et al. A call for clear and consistent communications regarding the role of pharmacogenetics in antidepressant pharmacotherapy. Clin Pharmacol Ther. 2020;107(1):50–2. https://doi.org/10.1002/cpt.1661.

74. Hicks JK, Swen JJ, Thorn CF, Sangkuhl K, Kharasch ED, Ellingrod VL, et al. Clinical Pharmacogenetics Implementation Consortium guideline for CYP2D6 and CYP2C19 genotypes and dosing of tricyclic antidepressants. Clin Pharmacol Ther. 2013;93(5):402–8. https://doi.org/10.1038/clpt.2013.2.

75. Kalow W. Debrisoquine/sparteine monooxygenase and other P450s in brain. Pharmacogenet Drug Metab. 1992:649–56.

76. Karam WG, Goldstein JA, Lasker JM, Ghanayem BI. Human CYP2C19 is a major omeprazole 5-hydroxylase, as demonstrated with recombinant cytochrome P450 enzymes. Drug Metab Dispos. 1996;24(10):1081–7.

77. Ohlsson Rosenborg S, Mwinyi J, Andersson M, Baldwin RM, Pedersen RS, Sim SC, et al. Kinetics of omeprazole and escitalopram in relation to the CYP2C19*17 allele in healthy subjects. Eur J Clin Pharmacol. 2008;64(12):1175–9. https://doi.org/10.1007/s00228-008-0529-z.
78. Hebert MF. Impact of pregnancy on maternal pharmacokinetics of medications. In: Mattison DR, editor. Clinical pharmacology during pregnancy. Academic; 2013. p. 17–39. https://doi.org/10.1016/B978-0-12-386007-1.00003-9.
79. Tornio A, Backman JT. Cytochrome P450 in pharmacogenetics: an update. In: Brøsen K, Damkier P, editors. Advances in pharmacology, vol. 83. Academic; 2018. p. 3–32. https://doi.org/10.1016/bs.apha.2018.04.007.
80. Sanford JC, Guo Y, Sadee W, Wang D. Regulatory polymorphisms in CYP2C19 affecting hepatic expression. Drug Metab Drug Interact. 2013;28(1):23–30. https://doi.org/10.1515/dmdi-2012-0038.
81. Fabbri C, Tansey KE, Perlis RH, Hauser J, Henigsberg N, Maier W, et al. Effect of cytochrome CYP2C19 metabolizing activity on antidepressant response and side effects: meta-analysis of data from genome-wide association studies. Eur Neuropsychopharmacol. 2018;28(8):945–54. https://doi.org/10.1016/j.euroneuro.2018.05.009.
82. Rudberg I, Hendset M, Uthus LH, Molden E, Refsum H. Heterozygous mutation in CYP2C19 significantly increases the concentration/dose ratio of racemic citalopram and escitalopram (S-citalopram). Ther Drug Monit. 2006;28(1):102–5. https://doi.org/10.1097/01.ftd.0000189899.23931.76.
83. Rudberg I, Hermann M, Refsum H, Molden E. Serum concentrations of sertraline and N-desmethyl sertraline in relation to CYP2C19 genotype in psychiatric patients. Eur J Clin Pharmacol. 2008;64(12):1181–8. https://doi.org/10.1007/s00228-008-0533-3.
84. Taylor C, Crosby I, Yip V, Maguire P, Pirmohamed M, Turner RM. A review of the important role of CYP2D6 in pharmacogenomics. Genes (Basel). 2020;11(11). https://doi.org/10.3390/genes11111295.
85. Yasukochi Y, Satta Y. Evolution of the CYP2D gene cluster in humans and four non-human primates. Genes Genet Syst. 2011;86(2):109–16. https://doi.org/10.1266/ggs.86.109.
86. Kalow W, Tang BK, Endrenyi L. Hypothesis: comparisons of inter- and intra-individual variations can substitute for twin studies in drug research. Pharmacogenetics. 1998;8(4):283–9. https://doi.org/10.1097/00008571-199808000-00001.
87. Niznik HB, Tyndale RF, Sallee FR, Gonzalez FJ, Hardwick JP, Inaba T, et al. The dopamine transporter and cytochrome P450IID1 (debrisoquine 4-hydroxylase) in brain: resolution and identification of two distinct [3H]GBR-12935 binding proteins. Arch Biochem Biophys. 1990;276(2):424–32.
88. Sangar MC, Anandatheerthavarada HK, Tang W, Prabu SK, Martin MV, Dostalek M, et al. Human liver mitochondrial cytochrome P450 2D6–individual variations and implications in drug metabolism. FEBS J. 2009;276(13):3440–53. https://doi.org/10.1111/j.1742-4658.2009.07067.x.
89. Yang Y, Botton MR, Scott ER, Scott SA. Sequencing the CYP2D6 gene: from variant allele discovery to clinical pharmacogenetic testing. Pharmacogenomics. 2017;18(7):673–85. https://doi.org/10.2217/pgs-2017-0033.
90. Jarvis JP, Peter AP, Shaman JA. Consequences of CYP2D6 copy-number variation for pharmacogenomics in psychiatry. Front Psychiatry. 2019;10(432). https://doi.org/10.3389/fpsyt.2019.00432.
91. Farooq M, Kelly EJ, Unadkat JD. CYP2D6 is inducible by endogenous and exogenous corticosteroids. Drug Metab Dispos. 2016;44(5):750–7. https://doi.org/10.1124/dmd.115.069229.
92. Shin JG, Kane K, Flockhart DA. Potent inhibition of CYP2D6 by haloperidol metabolites: stereoselective inhibition by reduced haloperidol. Br J Clin Pharmacol. 2001;51(1):45–52. https://doi.org/10.1046/j.1365-2125.2001.01313.x.
93. Ning M, Duarte JD, Rubin LH, Jeong H. CYP2D6 protein level is the major contributor to interindividual variability in CYP2D6-mediated drug metabolism in healthy human liver tissue. Clin Pharmacol Ther. 2018;104(5):974–82. https://doi.org/10.1002/cpt.1032.

94. Rutman MP, Horn JR, Newman DK, Stefanacci RG. Overactive bladder prescribing considerations: the role of polypharmacy, anticholinergic burden, and CYP2D6 drug–drug interactions. Clin Drug Investig. 2021;41(4):293–302. https://doi.org/10.1007/s40261-021-01020-x.

95. Bertilsson L, Dahl ML, Dalén P, Al-Shurbaji A. Molecular genetics of CYP2D6: clinical relevance with focus on psychotropic drugs. Br J Clin Pharmacol. 2002;53(2):111–22. https://doi.org/10.1046/j.0306-5251.2001.01548.x.

96. Bradford LD. CYP2D6 allele frequency in European Caucasians, Asians Africans and their descendants. Pharmacogenomics. 2002;3(2):229–43. https://doi.org/10.1517/14622416.3.2.229.

97. Gaedigk A, Simon S, Pearce R, Bradford L, Kennedy M, Leeder J. The CYP2D6 activity score: translating genotype information into a qualitative measure of phenotype. Clin Pharmacol Ther. 2008;83(2):234–42. https://doi.org/10.1038/sj.clpt.6100406.

98. Ingelman-Sundberg M. Genetic polymorphisms of cytochrome P450 2D6 (CYP2D6): clinical consequences, evolutionary aspects and functional diversity. Pharmacogenomics J. 2005;5(1):6–13. https://doi.org/10.1038/sj.tpj.6500285.

99. Crux NB, Elahi S. Human leukocyte antigen (HLA) and immune regulation: how do classical and non-classical HLA alleles modulate immune response to human immunodeficiency virus and hepatitis C virus infections? Front Immunol. 2017;8(832). https://doi.org/10.3389/fimmu.2017.00832.

100. Amstutz U, Ross CJ, Castro-Pastrana LI, Rieder MJ, Shear NH, Hayden MR, et al. HLA-A 31:01 and HLA-B 15:02 as genetic markers for carbamazepine hypersensitivity in children. Clin Pharmacol Ther. 2013;94(1):142–9. https://doi.org/10.1038/clpt.2013.55.

101. Fang H, Xu X, Kaur K, Dedek M, Zhu G-d, Riley BJ, et al. A screening test for HLA-B*15:02 in a large United States patient cohort identifies broader risk of carbamazepine-induced adverse events. Front Pharmacol. 2019;10(149). https://doi.org/10.3389/fphar.2019.00149.

102. Grover S, Kukreti R. HLA alleles and hypersensitivity to carbamazepine: an updated systematic review with meta-analysis. Pharmacogenet Genomics. 2014;24(2):94–112. https://doi.org/10.1097/FPC.0000000000000021.

103. Tangamornsuksan W, Scholfield N, Lohitnavy M. Association between HLA genotypes and oxcarbazepine-induced cutaneous adverse drug reactions: a systematic review and meta-analysis. J Pharm Pharm Sci. 2018;21(1):1–18. https://doi.org/10.18433/J36S7D.

104. Genin E, Chen DP, Hung SI, Sekula P, Schumacher M, Chang PY, et al. HLA-A*31:01 and different types of carbamazepine-induced severe cutaneous adverse reactions: an international study and meta-analysis. Pharmacogenomics J. 2014;14(3):281–8. https://doi.org/10.1038/tpj.2013.40.

105. Ksouda K, Affes H, Mahfoudh N, Chtourou L, Kammoun A, Charfi A, et al. HLA-A*31:01 and carbamazepine-induced DRESS syndrome in a sample of North African population. Seizure. 2017;53:42–6. https://doi.org/10.1016/j.seizure.2017.10.018.

106. Dean L. Carbamazepine therapy and HLA genotype. In: Pratt VM, Scott SA, Pirmohamed M, et al., editors. Medical genetics summaries. Bethesda (MD): National Center for Biotechnology Information (US); 2015.

107. Phillips EJ, Sukasem C, Whirl-Carrillo M, Müller DJ, Dunnenberger HM, Chantratita W, et al. Clinical Pharmacogenetics Implementation Consortium guideline for HLA genotype and use of carbamazepine and oxcarbazepine: 2017 update. Clin Pharmacol Ther. 2018;103(4):574–81. https://doi.org/10.1002/cpt.1004.

108. Le-Niculescu H, Roseberry K, Gill SS, Levey DF, Phalen PL, Mullen J, et al. Precision medicine for mood disorders: objective assessment, risk prediction, pharmacogenomics, and repurposed drugs. Mol Psychiatry. 2021;26(7):2776–804.

109. Oz MD, Baskak B, Uckun Z, Artun NY, Ozdemir H, Ozel TK, et al. Association between serotonin 2A receptor (HTR2A), serotonin transporter (SLC6A4) and brain-derived neurotrophic factor (BDNF) gene polymorphisms and citalopram/sertraline induced sexual dysfunction in MDD patients. Pharmacogenomics J. 2020;20(3):443–50. https://doi.org/10.1038/s41380-021-01061-w.

110. Margoob MA, Mushtaq D. Serotonin transporter gene polymorphism and psychiatric disorders: is there a link? Indian J Psychiatry. 2011;53(4):289–99. https://doi.org/10.4103/0019-5545.91901.

111. Kenna GA, Roder-Hanna N, Leggio L, Zywiak WH, Clifford J, Edwards S, et al. Association of the 5-HTT gene-linked promoter region (5-HTTLPR) polymorphism with psychiatric disorders: review of psychopathology and pharmacotherapy. Pharmacogenomics Pers Med. 2012;5:19–35. https://doi.org/10.2147/PGPM.S23462.

112. Serretti A, Kato M, De Ronchi D, Kinoshita T. Meta-analysis of serotonin transporter gene promoter polymorphism (5-HTTLPR) association with selective serotonin reuptake inhibitor efficacy in depressed patients. Mol Psychiatry. 2007;12(3):247–57. https://doi.org/10.1038/sj.mp.4001926.

113. Kato M, Fukuda T, Wakeno M, Fukuda K, Okugawa G, Ikenaga Y, et al. Effects of the serotonin type 2A, 3A and 3B receptor and the serotonin transporter genes on paroxetine and fluvoxamine efficacy and adverse drug reactions in depressed Japanese patients. Neuropsychobiology. 2006;53(4):186–95. https://doi.org/10.1159/000094727.

114. Kato M, Fukuda T, Wakeno M, Okugawa G, Takekita Y, Watanabe S, et al. Effect of 5-HT1A gene polymorphisms on antidepressant response in major depressive disorder. Am J Med Genet B Neuropsychiatr Genet. 2009;150b(1):115–23. https://doi.org/10.1002/ajmg.b.30783.

115. Hu X-Z, Rush AJ, Charney D, Wilson AF, Sorant AJM, Papanicolaou GJ, et al. Association between a functional serotonin transporter promoter polymorphism and citalopram treatment in adult outpatients with major depression. Arch Gen Psychiatry. 2007;64(7):783–92. https://doi.org/10.1001/archpsyc.64.7.783.

116. Noskova T, Pivac N, Nedic G, Kazantseva A, Gaysina D, Faskhutdinova G, et al. Ethnic differences in the serotonin transporter polymorphism (5-HTTLPR) in several European populations. Prog Neuropsychopharmacol Biol Psychiatry. 2008;32(7):1735–9. https://doi.org/10.1016/j.pnpbp.2008.07.012.

117. Goldman N, Glei DA, Lin Y-H, Weinstein M. The serotonin transporter polymorphism (5-HTTLPR): allelic variation and links with depressive symptoms. Depress Anxiety. 2010;27(3):260–9. https://doi.org/10.1002/da.20660.

118. Cao J, Hudziak JJ, Li D. Multi-cultural association of the serotonin transporter gene (SLC6A4) with substance use disorder. Neuropsychopharmacology. 2013;38(9):1737–47. https://doi.org/10.1038/npp.2013.73.

119. Fratelli C, Siqueira J, Silva C, Ferreira E, Silva I. 5HTTLPR Genetic variant and major depressive disorder: a review. Genes (Basel). 2020;11(11). https://doi.org/10.3390/genes1111 1260.

120. Murphy GM Jr, Hollander SB, Rodrigues HE, Kremer C, Schatzberg AF. Effects of the serotonin transporter gene promoter polymorphism on mirtazapine and paroxetine efficacy and adverse events in geriatric major depression. Arch Gen Psychiatry. 2004;61(11):1163–9. https://doi.org/10.1001/archpsyc.61.11.1163.

121. Kim H, Lim SW, Kim S, Kim JW, Chang YH, Carroll BJ, et al. Monoamine transporter gene polymorphisms and antidepressant response in Koreans with late-life depression. JAMA. 2006;296(13):1609–18. https://doi.org/10.1001/jama.296.13.1609.

122. Meyer JH, Kapur S, Eisfeld B, Brown GM, Houle S, DaSilva J, et al. The effect of paroxetine on 5-HT(2A) receptors in depression: an [(18)F]setoperone PET imaging study. Am J Psychiatry. 2001;158(1):78–85. https://doi.org/10.1176/appi.ajp.158.1.78.

123. Du D, Tang Q, Han Q, Zhang J, Liang X, Tan Y, et al. Association between genetic polymorphism and antidepressants in major depression: a network meta-analysis. Pharmacogenomics. 2020;21(13):963–74. https://doi.org/10.2217/pgs-2020-0037.

124. McMahon FJ, Buervenich S, Charney D, Lipsky R, Rush AJ, Wilson AF, et al. Variation in the gene encoding the serotonin 2A receptor is associated with outcome of antidepressant treatment. Am J Hum Genet. 2006;78(5):804–14. https://doi.org/10.1086/503820.

125. Lesser IM, Castro DB, Gaynes BN, Gonzalez J, Rush AJ, Alpert JE, et al. Ethnicity/race and outcome in the treatment of depression: results from STAR*D. Med Care. 2007;45(11):1043–51. https://doi.org/10.1097/MLR.0b013e3181271462.

126. Lucae S, Ising M, Horstmann S, Baune BT, Arolt V, Müller-Myhsok B, et al. HTR2A gene variation is involved in antidepressant treatment response. Eur Neuropsychopharmacol. 2010;20(1):65–8. https://doi.org/10.1016/j.euroneuro.2009.08.006.
127. Pérez V, Gilaberte I, Faries D, Alvarez E, Artigas F. Randomised, double-blind, placebo-controlled trial of pindolol in combination with fluoxetine antidepressant treatment. Lancet. 1997;349(9065):1594–7. https://doi.org/10.1016/S0140-6736(96)08007-5.
128. Isaac MT, Tome MB. Selective serotonin reuptake inhibitors plus pindolol. Lancet. 1997;350(9073):288–9. https://doi.org/10.1016/S0140-6736(05)62250-7.
129. Blier P, Bergeron R. The use of pindolol to potentiate antidepressant medication. J Clin Psychiatry. 1998;59(Suppl 5):16–25.
130. Yu YW, Tsai SJ, Liou YJ, Hong CJ, Chen TJ. Association study of two serotonin 1A receptor gene polymorphisms and fluoxetine treatment response in Chinese major depressive disorders. Eur Neuropsychopharmacol. 2006;16(7):498–503. https://doi.org/10.1016/j.euroneuro. 2005.12.004.
131. Hashimoto K, Sawa A, Iyo M. Increased levels of glutamate in brains from patients with mood disorders. Biol Psychiatry. 2007;62(11):1310–6. https://doi.org/10.1016/j.biopsych. 2007.03.017.
132. Shinohe A, Hashimoto K, Nakamura K, Tsujii M, Iwata Y, Tsuchiya KJ, et al. Increased serum levels of glutamate in adult patients with autism. Prog Neuropsychopharmacol Biol Psychiatry. 2006;30(8):1472–7. https://doi.org/10.1016/j.pnpbp.2006.06.013.
133. Paddock S, Laje G, Charney D, Rush AJ, Wilson AF, Sorant AJ, et al. Association of GRIK4 with outcome of antidepressant treatment in the STAR*D cohort. Am J Psychiatry. 2007;164(8):1181–8. https://doi.org/10.1176/appi.ajp.2007.06111790.
134. Perlis RH, Fijal B, Dharia S, Heinloth AN, Houston JP. Failure to replicate genetic associations with antidepressant treatment response in duloxetine-treated patients. Biol Psychiatry. 2010;67(11):1110–3. https://doi.org/10.1016/j.biopsych.2009.12.010.
135. Creese I, Burt DR, Snyder SH. Dopamine receptors and average clinical doses. Science. 1976;194(4264):546. https://doi.org/10.1126/science.194.4264.546.
136. Creese I, Burt DR, Snyder SH. Dopamine receptor binding predicts clinical and pharmacological potencies of antischizophrenic drugs. Science. 1976;192(4238):481–3. https://doi.org/ 10.1126/science.3854.
137. Burt DR, Creese I, Snyder SH. Properties of [3H]haloperidol and [3H]dopamine binding associated with dopamine receptors in calf brain membranes. Mol Pharmacol. 1976;12(5):800–12.
138. Enna SJ, Bennett JP Jr, Burt DR, Creese I, Snyder SH. Stereospecificity of interaction of neuroleptic drugs with neurotransmitters and correlation with clinical potency. Nature. 1976;263(5575):338–41. https://doi.org/10.1038/263338a0.
139. Perlis RH. Pharmacogenomic testing and personalized treatment of depression. Clin Chem. 2014;60(1):53–9. https://doi.org/10.1373/clinchem.2013.204446.
140. Kapur S, Zipursky R, Jones C, Remington G, Houle S. Relationship between dopamine D(2) occupancy, clinical response, and side effects: a double-blind PET study of first-episode schizophrenia. Am J Psychiatry. 2000;157(4):514–20. https://doi.org/10.1176/appi.ajp.157. 4.514.
141. Mamo D, Graff A, Mizrahi R, Shammi CM, Romeyer F, Kapur S. Differential effects of aripiprazole on D(2), 5-HT(2), and 5-HT(1A) receptor occupancy in patients with schizophrenia: a triple tracer PET study. Am J Psychiatry. 2007;164(9):1411–7. https://doi.org/10.1176/appi. ajp.2007.06091479.
142. Reynolds GP, Yao Z, Zhang X, Sun J, Zhang Z. Pharmacogenetics of treatment in first-episode schizophrenia: D3 and 5-HT2C receptor polymorphisms separately associate with positive and negative symptom response. Eur Neuropsychopharmacol. 2005;15(2):143–51. https://doi.org/10.1016/j.euroneuro.2004.07.001.

143. Malhotra AK, Goldman D, Buchanan RW, Rooney W, Clifton A, Kosmidis MH, et al. The dopamine D3 receptor (DRD3) Ser9Gly polymorphism and schizophrenia: a haplotype relative risk study and association with clozapine response. Mol Psychiatry. 1998;3(1):72–5. https://doi.org/10.1038/sj.mp.4000288.

144. Barlas IO, Cetin M, Erdal ME, et al. Lack of association between DRD3 gene polymorphism and response to clozapine in Turkish schizoprenia patients. Am J Med Genet B Neuropsychiatr Genet. 2009;150B(1):56–60. https://doi.org/10.1002/ajmg.b.30770.

145. Lane HY, Hsu SK, Liu YC, Chang YC, Huang CH, Chang WH. Dopamine D3 receptor Ser9Gly polymorphism and risperidone response. J Clin Psychopharmacol. 2005;25(1):6–11. https://doi.org/10.1097/01.jcp.0000150226.84371.76.

146. Van Tol HH, Wu CM, Guan HC, Ohara K, Bunzow JR, Civelli O, et al. Multiple dopamine D4 receptor variants in the human population. Nature. 1992;358(6382):149–52. https://doi.org/10.1038/358149a0.

147. Rao PA, Pickar D, Gejman PV, Ram A, Gershon ES, Gelernter J. Allelic variation in the D4 dopamine receptor (DRD4) gene does not predict response to clozapine. Arch Gen Psychiatry. 1994;51(11):912–7. https://doi.org/10.1001/archpsyc.1994.03950110072009.

148. Kohn Y, Ebstein RP, Heresco-Levy U, Shapira B, Nemanov L, Gritsenko I, et al. Dopamine D4 receptor gene polymorphisms: relation to ethnicity, no association with schizophrenia and response to clozapine in Israeli subjects. Eur Neuropsychopharmacol. 1997;7(1):39–43. https://doi.org/10.1016/s0924-977x(96)00380-x.

149. Depression. Available at: https://www.who.int/news-room/fact-sheets/detail/depression. Accessed 13 Nov 2022.

150. Li G, Fife D, Wang G, Sheehan JJ, Bodén R, Brandt L, et al. All-cause mortality in patients with treatment-resistant depression: a cohort study in the US population. Ann Gen Psychiatry. 2019;18:23. https://doi.org/10.1186/s12991-019-0248-0.

151. Bolton JM, Gunnell D, Turecki G. Suicide risk assessment and intervention in people with mental illness. BMJ. 2015;351: h4978. https://doi.org/10.1136/bmj.h4978.

152. Ang DC, Choi H, Kroenke K, Wolfe F. Comorbid depression is an independent risk factor for mortality in patients with rheumatoid arthritis. J Rheumatol. 2005;32(6):1013–9.

153. Antelman G, Kaaya S, Wei R, Mbwambo J, Msamanga GI, Fawzi WW, et al. Depressive symptoms increase risk of HIV disease progression and mortality among women in Tanzania. JAIDS. 2007;44(4). https://doi.org/10.1097/QAI.0b013e31802f1318.

154. Hasler G. Pathophysiology of depression: do we have any solid evidence of interest to clinicians? World Psychiatry. 2010;9(3):155–61. https://doi.org/10.1002/j.2051-5545.2010.tb00298.x.

155. Mrazek DA. Psychiatric pharmacogenomic testing in clinical practice. Dial Clin Neurosci. 2010;12(1):69–76. https://doi.org/10.31887/DCNS.2010.12.1/dmrazek.

156. Rush AJ, Trivedi MH, Wisniewski SR, Nierenberg AA, Stewart JW, Warden D, et al. Acute and longer-term outcomes in depressed outpatients requiring one or several treatment steps: a STAR*D report. Am J Psychiatry. 2006;163(11):1905–17. https://doi.org/10.1176/ajp.2006.163.11.1905.

157. Hampton LM, Daubresse M, Chang H-Y, Alexander GC, Budnitz DS. Emergency department visits by adults for psychiatric medication adverse events. JAMA Psychiat. 2014;71(9):1006–14. https://doi.org/10.1001/jamapsychiatry.2014.436.

158. Patient predictors of response to psychotherapy and pharmacotherapy. Findings in the NIMH treatment of depression collaborative research program. Am J Psychiatry. 1991;148(8):997–1008. https://doi.org/10.1176/ajp.148.8.997.

159. Tansey KE, Guipponi M, Hu X, Domenici E, Lewis G, Malafosse A, et al. Contribution of common genetic variants to antidepressant response. Biol Psychiatry. 2013;73(7):679–82. https://doi.org/10.1016/j.biopsych.2012.10.030.

160. Seripa D, Pilotto A, Paroni G, Fontana A, D'Onofrio G, Gravina C, et al. Role of the serotonin transporter gene locus in the response to SSRI treatment of major depressive disorder in late life. J Psychopharmacol. 2015;29(5):623–33. https://doi.org/10.1177/0269881115578159.

161. Manoharan A, Shewade DG, Rajkumar RP, Adithan S. Serotonin transporter gene (SLC6A4) polymorphisms are associated with response to fluoxetine in south Indian major depressive disorder patients. Eur J Clin Pharmacol. 2016;72(10):1215–20. https://doi.org/10.1007/s00 228-016-2099-9.

162. Camarena B, Álvarez-Icaza D, Hernández S, Aguilar A, Münch L, Martínez C, et al. Association study between serotonin transporter gene and fluoxetine response in Mexican patients with major depressive disorder. Clin Neuropharmacol. 2019;42(1):9–13. https://doi.org/10.1097/WNF.0000000000000315.

163. Ren F, Ma Y, Zhu X, Guo R, Wang J, He L. Pharmacogenetic association of bi- and triallelic polymorphisms of SLC6A4 with antidepressant response in major depressive disorder. J Affect Disord. 2020;273:254–64. https://doi.org/10.1016/j.jad.2020.04.058.

164. Kam H, Jeong H. Pharmacogenomic biomarkers and their applications in psychiatry. Genes (Basel). 2020;11(12). https://doi.org/10.3390/genes11121445.

165. Kao CF, Kuo PH, Yu YW, Yang AC, Lin E, Liu YL, et al. Gene-based association analysis suggests association of HTR2A with antidepressant treatment response in depressed patients. Front Pharmacol. 2020;11: 559601. https://doi.org/10.3389/fphar.2020.559601.

166. Yan P, Gao B, Wang S, Wang S, Li J, Song M. Association of 5-HTR2A -1438A/G polymorphism with anorexia nervosa and bulimia nervosa: a meta-analysis. Neurosci Lett. 2021;755: 135918. https://doi.org/10.1016/j.neulet.2021.135918.

167. Wan YS, Zhai XJ, Tan HA, Ai YS, Zhao LB. Associations between the 1438A/G, 102T/C, and rs7997012G/A polymorphisms of HTR2A and the safety and efficacy of antidepressants in depression: a meta-analysis. Pharmacogenomics J. 2021;21(2):200–15. https://doi.org/10.1038/s41397-020-00197-2.

168. Murphy LE, Fonseka TM, Bousman CA, Müller DJ. Gene-drug pairings for antidepressants and antipsychotics: level of evidence and clinical application. Mol Psychiatry. 2021. https://doi.org/10.1038/s41380-021-01340-6.

169. Whirl-Carrillo M, McDonagh EM, Hebert JM, Gong L, Sangkuhl K, Thorn CF, et al. Pharmacogenomics knowledge for personalized medicine. Clin Pharmacol Ther. 2012;92(4):414–7. https://doi.org/10.1038/clpt.2012.96.

170. Yuce-Artun N, Baskak B, Ozel-Kizil ET, Ozdemir H, Uckun Z, Devrimci-Ozguven H, et al. Influence of CYP2B6 and CYP2C19 polymorphisms on sertraline metabolism in major depression patients. Int J Clin Pharm. 2016;38(2):388–94. https://doi.org/10.1007/s11096-016-0259-8.

171. Saiz-Rodríguez M, Belmonte C, Román M, Ochoa D, Koller D, Talegón M, et al. Effect of polymorphisms on the pharmacokinetics, pharmacodynamics and safety of sertraline in healthy volunteers. Basic Clin Pharmacol Toxicol. 2018;122(5):501–11. https://doi.org/10.1111/bcpt.12938.

172. Bråten LS, Haslemo T, Jukic MM, Ingelman-Sundberg M, Molden E, Kringen MK. Impact of CYP2C19 genotype on sertraline exposure in 1200 Scandinavian patients. Neuropsychopharmacology. 2020;45(3):570–6. https://doi.org/10.1038/s41386-019-0554-x.

173. Milosavljević F, Bukvić N, Pavlović Z, Miljević Č, Pešić V, Molden E, et al. Association of CYP2C19 and CYP2D6 poor and intermediate metabolizer status with antidepressant and antipsychotic exposure: a systematic review and meta-analysis. JAMA Psychiat. 2021;78(3):270–80. https://doi.org/10.1001/jamapsychiatry.2020.3643.

174. Schwartz TL, Siddiqui UA, Stahl SM. Vilazodone: a brief pharmacological and clinical review of the novel serotonin partial agonist and reuptake inhibitor. Ther Adv Psychopharmacol. 2011;1(3):81–7. https://doi.org/10.1177/2045125311409486.

175. Stahl S. Essential psychopharmacology: the Prescriber's guide. 4th ed. Cambridge: Cambridge University Press; 2011.

176. Rabiner EA, Gunn RN, Wilkins MR, Sargent PA, Mocaer E, Sedman E, et al. Drug action at the 5-HT(1A) receptor in vivo: autoreceptor and postsynaptic receptor occupancy examined with PET and [carbonyl-(11)C]WAY-100635. Nucl Med Biol. 2000;27(5):509–13. https://doi.org/10.1016/s0969-8051(00)00120-7.

177. Bang-Andersen B, Ruhland T, Jørgensen M, Smith G, Frederiksen K, Jensen KG, et al. Discovery of 1-[2-(2,4-dimethylphenylsulfanyl)phenyl]piperazine (Lu AA21004): a novel multimodal compound for the treatment of major depressive disorder. J Med Chem. 2011;54(9):3206–21. https://doi.org/10.1021/jm101459g.

178. Pehrson AL, Cremers T, Bétry C, van der Hart MG, Jørgensen L, Madsen M, et al. Lu AA21004, a novel multimodal antidepressant, produces regionally selective increases of multiple neurotransmitters—a rat microdialysis and electrophysiology study. Eur Neuropsychopharmacol. 2013;23(2):133–45. https://doi.org/10.1016/j.euroneuro.2012.04.006.

179. Pehrson AL, Sanchez C. Serotonergic modulation of glutamate neurotransmission as a strategy for treating depression and cognitive dysfunction. CNS Spectr. 2014;19(2):121–33. https://doi.org/10.1017/S1092852913000540.

180. Mørk A, Montezinho LP, Miller S, Trippodi-Murphy C, Plath N, Li Y, et al. Vortioxetine (Lu AA21004), a novel multimodal antidepressant, enhances memory in rats. Pharmacol Biochem Behav. 2013;105:41–50. https://doi.org/10.1016/j.pbb.2013.01.019.

181. Stahl SM. Modes and nodes explain the mechanism of action of vortioxetine, a multimodal agent (MMA): blocking 5HT3 receptors enhances release of serotonin, norepinephrine, and acetylcholine. CNS Spectr. 2015;20(5):455–9. https://doi.org/10.1017/S1092852915000346.

182. Stahl SM. Modes and nodes explain the mechanism of action of vortioxetine, a multimodal agent (MMA): enhancing serotonin release by combining serotonin (5HT) transporter inhibition with actions at 5HT receptors (5HT1A, 5HT1B, 5HT1D, 5HT7 receptors). CNS Spectr. 2015;20(2):93–7. https://doi.org/10.1017/S1092852915000139.

183. Hvenegaard MG, Bang-Andersen B, Pedersen H, Jørgensen M, Püschl A, Dalgaard L. Identification of the cytochrome P450 and other enzymes involved in the in vitro oxidative metabolism of a novel antidepressant, Lu AA21004. Drug Metab Dispos. 2012;40(7):1357–65. https://doi.org/10.1124/dmd.112.044610.

184. Areberg J, Petersen KB, Chen G, Naik H. Population pharmacokinetic meta-analysis of vortioxetine in healthy individuals. Basic Clin Pharmacol Toxicol. 2014;115(6):552–9. https://doi.org/10.1111/bcpt.12256.

185. Dean L. Amitriptyline therapy and CYP2D6 and CYP2C19 genotype. In: Pratt VM, Scott SA, Pirmohamed M, et al., editors. Medical genetics summaries. Bethesda (MD): National Center for Biotechnology Information (US); 2017.

186. Ryu S, Park S, Lee JH, Kim YR, Na HS, Lim HS, et al. A study on CYP2C19 and CYP2D6 polymorphic effects on pharmacokinetics and pharmacodynamics of amitriptyline in healthy Koreans. Clin Transl Sci. 2017;10(2):93–101. https://doi.org/10.1111/cts.12451.

187. Shimoda K, Someya T, Yokono A, Morita S, Hirokane G, Takahashi S, et al. The impact of CYP2C19 and CYP2D6 genotypes on metabolism of amitriptyline in Japanese psychiatric patients. J Clin Psychopharmacol. 2002;22(4):371–8. https://doi.org/10.1097/00004714-200208000-00007.

188. Steimer W, Zöpf K, von Amelunxen S, Pfeiffer H, Bachofer J, Popp J, et al. Amitriptyline or not, that is the question: pharmacogenetic testing of CYP2D6 and CYP2C19 identifies patients with low or high risk for side effects in amitriptyline therapy. Clin Chem. 2005;51(2):376–85. https://doi.org/10.1373/clinchem.2004.041327.

189. Matthaei J, Brockmöller J, Steimer W, Pischa K, Leucht S, Kullmann M, et al. Effects of genetic polymorphism in CYP2D6, CYP2C19, and the organic cation transporter OCT1 on amitriptyline pharmacokinetics in healthy volunteers and depressive disorder patients. Front Pharmacol. 2021;12: 688950. https://doi.org/10.3389/fphar.2021.688950.

190. Kordou Z, Skokou M, Tsermpini EE, Chantratita W, Fukunaga K, Mushiroda T, et al. Discrepancies and similarities in the genome-informed guidance for psychiatric disorders amongst different regulatory bodies and research consortia using next generation sequencing-based clinical pharmacogenomics data. Pharmacol Res. 2021;167: 105538. https://doi.org/10.1016/j.phrs.2021.105538.

191. Morinobu S, Tanaka T, Kawakatsu S, Totsuka S, Koyama E, Chiba K, et al. Effects of genetic defects in the CYP2C19 gene on the N-demethylation of imipramine, and clinical outcome

of imipramine therapy. Psychiatry Clin Neurosci. 1997;51(4):253–7. https://doi.org/10.1111/j.1440-1819.1997.tb02593.x.

192. Bousman CA, Müller DJ, Ng CH, Byron K, Berk M, Singh AB. Concordance between actual and pharmacogenetic predicted desvenlafaxine dose needed to achieve remission in major depressive disorder: a 10-week open-label study. Pharmacogenet Genomics. 2017;27(1):1–6. https://doi.org/10.1097/FPC.0000000000000253.

193. Maciukiewicz M, Marshe VS, Hauschild AC, Foster JA, Rotzinger S, Kennedy JL, et al. GWAS-based machine learning approach to predict duloxetine response in major depressive disorder. J Psychiatr Res. 2018;99:62–8. https://doi.org/10.1016/j.jpsychires.2017.12.009.

194. Perlis RH, Fijal B, Dharia S, Houston JP. Pharmacogenetic investigation of response to duloxetine treatment in generalized anxiety disorder. Pharmacogenomics J. 2013;13(3):280–5. https://doi.org/10.1038/tpj.2011.62.

195. Kurose K, Hiratsuka K, Ishiwata K, Nishikawa J, Nonen S, Azuma J, et al. Genome-wide association study of SSRI/SNRI-induced sexual dysfunction in a Japanese cohort with major depression. Psychiatry Res. 2012;198(3):424–9. https://doi.org/10.1016/j.psychres.2012.01.023.

196. Kato M, Serretti A, Nonen S, Takekita Y, Wakeno M, Azuma J, et al. Genetic variants in combination with early partial improvement as a clinical utility predictor of treatment outcome in major depressive disorder: the result of two pooled RCTs. Transl Psychiatry. 2015;5(2): e513. https://doi.org/10.1038/tp.2015.6.

197. Jorenby DE, Leischow SJ, Nides MA, Rennard SI, Johnston JA, Hughes AR, et al. A controlled trial of sustained-release bupropion, a nicotine patch, or both for smoking cessation. N Engl J Med. 1999;340(9):685–91. https://doi.org/10.1056/NEJM199903043400903.

198. Schnoll RA, Lerman C. Current and emerging pharmacotherapies for treating tobacco dependence. Expert Opin Emerg Drugs. 2006;11(3):429–44. https://doi.org/10.1517/14728214.11.3.429.

199. Fava M, Rush AJ, Thase ME, Clayton A, Stahl SM, Pradko JF, et al. 15 years of clinical experience with bupropion HCl: from bupropion to bupropion SR to bupropion XL. Prim Care Companion J Clin Psychiatry. 2005;7(3):106–13. https://doi.org/10.4088/pcc.v07n0305.

200. Dhillon S, Yang LP, Curran MP. Spotlight on bupropion in major depressive disorder. CNS Drugs. 2008;22(7):613–7. https://doi.org/10.2165/00023210-200822070-00006.

201. Bondarev ML, Bondareva TS, Young R, Glennon RA. Behavioral and biochemical investigations of bupropion metabolites. Eur J Pharmacol. 2003;474(1):85–93. https://doi.org/10.1016/s0014-2999(03)02010-7.

202. Jefferson JW, Pradko JF, Muir KT. Bupropion for major depressive disorder: pharmacokinetic and formulation considerations. Clin Ther. 2005;27(11):1685–95. https://doi.org/10.1016/j.clinthera.2005.11.011.

203. Chen Y, Liu H-f, Liu L, Nguyen K, Jones EB, Fretland AJ. The in vitro metabolism of bupropion revisited: concentration dependent involvement of cytochrome P450 2C19. Xenobiotica. 2010;40(8):536–46. https://doi.org/10.3109/00498254.2010.492880.

204. Gaebler AJ, Schneider KL, Stingl JC, Paulzen M. Subtherapeutic bupropion and hydroxybupropion serum concentrations in a patient with CYP2C19*1/*17 genotype suggesting a rapid metabolizer status. Pharmacogenomics J. 2020;20(6):840–4. https://doi.org/10.1038/s41397-020-0169-y.

205. Zhu AZ, Cox LS, Nollen N, Faseru B, Okuyemi KS, Ahluwalia JS, et al. CYP2B6 and bupropion's smoking-cessation pharmacology: the role of hydroxybupropion. Clin Pharmacol Ther. 2012;92(6):771–7. https://doi.org/10.1038/clpt.2012.186.

206. The FDA Table of Pharmacogenetic Associations 2020. Available at: https://www.fda.gov/medical-devices/precision-medicine/table-pharmacogenetic-associations. Accessed 13 Nov 2022.

207. Timmer CJ, Sitsen JM, Delbressine LP. Clinical pharmacokinetics of mirtazapine. Clin Pharmacokinet. 2000;38(6):461–74. https://doi.org/10.2165/00003088-200038060-00001.

208. Chen K. Organization of MAO A and MAO B promoters and regulation of gene expression. Neurotoxicology. 2004;25(1–2):31–6. https://doi.org/10.1016/S0161-813X(03)00113-X.

209. Fiedorowicz JG, Swartz KL. The role of monoamine oxidase inhibitors in current psychiatric practice. J Psychiatr Pract. 2004;10(4):239–48. https://doi.org/10.1097/00131746-200 407000-00005.

210. Ionescu DF, Rosenbaum JF, Alpert JE. Pharmacological approaches to the challenge of treatment-resistant depression. Dial Clin Neurosci. 2015;17(2):111–26. https://doi.org/10. 31887/DCNS.2015.17.2/dionescu.

211. Tikkanen R, Auvinen-Lintunen L, Ducci F, Sjöberg RL, Goldman D, Tiihonen J, et al. Psychopathy, PCL-R, and MAOA genotype as predictors of violent reconvictions. Psychiatry Res. 2011;185(3):382–6. https://doi.org/10.1016/j.psychres.2010.08.026.

212. Qiu M, Zhang C, Dai Y, Zhang L, Wang Y, Peng W, et al. mRNA levels of MAOA and 5-HT2A receptor in patients with pathological internet use: correlations with comorbid symptoms. Front Psychiatry. 2021;12(1197). https://doi.org/10.3389/fpsyt.2021.667699.

213. Kennedy SH. Continuation and maintenance treatments in major depression: the neglected role of monoamine oxidase inhibitors. J Psychiatry Neurosci. 1997;22(2):127–31.

214. Becker ML, Visser LE, van Schaik RH, Hofman A, Uitterlinden AG, Stricker BH. OCT1 polymorphism is associated with response and survival time in anti-Parkinsonian drug users. Neurogenetics. 2011;12(1):79–82. https://doi.org/10.1007/s10048-010-0254-5.

215. Patel KR, Cherian J, Gohil K, Atkinson D. Schizophrenia: overview and treatment options. P T. 2014;39(9):638–45.

216. Driessen J, Baik SH, Zhang Y. Trends in off-label use of second-generation antipsychotics in the medicare population from 2006 to 2012. Psychiatr Serv. 2016;67(8):898–903. https://doi. org/10.1176/appi.ps.201500316.

217. Domino ME, Swartz MS. Special section on implications of CATIE: who are the new users of antipsychotic medications? Psychiatr Serv. 2008;59(5):507–14.

218. Moreno-Küstner B, Martín C, Pastor L. Prevalence of psychotic disorders and its association with methodological issues. A systematic review and meta-analyses. PLoS One. 2018;13(4):e0195687. https://doi.org/10.1371/journal.pone.0195687.

219. Dennis JA, Gittner LS, Payne JD, Nugent K. Characteristics of U.S. adults taking prescription antipsychotic medications, National Health and Nutrition Examination Survey 2013–2018. BMC Psychiatry. 2020;20(1):483. https://doi.org/10.1186/s12888-020-02895-4.

220. Arranz MJ, Salazar J, Hernández MH. Pharmacogenetics of antipsychotics: clinical utility and implementation. Behav Brain Res. 2021;401: 113058. https://doi.org/10.1016/j.bbr.2020. 113058.

221. Ahmed Z, Hao S, Williamson T, McMorris CA, Bousman CA. Psychotropic prescribing rates and pharmacogenomic testing implications for autism in the Canadian primary care sentinel surveillance network. Pharmacogenet Genomics. 2022;32(3):94–100. https://doi.org/10. 1097/FPC.0000000000000457.

222. Corponi F, Fabbri C, Serretti A. Pharmacogenetics in psychiatry. Adv Pharmacol. 2018;83:297–331. https://doi.org/10.1016/bs.apha.2018.03.003.

223. Jukic MM, Smith RL, Haslemo T, Molden E, Ingelman-Sundberg M. Effect of CYP2D6 genotype on exposure and efficacy of risperidone and aripiprazole: a retrospective, cohort study. Lancet Psychiatry. 2019;6(5):418–26. https://doi.org/10.1016/S2215-0366(19)300 88-4.

224. Li J, Hashimoto H, Meltzer HY. Association of serotonin$_{2C}$ receptor polymorphisms with antipsychotic drug response in schizophrenia. Front Psychiatry. 2019;10(58). https://doi.org/ 10.3389/fpsyt.2019.00058.

225. Nozawa M, Ohnuma T, Matsubara Y, Sakai Y, Hatano T, Hanzawa R, et al. The relationship between the response of clinical symptoms and plasma olanzapine concentration, based on pharmacogenetics: Juntendo University Schizophrenia Projects (JUSP). Ther Drug Monit. 2008;30(1):35–40. https://doi.org/10.1097/FTD.0b013e31816336fd.

226. Shimoda K, Someya T, Morita S, Hirokane G, Yokono A, Takahashi S, et al. Lack of impact of CYP1A2 genetic polymorphism (C/A polymorphism at position 734 in intron 1 and G/A polymorphism at position -2964 in the 5′-flanking region of CYP1A2) on the plasma concentration of haloperidol in smoking male Japanese with schizophrenia. Prog

Neuropsychopharmacol Biol Psychiatry. 2002;26(2):261–5. https://doi.org/10.1016/s0278-5846(01)00263-9.

227. Arranz MJ, Blanco JP, Samperiz BA. Pharmacogenetics of the efficacy of antipsychotic drugs in schizophrenia. In: Rybakowski JK, Serretti A, editors. Genetic influences on response to drug treatment for major psychiatric disorders. Cham: Springer; 2016. p. 1–20. https://doi.org/10.1007/978-3-319-27040-1_1.

228. Czerwensky F, Leucht S, Steimer W. CYP1A2*1D and *1F polymorphisms have a significant impact on olanzapine serum concentrations. Ther Drug Monit. 2015;37(2):152–60. https://doi.org/10.1097/FTD.0000000000000119.

229. Ivanova SA, Toshchakova VA, Filipenko ML, Fedorenko OY, Boyarko EG, Boiko AS, et al. Cytochrome P450 1A2 co-determines neuroleptic load and may diminish tardive dyskinesia by increased inducibility. World J Biol Psychiatry. 2015;16(3):200–5. https://doi.org/10.3109/15622975.2014.995222.

230. Ivanova SA, Filipenko ML, Vyalova NM, Voronina EN, Pozhidaev IV, Osmanova DZ, et al. CYP1A2 and CYP2D6 gene polymorphisms in schizophrenic patients with neuroleptic drug-induced side effects. Bull Exp Biol Med. 2016;160(5):687–90. https://doi.org/10.1007/s10517-016-3250-4.

231. Zai CC, Maes MS, Tiwari AK, Zai GC, Remington G, Kennedy JL. Genetics of tardive dyskinesia: promising leads and ways forward. J Neurol Sci. 2018;389:28–34. https://doi.org/10.1016/j.jns.2018.02.011.

232. Arranz MJ, Gonzalez-Rodriguez A, Perez-Blanco J, Penadés R, Gutierrez B, Ibañez L, et al. A pharmacogenetic intervention for the improvement of the safety profile of antipsychotic treatments. Transl Psychiatry. 2019;9(1):1–8. https://doi.org/10.1038/s41398-019-0511-9.

233. de Leon J. Personalizing dosing of risperidone, paliperidone and clozapine using therapeutic drug monitoring and pharmacogenetics. Neuropharmacology. 2020;168: 107656. https://doi.org/10.1016/j.neuropharm.2019.05.033.

234. Whiteford HA, Ferrari AJ, Degenhardt L, Feigin V, Vos T. The global burden of mental, neurological and substance use disorders: an analysis from the Global Burden of Disease Study 2010. PLoS ONE. 2015;10(2): e0116820. https://doi.org/10.1371/journal.pone.0116820.

235. Schmidt D, Elger CE. What is the evidence that oxcarbazepine and carbamazepine are distinctly different antiepileptic drugs? Epilepsy Behav. 2004;5(5):627–35. https://doi.org/10.1016/j.yebeh.2004.07.004.

236. Beydoun A, Kutluay E. Oxcarbazepine. Expert Opin Pharmacother. 2002;3(1):59–71. https://doi.org/10.1517/14656566.3.1.59.

237. Beydoun A, DuPont S, Zhou D, Matta M, Nagire V, Lagae L. Current role of carbamazepine and oxcarbazepine in the management of epilepsy. Seizure. 2020;83:251–63. https://doi.org/10.1016/j.seizure.2020.10.018.

238. Leckband SG, Kelsoe JR, Dunnenberger HM, George AL Jr, Tran E, Berger R, et al. Clinical Pharmacogenetics Implementation Consortium guidelines for HLA-B genotype and carbamazepine dosing. Clin Pharmacol Ther. 2013;94(3):324–8. https://doi.org/10.1038/clpt.2013.103.

239. Trachtenberg E, Vinson M, Hayes E, Hsu YM, Houtchens K, Erlich H, et al. HLA class I (A, B, C) and class II (DRB1, DQA1, DQB1, DPB1) alleles and haplotypes in the Han from southern China. Tissue Antigens. 2007;70(6):455–63. https://doi.org/10.1111/j.1399-0039.2007.00932.x.

240. Chang CC, Too CL, Murad S, Hussein SH. Association of HLA-B*1502 allele with carbamazepine-induced toxic epidermal necrolysis and Stevens-Johnson syndrome in the multi-ethnic Malaysian population. Int J Dermatol. 2011;50(2):221–4. https://doi.org/10.1111/j.1365-4632.2010.04745.x.

241. Pimtanothai N, Charoenwongse P, Mutirangura A, Hurley CK. Distribution of HLA-B alleles in nasopharyngeal carcinoma patients and normal controls in Thailand. Tissue Antigens. 2002;59(3):223–5. https://doi.org/10.1034/j.1399-0039.2002.590308.x.

242. Saito S, Ota S, Yamada E, Inoko H, Ota M. Allele frequencies and haplotypic associations defined by allelic DNA typing at HLA class I and class II loci in the Japanese population. Tissue Antigens. 2000;56(6):522–9. https://doi.org/10.1034/j.1399-0039.2000.560606.x.

243. Shekhani R, Steinacher L, Swen JJ, Ingelman-Sundberg M. Evaluation of current regulation and guidelines of pharmacogenomic drug labels: opportunities for improvements. Clin Pharmacol Ther. 2020;107(5):1240–55. https://doi.org/10.1002/cpt.1720.

244. Gomez-Sanchez CI, Carballo JJ, Riveiro-Alvarez R, Soto-Insuga V, Rodrigo M, Mahillo-Fernandez I, et al. Pharmacogenetics of methylphenidate in childhood attention-deficit/hyperactivity disorder: long-term effects. Sci Rep. 2017;7(1):10391. https://doi.org/10.1038/s41598-017-10912 y.

245. Brown JT, Bishop JR, Sangkuhl K, Nurmi EL, Mueller DJ, Dinh Jean C, et al. Clinical Pharmacogenetics Implementation Consortium guideline for cytochrome P450 (CYP)2D6 genotype and atomoxetine therapy. Clin Pharmacol Ther. 2019;106(1):94–102. https://doi.org/10.1002/cpt.1409.

246. Mandrioli R, Mercolini L, Raggi MA. Benzodiazepine metabolism: an analytical perspective. Curr Drug Metab. 2008;9(8):827–44. https://doi.org/10.2174/138920008786049258.

247. Nutt DJ, Malizia AL. New insights into the role of the GABA(A)-benzodiazepine receptor in psychiatric disorder. Br J Psychiatry. 2001;179:390–6. https://doi.org/10.1192/bjp.179.5.390.

Pharmacogenomics in Anesthesia

Dragan Primorac and Lidija Bach-Rojecky

Abstract

In everyday practice, anesthesiologists face challenges when optimizing anesthesia for their patients. Anesthetic and adjuvant drugs dose adjustments are particularly challenging because of inter-individual differences in the anesthetic drug doses which induce and maintain anesthesia, and different time-course for recovery. Beside procedure-related factors and pharmacological features of drugs, the patient's genetic makeup can influence overall anesthesia outcomes.

D. Primorac (✉)
St. Catherine Specialty Hospital, 10000 Zagreb, Croatia
e-mail: dragan.primorac@svkatarina.hr; draganprimorac2@gmail.com

University of Split School of Medicine, 21000 Split, Croatia

Josip Juraj Strossmayer University of Osijek Faculty of Medicine, 31000 Osijek, Croatia

University of Rijeka School of Medicine, 51000 Rijeka, Croatia

Josip Juraj Strossmayer University of Osijek Faculty of Dental Medicine and Health, 31000 Osijek, Croatia

Eberly College of Science, Penn State University, 517 Thomas Street, State College, PA 16803, USA

The Henry C. Lee College of Criminal Justice and Forensic Sciences, University of New Haven, West Haven, CT, USA

National Forensic Science University, Gandhinagar, Gujarat, India

College of Medicine and Forensics, Xi'an Jiaotong University, Xi'an, China

Medical School REGIOMED, 96450 Coburg, Germany

L. Bach-Rojecky
University of Zagreb Faculty of Pharmacy and Biochemistry, 10000 Zagreb, Croatia

D. Primorac
International Center For Applied Biological Sciences, 10000, Zagreb, Croatia

Therefore, applying pharmacogenomics (PGx) testing before the anesthesia procedure might be a way to increase anesthetic drugs' efficacy and safety. PGx can suggest dose adjustments, detect responders, and non-responders among patients, and predict the risk for some adverse reactions. General anesthesia commonly combines drugs, such as inhalational anesthetics, intravenous anesthetics, local anesthetics, sedatives, muscle relaxants, and opioid analgesics. For some of them, PGx testing is implemented into the clinical guidelines, while others still need evidence from intensive ongoing research.

Keywords

Pharmacogenomics • Anesthetics • Opioid analgesics • Sedatives • Muscle relaxants • Toxicity

1   Introduction

General anesthesia commonly combines various drugs, such as inhalational and intravenous anesthetics, hypnotic-sedative agents, muscle relaxants, opioid analgesics, and local anesthetics. Other drugs, like antiemetics, non-steroidal anti-inflammatory drugs, and proton pump inhibitors, are commonly used in the perioperative and postoperative periods [1].

In addition to various factors related to patients and anesthesia procedures (Fig. 1), variations in genes can influence anesthesia outcomes, as well. Polymorphisms in genes encoding for drugs' protein targets, transporters, metabolic enzymes, or other proteins associated with the higher risk for certain toxicities can change drugs' pharmacodynamics and pharmacokinetic characteristics, and make patients more prone to develop adverse effects [2].

General anesthetics are among the most dangerous drugs used in clinic. They have narrow therapeutic window, special pharmacokinetic features, and numerous side effects and risks. The majority of potentially fatal side effects are dose/concentration-dependent, such as hypotension, central nervous system (CNS) and respiratory depression [2, 3]. These risks are predictable since they are associated with drugs' pharmacological action. Inhalational anesthetics and muscle relaxant succinylcholine in some individuals can trigger a rare and potentially fatal hypermetabolic condition—malignant hyperthermia (MH). Studies established the genetic background of MH and guidelines based on the highest level of evidence suggest preventive PGx testing to determine patients with a susceptible genotype [4].

For other drugs used in the anesthesia, there is not enough evidence to associate certain genotypes with observed differences in efficacy and the risk for serious adverse effects. More evidence from clinical, real-world practice is needed, which is an ongoing process.

Recently, several comprehensive review papers have been published related to the role of PGx in anesthesiology [1–3]. Here, we briefly overview gene variants and their possible influence on the therapeutic effects of the major drug classes used in anesthesiology.

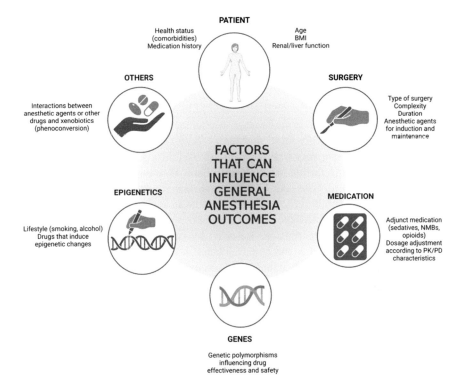

Fig. 1 Factors that can influence anesthesia outcomes (made by authors according to Ref. [2]). *Legend: BMI—body mass index; NMBs—neuromuscular blockers; PK/PD—pharmacokinetics/ pharmacodynamics*

2   Volatile (Inhalational) Anesthetics

Volatile anesthetics, like isoflurane, desflurane, and sevoflurane, differ in their physicochemical properties, potency, solubility in blood and tissues, and the time needed for induction and recovery from anesthesia [1, 2].

Inhalational anesthetics have specific pharmacokinetic characteristics: they are rapidly absorbed from the lungs into the systemic circulation and distributed into tissues due to high solubility in lipids and fast diffusion through physiological barriers. Depending on the concentration, they interfere with the function of diverse membrane proteins, such as nicotinic receptors for acetylcholine, GABA-A receptors for gamma-aminobutyric acid (GABA), N-methyl-D-aspartate (NMDA) receptor for the excitatory neurotransmitter glutamate, serotonin 5-HT3 receptor, as well as voltage-gated sodium, potassium, and calcium channels [2].

These diverse and complex targeted macromolecules often consist of several protein subunits encoded by various genes, whose variations, for now in theory, might influence the anesthesia outcome. Also, inhalational anesthetics are minimally metabolized and are primarily excreted by the lungs, thus eliminating the variations in metabolic enzymes or transporters as factors influencing their therapeutic effects and risks.

The main differences between desflurane, isoflurane, and sevoflurane are briefly described in the following text. Because desflurane and sevoflurane induce rapid induction and fast recovery from anesthesia, they can be applied for outpatient surgery. Desflurane has very low fat-to-blood solubility and is suitable for obese patients during a long-lasting surgical procedure. However, it can cause adverse effects in the upper airways and is not appropriate for the induction of anesthesia [2]. Neither isoflurane is suitable for anesthesia induction because of airway irritation due to its unpleasant odor. Isoflurane also reduces systemic vascular resistance and causes hypotension, followed by compensatory sympathetic activation, transient tachycardia, and hypertension [2]. Both anesthetics are minimally metabolized and are primarily exhaled via the lungs.

Sevoflurane has some benefits over desflurane and isoflurane. For example, it is not an irritant of the airways, it relaxes bronchial smooth muscles and has no effect on cardiac function or heart rhythm [5]. Around 5% of the inhaled dose is metabolized in the liver via CYP2E1 to hexafluoroisopropanol and fluoride. There is a theoretical risk of kidney injury induced by fluoride, but clinically relevant data related to potential sevoflurane nephrotoxicity is missing [2].

The most important genetically mediated safety risk of volatile anesthetics is malignant hyperthermia. In susceptible individuals, volatile anesthetics may cause the release of calcium from the sarcoplasmic reticulum into the cytoplasm of skeletal muscle cells, with consequent increased cellular metabolism, glycogenolysis, and skeletal muscles contractures, all of which result in heat overproduction, increased lactate level, and with acidosis. The occurrence of MH is possible during anesthesia or up to an hour after the use of inhalational agents was ceased [4, 6].

The genetic background of this serious hypermetabolic condition was determined, with two genes playing the major role, *RYR1*, and *CACNA1S*. MH susceptibility is inherited in an autosomal dominant pattern. RYR1 is a calcium channel at the membrane of the sarcoplasmic reticulum, which mediates calcium release from the intracellular depo into the cytoplasm. Another associated regulator protein of intracellular calcium is the L-type calcium channel located on the plasma membrane. A sum of 50 variants in both the *RYR1* and *CACNA1S* genes are associated with MH susceptibility [4, 6].

Based on accumulated evidence, the Clinical Pharmacogenetics Implementation Consortium (CPIC) and European Malignant Hyperthermia Group recommend avoiding inhalational anesthetics in MH-susceptible patients based on the results of PGx testing [4, 6].

Nitrous oxide (N_2O) gas is a weak anesthetic (it has minimal alveolar concentration >100%) and is thus usually combined with other inhalational anesthetics because it diminishes their concentrations necessary for optimal general anesthesia.

It exerts a strong analgesic effect mediated by opioid and adrenergic neurotransmitter systems activation [2]. It can also increase blood pressure due to sympathetic nervous system stimulation. N_2O rapidly enters body cavities but cannot escape fast enough, thus leading to increased pressure in body cavities [7].

N_2O can increase homocysteine levels because the remethylation of homocysteine to methionine is inhibited, due to the irreversible oxidation of the cobalt in vitamin B12, a cofactor for the enzyme methionine synthase. Hyperhomocysteinemia is especially important in patients deficient in methylenetetrahydrofolate reductase (MTHFR) caused by *MTHFR* gene polymorphisms. *MTHFR* 677 C>T or 1298 A>C (with a prevalence of both SNPs of 20% in the Western European population) significantly increases the risk for hyperhomocysteinemia in homozygous carriers after N_2O application [8].

3   Intravenous Anesthetics

Propofol, etomidate, ketamine, and thiopental are used for the induction and maintenance of general anesthesia. These lipophilic small drug molecules after intravenous application show an excellent distribution to the CNS with fast redistribution to peripheral tissues. Therefore, the onset of anesthesia is fast, accompanied by fast recovery as well. Although these drugs share some pharmacological features, they significantly differ in pharmacodynamic profile, pharmacokinetics, adverse effects, and effects on peripheral organs [1, 2]. Understanding their peculiarities and differences should guide clinicians on which drug to use in a specific clinical setting. Patient characteristics, like age, health status, and concomitant medications, also affect the choice of optimal anesthetic drug. Among endogenous factors, the role of genetics is drawing much attention. Investigations of specific genotypes that could influence anesthetic drug efficacy and safety are still underway, and data are continuously collected. For now, there are no evidence-based pharmacogenomics recommendations for either drug in the class [2].

Propofol differs from other drugs because of its wider effects. It exerts sedative-hypnotic, but also anxiolytic, anticonvulsant, anti-inflammatory, antiemetic, antioxidative, and possibly neuroprotective actions [2]. Propofol primarily activates GABA-A receptors, while blockade of NMDA receptors and interference with calcium channels might also contribute to its central depressant effect. Despite its wide use, clinicians are encountering inter-individual differences in doses for anesthesia induction and maintenance, and the time to onset and recover from anesthesia. These variations might be a consequence of variants in genes encoding for propofol molecular targets or enzymes involved in its biotransformation [2, 9]. One study suggested an association of polymorphism in the gene encoding for serotonin 5HT2A receptor subtype (SNP rs6313) and the dose required for anesthesia and time to recovery. Carriers of the minor allele (G) required a lower propofol dose, and the time to induce anesthesia in those patients is reduced by 40% [9]. An association of SNPs in genes *GABRA1* (rs2279020) encoding alfa-1 receptor subunit and *SCN9A* (rs6746030) encoding sodium channel with a depth of anesthesia has also been proposed [9]. Additionally, several polymorphisms have been associated with the risk of cardiovascular side effects after propofol application, especially mutations in *GABRA1* (rs2279020), *GABRA2* (rs11503014), and *CHRM2* (rs1824024) encoding cholinergic muscarinic receptor [9].

Genes encoding for metabolic enzymes have also been investigated since propofol undergoes an extensive metabolic transformation. For 70% of propofol, enzyme uridine 5′-diphosphate (UDP) glucuronosyltransferase is essential for transformation to hydrophilic glucuronide metabolite, while the other 30% first undergo hydroxylation via CYP2B6 and to a minor extent CYP2C9 [2]. The most investigated metabolic enzyme is the highly polymorphic *CYP2B6* gene. One study showed that SNP rs3745274 GT and TT genotypes are connected to the reduced propofol metabolism rate, which allows a decreased dose of propofol, as compared to patients with the GG genotype [10]. Pharmacokinetic model-based dosing simulations suggested that *CYP2B6* SNP rs2279343 affects the toxicity of propofol in elderly patients with AA and AG genotypes. Those patients will need a 50% lower propofol dose to reduce the risk of adverse effects due to overdosing [11]. Further evidence for *CYP2B6* gene polymorphisms and other genes potentially related to propofol's efficacy and safety is needed.

Etomidate exerts anesthetic effect by activation of GABA-A receptors. It also reduces cortisol and aldosterone synthesis in the adrenal gland by inhibiting the enzyme 11-β-hydroxylase. This effect may have a negative impact on severely ill patients with sepsis or septic shock [12]. Etomidate is the anesthetic of choice in patients with cardiovascular risk because of its favorable effect on the cardiovascular system. Its biotransformation does not include CYP enzymes but hepatic esterases, which catalyze hydrolysis reactions to inactive metabolites excreted by urine [2]. The investigations suggested that some mutations in genes encoding GABA-A receptor subunits β2, β3, and γ affect etomidate binding affinity, but the clinical relevance of these findings is not yet established [13].

Ketamine blocks glutamate NMDA receptors in a non-competitive manner, although it has other pharmacological targets for which it binds with a lower affinity. In sub-anesthetic doses, it exerts a rapid antidepressant effect. In higher doses, it induces hypnosis, analgesia, and amnesia, preserves breathing and airway reflexes, has a moderate bronchodilatory effect, and increases the heart rate, blood pressure, and cardiac output [14]. However, multiple adverse effects and risks, which include muscular discoordination, seizure, hypothermia, behavioral changes, hallucinations, delusions, etc., limit its use as an anesthetic [2, 14].

It is extensively metabolized by CYP3A4 (major route) and to a lesser extent by CYP2B6 to the pharmacologically active norketamine, which is further conjugated to form glucuronidated metabolites [2]. One study associated *the CYP2B6* *6 allele with a higher incidence of adverse effects in chronic pain patients because of the decreased clearance of ketamine compared to patients with the *CYP2B6* *1/*6 and *1/*1 haplotypes [15].

Barbiturate thiopental induces rapid onset of sedative and hypnotic effects, with ultra-short duration used for induction of anesthesia. After prolonged infusion, it accumulates in the fat tissue with a very slow elimination rate, which negatively influences complete recovery from anesthesia [2]. Its main pharmacodynamic mechanism includes the activation of GABA-A receptors, with additional targets of minor significance (like nicotinic acetylcholine receptor and Ca^{2+}-ATPase). It is extensively metabolized in the liver to active and inactive metabolites. Despite its long history of use, there is no data about the potential role of specific pharmacogenes in its anesthetic profile [1, 2].

4   Sedatives

In contrast to barbiturates, benzodiazepines, like diazepam and midazolam, show better pharmacological characteristics and improved safety. They act as positive allosteric modulators of GABA-A receptors leading to increased receptor affinity for GABA with more frequent chloride channel opening and a pronounced central depressant effect. Drugs in this large class differ in their affinities for the binding sites on the receptor complex, selectivity for the receptor subunits, and potency [16]. They are all lipophilic, with large volumes of distribution, and plasma protein binding, but differ in biotransformation rate and the duration of action. Some benzodiazepines are metabolized by CYP3A4 and CYP2C19 enzymes, while others (like oxazepam and lorazepam) primarily undergo conjugation reactions catalyzed by UDP-glucuronosyltransferase (UGT) [2]. This class of drugs is generally well tolerated, but some patients are at higher risk for adverse reactions. Elderly patients, because of a lower amount of fatty tissue and decreased renal and liver function, exert slower drug elimination and are at increased risk of prolonged sedation and CNS depression [16]. In order to find genetic predictors of possible drugs' higher risk of toxicity, research has focused on polymorphisms of GABA-A receptor subunits, especially on those genes that encode for α subunits (α1-α6). For example, patients with AA genotype on rs4263535 in the *GABRA1* gene (coding for α1 subunit) are at increased risk of deep sedation, but more studies are needed to confirm the clinical significance of this observation [17].

Regarding metabolizing enzymes CYP3A4 and CYP2C19, it was found that *CYP2C19*2* and **3* alleles are associated with reduced diazepam metabolism, resulting in prolonged recovery from anesthesia and an increased risk of CNS depression [18].

While polymorphisms in *CYP3A4* and *CYP3A5* genes have no evidence to influence midazolam effects, one study found that patients with SNP rs4263535 in *GABRA1* which are AA carriers require a lower dose of midazolam to avoid profound sedation during the surgery [17].

Dexmedetomidine is used for sedation in intensive care units, for procedural sedation, as an adjunct during anesthesia, and for the treatment of agitated patients. These effects are mediated by selective activation of pre- and post-synaptic α2A adrenergic receptors in *locus coeruleus*. While studies did not demonstrate any relevant gene variations affecting the pharmacokinetics of dexmedetomidine [2], certain variants in the gene encoding for α2A receptor (*ADRA2A*) had shown an association with drug efficacy. For example, SNP rs1800544 genotypes GG or GC are connected to decreased sedative response if compared to the CC genotype [19], but this needs further confirmation.

5 Local Anesthetics

Local anesthetics prevent nerve impulse transmission by blocking the sodium current into the cell after binding in the inner pore of the Na(v)1.7 sodium channels in excitable tissues. Drugs show frequency-dependent and voltage-dependent binding affinity, meaning they bind with greater affinity for channels that open more frequently when resting membrane potential is more positive. Based on chemical structure, local anesthetics are either esters or amides, which differ in physicochemical and pharmacological properties, and duration of action [1]. They can be absorbed into the systemic circulation after local application, inducing concentration-dependent adverse effects because of interference with impulse generation and conduction. Amides, like lidocaine, bupivacaine, and levobupivacaine, are metabolized in the liver by CYP3A4, while the elimination of esters tetracaine and procaine depends on plasma/tissue butyrylcholinesterase activity [1].

A limited number of studies investigated potential pharmacogenes related to the efficacy and risks of these drugs. One in vitro experiment has shown that Asn395Lys mutation in the *SCN9A* gene encoding for the sodium voltage-gated channel alpha subunit 9 could contribute to resistance to lidocaine [20]. At present, no clinical studies have been conducted to support the significance of this variation.

It was recognized that enzymatic disorder of the red blood cells characterized by glucose-6-phosphate dehydrogenase (G6PD) deficiency, due to *G6PD* gene variants, can increase the risk for acute hemolysis after local anesthetics applications. G6PD is necessary for the maintenance of reduced glutathione within the cell, thus protecting cells from oxidative stress damage. Based on collected data, PharmGKB recommends that patients with G6PD deficiency are advised against the use of local anesthetics with a known risk of methemoglobinemia, like benzocaine, prilocaine, lidocaine, and articaine [21].

6 Neuromuscular Blocking Drugs

Neuromuscular blocking drugs (NMBs) are used to facilitate endotracheal intubation, optimize surgical conditions, and assist with mechanical ventilation. NMBs can cause various adverse effects, like cardiovascular, autonomic, and histamine-related, with acute respiratory complications postoperatively [22].

NMBs divide into two groups, nondepolarizing (mivacurium, [cis]atracurium, rocuronium, and vecuronium) and depolarizing (succinylcholine, also known as suxamethonium). The nondepolarizing drugs are competitive antagonists of a nicotinic acetylcholine receptor (nAChR), while depolarizing bind as acetylcholine, first activating the receptor and increasing sodium current into the cell, followed by receptor desensitization [2]. After binding to nAChR, both drug classes block inward sodium current and prevent muscle cell action potential generation.

Drugs show chemical and pharmacological diversities, which influences differences in time of onset, and duration of action. Advanced age, female sex, decrease in hepatic blood flow during surgery, smoking, and ethnic background can influence the pharmacological features of NMBs and explain inter-individual differences in clinical response after their application [22].

Several reports have demonstrated variabilities in the duration of action of rocuronium. Since its elimination mostly relies on biliary excretion (around 70%) of the unchanged drug, transport protein organic anion transporting polypeptide 1A2 and B1 (OATP1A2, OATP1B1) gained some attention. SNP rs3834939 in the *SLOC1A2* gene that encodes OATP1A2 is particularly interesting as it affects rocuronium elimination. Patients with −189_−188InsA, −/A, and A/A genotypes may have compromised rocuronium clearance compared to those with −/− genotypes, with potentially prolonged blocking action and recovery time [23]. In addition, the *ABCB1* TT genotype on rs1128503 and *SLCO1B1* AG and GG genotypes on rs2306283 decrease the hepatic clearance of rocuronium, which can cause its accumulation, and influence the duration of action and recovery [24].

Succinylcholine (SCH) is usually used to facilitate rapid sequence intubation because of its rapid onset and short duration of action. However, it can cause prolonged neuromuscular blockade, leading to postanesthetic apnea and possibly respiratory depression and death. This is estimated to occur in approximately 1 in 1800 applications [25].

The enzyme butyrylcholinesterase (BChE) hydrolyses SCH to succinylmonocholine, succinic acid, and choline. At least 75 genetic variants of the *BCHE* gene have been identified that cause enzyme deficiency. The most common and significant variants are A—atypical, K—Kalow, F—fluoride, and S—silent. One study predicted that approximately 0.06% of individuals have severe BChE deficiency, 8% moderate, and 29% mild enzyme deficiency [24]. The published evidence indicates that patients with moderate BChE deficiency are at risk of prolonged SHC-induced neuromuscular blockade [26]. According to PharmGKB (https://www.pharmgkb.org/labelAnnotation/PA166122970), FDA, as well as Health Canada, it is recommended that SCH "should be used with caution, if at all, in patients known to be or suspected of being homozygous for the atypical plasma cholinesterase gene" [26]. As with SCH, the same recommendation exists for mivacurium.

SCH shares the risk for malignant hyperthermia with inhalational anesthetics, with the same genetic susceptibility in the background, as described earlier [4]. Therefore, in patients with SNPs in the *RYR1* or *CACNA1S* genes, SCH application should be avoided.

7   Opioid Analgesics

Although opioid analgesic drugs are widely used to prevent and treat peri- and postoperative pain, the focus of this chapter will be on drugs used during anesthesia. Synthetic opioids fentanyl and its analogs alfentanil, remifentanil, and sufentanil are commonly used because of their strong analgesic effect with decreased pain-evoked hemodynamic changes. These drugs can cause various central and peripheral opioid-related adverse effects with potentially fatal respiratory depression in larger doses [1, 27].

Sufentanil is the most potent, while alfentanil has around 1/4 to 1/10 the potency of fentanyl. Fentanyl and sufentanil have a short time to peak analgesia and short-lasting effect after small bolus doses, while recovery after prolonged administration varies considerably. Since remifentanil has the shortest duration of action (<10 min) and a low potential for accumulation, it is suitable for brief painful procedures [2].

These drugs activate opioid receptors after high-affinity binding, especially the μ-receptor (or MOR) subtype in the CNS and at the periphery. Studies have shown that the variability in the analgesia might to some extent be affected by genetic variants in the *OPRM1* gene encoding MOR, *ABCB1* encoding P-gp transporter, and *COMT* encoding catechol-O-methyltransferase enzyme which metabolizes catecholamines. Over 100 allelic variants of *OPRM1* that could potentially influence opioid analgesia have been identified. One of the most studied SNPs is rs1799971 (118 A>G). The frequency of this variant is high among individuals of Asian ancestry (35–50%), followed by individuals of European (15.4%), Hispanic (14%), and African ancestry (4.7%) [28].

Since reduced COMT activity is associated with the upregulation of opioid receptors, polymorphisms of the *COMT* gene have been suggested to influence analgesic efficacy. The most studied functional SNP of *COMT* is rs4680, which reduces enzyme activity [29], but there is not enough evidence for its connection with opioid efficacy or safety risks.

Fentanyl, alfentanil, and sufentanil are metabolized by CYP3A4 (fentanyl via CYP3A5 in addition) in the liver, followed by conjugation, while remifentanil undergoes metabolism by nonspecific plasma and tissue esterases. Some studies indicated that polymorphisms of the *CYP3A4* gene could influence the effects of these drugs. For example, patients homozygous for the *1G allele require higher doses of fentanyl to achieve adequate analgesia [30, 31]. Of other potential gene polymorphisms, weak evidence correlates the *ABCB1* rs1045642 AA genotype with a lower fentanyl dose requirement, but this needs further proof in a larger cohort of patients [2].

As for remifentanil, one study found that mutation (A→G) at *ABCB1* rs1045642 site leads to higher consumption of remifentanil, lower analgesic efficacy, longer analepsia duration, and poorer postoperative recovery [32].

Due to a lack of strong evidence, only two drugs (codeine and tramadol) to treat postoperative pain have evidence-based guidelines that suggest dosage adjustments according to the patient's genotype (related to *CYP2D6* gene) [33]. While waiting for more evidence regarding genotype-guided pain therapy, all efforts should be made to secure optimal analgesia with an acceptable adverse effects profile.

8   Conclusion

To secure effective and safe anesthesia and fast recovery with minimal patient suffering during preoperative and postoperative periods, various drugs from different pharmacotherapy classes are used. Taking into consideration all relevant patient-related factors, anesthetic procedure-related specificities, and drugs' pharmacological characteristics, evidence-based pharmacogenomics implementation will further improve anesthesia care and optimize clinical outcomes.

References

1. Bach-Rojecky L, Čutura T, Lozić M, Husedžinović Kliškinjić I, Matišić V, Primorac D. Personalized anesthetic pharmacology. In: Dabbagh A, editor. Personalized medicine in anesthesia, pain and perioperative medicine. Switzerland: Springer; 2021.
2. Bach-Rojecky L, Vađunec D, Lozić M, Žunić K, Špoljar GG, Čutura T, et al. Challenges in anesthesia personalization resolving the pharmacogenomics puzzle. Per Med. 2019;16(6):511–25. https://doi.org/10.2217/pme-2019-0056.
3. Xie S, Ma W, Guo Q, Liu J, Li W, McLeod HL, He Y. The pharmacogenetics of medications used in general anesthesia. Pharmacogenomics. 2018;19(3):285–98. https://doi.org/10.2217/pgs-2017-0168.
4. Gonsalves SG, Dirksen RT, Sangkuhl K, Pulk R, Alvarellos M, Vo T, et al. Clinical Pharmacogenetics Implementation Consortium (CPIC) guideline for the use of potent volatile anesthetic agents and succinylcholine in the context of RYR1 or CACNA1S genotypes. Clin Pharmacol Ther. 2019;105(6):1338–44. https://doi.org/10.1002/cpt.1319.
5. Li F, Yuan Y. Meta-analysis of the cardioprotective effect of sevoflurane versus propofol during cardiac surgery. BMC Anesthesiol. 2015;15:128. https://doi.org/10.1186/s12871-015-0107-8.
6. Rüffert H, Bastian B, Bendixen D, Girard T, Heiderich S, Hellblom A, et al. Consensus guidelines on perioperative management of malignant hyperthermia suspected or susceptible patients from the European Malignant Hyperthermia Group. Br J Anaesth. 2021;126(1):120–30. https://doi.org/10.1016/j.bja.2020.09.029.
7. Munson ES. Transfer of nitrous oxide into body air cavities. Br J Anesth. 1974;46:202–9.
8. Nagele P, Zeugswetter B, Wiener C, Burger H, Hüpfl M, Mittlböck M, Födinger M. Influence of methylenetetrahydrofolate reductase gene polymorphisms on homocysteine concentrations after nitrous oxide anesthesia. Anesthesiology. 2008;109(1):36–43. https://doi.org/10.1097/ALN.0b013e318178820b.
9. Zhong Q, Chen X, Zhao Y, Liu R, Yao S. Association of polymorphisms in pharmacogenetic candidate genes with propofol susceptibility. Sci Rep. 2017;7(1):3343. https://doi.org/10.1038/s41598-017-03229-3.
10. Mourão AL, de Abreu FG, Fiegenbaum M. Impact of the cytochrome P450 2B6 (CYP2B6) gene polymorphism c.516G>T (rs3745274) on propofol dose variability. Eur J Drug Metab Pharmacokinet. 2016;41(5):511–5. https://doi.org/10.1007/s13318-015-0289-y.
11. Eugene AR. CYP2B6 genotype guided dosing of propofol anesthesia in the elderly based on nonparametric population pharmacokinetic modeling and simulations. Int J Clin Pharmacol Toxicol. 2017;6(1):242–9.

12. Wagner CE, Bick JS, Johnson D, Ahmad R, Han X, Ehrenfeld JM, et al. Etomidate use and postoperative outcomes among cardiac surgery patients. Anesthesiology. 2014;120(3):579–89. https://doi.org/10.1097/ALN.0000000000000087.
13. Desai R, Ruesch D, Forman A. Gamma-amino butyric acid type A receptor mutations at beta2N265 alter etomidate efficacy while preserving basal and agonist-dependent activity. Anesthesiology. 2009;111(4):774–84. https://doi.org/10.1097/ALN.0b013e3181b55fae.
14. Borsato GS, Siegel JL, Rose MQ, Ojard M, Feyissa AM, Quinones-Hinojosa A, et al. Ketamine in seizure management and future pharmacogenomic considerations. Pharmacogenomics J. 2020;20(3):351–4. https://doi.org/10.1038/s41397-019-0120-2.
15. Li Y, Jackson KA, Slon B Hardy JR, Franco M, William L, et al. CYP2B6*6 allele and age substantially reduce steady-state ketamine clearance in chronic pain patients: impact on adverse effects. Br J Clin Pharmacol. 2015;80(2):276–84. https://doi.org/10.1111/bcp.12614.
16. Griffin CE 3rd, Kaye AM, Bueno FR, Kaye AD. Benzodiazepine pharmacology and central nervous system-mediated effects. Ochsner J. 2013;13(2):214–23.
17. Choi YJ, Lee SY, Yang KS, Park JY, Yoon SZ, Yoon SM. Polymorphism rs4263535 in GABRA1 intron 4 was related to deeper sedation by intravenous midazolam. J Int Med Res. 2015;43(5):686–98. https://doi.org/10.1177/0300060515587580.
18. Inomata S, Nagashima A, Itagaki F, Homma M, Nishimura M, Osaka Y, et al. CYP2C19 genotype affects diazepam pharmacokinetics and emergence from general anesthesia. Clin Pharmacol Ther. 2005;78(6):647–55. https://doi.org/10.1016/j.clpt.2005.08.020.
19. Yağar S, Yavaş S, Karahalil B. The role of the ADRA2A C1291G genetic polymorphism in response to dexmedetomidine on patients undergoing coronary artery surgery. Mol Biol Rep. 2011;38(5):3383–9. https://doi.org/10.1007/s11033-010-0446-y.
20. Cohen M, Sadhasivam S, Vinks AA. Pharmacogenetics in perioperative medicine. Curr Opin Anaesthesiol. 2012;25(4):419–27. https://doi.org/10.1097/ACO.0b013e3283556129.
21. Elyassi AR, Rowshan HH. Perioperative management of the glucose-6-phosphate dehydrogenase deficient patient: a review of literature. Anesth Prog. 2009;56(3):86–91. https://doi.org/10.2344/0003-3006-56.3.86.
22. Renew JR, Ratzlaff R, Hernandez-Torres V, Brull SJ, Prielipp RC. Neuromuscular blockade management in the critically Ill patient. J Intensive Care. 2020;8:37. https://doi.org/10.1186/s40560-020-00455-2.
23. Costa ACC, Coelho EB, Lanchote VL, Correia BV, Abumansur JT, Lauretti GR, de Moraes NV. The SLCO1A2-189-188InsA polymorphism reduces clearance of rocuronium in patients submitted to elective surgeries. Eur J Clin Pharmacol. 2017;73(8):957–63. https://doi.org/10.1007/s00228-017-2243-1.
24. Ahlström S, Bergman P, Jokela R, Ottensmann L, Ahola-Olli A, Pirinen M, et al. First genome-wide association study on rocuronium dose requirements shows association with SLCO1A2. Br J Anaesth. 2021;126(5):949–57. https://doi.org/10.1016/j.bja.2021.01.029.
25. Schaefer MS, Hammer M, Santer P, Grabitz SD, Patrocinio M, Althoff FC, et al. Succinylcholine and postoperative pulmonary complications: a retrospective cohort study using registry data from two hospital networks. Br J Anaesth. 2020;125(4):629–36. https://doi.org/10.1016/j.bja.2020.05.059.
26. Zhu GD, Dawson E, Huskey A, Gordon RJ, Del Tredici AL. Genetic testing for BCH variants identifies patients at risk of prolonged neuromuscular blockade in response to succinylcholine. Pharmgenomics Pers Med. 2020;13:405–14. https://doi.org/10.2147/PGPM.S263741.
27. Vieira CM, Fragoso RM, Pereira D, Medeiros R. Pain polymorphisms and opioids: an evidence based review. Mol Med Rep. 2019;19:1423–34. https://doi.org/10.3892/mmr.2018.9792.
28. Levran O, Kreek MJ. Population-specific genetic background for the OPRM1 variant rs1799971 (118A>G): implications for genomic medicine and functional analysis. Mol Psychiatry. 2021;26(7):3169-77. https://doi.org/10.1038/s41380-020-00902-4.
29. Kambur O, Männistö PT. Catechol-O-methyltransferase and pain. Int Rev Neurobiol. 2010;95:227–79. https://doi.org/10.1016/B978-0-12-381326-8.00010-7.

30. Dong ZL, Li H, Chen QX, Hu Y, Wu SJ, Tang LY, et al. Effect of CYP3A4*1G on the fentanyl consumption for intravenous patient-controlled analgesia after total abdominal hysterectomy in Chinese Han population. J Clin Pharm Ther. 2012;37(2):153–6. https://doi.org/10.1111/j. 1365-2710.2011.01268.x.

31. Yan Q, Su Y, Gao L, Ding N, Zhang HY, EW, Wang Y, et al. Impact of CYP3A4*1G polymorphism on fentanyl analgesia assessed by analgesia nociception index in chinese patients undergoing hysteroscopy. Chin Med J (Engl). 2018;131(22):2693–8. https://doi.org/10.4103/ 0366-6999.243934.

32. Wang W, Zhou Q, Yuan C. Influence of (ATP)-binding cassette transporter subfamily B member 1 (ABCB1) gene polymorphism on the efficacy of remifentanil. Med Sci Monit. 2019;25:5258–62. https://doi.org/10.12659/MSM.914921.

33. Primorac D, Höppner W, editors. Pharmacogenetics in clinical practice: experience with 55 commonly used drugs. Zagreb, Hamburg, Philadelphia: St. Catherine Specialty Hospital, Bioglobe GmbH, ISABS; 2022. Available from: https://www.stcatherine.com/centre-of-excellence/10/individualized-and-preventive-medicine/pharmacogenomics/69. Accessed 2 Mar 2022.

Pharmacogenomics in Cardiovascular Diseases

Adrijana Kekic

Abstract

Pharmacogenomics has a potential to improve and individualize treatment of cardiovascular diseases. In the past couple of decades, strong evidence emerged to inform PGx guided drug prescribing, dose selection, and clinical implementation of some common cardiovascular drug classes such as anticoagulants, antiplatelets, and statins. This chapter discusses evidence, including several clinical trials, treatment algorithms, genetic variants with demonstrated clinical impact and guidelines related to these drug and other cardiovascular drug classes.

Keywords

Cardiology · Cardiovascular drugs · Clopidogrel · Warfarin · Statins · Pharmacogenetics · Pharmacogenomics

1 Introduction

The role of pharmacogenomics in cardiovascular disease management is growing. Decreases in the cost of pharmacogenetics testing, shift from reactive to pre-emptive testing of multiple genes, increase in implementation efforts, improvements in clinical decision support, innovations in research design, and other factors hold promise in further advancing personalized medicine [1, 2]. This is evident by ongoing global initiatives of PGx implementation [3–5].

Strong evidence informs drug prescribing and genotype-guided dosing recommendations with warfarin, clopidogrel, and statins. Their pharmacogenetic testing has been successfully implemented in clinical practices. Data strongly

A. Kekic (✉)

Department of Pharmacy, Center for Individualized Medicine, Mayo Clinic, Phoenix, AZ, USA

e-mail: Kekic.adrijana@mayo.edu

© The Author(s), under exclusive license to Springer Nature Switzerland AG 2023
D. Primorac et al. (eds.), *Pharmacogenomics in Clinical Practice*,
https://doi.org/10.1007/978-3-031-45903-0_11

supports clopidogrel-*CYP2C19* association to predict the effectiveness of clopidogrel after percutaneous coronary intervention (PCI), warfarin-*CYP2C9/VKORC1* associations to guide initial dosing of warfarin, and simvastatin-*SLCO1B1* association to predict individuals at increased risk of simvastatin-induced myopathy [5]. Currently, other cardiovascular drugs have limited data to guide drug and dose selections based on their drug-gene pairs.

One of the challenges in bringing PGx testing to beside and beyond is discordance in recommendations. The US Food and Drug Administration (FDA), the European Medical Agencies (EMA/FM), and other regulatory authorities include pharmacogenetic information in their drug labels with a significant discrepancy between them [6]. The FDA-examined associations can be found on their website in the Table of Pharmacogenomic Biomarkers in Drug Labeling (last updated in May 2021) [7]. There are currently 298 FDA-approved drugs with pharmacogenetic biomarkers in drug labels. The majority are oncology drugs ($n = 102$) with both somatic (non-inherited) and germline (inherited) biomarkers. Most other drugs are with germline biomarkers and include psychiatry ($n = 35$), infectious disease ($n = 30$), neurology ($n = 27$), anesthesiology ($n = 16$), cardiology ($n = 13$ cardiology drugs and $n = 6$ drugs with the risk of QTc prolongation). See Table 1 for drugs in cardiovascular medicine with PGx biomarkers in their FDA drug labels. The table includes typical cardiovascular and non-cardiovascular drugs with the risk of QTc prolongation based on drug-gene interactions evidence from many trials and studies.

Several professional societies contribute to clinical recommendations for many drug-gene pairs, and their guidelines are annotated in the Pharmacogenomics Knowledgebase (PharmGKB) [8]. Most of the assessments are done by the Clinical Pharmacogenetics Implementation Consortium (CPIC) and the Royal Dutch Association for the Advancement of Pharmacy-Pharmacogenetics Working Group (DPWG), with contributions from the Canadian Pharmacogenomics Network for Drug Safety (CPNDS), The French National Network of Pharmacogenetics (RNPGx), and others. These evidence-based recommendations are crucial for clinicians implementing PGx in their clinical practice to better predict drug response phenotypes and individualize drug therapy for their patients (see Table 2).

Consistency between PGx professional society guidelines helps build clinical decision support to guide clinicians at the point of prescribing. However, discordance exists for several drugs, including cardiovascular such as clopidogrel, statins, and warfarin [6, 9]. Guidelines for each drug are explored further in this chapter.

2   Clopidogrel

Pharmacogenetics

Clopidogrel, prasugrel, and ticagrelor are oral antiplatelet drugs in the class of P2Y12 purine receptor blockers or inhibitors. Worldwide, clopidogrel remains the most widely prescribed P2Y12 inhibitor for the prevention of thrombotic events

Table 1 PGx Associations for CV drugs. Adopted from the FDA [7]

Drug	Gene	Phenotype	Description of a drug-gene interaction
I. *PGx associations with evidence to support therapeutic management recommendations (cardiovascular drugs and drugs with the risk of QTc prolongation)*			
Clopidogrel	CYP2C9	IM, PM	Results in lower systemic active metabolite concentrations, lower antiplatelet response, and may result in higher cardiovascular risk. Consider the use of another platelet P2Y12 inhibitor
Propafenone	CYP2D6		Results in higher systemic concentrations and higher adverse reaction risk (arrhythmia). Avoid use in poor metabolizers taking a CYP3A4 inhibitor
Warfarin	CYP2C9	IM, PM	Alters systemic concentrations and dosage requirements. Select initial dosage, considering clinical and genetic factors. Monitor and adjust dosages based on INR
	CYP4F2	V433M variant	May affect dosage requirements. Monitor and adjust doses based on INR
	VKORC1	−1639G>A variant carriers	Alters dosage requirements. Select initial dosage, considering clinical and genetic factors. Monitor and adjust dosages based on INR
Deutetrabenazine	CYP2D6	PM	Results in higher systemic concentrations and adverse reaction risk (QT prolongation). The maximum recommended dosage should not exceed 36 mg (maximum single dose of 18 mg)
Eliglustat	CYP2D6	UR NM IM PM	Alters systemic concentrations, effectiveness, and adverse reaction risk (QT prolongation). Indicated for normal, intermediate, and poor metabolizer patients. Ultrarapid metabolizers may not achieve adequate concentrations to achieve a therapeutic effect. The recommended dosages are based on CYP2D6 metabolizer status. Co-administration with strong CYP3A inhibitors is contraindicated in intermediate and poor CYP2D6 metabolizers. Refer to FDA labeling for specific dosing recommendations

(continued)

Table 1 (continued)

Drug	Gene	Phenotype	Description of a drug-gene interaction
Iloperidone	CYP2D6	PM	Results in higher systemic concentrations and higher adverse reaction risk (QT prolongation). Reduce dosage by 50%
Thioridazine	CYP2D6	PM	Results in higher systemic concentrations and higher adverse reaction risk (QT prolongation). Predicted effect based on experience with CYP2D6 inhibitors. Contraindicated in poor metabolizers
II. *PGx associations with data of potential impact on drug safety or response*			
Carvedilol	CYP2D6	PM	Results in higher systemic concentrations and higher adverse reaction risk (dizziness)
Procainamide	NAT (nonspecific)	PM	Alters systemic parent drug and metabolite concentrations. May result in higher adverse reaction risk
Simvastatin	SLCO1B1	521 TC or 521 CC (intermediate or poor function transporters)	Results in higher systemic concentrations and higher adverse reaction risk (myopathy). The risk of adverse reaction (myopathy) is higher for patients on 80 mg than for those on lower doses
Efavirenz	CYP2B6	PM	Results in higher systemic concentrations and higher adverse reaction risk (QT prolongation)
Tolterodine	CYP2D6	PM	Results in higher systemic concentrations and higher adverse reaction risk (QT prolongation)
III. *PGx associations with data of potential impact to only pharmacokinetics*			
Atorvastatin	SLCO1B1	521 CC (poor function)	May result in higher systemic concentrations
Hydralazine	NAT	PM	Results in higher systemic concentrations
Metoprolol	CYP2D6	PM	Results in higher systemic concentrations
Nebivolol	CYP2D6	PM	May result in higher systemic concentrations
Propranolol	CYP2D6	PM	May affect systemic concentrations
Rosuvastatin	SLCO1B1	521 CC (poor function)	Results in higher systemic concentrations

Legend CYP cytochrome P450, NAT (n-acetyltransferase), SLCO1B1 (solute organic anion transporting peptide 1B1)
NM normal metabolizer, *IM* intermediate metabolizer, *RM* rapid metabolizer, *UM* ultra-rapid metabolizer

Table 2 Cardiovascular drugs with drug-gene pairs and genotype-based recommendations as annotated by PharmGKB (highest level of recommendation). Adopted from Davila–Fajardo et al. [10] and expanded

Class	Drug	Genes (variants)	Guidelines	Level	Drug label annotations
Antiplatelet	Clopidogrel	*CYP2C19* (*1–*6, *8, *17)	CPIC DPWG RNPGx	1A	EMA FDA HDSC PMDA Swissmedic
Anticoagulant	Warfarin	*CYP2C9* (*1–*6, *8, *11)	CPIC CPNDS DPWG RNPGx	1A	FDA HCSC Also includes *PROC, PROS1*
		VKORC1 (rs9923231)	CPIC DPWG	1A	
		rs12777823	CPIC	1A	
		CYP4F2 (rs2108622)	CPIC	1A	
	Acenocoumarol	*CYP2C9* (*1, *2, *3)	DPWG RNPGx	1B	Swissmedic
		VKORC1 (rs9923231)	DPWG RNPGx	1A	
Antilipid	Simvastatin	*SLCO1B1* (*1, *5, rs4149056)	CPIC DPWG RNPGx [11]	1A	R: Swissmedic recommend testing I: FDA
	Atorvastatin	*SLCO1B1* (rs4149056)	DPWG		R: Swissmedic I: FDA, HCSC, PMDA
Antihypertensive	Flecainide	CYP2D6 (*1, *4, *5, *10, *21, *36)	DPWG	1A	
	Propafenone	CYP2D6 (*1, *2, *5, *10, *36)	DPWG	1A	A: FDA, HCSCA Swissmedic
	Metoprolol	CYP2D6 (*1–*6, *9, *10, *17, *29, *31, *35, *41)	DPWG	1A	A: HDSC, Swissmedic I: FDA

in patients with acute coronary syndrome (ACS) and/or stroke [12–14]. However, in patients with ACS, guidelines prefer prasugrel and ticagrelor over clopidogrel, based on their superior efficacy in clinical trials [15, 16]. Concerns exist with limited universal use of prasugrel and ticagrelor due to higher cost, increased risk of bleeding, and higher discontinuation rates compared to clopidogrel [15–17].

But, concerns also exist due to significant interindividual differences observed in response to clopidogrel, including non-responsiveness or resistance [18], not seen in clinical trials with prasugrel and ticagrelor. However, earlier clinical trials with clopidogrel did not consider a common *CYP2C19* genetic variability associated with reduced levels of enzyme activity and reduced efficacy of clopidogrel. Recent evidence suggests that clopidogrel can be an effective antiplatelet if full enzyme activity is present in patients who have undergone stent implementation after the percutaneous coronary intervention (PCI) [19].

Dual therapy with acetylsalicylic acid and one of the P2Y12 inhibitors (clopidogrel, prasugrel, or ticagrelor) is the standard of care in patients following (PCI) to reduce the risk of major adverse cardiovascular events (MACE) [20].

Clopidogrel is a thienopyridine prodrug that lacks antiplatelet activity until converted into an active metabolite. It is the active metabolite that irreversibly inhibits the P2Y12 receptor, resulting in antiplatelet activity. This bioactivation to the active metabolite is a two-oxidative step process involving many hepatic CYP450 enzymes, CYP2C19 being crucial [21, 22].

CYP2C19 is encoded by *CYP2C19* located on chromosome 10q23.23. *CYP2C19* is a highly polymorphic gene with over 40 genetic variants that correspond to about 35 enzyme isoforms [23]. Currently, only three of *CYP2C19* alleles (*2, *3, *17) are recommended as essential for clinical testing by the US Association of Molecular Pathology. The recommendation is based on their PGx Working Group's assessment that considered allelic frequencies in different populations, ethnicities, and other technical factors [24, 25].

Enzyme function of CYP2C19, as influenced by *CYP2C19* allelic variants, can range from no enzyme function (*2, *3 alleles) to increased enzyme function (*17 allele). Alleles *2 (12–35%) and *17 (3–21%) are common in the general population while *3 is very rare and found predominantly in Asians at 10% prevalence. No enzyme function is found in 30% of the population (especially in East Asia, Oceania, etc.) and can correlate to either intermediate metabolizer (IM) (*1/*2, *1/*3) or poor metabolizer (PM) phenotypes [25, 26]. These phenotypes affect the pharmacokinetics and pharmacodynamics of clopidogrel and are associated with inadequate response to the drug [27–33]. The same effects were not found with prasugrel nor ticagrelor, making them preferred alternatives compared to safety concerns with clopidogrel dose escalation [29, 33–35]. Increased enzyme function is found in up to 30% of the population (especially in Mediterranean South Europe, Middle East, etc.) and can correlate to either rapid metabolizer (RM) or ultra-rapid metabolizer (UM) phenotypes [25, 26]. Although its clinical impact is still unclear, *17 allele (rs12248560) was found to be associated with lower on-treatment platelet aggregation [36], better platelet response to clopidogrel [37], and more recently, an increased risk of bleeding, especially in patients with atrial fibrillation and acute coronary syndrome that require double or triple rivaroxaban and clopidogrel treatment [38].

CYP2C19 was the key genomic contributor of interindividual variants in clopidogrel's response in a 2009 GWAS by Shuldiner et al. [39]. They explored *ABCB1*,

CES1, ITGB3, PON1, and *P2RY12* to assess their influence on clopidogrel. Currently, evidence is mixed with studies reporting contradictory findings [30, 40–46]. *CES1* evidence looks the most promising. Carboxylesterase 1 (CES1) hydrolyses clopidogrel to an inactive metabolite, and it accounts for almost 85% of its hepatic metabolism. Lewis et al. showed that *CES1* polymorphism Gly143Glu (rs71647871) was associated with reduced CES1 activity (less hydrolysis to inactive metabolite), increased clopidogrel active metabolite, and greater clopidogrel response [47]. The same author published findings from another study, this time a multicenter, and international study of 3391 Caucasian patients. Citing a small percentage of other non-genetic factors on variations in clopidogrel response, their objective was to assess the role of 31 candidate SNPs, including *CES1,* and evaluate their effect on cardiovascular (CVE) risk. They found several polymorphisms, including *CES1,* that impact clopidogrel, suggesting that PGx polygenic response score (PGxRS) is likely a more superior predictive model compared to a single drug-gene pair model [48].

Evidence
Dual antiplatelet therapy with aspirin and clopidogrel is shown to prevent recurring ischemic events after an ACS or a PCI [49]. Yet, many patients on dual therapy experience recurring ischemic or thrombotic events. Several studies examined the role of genetic variants on clopidogrel response variability and recurring events, including major adverse cardiac events (MACE) such as death and stroke. Their study designs vary and include clinical and non-clinical studies, clinical trials, meta-analyses, real-world data, and cost-effectiveness studies. Combined, their findings support evidence for genotype-guided prescribing of clopidogrel in ACS and PCI, although with some caveats further elaborated in the following paragraphs.

Large-scale studies in high-risk populations from 2009 and 2010 examined the clinical impact of genetic variants on clopidogrel-treated patients with coronary artery disease (CAD) of mostly European ancestry. Genetic post-hoc substudies of TRINTON 38 and PLATO trials also evaluated the association between *CYP2C19* genotype and cardiovascular events and outcomes.

In 2007, TRITON-TIMI 38 trial compared prasugrel versus clopidogrel in over 13,000 patients with ACS-PCI-stent [50]. Prasugrel increased bleeding risk but reduced cardiovascular risks (percentage of CV death, ACS, or stroke) compared to clopidogrel. Three genetic post-hoc studies of TRITON-TIMI 38 followed. In 2009, Mega et al. found that patients with *CYP2C19* loss-of-function (LOF) allele had a higher risk of CV death compared to non-carriers (HR 1.53, 95% CI: 1.07–2.19, $p = 0.01$) [51]. They were also at higher risk of stent thrombosis (HR = 3.09, 95% CI: 1.19–8.00, $p = 0.02$) compared to normal metabolizers (NMs). In the subsequent study, they examined the effect of the *ABCB1* genotype either alone or with *CYP2C19* on CV outcomes. They found that patients who did had at-risk alleles with either *ABCB1* 3435C>T (TT genotype) or *CYP2C9* LOF allele had an increased rate of MACE at 15 months compared to those without at-risk alleles [30, 51]. A third post-doc by Sorich et al. [50] also found that clopidogrel-treated patients with *CYP2C19* LOF allele had a higher risk of MCAE at 15 months compared to non-carriers.

In 2009, the PLATO trial compared ticagrelor versus clopidogrel in patients with ACS (only 64% had PCI). The following year, Wallentin et al. [32] performed a genetic post-hoc of clopidogrel-treated patients and found an increased rate of CV events in *CYP2C19* LOF allele carriers in the first 30 days of the treatment, but not beyond.

High-risk young patients: A cohort study by Collete et al. [52] included 259 patients younger than 45 years of age diagnosed with their first ACS (myocardial infarction) and treated with clopidogrel for at least one month. They assessed if *CYP2C9*2* loss-of-function allele in intermediate and poor metabolizers (IMs and PMs) was associated with the long-term prognosis of patients chronically treated with clopidogrel. The primary endpoint was MACE composite (cardiovascular death, ACS, urgent PCI) and the key secondary endpoint was stent prognosis. Patients were followed every 6 months for beyond 4 years with a median clopidogrel exposure time of 1.07 years (IQR 0.28–3.0). The primary endpoint was observed more frequently in patients with *CYP2C9** (LOF) compared to no LOF (15 vs. 11 events, HR 3.69 [95% CI 1.69–8.05], $p = 0.0005$). The secondary endpoint was also higher in patients with LOF allele compared to no LOF allele (eight vs. four events, HR 6.02 [1.81–20.04], and $p = 0.0009$). Even after the multivariable analysis, the *CYP2C9*2* variant was the lone and independent predictor of cardiovascular events (HR 4.04 [1.81–9.02] and $p = 0.0006$).

In a larger study of 2208 patients with an acute MI receiving clopidogrel, Simon et al. [40] explored the association between several pharmacogenes and cardiovascular outcomes. They examined the link between alleles that affect clopidogrel's pharmacokinetics (*ABCB1, CYP2C19,* and *CYP3A4*) and pharmacodynamics (*P2RY12* and *ITGB3*) to the risk of death from any cause, non-fatal stroke, or myocardial infarction (MACE) during 1 year of follow-up. Patients with *ABCB1* (TT) genotype were at higher risk of CV events compared to CC genotype (15.5% vs. 10.7%; adjusted HR = 1.72, CI 95% CI: 1.20–2.47). Patients with *CYP2C19* LOF alleles (IM or PM) had 3.58 times higher risk of MACE compared to those with no LOF alleles (NM).

A genome-wide association study by Shuldiner et al., Pharmacogenomics of Antiplatelet Intervention (PAPI) Study, sought to identify variants that influence response to clopidogrel [39]. The investigators administered clopidogrel for 7 days to 429 healthy Amish people to measure response using ex vivo platelet aggregometry. These and other large-scale studies all showed an increased risk of MACE after PCI in ACS patients treated with clopidogrel who carried LOF allele (were IM or PM) compared to patients without LOF allele (NM) [29, 53].

In 2010, Mega et al. [31] performed a meta-analysis of nine studies totaling 9,685 clopidogrel-treated patients (91% with PCI) and found that the risk of MACE was significantly higher in *CYP2C19* LOF allele carriers such as IMs (HR 1.55, 95% CI 1.11–2.17) or PMs (HR1.76, 95% CI 1.24–2.50) compared to NMs.

A subsequent meta-analysis confirmed higher rates of MACE in *CYP2C19* IMs or PMs treated with clopidogrel compared to NMs [53–56]. What followed were several clinical studies and randomized controlled trials.

Randomized controlled trials (RCT) investigated *CYP2C19* guided antiplatelet therapy and cardiovascular outcomes. The earliest of them was a 2013 trial by Xie et al. [57]. They enrolled 600 patients with CAD and PCI with stent implementation. Patients were randomized to either personalized genotype-guided therapy (intervention) or conventional therapy with clopidogrel (control). The incidence of MACE, as the primary endpoint, was 2.66% ($p < 0.01$) for the intervention group versus 9.03% for the control group. There was no difference in bleeding events between the groups.

The PHARMCLO RCT in 2018 remains the largest trial to evaluate the genotype-guided selection of an antiplatelet drug at the bedside. This prospective, multicenter RCT in Italy, enrolled 888 hospitalized patients with ACS (STEMI or non-STEMI, and the majority had PCI) between 2013 and 2015. Patients were randomized to either genotype-guided prescribing using ST Q3 system (*ABCB1*, *CYP2C9*2*, and *CYP2C19*7*) or standard treatment. MACE was the primary endpoint. The study was stopped at only 25% enrollment due to "lack of in vitro diagnostic certification of the genotyping instrument." Even though only a quarter of the study participant got enrolled, the primary endpoint was 15.9% in the intervention (genotype-guided arm) versus 25.9% in the control arm (HR:0.58; 95% CI: 0.43–0.78; $p < 0.001$) [58].

In 2019, Claassens et al. [19] published findings from their multicenter RCT that started in 2011 in the Netherlands, called cost-effectiveness of genotype-guided treatment with antiplatelet drugs in STEMI patients: optimization of treatment (POPular Genetics). They compared genotype-guided therapy ($n = 1242$) versus standard therapy with either ticagrelor or prasugrel ($n = 1246$). The goal was to evaluate the efficacy, safety, and cost-effectiveness of *CYP2C19* genotype-guided treatment. Prasugrel or ticagrelor were used in IMs and PMs (carries of *2 or *3 alleles) and clopidogrel in non-carriers of the alleles. Incidence of all-cause death, MI, stent thrombosis, stroke, or major bleeding was 5.1% compared to 5.9% in the control or standard therapy arm ($p < 0.001$ for non-inferiority). Major and minor bleeding was lower in the GGT arm at 9.8% compared to 12.5% in the standard therapy arm of the study (HR:0.78, 95% CI0.61–0.98, $P = 0.04$) [19].

In 2020, a much-anticipated RCT TAILOR-PCI published its results [59]. Study design differed from POPular Genetics in respect to the diagnosis of the population studied and intervention. TAILOR-PCI included patients with either stable ACS or ACS undergoing PCI-stent. Patients were randomized into either *CYP2C19* genotype-guided therapy arm ($n = 903$) or conventional therapy with clopidogrel arm, irrespective of *CYP2C19* genotype ($n = 946$). Like in the prior RCT [60], only those without LOF allele (NM, RM, and UM) received clopidogrel. Both primary and secondary endpoints nearly missed the threshold for statistical significance ($p = 0.06$ and $p = 0.05$). The primary endpoint of MACE occurred in 4.0% of the GGT arm compared to 5.9% of the conventional group arm (HR 0.66, 95%

CI 0.43–1.02, $P = 0.06$). However, post-hoc analysis showed a favorable outcome in the GGT arm with a reduction in the rate of events in the first 90 days ($p = 0.001$) which means that in patients with ACS post-PCI, early genotype-guided therapy (first 90 days) offers the greatest clinical benefit.

Clinical Guidelines

A high level of evidence exists for genotype-guided therapy in high-risk patients treated with clopidogrel for reduction of CV events, as discussed in previous paragraphs. The DPWG, CPIC, and RNPGx have guidelines for clopidogrel-*CYP2C19* pair although with discordance [9, 11, 25]. There is a consensus between the CPIC and the DPWG guidelines that label clopidogrel-*CYP2C19* interaction as 1A per PharmGKB (their highest level of evidence score that is supported by RCTs, systematic reviews, and meta-analysis), especially in ACS patient post-PCI-stent [9, 25, 61]. Both recommend an alternative for clopidogrel in *CYP2C19* loss of function allele carriers such as IMs or PMs due to an increased risk for reduced response to clopidogrel (diminished antiplatelet effect). Specifically, the CPIC recommends prasugrel or ticagrelor over clopidogrel in CYP2C19 IMs and PMs with an acute coronary syndrome undergoing percutaneous coronary intervention. The DPWG recommends prasugrel or ticagrelor as alternatives to clopidogrel 75 mg for CYP2C19 IMs treated for PCI, stroke, or transient ischemic attack (TIA), or clopidogrel 150 mg daily dose. They recommend prasugrel or ticagrelor over clopidogrel for CYP2C19 PMs treated for the same indications. For other indications, the DPWG recommends no action for IMs and suggests measuring platelet function testing and choosing prasugrel or ticagrelor in case of high treatment reactivity in PM patients.

With mounting evidence leading to 2010, the FDA revised a boxed warning to clopidogrel's drug label to warn of reduced drug efficacy seen in PMs, needing an alternative P2Y12 inhibitor [62]. The FDA evaluated evidence behind drug-gene interactions and compiled them in their table of pharmacogenomics associations that include both CYP2C19 IMs and PMs [7]. Additionally, drug labels with pharmacogenetic information are approved by the EMA, Swissmedic, PMDA, and HCSC.

Clinical guidelines contradict both genotype-based guidelines (CPIC, DPWG) and drug label recommendations from the FDA and EMA for the treatment of ACS. The American College of Cardiology/American Heart Association (ACC/AHA) was published in 2016 and before RCTs in [57, 59, 60]. This could account for why they currently recommend against routine genotyping for all patients undergoing PCI-stent, although they suggest testing in high-risk patients. For high-risk patients who are LOF allele carriers, ACC/AHA recommends prasugrel or ticagrelor, echoing the CPIC recommendations [63].

Evidence-based guidelines are one of the key elements of successful implementation of pharmacogenetics knowledge in clinical practice to optimize and individualize drug therapy outcomes. Despite discord in guidelines and other challenges, pharmacogenetic testing continues to be implemented [1, 64]. *CYP2C19* testing for genotype-guided therapy with clopidogrel continues to be one of the most common PGx testings [5].

It is important to note that other clinical factors and biomarkers may contribute to variability in clopidogrel's response.

Clopidogrel Highlights

- **Drug**: Clopidogrel is a prodrug that requires a functional CYP2C19 to become an active antiplatelet drug.
- **Genetics**: Approximately, 5–30% of the global population carries a *CYP2C19* LOF allele associated with an increased risk of MACE.
- **Evidence**: The greatest benefit is with early genotype-guided treatment (first 90 days) in high-risk patients with ACS-post PCI with a *CYP2C19* LOF allele.
- **Guidelines**: Genotype-guided therapy guidelines exist for clopidogrel-CYP2C19.
- **Future**: Polygenic risk score is likely more important than any single gene alone.

3   Anticoagulant Drugs

3.1   Warfarin

Drug

Warfarin is an anticoagulant drug used widely to prevent and treat blood clots [65]. Discovered and named after Wisconsin Alumni Research Foundation ("-arin" added to reflect drug class), it was initially used as a rodenticide [66]. Eventually, clinical evidence of its blood-thinning benefits in humans emerged, making it one of the most used drugs worldwide. It is FDA approved for prophylaxis and treatment of venous thrombosis (VT) and its complications such as pulmonary embolism (PE) [67], thromboembolic complications from atrial fibrillation, cardiac valve replacement, and from genetic factors such as protein C and S deficiency or Factor V Leiden [68], and reduction in the risk of death from recurrent myocardial infarction and thromboembolic events such as stroke in high-risk patients [69]. Its FDA off-label uses include secondary prevention of recurrent stroke and transient ischemic attacks [70, 71]. Adequate dosing is crucial for optimal therapeutic response.

Great variability in dose-drug response is associated with a significant risk of thromboembolism if the dose is low and risk of bleeding if the dose is high. Warfarin has a narrow therapeutic index that requires frequent laboratory monitoring of international normalized ratio (INR) to help measure how quickly blood clots, known as prothrombin time (PT). An INR goal for most patients is 2.0–3.0 and for some, such as patients with a mechanical heart valve, that goal is higher at 2.5–3.5 [70, 72]. Empiric dosing to meet the goal is based on many patient-specific factors such as age, underlying condition, presence of other medications, etc. However, these factors account for only 12–22% of the dose variably. In addition to its narrow therapeutic index, wide interindividual variability in warfarin's response algorithms [73, 74] are built that incorporates clinical and genetic factors to help guide drug dosing, especially when initiating warfarin treatment.

Warfarin is a racemic mixture of R and S-enantiomer. The mixture is metabolized by hepatic CYP2C9, CYP1A2, and CYP3A4. S-enantiomer is 2.7–3.8 times more potent than R, and it is mainly metabolized by CYP2C9 [75, 76].

Pharmacogenetics

CYP2C9 and *VKORC1* are two main genes with variants found to majorly contribute to variability in warfarin's dose requirement and drug response.

CYP4F2 was also found to contribute but minorly. *CYP2C9* is a polymorphic gene with many allelic variants. Robust evidence from earlier pharmacogenetics studies showed that *2 and *3 carriers have a reduced enzymatic activity and required reduced dose, especially in Caucasian and Asian populations studied and that the genotype-guided dosing could improve time to stable, therapeutic INR, and reduce adverse events [77, 78]. However, they could not account for the lower dose requirements observed in African Americans when compared to European Americans [79]. Subsequent studies explored this further and found *5, *6, *8, and *11 alleles were exclusive to the population of African ancestry. These alleles, like *2 and *3 (the most common in populations of European ancestry), also have a reduced enzymatic activity associated with reduced clearance of S-enantiomer (more potent metabolite) and reduced dose requirements [80–82]. A study in 2010 by Cavallari et al. [73] enrolled 226 patients who were mostly female (71%). Carriers of *2, *3, *6, *8, or *11 had significantly lower warfarin dose requirements compared to non-carriers. A 2020 meta-analysis of 48 studies by Asiimwe et al. [83] examined genetic factors influencing warfarin dose in black African patients. Dose reduction was dependent on a *CYP2C9* allele in the following severity order of a weekly dose reduction: dose reduced by 13.4 mg/week for *5 (rs28371686) carriers > 12.5 mg for *3 (rs1057910) > 8.1 mg for *6 (rs9332131) > 6.8 mg for *2 (rs1799853) and 5.3 mg for *11 (rs28371685).

Warfarin targets and inhibits an enzyme called vitamin K reductase complex 1 encoded by synonymous *VKORC1*. The enzyme regenerates vitamin K hydroquinone, a cofactor for the posttranslational activation of vitamin K–dependent clotting proteins II, VII, IX, and X, as well as the anticoagulant proteins C, S, and Z [84]. *VKORC1* mutations were associated with reduced enzyme activity and warfarin dosing requirement [85, 86]. The genetic effects of *VKORC1* and *CYP2C9* in African and Asian populations are concordant with those seen in Europeans; however, the frequency distribution of allelic variants can vary considerably between major populations [87].

Evidence

Several differently designed clinical trials examined outcomes and efficacy of genotype-guided warfarin dosing (Table 3). They were multicenter, randomized

Table 3 Summary of clinical trials, examined outcomes, and efficacy of genotype-guided warfarin dosing

Study and year (references)	Intervention group	Control group	Follow-up	Genetic variants	Primary endpoint	Outcomes (intervention vs. control)
Pirmohamed EU-PACT 2013 [89]	AF (72.1%) VF (27.9%) European (98.5%)	Fixed-dose strategy based on age	12 weeks	CYP2C9 (*2, *3) VKORC1 −1639G>A	% TTR	67.4% versus 60.3% (p < 0.001)
Kimmel COAG 2013 [90]	AF (23%) DVT or PE (56%) 33% non-European (27% African-American and 6% Hispanic)	Clinical algorithm dosing	4 weeks	CYP2C9 (*2, *3) VKORC1 −1639G>A	% TTR	All patients: 45.2% versus 45% (p = 0.91) African patients: 35.2% versus 43.5% (p = 0.01)
Gage (GIFT) 2017 [93]	Hip or knee arthroplasty > 65 years old European (91%)	Clinical algorithm dosing	30 days 60 days	CYP2C9 (*2, *3) VKORC1 −1639G>A CYP4F2*3	Composite (major bleeding, INR > 4, VT, death)	At least one PEP: 10.8% versus 14.7% (RR 0.7, 95% CI 0.56–0.95, p = 0.02)

controlled trials that used genotype-based algorithms that tested CYP2C9*2, *3, and VKORC1 variants. The later trial, GIFT [88], also genotyped the CYP4F2*3 variant. Two earlier trials from 2013, the European Pharmacogenetics of Anticoagulant Therapy (EU-PACT) by Pirmohamed [89] and Clarification of Optimal Anticoagulation through Genetics (COAG) by Kimmel [90], published contradictory findings.

Primohamed et al. [89] prospectively compared the effects of genotype-guided dosing versus standard dosing in patients starting warfarin therapy. Of 455 recruited patients with AF and VT, the majority (98%) were white Europeans from Sweden and UK. Point of care testing was used to genotype three alleles: CYP2C9 *2, CYP2C9*3, and VKROC1 (−1639G>A). The intervention period was the first 5 days of initiating warfarin therapy. A 3-day loading dose was used in the control group. The primary outcome was the percentage time in the therapeutic range (INR 2.0–3.0) during the first 12 weeks of starting warfarin. A difference in the primary outcome (%TTN) was observed and favored the intervention group compared to the control group (67.4% vs. 60.3%, p < 0.001). Also, less time was needed to reach a therapeutic INR in the genotype group compared to the control group (21 days vs. 29 days, p < 0.001). Although the median number of additional INR measurements did not differ between the groups, genotype-based dosing increased the time in the therapeutic range by 7.1% and reduced the incidence of supratherapeutic dosing.

In a double-blinded RCT, Kimmel et al. [90] recruited 1015 patients (inpatients and outpatients) across 18 clinical centers in the United States. Most patients had AF (23%) or DVT/PE (56%), and about 33% were non-European (27% Black and 6% Hispanic). The intervention period was the first five days of warfarin therapy. The investigators used a genotype-guided warfarin-dosing algorithm (*VKROC1, CYP2C9*2, *3*) in the intervention group and a clinically based dosing algorithm (clinical variables only) in the control group. No loading dose was used in the control group for this study compared to EU-PACT. The primary outcome was also the percentage time in therapeutic range (TTR) from day 4 or 5 through day 28. In genotype-based dosing %, TTR was 45.2 and 45%. However, compared to the EU-PACT finding, the COAG investigators concluded they found no benefit using genotype-based versus clinically based dosing algorithm.

A systemic review by Shaw et al. [91] examined the association between warfarin therapy and genetic variants (*VKORC1, CYP2C9*) and evaluated differences between EU-PACT and COAG. They found several differences, including population studied (2% non-European in EU-PACT vs. 33% non-European in COAG), different indication and warfarin dose required (AF, VT in EU-PACT vs. AF and DVT or PE in COAG), length of follow-up time (only 4 weeks in COAG vs. 12 weeks in EU-PACT), the difference in doing in the control group (a loading dose used in COAG, but not in EU-PACT), and availability of genotype results (approximately 2 h in EU-PACT vs. 55% not available for the first dose in COAG). It is important to recognize that neither trial tested for variants of clinical impact (*CYP2C9*5, *6, *8,* and *11*) in patients of African ancestry, which could have resulted in overdosing. A 2015 cohort study by Drozda et al. [92] showed that failure to account for alleles important in African Americans (*CYP2C9*5, *6, 8*,* and *11*) leads to significant dosing errors. This is exactly what was observed in the COAG trial as well, where patients of African ancestry had worse anticoagulant control in the genotype group compared to the control.

Following EU-PACT and COAG trials in 2013, results of another randomized control trial were published in 2017 (Table 3), known as the GIFT (Genetic Informatics Trial) [93]. Their investigators wanted to know if genotype-guided dosing of warfarin prevents adverse drug events, citing that warfarin accounts for more drug-related emergency department visits in older adults than any other medication [94, 95]. To answer this, they enrolled 1650 patients from the United States over the age of 65 undergoing elective hip or knee arthroplasty. Genotype-guided warfarin dosing (intervention group) was compared to clinically guided dosing (control group). Patients were genotyped for *CYP2C9* (*2, *3*), *VKORC1* ($-1639G>A$), and *CYP4F2*3* (V433M), the last being an allele not included in the previous two RCTs. The majority were female (63.6%) and white (91.0%) and received at least one dose of warfarin (96.8%). Genotype-guided doing compared to clinically guided dosing reduced the rate of at least 1 composite endpoint (major bleeding, INR of 4 or greater, venous thromboembolism, or death) by about 4% (10.8% vs.

14.7%). The rate of either major or non-major bleeding was also reduced, 7.1% in the intervention group compared to 9.4% in the control group.

Meta-Analysis

Following EU-PACT and COAG trials, many have been assessed and published on different genotype-based dosing algorithms. Several meta-analyses followed, some with contradictory conclusions. For example, a meta-analysis of nine RTCs ($n = 1952$ patients) by Goulding et al. found a statistically significant reduction in bleeding and thromboembolism in the genotype-based dosing group compared to the control. They concluded that the genotype-based algorithm could improve clinical effectiveness [96].

Similar results favoring genotype-based dosing were reported by Tang et al. [97] in a meta-analysis of ten studies ($n = 5299$ patients), nine were RCTs, and one was a cohort study. Genotype-guided dosing group had better clinical outcomes: a higher % TTR compared to the control group, reduced major bleeding risk (RR 0.47, 95% CI 0.24–0.91, $p = 0.02$), and reduced risk of thromboembolic events by 21% compared to the control group (RR = 0.79, 95% CI 0.38–1.63).

Contrary to Tang et al., a 2015 meta-analysis of several clinical trials ($n = 1910$) by Liao et al. [98] did not find any difference in the incidence of adverse effects (RR 0.94, 95% CI 0.84–1.04, and $p = 0.647$) and death (RR 1.36. 95% CI 0.46–4.05, and $p = 0.328$) between the two groups. Same year another meta-analysis by Shi et al. [99] of 11 trials and 2678 patients, showed no difference between the two groups in respect to the TTR. However, GGD group had significantly shorter time to maintenance dose (MD $= -8.80$; 95% CI: -11.99 to -5.60; $p < 0.00001$), the time to first therapeutic INR (MD $= -2.80$; 95% CI: -3.45 to -2.15; < 0.00001), significantly reduced the risk of adverse events (RR $= 0.86$; 95% CI: 0.75–0.99; $p = 0.03$), and major bleeding (RR $= 0.36$; 95% CI: 0.15–0.89, and $p = 0.03$).

Algorithm and Guidelines

Several genotype-based dosing algorithms have been investigated and published for warfarin [77, 100–105]. Most include clinical factors and genetic variants.

One of the first warfarin genotype-based dosing algorithms was published in 2008 by Gage et al. [88]. It included clinical factors (age, body surface area, drugs such as amiodarone and simvastatin, gender, race, and target INR) and genetic variants CYP2C9*2 and *3. Not long after, they added smoking, drug indication, and VKROC1 1639G>A genetic variant.

The International Warfarin Pharmacogenetics Consortium (IWPC) is another algorithm to guide initial warfarin dosing. It also considers CYP2C9 inducers (carbamazepine, phenytoin, and rifampin). Both Gage and the IWPC algorithms give similar dosing estimates although there are differences in variants: Gage algorithm includes CYP2C9*5 and *6 (of impact in patients of African descent) and CYP4F2*3 [100, 106].

Overall, it is estimated that these algorithms account for 50% of the dose variation [88, 107]. A retrospective cohort study of 1378 patients from three anticoagulation centers in the US found that warfarin dose prediction using a genotype-based algorithm was significantly more accurate ($p < 0.001$) compared to all other methods of empiric dosing (37%; odds ratio [OR]: 2.2), clinical algorithm (39%; OR: 2.2), warfarin label (43%; OR: 1.8), and genotype mean dose table (44%; OR: 1.9) [107].

The CPIC guideline for pharmacogenetics-guided warfarin dosing was updated in 2017. It included the *CYP4F2*3* (rs2108622) variant, which found to significantly contribute to warfarin dosing variability in the Italian population [108]. Borgiani et al. showed that this variant accounted for 7% of the mean weekly dose and that 60.5% of interindividual variability could be explained by *CYP2C9*, *CYP4F2*, and *VKORC1* genetic variants, age, and weight. If *CYP4F2*3* variant is detected, a dose increase of 5 to 10% is recommended ("optional" recommendation only by the CPIC) [106].

Cost-Effectiveness
Every year about 2 million people in the US start warfarin therapy, yet more than a third fail to respond to their initial dose. Estimated 43,000 ER visits in the US are due to adverse drug events from warfarin, second only to insulin [109]. Dosing warfarin has its challenges. If dosed high, it can lead to bleeding. If dosed low, it can lead to increased risk for stroke. Considering genetic contribution to variability in warfarin drug response, the American Enterprise Institute for Public Health Research (AEI)-Brookings Report estimates that implementation of routine genetic testing could reduce the number of warfarin-related major bleeding events by 85,000 and reduce strokes by 17,000 annually in the United States, resulting in a reduction of $1.1 billion annually in health care spending [110].

In 1993, Ladenfeld and Beyth [111] reported a risk of bleeding to be five times more (0.6–9.6%) in patients taking warfarin compared to patients not taking warfarin. The risk of bleeding was up to ten times higher during the first month than in the first year of warfarin therapy. Advanced age, female sex, prior history of bleeding events, and comorbidities (hypertension, cerebrovascular disease, atrial fibrillation, heart disease, renal insufficiency, liver disease, and alcoholism) are considered as some of the most significant risk factors. In 2007, Leigh and White [112] used a semi-Markov model to assess the cumulative cost associated with warfarin-related adverse drug events (bleeding and stroke). In a hypothetical cohort of 10,000 patients over the age of 70 years treated with warfarin for atrial fibrillation, they estimated the cost to be $18.3 million per 10,000 patients over five years. Others have examined the cost-effectiveness of warfarin GGD related to reduced bleeding events and improved quality-adjusted-life-years (QALYs). A couple of studies from 2009 assessed the cost-effectiveness of GGD in patients with atrial fibrillation. A 2009 meta-analysis by Eckman et al. [113] found that when starting warfarin therapy, GGD versus standard dosing may be cost-effective only for those patients at high risk of bleeding, but not for other patients. In addition to small cohorts, included studies did not consider other clinically meaningful measurements of effectiveness (besides the number of bleeding events), such as the number of dose adjustments, time to stable, and therapeutic INR (more precise starting dose).

3.2   Acenocoumarol

Acenocoumarol is a vitamin K epoxide inhibitor used for the prevention of throm-boembolic and bleeding events. Compared to warfarin, it has a shorter half-life [114]. Evidence from the 2021 PLECTRUM Study by Menichelli et al. [115] points to a lower anticoagulant quality of acenocoumarol compared to warfarin regardless of sex, age, or INR range. Like warfarin, genetic variants in *CYP2C9* and *VKORC1* are associated with drug variability and efficacy [116–118]. In one of the first RCT (2012) to compare genotype-guided dosing algorithm versus stan-dard dosing in VTE, Carcas et al. [119] developed and published an algorithm in 2012 that included *CYP2C9, CYP4F2, VKORC* (and ApoE) variants. A 2020 discovery cohort study by Roco et al. [118] genotyped 304 Chilean patients. They aimed to develop an algorithm that combined clinical factors and genetic variants to explain the variability of acenocoumarol dose. The genetic variants *VKORC1* (rs9923231), *CYP2C9*2* (rs1799853), and *CYP2C9*3* (rs10579910) had a greater impact (37%) on dose variability than clinical variants such age, sex, BMI, and initial INR (19%).

3.3   Direct Oral Anticoagulants

Direct oral anticoagulants (DOACs) emerged as alternatives to warfarin for the prevention of thrombosis [120]. In 2010 the FDA first approved **dabigatran**, fol-lowed by **rivaroxaban, apixaban, edoxaban, and betrixaban** in later years. Trials with DOACs showed superiority or non-inferiority compared to warfarin or low molecular weight heparins in reducing the risk of thromboembolism and bleeding [121–123].

DOACs are grouped into two main classes: oral direct Xa inhibitors (apixaban, betrixaban, edoxaban, and rivaroxaban) and direct thrombin inhibitors (dabiga-tran). Compared to DOACs, warfarin requires frequent drug monitoring due to its narrow therapeutic index and wide interindividual difference in drug response with variations in dose requirements up to 20-fold [124]. In addition to the less fre-quent need for drug monitoring and less variability in response, other advantages of DOACs over warfarin include quicker onset and offset, fewer drug-drug inter-actions, and no major drug-food interactions [125]. Due to these factors, DOACs prescriptions continue to surpass those for warfarin in the US [126].

Pharmacogenetics and Evidence

Disproportionately more pharmacogenetic studies were done with warfarin than with DOCAs. While there are genotype-based guidelines for warfarin, none are yet available for DOACs due to the low level of evidence between DOAC's drug-gene pairs to back them up. Several pharmacogenetic studies identified polymorphisms associated with DOAC metabolism and altered serum concentrations. However, their clinical significance remains unclear [127].

Evidence

Interindividual variability observed with DOACs is thought to be related to polymorphism of genes that encode proteins involved in DOACs metabolism (*CES1, CYP3A4, CYP3A5, and UGT*s) and transport (*ABCB1 and ABCG2*).

Dabigatran etexilate is a prodrug converted by esterases to its active metabolite, dabigatran. In vivo and in *vitro* studies showed that CYP enzymes do not contribute to the metabolism of dabigatran etexilate or dabigatran [128, 129]. Instead, P-glycoprotein plays a role as a drug efflux transporter of dabigatran etexilate [130]. This protein is a member of the adenosine triphosphate-binding cassette transporter superfamily, encoded by a polymorphic *ABCB1* gene associated with altered plasma concentration of its substrates, including dabigatran and rivaroxaban [131, 132]. However, the presence of P-gp inhibitors such as clarithromycin affected the pharmacokinetics of dabigatran and rivaroxaban more than *ABCB1* polymorphisms in healthy males [132]. In a recent study from 2020 by Zubair et al. [133], women showed higher exposure to dabigatran than men. Concomitant use of pantoprazole and genetic variants in *SLC22A1, CYP2D6,* and CYP3A5 genes showed altered dabigatran pharmacokinetics and more adverse drug events in women compared to men [133].

Rivaroxaban is primarily metabolized by CYP3A4, CYP3A5, and CYP2J. It does not induce or inhibit CYP450, but co-administration with potent CYP450 inducers and P-glycoprotein inducers (carbamazepine, phenytoin, rifampin, St. John's wort, etc.) reduces its plasma concentration. In a 2018 study by Sychev et al., CYP3A4 activity affected rivaroxaban plasma concentration [134] but their follow-up study in 2019 did not replace these findings, and instead showed no difference in with *CYP3A4*22 (rs35599367) polymorphism associated with reduced enzyme function [38].

Rivaroxaban is transported by P-glycoprotein and the breast cancer resistance protein (BCRP), encoded by *ABCB1*. In 2016, Lorenzinin et al. reported rivaroxaban-induced bleeding in a patient with homozygous *ABCB1* TT genotype for rs2032582 and rs1045642 [135]. However, the Gouin-Thibault study of healthy participants in 2017 found no association between these two variants and peak plasma concentration [132].

Apixaban is metabolized mainly by CYP3A4 and CYP3A5, while other enzymes also contribute (CYP1A2, CYP2C8, CYP2C9, CYP2C19, CYP2J2M SULT1A1, SULT1A2, and SULT1A4) [136, 137]. Co-administration of potent CYP3A4/5 and P-glycoprotein inhibitors increase its plasma concentration by two-fold, while co-administration of potent CYP3A4/5 and P-glycoprotein inducers reduced its plasma concentration [138]. Pharmacogenetic studies showed a stronger association between drug transporter than CYP450 enzymes. In a 2016 study by Dimatteo et al., *ABCB1* rs4148738 was associated with increased peak plasma concentration ($p < 0.05$) [139]. A 2017 Ueshima et al. study showed dose increase of apixaban in Japanese patients with *CYP3A5*1/*3* or *3/*3* (rs776746) and *ABCG2* 421A>A (rs2231142) genotypes compared to *CYP3A5*1/ *1* and *ABCG2* 421C>C genotypes, respectively; variants 1236C>T (rs1128503), 2677G>T (rs2032582), and 3435C>T (rs1045642) of the *ABCB1* gene had no impact on this ratio [140]. A recent 2020 study by Gulilat et al. found that Caucasian patients with atrial fibrillation who had *ABCG2* 421C>A variants had higher peak and trough levels of apixaban [141]. The effect of sulfotransferase *SULTA1A1* and their polymorphisms has not been elucidated [137].

Edoxaban is mainly metabolized by CES1 and transported by P-glycoprotein. Although several polymorphisms are identified with genes that encode these enzymes, only one study explored their effect on edoxaban drug concentration rs1045642 (3435C>T) variants of *ABCB1* and rs4149056 (521T>C) of *SLCO1B1* [142]. None of the variants altered the drug's pharmacokinetics.

Betrixaban is not metabolized by CYPs but rather hydrolyzed to inactive metabolites. Like other DOACs, it is also transported by P-glycoprotein, encoded by the *ABCB1* gene [143]. It is possible that genetic variants of *ABCB1* could affect and alter its plasma concentration. Currently, there is no data available on such association.

Guidelines

There are no recommendations for DOAC's drug-gene pairs in respect to *ABCB1*, *ABCG2*, *CES1*, *CYP3A4*, and *CYP3A5* due to a low level of evidence and conflicting results. The DAPHNE clinical trial at University Hospitals of Geneva is underway. Investigators aim to assess the impact of *ABCB1*, *CYP3A4*, *CYP3A5*, and *CYP3A7* genes on the pharmacokinetics of apixaban and rivaroxaban [138]. Results of this trial as well as future RCT could help inform prescribing of PGx tests and these agents.

---

4   Antilipid Drugs

Drugs

Cardiovascular diseases (CVDs) are the leading cause of global mortality and a major contributor to global disability [144]. Statins are among the most prescribed medications worldwide due to their efficacy in preventing adverse cardiovascular outcomes associated with CVDs [145, 146]. They are used in combination with lifestyle to lower cholesterol production and reduce dyslipidemia complications such as stroke. Statins reduce LDL cholesterol by inhibiting HMG-CoA reductase, the rate-limiting enzyme for making cholesterol [147]. Decades of use emphasize their clinical benefit, but long-term safety concerns continue to emerge (hepatotoxicity, muscle toxicity, cognitive impairment, new onset of diabetes, etc.). Current evidence suggests that the benefits of statins still outweigh their potential risks [148, 149].

Both drug differences in the class and interindividual differences contribute to large variability in clinical response to statins [146, 147, 149–151]. Statins differ in their affinity for the drug-metabolizing enzyme, drug transporters, and solubility in either lipid medium or water [152, 153]. Lipophilic statins (atorvastatin, fluvastatin, lovastatin, pitavastatin, and simvastatin) are metabolized by CYPs and have wide distribution into many tissues. Hydrophilic statins (pravastatin and rosu-vastatin) do not require major metabolism by CYPs. However, they have greater hepatic specificity due to an active transport into hepatic cells. This is thought to be associated with fewer side effects in extrahepatic tissues compared to lipophilic statins [147, 153].

Although well-tolerated, 10–25% of patients report statin-associated muscle symptoms (SAMS), 5–10% report mild myalgias, and only 1 out of 100,000 patients (0.001%) report statin-induced necrotizing autoimmune myopathy [154]. For some patients, these adverse drug events may lead to statin intolerance, defined as the inability to tolerate two or more statins [150, 155]. Increased reporting of serious side effects, especially muscle toxicity (myalgia, myopathy, and rhabdomy-olysis), has led to a decline in prescribing of simvastatin [156]. It is estimated that 1–5% of patients experience simvastatin-induced myopathy which risk being the highest at daily doses over 80 mg [157]. Findings from A to Z [158] and SEARCH [159] trials support such statistics and have led to a drug label change by the FDA in 2011, which restricted the maximum approved daily dose of simvastatin to 80 mg [160]. Atorvastatin and rosuvastatin also have pharmacogenomics biomarkers in their labels.

Pharmacogenetics and Evidence
Simvastatin is primarily metabolized by CYP34A with notable contributions from CYP3A5, CYP2C9, and CYP2C19. It is transported by an efflux protein, encoded by *SLCO1B* [161]. *SLCO1B1* is a gene that encodes for organic anion transporting peptide 1B1 (OATP1B1), involved in the transport of many substrates, including simvastatin, into hepatic cells [162]. The strongest evidence of genetic variants and muscle toxicity association was found with the *SLCO1B1* c.521T>C (rs4149056) variant assigned to *5 and *17 haplotypes [163]. This variant is associated with decreased function of OATP1 transporter and reduced simvastatin transport into the liver. Reduced transport can lead to higher plasma concentrations of simvastatin associated with an increased risk of side effects such as myopathy [151].

The STRENGTH pharmacogenetic study evaluated statin efficacy and safety. A total of 509 study participants were randomized to first low dose and then a high dose of atorvastatin, simvastatin, and pravastatin. Seven reduced function alleles of *CYP2D6, CYP2C8, CYP2C9, CYP34A*, and *SLCO1C1* were investigated for asso-ciation with the composite adverse events (CAE), like discontinuation due to any side effects of creatinine kinase > 3 times baseline during follow-up. *SLCO1B1*5* (percent with $\geq$ 1 allele in CAE vs. no CAE groups, 37% vs. 25%, $p = 0.03$) and female sex (percent female in CAE vs. no CAE groups, 66% vs. 50%, $p < 0.01$) were associated with mild statin-induced adverse effects. The C allele was associated with an increased risk of adverse drug events (ADEs) in patients with hypercholesteremia when treated with atorvastatin, pravastatin, or simvastatin [164].

A 2015 meta-analysis of case–control studies by Hou et al. [165] inves-tigated the evidence of an association between genetic variants of *SLCO1B1* and statin-related myopathy. They concluded that evidence of association exists between *SLCO1B1* gene 521T>C polymorphism (C allele) and increased risk of statin-related myopathy, especially for patients taking simvastatin.

Similar association was found in a 2018 meta-analysis by Xiang et al. of 3265 myopathy patients from 14 studies [166]. *SLCO1B1* 521T>C variant or C allele was associated with significantly higher risk of drug-induced myopathy especially for simvastatin OR: 2.35; 95% CI: 1.08–5.12; $P = 0.032$), rosuvastatin (OR: 1.69; 95% CI: 1.07–2.67; $P = 0.024$), and cerivastatin (OR: 1.95; 95% CI: 1.47–2.57; $P < 0.001$) compared to T allele.

Atorvastatin is a lipophilic statin, metabolized by CYP3A4 [147]. The FDA-approved label includes a PGx biomarker with comments of increased exposure due to inhibition of CYP3A4 and/or transporters (BCRP, SLCO1B1/SLCO1B3), and P-glycoprotein (ABCB1). The DPWG recommends an alternative drug in patients with the *SLCO1B1* T521>C allele and with additional significant risk factors for statin-induced myopathy [163]. In a 2020 GWAS study, Turner et al. found strong associations between rs4149056 and circulating atorvastatin levels and muscle-related side effects in atorvastatin-treated patients with non-ST-segment elevation ACS [167]. But evidence lacks to inform genotype-based guidance when prescribing atorvastatin.

Rosuvastatin is a hydrophilic statin, metabolized by CYP2C9, CYP2C19, and generally well tolerated. Only eight cases of rhabdomyolysis induced by rosuvastatin and ticagrelor have been reported in the literature and described by Vrkic Kirhmajer et al. in [168]. A case report by Calderon-Ospina et al. published in 2020, described a 65-year-old female patient with rosuvastatin-induced rhabdomyolysis (RIR) and familial hypercholesteremia. They acknowledged her other risk factors for RIR (age, female sex, excessive dose of rosuvastatin, and renal impairment). However, their findings indicate a polygenic nature of rosuvastatin side effects. Whole-exome sequencing assessed 160 genes involved in drug metabolism or inherited myopathies. A total of 19 genomic variants in 14 genes were identified, including three rare and potentially pathogenic variants in *CYP2I9, NPC1L1*, and *OBSCN* genes [169].

Most recently in 2021, Dagli Hernandez et al. published a case report of another 65-year-old female with familial hypercholesteremia who developed both late responses to rosuvastatin and myalgia while on treatment. Her adherence was similar between visits with no significant drug interactions. Authors attributed her drug response to low function alleles of *SLCO1B1*1B/*5, *SLCO1B3* (rs4149117 and rs7311358), no function activity allele *CYP3A5*3, and low function *ABCB1* rs2287622 allele [170].

Pravastatin is a hydrophilic statin not dependent on CYPs for its metabolism. There is no prescribing information based on drug-gene pairs (*SLCO1C1, ABCB1, ABCC2*, etc.). The highest level of evidence is with the *SLCO1B1* rs4149056 variant and pharmacokinetics of pravastatin (level 2A) and *KIF6* (kinesin-like protein) and drug efficacy in coronary disease and myocardial infarction (level 2B) [171]. *SLCO1B1* rs4149056 allele was associated with a significant decrease in pravastatin clearance in healthy Chinese study volunteers. Similar results were seen in European Americans and African Americans [172]. A cohort study of healthy

Finnish men showed that the same allele was associated with increased mean peak concentration and AUC in the homozygous rs4149056 CC genotype [173]. They contrasted hydrophilic pravastatin with lipophilic fluvastatin and found that *SLCO1B1* polymorphism greatly affected the pharmacokinetics of pravastatin but not fluvastatin and more so in men than in women.

Guidelines

CPIC first addressed SLCO1B1 LOF alleles and simvastatin-induced myopathy in 2012 guidelines, then in 2014 updated guidelines [163]. The updated guidelines recommended that LOF carriers (521T>C or rs4149056T>C or *5 allele) taking simvastatin use a lower dose (< 20 mg daily dose) or an alternative statin such as rosuvastatin or pravastatin. Due to emerging evidence, CPIC updated and published guidelines again in February 2022 with several changes (175).

The fist change involves *SLCO1B1* and impact to all statins. There is strong evidence that *SLCO1B1* mediates transport of all statins with varying degree that is drug-dependent. The most impacted is simvastatin, followed by other lipophilic statins (atorvastatin, lovastatin, and pitavastatin). Hydrophilic statins (pravastatin and rosuvastatin) seem to be impacted the least. The 2022 CPIC statin guidelines leverage presence of LOF allele (rs4149056T>C) recommending that poor and decreased function SLC01B1 phenotypes initiate with low dose statin regardless of the drug.

The second change is the addition of two drug-gene pairs, *ABCG2*-rosuvastatin and *CYP2C9*-fluvastatin. *ABCG2* encodes an efflux transporter (BCRP), primarily found in liver and kidneys. Decreased function allele *ABCG2* 421C>A (rs2231142) increases rosuvastatin concentration. Therefore, the guidelines recommend to either consider a daily dose less than 20mg or an alternative if higher dose (> 20 mg) is clinically indicated. Evidence points to moderate association between CYP2C9 LOF alleles and fluvastatin dose. Specifically for IMs (activity score of 1–1.5), they recommend avoiding doses above 40mg daily and for PMs (activity score 0–0.5) avoiding doses above 20 mg daily of fluvastatin.

The DPWG guidelines were updated in August 2020 for *SLCO1B1* and atorvastatin and simvastatin. For *LOF* allele or rs4149056T>C, they recommend that total daily dose not exceed 40 mg or switching to an alternative statin and to monitor for statin-associated musculoskeletal symptoms (SAMS) [174].

Although both CPIC and DPWG acknowledge potential benefits of pre-emptive testing of these genes to reduce the incidence of SAMS, they do not recommend drug statin avoidance or discontinuation based on these genetic test results, especially if the statin therapy is clinically indicated and based on shared decision-making between the patient and provider.

5   Other CV Drugs

5.1   Antiarrhythmics

Three drugs in this class with the PGx biomarkers are flecainide, procainamide, and propafenone. All three are metabolized by CYP2D6, especially flecainide and propafenone. Changes in QTc interval in respect to *CYP2D6* genotype were observed in a 2010 study of healthy Korean male individuals after flecainide administration [175]. In a 2015 study by Doki et al., a lower serum ratio of S- to R-flecainide was seen in CYP2D6 reduced activity in Japanese patients with supraventricular tachycardia [176].

The FDA drug label for propafenone warns of higher drug levels and risk of arrhythmias in CYP2D6 PMs taking CYP3A4 inhibitors. The only genotype-based guidelines currently come from the DPWG. They recommend reducing the dose of flecainide by 50% for CYP2D6 PMs and by 25% for CYP2D6 IMs with indications other than Brugada syndrome. They also recommend reducing propafenone dose by 70% in CYP2D6 PMs or using an alternative for CYP2D6 IMs and UMs [177].

5.2   Beta-Blockers

Drugs and pharmacogenetics. Beta-blockers are widely used for the treatment of CVD and the management of non-CVDs. Carvedilol, metoprolol, nebivolol, and propranolol have PGx biomarkers in the FDA's Table of Pharmacogenetic Associations (last updated May 2021). These and timolol are metabolized by CYP2D6. Although CYP2D6 polymorphisms were shown to alter their drug levels, evidence is not strong to guide prescribing (CPIC level B/C, PharmGKB level 2–3) [74].

The CPIC guidelines have limited prescribing information. The DPWG gives guidance on dose adjustment and prescribing for metoprolol-treated patients. For those who have reduced or no function *CYP2D6* alleles (IMs and PMs), they recommend dose reduction by no more than 25% or 50% of the standard dose, in the event of symptomatic bradycardia, or if a gradual reduction in heart rate is needed. For patients with increased function *CYP2D6* alleles (UMs), they recommend either increasing the dose to 2.5 times the standard dose or using an alternative (based on effectiveness and side effects) [178, 179]. No recommendations based on the *CYP2D6* genotype are available for atenolol, bisoprolol, carvedilol, nebivolol, and the rest of the beta-blockers, by CPIC, DPWG, or other professional societies. Many pharmacogenetic studies explored the role of polymorphism in pharmacodynamics and pharmacokinetics genes. Certain variants of drug target genes suggest protection in heart failure and hypertension, while drug-metabolizing *CYP2D6* variants affect drug levels of some beta-blockers [74].

Pharmacogenetics and Evidence

Metoprolol succinate is a lipophilic β_1-selective β-blocker used for heart fail-ure based on the benefits observed in an international, multicenter, double-blind, randomized, and placebo-controlled trial of 3991 patients, called MERIT-HF (Metoprolol CR/XL Randomized Intervention Trial in Congestive Heart Failure) [180]. Initial pharmacogenetic substudies explored the β_1 adrenergic receptor poly-morphisms but found no significant association with adverse effects in heart failure [181, 182]. However, assessment of drug target studies suggests an enhanced benefit from a beta-blocker therapy in patients with polymorphisms of pharma-codynamic genes *ADRB1* and *GRK5* [183]. Both genes encode for the G-protein coupled receptors, the target of action of beta-blockers, and their cardiovascular benefits.

For example, greater efficacy of a beta-blocker was seen in patients with *ADRB1* Arg389Arg (rs1801253) and Ser49Gly (rs1801252) genotypes. Both are associ-ated with decreased receptor activity and signal transduction. Compared to other genotypes, these patients show decreased diastolic blood pressure response and a greater reduction from a beta-blocker therapy in atrial fibrillation, heart failure, and hypertension [184–186].

G-protein-coupled receptor kinase 5 (GRK5) quiets signaling between β_1 and β_2 adrenergic receptors. Regardless of beta-blocker use, *GRK5* Gln41Leu (rs2230345) variant increases the GRK5 receptor function and is associated with reduced mor-tality in patients with heart failure [187]. In 2011, Lobmeyer et al. observed the *GRK5* Gln41Leu allele was more common in Blacks (MAF = 0.227) than in Hispanics (MAF = 0.061) and Whites (MAF = 0.021). *GRK5* Gln41Leu was pro-tective in patients with hypertension treated with atenolol or hydrochlorothiazide, without affecting response to either drug [188].

A stronger association was observed between *CYP2D6* polymorphism and the pharmacokinetics of beta-blockers. In 2014, Hall et al. did a post-hoc PGx sub-study in a subpopulation of the MERIT-HF. They aimed to assess the effect of the *CYP2D6*4* allele on pharmacokinetics in metoprolol-treated patients with sys-tolic heart failure. *CYP2D6*4* is a null allele (no enzyme activity) with an allelic frequency of 20% in Caucasian Europeans [189, 190]. Among 605 patients, 313 patients were randomized to the metoprolol treatment arm, the majority being men (78.9%). Of those in the treatment arm, 112 patients (35.8%) had *CYP2D6*1/*4* genotype (IM phenotype) and 12 patients (3.8%) had *CYP2D6 *4/*4* genotype (PM phenotype). A 2017 study by Luzum et al. examined if the *CYP2D6*4* LOF allele was associated with a beta-blocker (carvedilol or metoprolol) maintenance dose in patients with heart failure. Most patients were male (60%) and of European descent (90%). CYP2D6 metabolizes both drugs, carvedilol to active metabolite and metoprolol to the less active metabolite. *CYP2D6*4* was associated with lower maintenance dose of metoprolol (OR 0.13 [95% CI 0.02–0.75] $p = 0.023$), and higher maintenance dose of carvedilol (OR 2.94 [95% CI 0.84–10.30] $p = 0.093$) [191].

Data from several studies found *CYP2D6* variants increase side effects of beta-blockers, such as bradycardia, but evidence lacks to support the association between *CYP2D6* variants and blood pressure control or reduction in cardiovascular risks [178].

6   Conclusion

Evidence supports PGx testing with drugs used for the management of cardiovascular diseases. The genotype-based guidelines exist that are based on multiple randomized controlled trials and other studies. The strongest evidence with high concordance among guidelines exists for clopidogrel-*CYP2C19* (drug response), warfarin-*CYP2C9/VKORC1* (drug response), and simvastatin-*SLCO1B1* (statin-induced myopathy). Evidence continues to expand with other cardiovascular drugs. While the majority of PGx studies have been done with pharmacokinetic genes, especially *CYP2C9* (warfarin), *CYP2D19* (clopidogrel), and *CYP2D6* (beta-blockers, antiarrhythmics), some interesting and promising results have come from drug targets studies concerning cardiovascular risks and benefits.

Treating cardiovascular diseases is complex/challenging. The heterogeneity of CVDs is compounded by the increasing number of drugs used for their management and the intricacies of drug interactions. Additionally, a variety of patient-specific factors also influences treatment outcomes and adds to the complexity of selecting an optimal drug and dose for each patient. Emerging technologies such as artificial intelligence and machine learning hold promise in stratifying patients based on their clinical phenotypes and matching the best drug therapy for each patient.

References

1. Giri J, Moyer AM, Bielinski SJ, Caraballo PJ. Concepts driving pharmacogenomics implementation into everyday healthcare. Pharmacogenomics Pers Med. 2019;12:305–18. https://doi.org/10.2147/PGPM.S193185.
2. Krebs K, Milani L. Translating pharmacogenomics into clinical decisions: do not let the perfect be the enemy of the good. Human Gen. 2019;13(1):39. https://doi.org/10.1186/s40246-019-0229-z.
3. Dunnenberger HM, Crews KR, Hoffman JM, Caudle KE, Broeckel U, Howard SC, et al. Preemptive clinical pharmacogenetics implementation: current programs in five US medical centers. Annu Rev Pharmacol Toxicol. 2015;55:89–106. https://doi.org/10.1146/annurev-pharmtox-010814-124835.
4. van der Wouden CH, Cambon-Thomsen A, Cecchin E, Cheung KC, Dávila-Fajardo CL, Deneer VH, et al. Implementing pharmacogenomics in Europe: design and implementation strategy of the ubiquitous pharmacogenomics consortium. Clin Pharmacol Ther. 2017;101(3):341–58. https://doi.org/10.1002/cpt.602.
5. Volpi S, Bult CJ, Chisholm RL, Deverka PA, Ginsburg GS, Jacob HJ, et al. Research directions in the clinical implementation of pharmacogenomics: an overview of US programs and projects. Clin Pharmacol Ther. 2018;103(5):778–86. https://doi.org/10.1002/cpt.1048.

6. Shekhani R, Steinacher L, Swen JJ, Ingelman-Sundberg M. Evaluation of current regulation and guidelines of pharmacogenomic drug labels: opportunities for improvements. Clin Pharmacol Ther. 2020;107(5):1240–55. https://doi.org/10.1002/cpt.1720.

7. The FDA Table of Pharmacogenetic Associations 2020.

8. Klein TE, Chang JT, Cho MK, Easton KL, Fergerson R, Hewett M, et al. Integrating genotype and phenotype information: an overview of the PharmGKB project. Pharmacogenomics J. 2001;1(3):167–70. https://doi.org/10.1038/sj.tpj.6500035.

9. Abdullah-Koolmees H, van Keulen AM, Nijenhuis M, Deneer VHM. Pharmacogenetics guidelines: overview and comparison of the DPWG, CPIC, CPNDS, and RNPGx guidelines. Front Pharmacol. 2020;11:595219. https://doi.org/10.3389/fphar.2020.595219.

10. Dávila-Fajardo CL, Díaz-Villamarín X, Antúnez-Rodríguez A, Fernández-Gómez AE, García-Navas P, Martínez-González LJ, et al. Pharmacogenetics in the treatment of cardiovascular diseases and its current progress regarding implementation in the clinical routine. Genes 2019;10(4). https://doi.org/10.3390/genes10040261.

11. Lamoureux F, Duflot T. Pharmacogenetics in cardiovascular diseases: state of the art and implementation-recommendations of the French National Network of Pharmacogenetics (RNPGx). Therapie. 2017;72(2):257–67. https://doi.org/10.1016/j.therap.2016.09.017.

12. Kitzmiller JP, Groen DK, Phelps MA, Sadee W. Pharmacogenomic testing: relevance in medical practice: why drugs work in some patients but not in others. Cleve Clin J Med. 2011;78(4):243–57. https://doi.org/10.3949/ccjm.78a.10145.

13. Adams RJ, Albers G, Alberts MJ, Benavente O, Furie K, Goldstein LB, et al. Update to the AHA/ASA recommendations for the prevention of stroke in patients with stroke and transient ischemic attack. Stroke. 2008;39(5):1647–52. https://doi.org/10.1161/STROKEAHA. 107.189063.

14. Steinhubl SR, Berger PB, Mann JT III, Fry ETA, DeLago A, Wilmer C, et al. Early and sustained dual oral antiplatelet therapy following percutaneous coronary intervention a randomized controlled trial. JAMA. 2002;288(19):2411–20. https://doi.org/10.1001/jama.288. 19.2411.

15. Wallentin L, Becker RC, Budaj A, Cannon CP, Emanuelsson H, Held C, et al. Ticagrelor versus clopidogrel in patients with acute coronary syndromes. N Eng J Med. 2009;361(11):1045–57. https://doi.org/10.1056/NEJMoa0904327.

16. Wiviott SD, Braunwald E, McCabe CH, Montalescot G, Ruzyllo W, Gottlieb S, et al. Prasugrel versus clopidogrel in patients with acute coronary syndromes. N Eng J Med. 2007;357(20):2001–15. https://doi.org/10.1056/NEJMoa0706482.

17. Dayoub EJ, Seigerman M, Tuteja S, Kobayashi T, Kolansky DM, Giri J, et al. Trends in platelet adenosine diphosphate P2Y12 receptor inhibitor use and adherence among antiplatelet-naive patients after percutaneous coronary intervention, 2008–2016. JAMA Intern Med. 2018;178(7):943–50. https://doi.org/10.1001/jamainternmed.2018.0783.

18. Snoep JD, Hovens MM, Eikenboom JC, van der Bom JG, Jukema JW, Huisman MV. Clopidogrel nonresponsiveness in patients undergoing percutaneous coronary intervention with stenting: a systematic review and meta-analysis. Am Heart J. 2007;154(2):221–31. https://doi.org/10.1016/j.ahj.2007.04.014.

19. Claassens DMF, Vos GJA, Bergmeijer TO, Hermanides RS, van 't Hof AWJ, van der Harst P, et al. A genotype-guided strategy for oral P2Y(12) inhibitors in primary PCI. N Engl J Med. 2019;381(17):1621–31. https://doi.org/10.1056/NEJMoa1907096.

20. Levine GN, Bates ER, Bittl JA, Brindis RG, Fihn SD, Fleisher LA, et al. 2016 ACC/AHA guideline focused update on duration of dual antiplatelet therapy in patients with coronary artery disease: a report of the American College of Cardiology/American Heart Association Task Force on Clinical Practice Guidelines. J Thorac Cardiovasc Surg. 2016;152(5):1243–75. https://doi.org/10.1016/j.jacc.2016.03.513.

21. Kazui M, Nishiya Y, Ishizuka T, Hagihara K, Farid NA, Okazaki O, et al. Identification of the human cytochrome P450 enzymes involved in the two oxidative steps in the bioactivation of clopidogrel to its pharmacologically active metabolite. Drug Metab Dispos. 2010;38(1):92–9. https://doi.org/10.1124/dmd.109.029132.

22. Sangkuhl K, Klein TE, Altman RB. Clopidogrel pathway. Pharmacogenet Genom. 2010;20(7):463–5. https://doi.org/10.1097/FPC.0b013e3283385420.
23. Gaedigk A, Ingelman-Sundberg M, Miller NA, Leeder JS, Whirl-Carrillo M, Klein TE. The pharmacogene variation (PharmVar) consortium: incorporation of the human cytochrome P450 (CYP) allele nomenclature database. Clin Pharmacol Ther. 2018;103(3):399–401. https://doi.org/10.1002/cpt.910.
24. Pratt VM, Cavallari LH, Del Tredici AL, Hachad H, Ji Y, Kalman LV, et al. Recommendations for clinical warfarin genotyping allele selection a report of the Association for Molecular Pathology and the College of American Pathologists. J Mol Diagn. 2020;22(7):847–59. https://doi.org/10.1016/j.jmoldx.2020.04.204.
25. Scott SA, Sangkuhl K, Stein CM, Hulot JS, Mega JL, Roden DM, et al. Clinical pharmacogenetics implementation consortium guidelines for CYP2C19 genotype and clopidogrel therapy: 2013 update. Clin Pharmacol Ther. 2013;94(3):317–23. https://doi.org/10.1038/clpt.2013.105.
26. Fricke-Galindo I, Céspedes-Garro C, Rodrigues-Soares F, Naranjo ME, Delgado Á, de Andrés F, et al. Interethnic variation of CYP2C19 alleles, 'predicted' phenotypes and 'measured' metabolic phenotypes across world populations. Pharmacogenomics J. 2016;16(2):113–23. https://doi.org/10.1038/tpj.2015.70.
27. Brandt JT, Close SL, Iturria SJ, Payne CD, Farid NA, Ernest CS, et al. Common polymorphisms of CYP2C19 and CYP2C9 affect the pharmacokinetic and pharmacodynamic response to clopidogrel but not prasugrel. J Thromb Haemost. 2007;5(12):2429–36. https://doi.org/10.1111/j.1538-7836.2007.02775.x.
28. Umemura K, Furuta T, Kondo K. The common gene variants of CYP2C19 affect pharmacokinetics and pharmacodynamics in an active metabolite of clopidogrel in healthy subjects. J Thromb Haemost. 2008;6(8):1439–41. https://doi.org/10.1111/j.1538-7836.2008.03050.x.
29. Mega JL, Close SL, Wiviott SD, Shen L, Hockett RD, Brandt JT, et al. Cytochrome P450 genetic polymorphisms and the response to prasugrel relationship to pharmacokinetic, pharmacodynamic, and clinical outcomes. Circulation. 2009;119(19):2553-U44. https://doi.org/10.1161/CIRCULATIONAHA.109.851949.
30. Mega JL, Close SL, Wiviott SD, Shen L, Walker JR, Simon T, et al. Genetic variants in ABCB1 and CYP2C19 and cardiovascular outcomes after treatment with clopidogrel and prasugrel in the TRITON-TIMI 38 trial: a pharmacogenetic analysis. Lancet. 2010;376(9749):1312–9. https://doi.org/10.1016/S0140-6736(10)61273-1.
31. Mega JL, Simon T, Collet JP, Anderson JL, Antman EM, Bliden K, et al. Reduced-function CYP2C19 genotype and risk of adverse clinical outcomes among patients treated with clopidogrel predominantly for PCI a meta-analysis. JAMA. 2010;304(16):1821–30. https://doi.org/10.1001/jama.2010.1543.
32. Wallentin L, James S, Storey RF, Armstrong M, Barratt BJ, Horrow J, et al. Effect of CYP2C19 and ABCB1 single nucleotide polymorphisms on outcomes of treatment with ticagrelor versus clopidogrel for acute coronary syndromes: a genetic substudy of the PLATO trial. Lancet. 2010;376(9749):1320–8. https://doi.org/10.1016/S0140-6736(10)61274-3.
33. Mega JL, Hochholzer W, Frelinger AL, Kluk MJ, Angiolillo DJ, Kereiakes DJ, et al. Dosing clopidogrel based on CYP2C19 genotype and the effect on platelet reactivity in patients with stable cardiovascular disease. JAMA. 2011;306(20):2221–8. https://doi.org/10.1001/jama.2011.1703.
34. Price MJ, Murray SS, Angiolillo DJ, Lillie E, Smith EN, Tisch RL, et al. Influence of genetic polymorphisms on the effect of high-and standard-dose clopidogrel after percutaneous coronary intervention the GIFT (genotype information and functional testing) study. J Am Coll Cardiol. 2012;59(22):1928–37. https://doi.org/10.1016/j.jacc.2011.11.068.
35. Carreras ET, Hochholzer W, Frelinger AL, Nordio F, O'Donoghue ML, Wiviott SD, et al. Diabetes mellitus, CYP2C19 genotype, and response to escalating doses of clopidogrel Insights from the ELEVATE-TIMI 56 trial. Thromb Haemost. 2016;116(1):69–77. https://doi.org/10.1160/TH15-12-0981.

36. Sibbing D, Koch W, Gebhard D, Schuster T, Braun S, Stegherr J, et al. Cytochrome 2C19*17 allelic variant, platelet aggregation, bleeding events, and stent thrombosis in clopidogrel-treated patients with coronary stent placement. Circulation. 2010;121(4):512–8. https://doi.org/10.1161/CIRCULATIONAHA.109.885194.

37. Frére C, Cuisset T, Gaborit B, Alessi MC, Hulot JS. The CYP2C19*17 allele is associated with better platelet response to clopidogrel in patients admitted for non-ST acute coronary syndrome. J Thromb Haemost. 2009;7(8):1409–11. https://doi.org/10.1111/j.1538-7836.2009.03500.x.

38. Sychev DA, Baturina OA, Mirzaev KB, Rytkin E, Ivashchenko DV, Andreev DA, et al. CYP2C19*17 may increase the risk of death among patients with an acute coronary syndrome and non-valvular atrial fibrillation who receive clopidogrel and rivaroxaban. Pharmgenomics Pers Med. 2020;13:29–37. https://doi.org/10.2147/PGPM.S234910.

39. Shuldiner AR, O'Connell JR, Bliden KP, Gandhi A, Ryan K, Horenstein RB, et al. Association of Cytochrome P450 2C19 genotype with the antiplatelet effect and clinical efficacy of clopidogrel therapy. JAMA. 2009;302(8):849–58. https://doi.org/10.1001/jama.2009.1232.

40. Simon T, Verstuyft C, Mary-Krause M, Quteineh L, Drouet E, Meneveau N, et al. Genetic determinants of response to clopidogrel and cardiovascular events. N Engl J Med. 2009;360(4):363–75. https://doi.org/10.1056/NEJMoa0808227.

41. Zhai YJ, He HR, Ma XC, Xie J, Meng T, Dong YL, et al. Meta-analysis of effects of ABCB1 polymorphisms on clopidogrel response among patients with coronary artery disease. Eur J Clin Pharmacol. 2017;73(7):843–54. https://doi.org/10.1007/s00228-017-2235-1.

42. Bauer T, Bouman HJ, van Werkum JW, Ford NF, ten Berg JM, Taubert D. Impact of CYP2C19 variant genotypes on clinical efficacy of antiplatelet treatment with clopidogrel: systematic review and meta-analysis. BMJ. 2011;343. https://doi.org/10.1136/bmj.d4588.

43. Mega JL, Close SL, Wiviott SD, Man M, Duvvuru S, Walker JR, et al. PON1 Q192R genetic variant and response to clopidogrel and prasugrel: pharmacokinetics, pharmacodynamics, and a meta-analysis of clinical outcomes. J Thromb Thrombolysis. 2016;41(3):374–83. https://doi.org/10.1007/s11239-015-1264-9.

44. Hulot JS, Collet JP, Cayla G, Silvain J, Allanic F, Bellemain-Appaix A, et al. CYP2C19 but not PON1 genetic variants influence clopidogrel pharmacokinetics, pharmacodynamics, and clinical efficacy in post-myocardial infarction patients. Circ Cardiovasc Intervent. 2011;4(5):422–8. https://doi.org/10.1161/CIRCINTERVENTIONS.111.963025.

45. Lewis JP, Fisch AS, Ryan K, O'Connell JR, Gibson Q, Mitchell BD, et al. Paraoxonase 1 (PON1) gene variants are not associated with clopidogrel response. Clin Pharmacol Ther. 2011;90(4):568–74. https://doi.org/10.1038/clpt.2011.194.

46. Li M, Wang H, Xuan L, Shi X, Zhou T, Zhang N, et al. Associations between P2RY12 gene polymorphisms and risks of clopidogrel resistance and adverse cardiovascular events after PCI in patients with acute coronary syndrome. Medicine. 2017;96(14). https://doi.org/10.1097/MD.0000000000006553.

47. Lewis JP, Horenstein RB, Ryan K, O'Connell JR, Gibson Q, Mitchell BD, et al. The functional G143E variant of carboxylesterase 1 is associated with increased clopidogrel active metabolite levels and greater clopidogrel response. Pharmacogenet Genomics. 2013;23(1):1–8. https://doi.org/10.1097/FPC.0b013e32835aa8a2.

48. Lewis JP, Backman JD, Reny JL, Bergmeijer TO, Mitchell BD, Ritchie MD, et al. Pharmacogenomic polygenic response score predicts ischaemic events and cardiovascular mortality in clopidogrel-treated patients. Euro Heart J-Cardiovascular Pharmacother. 2020;6(4):203–10. https://doi.org/10.1093/ehjcvp/pvz045.

49. Smith Sidney C, Allen J, Blair Steven N, Bonow Robert O, Brass Lawrence M, Fonarow Gregg C, et al. AHA/ACC guidelines for secondary prevention for patients with coronary and other atherosclerotic vascular disease: 2006 update. J Am Coll Cardiol. 2006;47(10):2130–9. https://doi.org/10.1161/CIRCULATIONAHA.106.174516.

50. Sorich MJ, Vitry A, Ward MB, Horowitz JD, McKinnon RA. Prasugrel vs. clopidogrel for cytochrome P450 2C19-genotyped subgroups: integration of the TRITON-TIMI 38 trial data. J Thromb Haemost. 2010;8(8):1678–84.

51. Mega JL, Close SL, Wiviott SD, Shen L, Hockett RD, Brandt JT, et al. Cytochrome P-450 polymorphisms and response to clopidogrel. N Engl J Med. 2009;360(4):354–62. https://doi.org/10.1056/NEJMoa0809171.
52. Collet JP, Hulot JS, Pena A, Villard E, Esteve JB, Silvain J, et al. Cytochrome P450 2C19 polymorphism in young patients treated with clopidogrel after myocardial infarction: a cohort study. Lancet. 2009;373(9660):309–17. https://doi.org/10.1016/S0140-6736(08)61845-0.
53. Combescure C, Fontana P, Mallouk N, Berdague P, Labruyere C, Barazer I, et al. Clinical implications of clopidogrel non-response in cardiovascular patients: a systematic review and meta-analysis. J Thromb Haemost. 2010;8(5):923–33. https://doi.org/10.1111/j.1538-7836.2010.03809.x.
54. Hulot JS, Collet JP, Silvain J, Pena A, Bellemain-Appaix A, Barthelemy O, et al. Cardiovascular risk in clopidogrel-treated patients according to cytochrome P450 2C19*2 loss-of-function allele or proton pump inhibitor coadministration a systematic meta-analysis. J Am Coll Cardiol. 2010;56(2):134–43. https://doi.org/10.1016/j.jacc.2009.12.071.
55. Zabalza M, Subirana I, Sala J, Lluis-Ganella C, Lucas G, Tomas M, et al. Meta-analyses of the association between cytochrome CYP2C19 loss- and gain-of-function polymorphisms and cardiovascular outcomes in patients with coronary artery disease treated with clopidogrel. Heart. 2012;98(2):100–8. https://doi.org/10.1136/hrt.2011.227652.
56. Sorich MJ, Rowland A, McKinnon RA, Wiese MD. CYP2C19 genotype has a greater effect on adverse cardiovascular outcomes following percutaneous coronary intervention and in Asian populations treated with clopidogrel a meta-analysis. Circ Cardiovasc Genet. 2014;7(6):895-U387. https://doi.org/10.1161/CIRCGENETICS.114.000669.
57. Xie X, Ma YT, Yang YN, Li XM, Zheng YY, Ma X, et al. Personalized antiplatelet therapy according to CYP2C19 genotype after percutaneous coronary intervention: a randomized control trial. Int J Cardiol. 2013;168(4):3736–40. https://doi.org/10.1016/j.ijcard.2013.06.014.
58. Notarangelo FM, Maglietta G, Bevilacqua P, Cereda M, Merlini PA, Villani GQ, et al. Pharmacogenomic approach to selecting antiplatelet therapy in patients with acute coronary syndromes the PHARMCLO trial. J Am Coll Cardiol. 2018;71(17):1869–77. https://doi.org/10.1016/j.jacc.2018.02.029.
59. Pereira NL, Farkouh ME, So D, Lennon R, Geller N, Mathew V, et al. Effect of genotype-guided oral P2Y12 inhibitor selection vs conventional clopidogrel therapy on ischemic outcomes after percutaneous coronary intervention: the TAILOR-PCI randomized clinical trial. JAMA. 2020;324(8):761–71. https://doi.org/10.1001/jama.2020.12443.
60. Bergmeijer TO, Janssen PW, Schipper JC, Qaderdan K, Ishak M, Ruitenbeek RS, et al. CYP2C19 genotype-guided antiplatelet therapy in ST-segment elevation myocardial infarction patients-rationale and design of the patient outcome after primary PCI (POPular) genetics study. Am Heart J. 2014;168(1):16-22.e1. https://doi.org/10.1016/j.ahj.2014.03.006.
61. Scott SA, Sangkuhl K, Gardner EE, Stein CM, Hulot JS, Johnson JA, et al. Clinical pharmacogenetics implementation consortium guidelines for cytochrome P450–2C19 (CYP2C19) genotype and clopidogrel therapy. Clin Pharmacol Ther. 2011;90(2):328–32. https://doi.org/10.1038/clpt.2011.132.
62. Holmes DR, Dehmer GJ, Kaul S, Leifer D, O'Gara PT, Stein CM. ACCF/AHA clopidogrel clinical alert: approaches to the FDA "boxed warning" a report of the American College of Cardiology Foundation Task Force on Clinical Expert Consensus Documents and the American Heart Association. J Am Coll Cardiol. 2010;56(4):321–41. https://doi.org/10.1161/CIR.0b013e3181ee08ed.
63. Levine GN, Bates ER, Bittl JA, Brindis RG, Fihn SD, Fleisher LA, et al. 2016 ACC/AHA guideline focused update on duration of dual antiplatelet therapy in patients with coronary artery disease. J Thor Cardiovasc Surg. 2016;152(5):1243–75. https://doi.org/10.1016/j.jtcvs.2016.07.044.
64. Weitzel KW, Elsey AR, Langaee TY, Burkley B, Nessl DR, Obeng AO, et al. Clinical pharmacogenetics implementation: approaches, successes, and challenges. Am J Med Genet C Semin Med Genet. 2014;166c(1):56–67. https://doi.org/10.1002/ajmg.c.31390.

65. Ageno W, Gallus AS, Wittkowsky A, Crowther M, Hylek EM, Palareti G. Oral anticoagulant therapy: antithrombotic therapy and prevention of thrombosis, 9th ed: American College of Chest Physicians Evidence-Based Clinical Practice Guidelines. Chest. 2012;141(2 Suppl):e44S-e88S. https://doi.org/10.1378/chest.11-2292.

66. Pirmohamed M. Warfarin: almost 60 years old and still causing problems. Br J Clin Pharmacol. 2006;62(5):509–11. https://doi.org/10.1111/j.1365-2125.2006.02806.x.

67. Kearon C, Akl EA, Comerota AJ, Prandoni P, Bounameaux H, Goldhaber SZ, et al. Antithrombotic therapy for VTE disease: antithrombotic therapy and prevention of thrombosis, 9th ed: American College of Chest Physicians Evidence-Based Clinical Practice Guidelines. Chest. 2012;141(2 Suppl):e419S-e96S. https://doi.org/10.1378/chest.11-2301.

68. You JJ, Singer DE, Howard PA, Lane DA, Eckman MH, Fang MC, et al. Antithrombotic therapy for atrial fibrillation: antithrombotic therapy and prevention of thrombosis, 9th ed: American College of Chest Physicians Evidence-Based Clinical Practice Guidelines. Chest. 2012;141(2 Suppl):e531S-e75S. https://doi.org/10.1378/chest.11-2304.

69. Lansberg MG, O'Donnell MJ, Khatri P, Lang ES, Nguyen-Huynh MN, Schwartz NE, et al. Antithrombotic and thrombolytic therapy for ischemic stroke: antithrombotic therapy and prevention of thrombosis, 9th ed: American College of Chest Physicians Evidence-Based Clinical Practice Guidelines. Chest. 2012;141(2 Suppl):e601S-e36S. https://doi.org/10.1378/chest.11-2302.

70. Whitlock RP, Sun JC, Fremes SE, Rubens FD, Teoh KH. Antithrombotic and thrombolytic therapy for valvular disease: antithrombotic therapy and prevention of thrombosis, 9th ed: American College of Chest Physicians Evidence-Based Clinical Practice Guidelines. Chest. 2012;141(2 Suppl):e576S-e600S. https://doi.org/10.1378/chest.11-2305.

71. Robinson AA, Trankle CR, Eubanks G, Schumann C, Thompson P, Wallace RL, et al. Off-label use of direct oral anticoagulants compared with warfarin for left ventricular thrombi. JAMA Cardiol. 2020;5(6):685–92. https://doi.org/10.1001/jamacardio.2020.0652.

72. Holbrook A, Schulman S, Witt DM, Vandvik PO, Fish J, Kovacs MJ, et al. Evidence-based management of anticoagulant therapy: antithrombotic therapy and prevention of thrombosis, 9th ed: American College of Chest Physicians Evidence-Based Clinical Practice Guidelines. Chest. 2012;141(2 Suppl):e152S-e84S. https://doi.org/10.1378/chest.11-2295.

73. Cavallari LH, Langaee TY, Momary KM, Shapiro NL, Nutescu EA, Coty WA, et al. Genetic and clinical predictors of warfarin dose requirements in African Americans. Clin Pharmacol Ther. 2010;87(4):459–64. https://doi.org/10.1038/clpt.2009.223.

74. Duarte JD, Cavallari LH. Pharmacogenetics to guide cardiovascular drug therapy. Nat Rev Cardiol. 2021;18(9):649–65. https://doi.org/10.1038/s41569-021-00549-w.

75. Choonara IA, Haynes BP, Cholerton S, Breckenridge AM, Park BK. Enantiomers of warfarin and vitamin K1 metabolism. Br J Clin Pharmacol. 1986;22(6):729–32. https://doi.org/10.1111/j.1365-2125.1986.tb02966.x.

76. Rettie AE, Korzekwa KR, Kunze KL, Lawrence RF, Eddy AC, Aoyama T, et al. Hydroxylation of warfarin by human cDNA-expressed cytochrome P-450: a role for P-4502C9 in the etiology of (S)-warfarin-drug interactions. Chem Res Toxicol. 1992;5(1):54–9. https://doi.org/10.1021/tx00025a009.

77. Anderson JL, Horne BD, Stevens SM, Grove AS, Barton S, Nicholas ZP, et al. Randomized trial of genotype-guided versus standard warfarin dosing in patients initiating oral anticoagulation. Circulation. 2007;116(22):2563–70. https://doi.org/10.1161/CIRCULATIONAHA.107.737312.

78. Wen MS, Chang KC, Lee TH, Chen YF, Hung KC, Chang YJ, et al. Pharmacogenetic dosing of warfarin in the Han-Chinese population: a randomized trial. Pharmacogenomics. 2017;18(3):245–53. https://doi.org/10.2217/pgs-2016-0154.

79. Limdi N, McGwin G, Goldstein JA, Beasley TM, Arnett DK, Adler BK, et al. Influence of CYP2C9 and VKORC1 1173C/T genotype on the risk of hemorrhagic complications in African-American and European-American patients on warfarin. Clin Pharmacol Ther. 2008;83(2):312–21. https://doi.org/10.1038/sj.clpt.6100290.

80. Scordo MG, Pengo V, Spina E, Dahl ML, Gusella M, Padrini R. Influence of CYP2C9 and CYP2C19 genetic polymorphisms on warfarin maintenance dose and metabolic clearance. Clin Pharmacol Ther. 2002;72(6):702–10. https://doi.org/10.1067/mcp.2002.129321.

81. Allabi AC, Gala JL, Horsmans Y, Babaoglu MO, Bozkurt A, Heusterspreute M, et al. Functional impact of CYP2C*5, CYP2C9*6, CYP2C9*8, and CYP2C9*11 in vivo among black Africans. Clin Pharmacol Ther. 2004;76(2):113–8. https://doi.org/10.1016/j.clpt.2004.04.001.

82. Liu Y, Jeong H, Takahashi H, Drozda K, Patel SR, Shapiro NL, et al. Decreased warfarin clearance associated with the CYP2C9 R150H (*8) polymorphism. Clin Pharmacol Ther. 2012;91(4):660–5. https://doi.org/10.1038/clpt.2011.269.

83. Asiimwe IG, Zhang EJ, Osanlou R, Krause A, Dillon C, Suarez-Kurtz G, et al. Genetic factors influencing warfarin dose in black-African patients: a systematic review and meta-analysis. Clin Pharmacol Ther. 2020;107(6):1420–33. https://doi.org/10.1002/cpt.1755.

84. Kamali F, Wynne H. Pharmacogenetics of warfarin. Ann Rev Med. 2010;61(1):63–75. https://doi.org/10.1146/annurev.med.070808.170037.

85. D'Andrea G, D'Ambrosio RL, Di Perna P, Chetta M, Santacroce R, Brancaccio V, et al. A polymorphism in the VKORC1 gene is associated with an interindividual variability in the dose-anticoagulant effect of warfarin. Blood. 2005;105(2):645–9. https://doi.org/10.1182/blood-2004-06-2111.

86. Bader LA, Elewa H. The impact of genetic and non-genetic factors on warfarin dose prediction in MENA region: a systematic review. PLoS ONE. 2016;11(12):e0168732. https://doi.org/10.1371/journal.pone.0168732.

87. Fung E, Patsopoulos NA, Belknap SM, O'Rourke DJ, Robb JF, Anderson JL, et al. Effect of genetic variants, especially CYP2C9 and VKORC1, on the pharmacology of warfarin. Semin Thromb Hemost. 2012;38(8):893–904. https://doi.org/10.1055/s-0032-1328891.

88. Gage B, Eby C, Johnson J, Deych E, Rieder M, Ridker P, et al. Use of pharmacogenetic and clinical factors to predict the therapeutic dose of warfarin. Clin Pharmacol Ther. 2008;84(3):326–31. https://doi.org/10.1038/clpt.2008.10.

89. Pirmohamed M, Burnside G, Eriksson N, Jorgensen AL, Toh CH, Nicholson T, et al. A randomized trial of genotype-guided dosing of warfarin. Engl J Med. 2013;369(24):2294–303. https://doi.org/10.1056/NEJMoa1311386.

90. Kimmel SE, French B, Kasner SE, Johnson JA, Anderson JL, Gage BF, et al. A pharmacogenetic versus a clinical algorithm for warfarin dosing. N Engl J Med. 2013;369(24):2283–93. https://doi.org/10.1056/NEJMoa1310669.

91. Shaw K, Amstutz U, Kim RB, Lesko LJ, Turgeon J, Michaud V, et al. Clinical practice recommendations on genetic testing of CYP2C9 and VKORC1 variants in warfarin therapy. Ther Drug Monit. 2015;37(4):428–36. https://doi.org/10.1097/FTD.0000000000000192.

92. Drozda K, Wong S, Patel SR, Bress AP, Nutescu EA, Kittles RA, et al. Poor warfarin dose prediction with pharmacogenetic algorithms that exclude genotypes important for African Americans. Pharmacogenet Genom. 2015;25(2):73–81. https://doi.org/10.1097/FPC.0000000000000108.

93. Gage BF, Bass AR, Lin H, Woller SC, Stevens S, Al-Hammadi N, et al. Effect of genotype-guided warfarin dosing on clinical events and anticoagulation control among patients undergoing hip or knee arthroplasty the GIFT randomized clinical trial. JAMA. 2017;318(12):1115–24. https://doi.org/10.1001/jama.2017.11469.

94. Budnitz DS, Lovegrove MC, Shehab N, Richards CL. Emergency hospitalizations for adverse drug events in older Americans. N Engl J Med. 2011;365(21):2002–12. https://doi.org/10.1056/NEJMsa1103053.

95. Shehab N, Lovegrove MC, Geller AI, Rose KO, Weidle NJ, Budnitz DS. US emergency department visits for outpatient adverse drug events, 2013–2014. JAMA. 2016;316(20):2115–25. https://doi.org/10.1001/jama.2016.16201.

96. Goulding R, Dawes D, Price M, Wilkie S, Dawes M. Genotype-guided drug prescribing: a systematic review and meta-analysis of randomized control trials. Br J Clin Pharmacol. 2015;80(4):868–77. https://doi.org/10.1111/bcp.12475.

97. Tang Q, Zou H, Guo C, Liu Z. Outcomes of pharmacogenetics-guided dosing of warfarin: a systematic review and meta-analysis. Int J Cardiol. 2014;175(3):587–91. https://doi.org/10.1016/j.ijcard.2014.06.031.

98. Liao Z, Feng S, Ling P, Zhang G. Meta-analysis of randomized controlled trials reveals an improved clinical outcome of using genotype plus clinical algorithm for warfarin dosing. J Thromb Thrombol. 2015;39(2):228–34. https://doi.org/10.1007/s11239-014-1099-9.

99. Shi C, Yan W, Wang G, Wang F, Li Q, Lin N. Pharmacogenetics-based versus conventional dosing of warfarin: a meta-analysis of randomized controlled trials. PLoS ONE. 2015;10(12):e0144511. https://doi.org/10.1371/journal.pone.0144511.

100. Johnson EG, Horne BD, Carlquist JF, Anderson JL. Genotype-based dosing algorithms for warfarin therapy: data review and recommendations. Mol Diagn Ther. 2011;15(5):255–64. https://doi.org/10.1007/BF03256417.

101. Wu AH. Use of genetic and nongenetic factors in warfarin dosing algorithms. Pharmacogenomics. 2007;8(7):851–61. https://doi.org/10.2217/14622416.8.7.851.

102. Kaye JB, Schultz LE, Steiner HE, Kittles RA, Cavallari LH, Karnes JH. Warfarin pharmacogenomics in diverse populations. Pharmacotherapy. 2017;37(9):1150–63. https://doi.org/10.1002/phar.1982.

103. Sasano M, Ohno M, Fukuda Y, Nonen S, Hirobe S, Maeda S, et al. Verification of pharmacogenomics-based algorithms to predict warfarin maintenance dose using registered data of Japanese patients. Eur J Clin Pharmacol. 2019;75(7):901–11. https://doi.org/10.1007/s00228-019-02656-7.

104. Tavares LC, Marcatto LR, Santos P. Genotype-guided warfarin therapy: current status. Pharmacogenomics. 2018;19(7):667–85. https://doi.org/10.2217/pgs-2017-0207.

105. Chumnumwat S, Yi K, Lucksiri A, Nosoongnoen W, Chindavijak B, Chulavatnatol S, et al. Comparative performance of pharmacogenetics-based warfarin dosing algorithms derived from Caucasian, Asian, and mixed races in Thai population. Cardiovasc Ther. 2018;36(2). https://doi.org/10.1111/1755-5922.12315.

106. Johnson J, Caudle K, Gong L, Whirl-Carrillo M, Stein C, Scott S, et al. Clinical pharmacogenetics implementation consortium (CPIC) guideline for pharmacogenetics-guided warfarin dosing: 2017 update. Clin Pharmacol Ther. 2017;102(3):397–404. https://doi.org/10.1002/cpt.668.

107. Finkelman BS, Gage BF, Johnson JA, Brensinger CM, Kimmel SE. Genetic warfarin dosing: tables versus algorithms. J Am Coll Cardiol. 2011;57(5):612–8. https://doi.org/10.1016/j.jacc.2010.08.643.

108. Borgiani P, Ciccacci C, Forte V, Sirianni E, Novelli L, Bramanti P, et al. CYP4F2 genetic variant (rs2108622) significantly contributes to warfarin dosing variability in the Italian population. Pharmacogenomics. 2009;10(2):261–6. https://doi.org/10.2217/14622416.10.2.261.

109. McWilliam A, Lutter R, Nardinelli C. Healthcare impact of personalized medicine using genetic testing: an exploratory analysis for warfarin. Per Med. 2008;5(3):279–84. https://doi.org/10.2217/17410541.5.3.279.

110. Moyer TP, O'Kane DJ, Baudhuin LM, Wiley CL, Fortini A, Fisher PK, et al. Warfarin sensitivity genotyping: a review of the literature and summary of patient experience. Mayo Clin Proc. 2009;84(12):1079–94. https://doi.org/10.4065/mcp.2009.0278.

111. Landefeld CS, Beyth RJ. Anticoagulant-related bleeding: clinical epidemiology, prediction, and prevention. Am J Med. 1993;95(3):315–28. https://doi.org/10.1016/0002-9343(93)90285-w.

112. Leigh JP, White RH. An economic model of adverse events and costs for oral anticoagulants used for atrial fibrillation. Curr Med Res Opin. 2007;23(9):2071–81. https://doi.org/10.1185/030079907X210822.

113. Eckman MH, Rosand J, Greenberg SM, Gage BF. Cost-effectiveness of using pharmacogenetic information in warfarin dosing for patients with nonvalvular atrial fibrillation. Ann Intern Med. 2009;150(2):73–83. https://doi.org/10.7326/0003-4819-150-2-200901200-00005.

114. Stehle S, Kirchheiner J, Lazar A, Fuhr U. Pharmacogenetics of oral anticoagulants: a basis for dose individualization. Clin Pharmacokinet. 2008;47(9):565–94. https://doi.org/10.2165/00003088-200847090-00002.
115. Menichelli D, Poli D, Antonucci E, Cammisotto V, Testa S, Pignatelli P, et al. Comparison of anticoagulation quality between acenocoumarol and warfarin in patients with mechanical prosthetic heart valves: insights from the nationwide PLECTRUM study. Molecules. 2021;26(5). https://doi.org/10.3390/molecules26051425.
116. Bodin L, Verstuyft C, Tregouet DA, Robert A, Dubert L, Funck-Brentano C, et al. Cytochrome P450 2C9 (CYP2C9) and vitamin K epoxide reductase (VKORC1) genotypes as determinants of acenocoumarol sensitivity. Blood. 2005;106(1):135–40. https://doi.org/10.1182/blood-2005-01-0341.
117. Teichert M, van Schaik RH, Hofman A, Uitterlinden AG, de Smet PA, Stricker BH, et al. Genotypes associated with reduced activity of VKORC1 and CYP2C9 and their modification of acenocoumarol anticoagulation during the initial treatment period. Clin Pharmacol Ther. 2009;85(4):379–86. https://doi.org/10.1038/clpt.2008.294.
118. Roco A, Nieto E, Suárez M, Rojo M, Bertoglia MP, Verón G, et al. A Pharmacogenetically guided acenocoumarol dosing algorithm for chilean patients: a discovery cohort study. Front Pharmacol. 2020;11(325). https://doi.org/10.3389/fphar.2020.00325.
119. Carcas AJ, Borobia AM, Velasco M, Abad-Santos F, Díaz MQ, Fernández-Capitán C, et al. Efficiency and effectiveness of the use of an acenocoumarol pharmacogenetic dosing algorithm versus usual care in patients with venous thromboembolic disease initiating oral anticoagulation: study protocol for a randomized controlled trial. Trials. 2012;13:239. https://doi.org/10.1186/1745-6215-13-239.
120. Aronis KN, Hylek EM. Evidence gaps in the era of non–vitamin K oral anticoagulants. J Am Heart Assoc. 2018;7(3):e007338. https://doi.org/10.1161/JAHA.117.007338.
121. Ruff CT, Giugliano RP, Braunwald E, Hoffman EB, Deenadayalu N, Ezekowitz MD, et al. Comparison of the efficacy and safety of new oral anticoagulants with warfarin in patients with atrial fibrillation: a meta-analysis of randomised trials. Lancet. 2014;383(9921):955–62. https://doi.org/10.1016/S0140-6736(13)62343-0.
122. van der Hulle T, Kooiman J, den Exter PL, Dekkers OM, Klok FA, Huisman MV. Effectiveness and safety of novel oral anticoagulants as compared with vitamin K antagonists in the treatment of acute symptomatic venous thromboembolism: a systematic review and meta-analysis. J Thromb Haemost. 2014;12(3):320–8. https://doi.org/10.1111/jth.12485.
123. Kapoor A, Ellis A, Shaffer N, Gurwitz J, Chandramohan A, Saulino J, et al. Comparative effectiveness of venous thromboembolism prophylaxis options for the patient undergoing total hip and knee replacement: a network meta-analysis. J Thromb Haemost. 2017;15(2):284–94. https://doi.org/10.1111/jth.13566.
124. Wadelius M, Chen LY, Lindh JD, Eriksson N, Ghori MJR, Bumpstead S, et al. The largest prospective warfarin-treated cohort supports genetic forecasting. Blood. 2009;113(4):784–92. https://doi.org/10.1182/blood-2008-04-149070.
125. Rose DK, Bar B. Direct oral anticoagulant agents: pharmacologic profile, indications, coagulation monitoring, and reversal agents. J Stroke Cerebrovasc Dis. 2018;27(8):2049–58. https://doi.org/10.1016/j.jstrokecerebrovasdis.2018.04.004.
126. Zhu JY, Alexander GC, Nazarian S, Segal JB, Wu AW. Trends and variation in oral anticoagulant choice in patients with atrial fibrillation, 2010–2017. Pharmacotherapy. 2018;38(9):907–20. https://doi.org/10.1002/phar.2158.
127. Tseng AS, Patel RD, Quist HE, Kekic A, Maddux JT, Grilli CB, et al. Clinical review of the pharmacogenomics of direct oral anticoagulants. Cardiovasc Drugs Ther. 2018;32(1):121–6. https://doi.org/10.1007/s10557-018-6774-1.
128. Blech S, Ebner T, Ludwig-Schwellinger E, Stangier J, Roth W. The metabolism and disposition of the oral direct thrombin inhibitor, dabigatran, in humans. Drug Metab Dispos. 2008;36(2):386–99. https://doi.org/10.1124/dmd.107.019083.

129. Stangier J. Clinical pharmacokinetics and pharmacodynamics of the oral direct thrombin inhibitor dabigatran etexilate. Clin Pharmacokinet. 2008;47(5):285–95. https://doi.org/10.2165/00003088-200847050-00001.

130. Stangier J, Clemens A. Pharmacology, pharmacokinetics, and pharmacodynamics of dabigatran etexilate, an oral direct thrombin inhibitor. Clin Appl Thromb Hemost. 2009;15(Suppl 1):9s–16s. https://doi.org/10.1177/1076029609343004.

131. Chinn LW, Kroetz DL. ABCB1 pharmacogenetics: progress, pitfalls, and promise. Clin Pharmacol Ther. 2007;81(2):265–9. https://doi.org/10.1038/sj.clpt.6100052.

132. Gouin-Thibault I, Delavenne X, Blanchard A, Siguret V, Salem JE, Narjoz C, et al. Interindividual variability in dabigatran and rivaroxaban exposure: contribution of ABCB1 genetic polymorphisms and interaction with clarithromycin. J Thromb Haemost. 2017;15(2):273–83. https://doi.org/10.1111/jth.13577.

133. Zubiaur P, Saiz-Rodríguez M, Ochoa D, Navares-Gómez M, Mejía G, Román M, et al. Effect of sex, use of pantoprazole and polymorphisms in SLC22A1, ABCB1, CES1, CYP3A5 and CYP2D6 on the pharmacokinetics and safety of dabigatran. Adv Ther. 2020;37(8):3537–50. https://doi.org/10.1007/s12325-020-01414-x.

134. Sychev DA, Vardanyan A, Rozhkov A, Hachatryan E, Badanyan A, Smirnov V, et al. CYP3A activity and rivaroxaban serum concentrations in russian patients with deep vein thrombosis. Genet Test Mol Biomarkers. 2018;22(1):51–4. https://doi.org/10.1089/gtmb.2017.0152.

135. Ing Lorenzini K, Daali Y, Fontana P, Desmeules J, Samer C. Rivaroxaban-induced hemorrhage associated with ABCB1 genetic defect. Front Pharmacol. 2016;7:494. https://doi.org/10.3389/fphar.2016.00494.

136. O'Connor CT, Kiernan TJ, Yan BP. The genetic basis of antiplatelet and anticoagulant therapy: a pharmacogenetic review of newer antiplatelets (clopidogrel, prasugrel and ticagrelor) and anticoagulants (dabigatran, rivaroxaban, apixaban and edoxaban). Expert Opin Drug Metab Toxicol. 2017;13(7):725–39. https://doi.org/10.1080/17425255.2017.1338274.

137. Kanuri SH, Kreutz RP. Pharmacogenomics of novel direct oral anticoagulants: newly identified genes and genetic variants. J Personal Med. 2019;9(1):7. https://doi.org/10.3390/jpm9010007.

138. Raymond J, Imbert L, Cousin T, Duflot T, Varin R, Wils J, et al. Pharmacogenetics of direct oral anticoagulants: a systematic review. J Personal Med. 2021;11(1):37. https://doi.org/10.3390/jpm11010037.

139. Dimatteo C, D'Andrea G, Vecchione G, Paoletti O, Tiscia GL, Santacroce R, et al. ABCB1 SNP rs4148738 modulation of apixaban interindividual variability. Thromb Res. 2016;145:24–6. https://doi.org/10.1016/j.thromres.2016.07.005.

140. Ueshima S, Hira D, Fujii R, Kimura Y, Tomitsuka C, Yamane T, et al. Impact of ABCB1, ABCG2, and CYP3A5 polymorphisms on plasma trough concentrations of apixaban in Japanese patients with atrial fibrillation. Pharmacogenet Genom. 2017;27(9):329–36. https://doi.org/10.1097/FPC.0000000000000294.

141. Gulilat M, Keller D, Linton B, Pananos AD, Lizotte D, Dresser GK, et al. Drug interactions and pharmacogenetic factors contribute to variation in apixaban concentration in atrial fibrillation patients in routine care. J Thromb Thrombolysis. 2020;49(2):294–303. https://doi.org/10.1007/s11239-019-01962-2.

142. Ašić A, Marjanović D, Mirat J, Primorac D. Pharmacogenetics of novel oral anticoagulants: a review of identified gene variants & future perspectives. Pers Med. 2018;15(3):209–21. https://doi.org/10.2217/pme-2017-0092.

143. Palladino M, Merli G, Thomson L. Evaluation of the oral direct factor Xa inhibitor—betrixaban. Exp Opin Investig Drugs. 2013;22(11):1465–72. https://doi.org/10.1517/13543784.2013.825605.

144. Roth GA, Mensah GA, Johnson CO, Addolorato G, Ammirati E, Baddour LM, et al. Global Burden of cardiovascular diseases and risk factors, 1990–2019: update from the GBD 2019 study. J Am Coll Cardiol. 2020;76(25):2982–3021. https://doi.org/10.1016/j.jacc.2020.11.010.

145. Postmus I, Verschuren JJ, de Craen AJ, Slagboom PE, Westendorp RG, Jukema JW, et al. Pharmacogenetics of statins: achievements, whole-genome analyses and future perspectives. Pharmacogenomics. 2012;13(7):831–40. https://doi.org/10.2217/pgs.12.25.
146. Kapur NK, Musunuru K. Clinical efficacy and safety of statins in managing cardiovascular risk. Vasc Health Risk Manag. 2008;4(2):341–53. https://doi.org/10.2147/vhrm.s1653.
147. Egom EE, Hafeez H. Biochemistry of statins. Adv Clin Chem. 2016;73:127–68. https://doi.org/10.1016/bs.acc.2015.10.005.
148. Cholesterol Treatment Trialists C. Efficacy and safety of more intensive lowering of LDL cholesterol: a meta-analysis of data from 170 000 participants in 26 randomised trials. The Lancet. 2010;376(9753):1670–81. https://doi.org/10.1016/S0140-6736(10)61350-5.
149. Adhyaru BB, Jacobson TA. Safety and efficacy of statin therapy. Nat Rev Cardiol. 2018;15(12):757–69. https://doi.org/10.1038/s41569-018-0098-5.
150. Stroes ES, Thompson PD, Corsini A, Vladutiu GD, Raal FJ, Ray KK, et al. Statin-associated muscle symptoms: impact on statin therapy—European atherosclerosis society consensus panel statement on assessment, aetiology and management. Eur Heart J. 2015;36(17):1012–22. https://doi.org/10.1093/eurheartj/ehv043.
151. Hirota T, Fujita Y, Ieiri I. An updated review of pharmacokinetic drug interactions and pharmacogenetics of statins. Exp Opin Drug Metab Toxicol. 2020;16(9):809–22. https://doi.org/10.1080/17425255.2020.1801634.
152. Canestaro WJ, Austin MA, Thummel KE. Genetic factors affecting statin concentrations and subsequent myopathy: a HuGENet systematic review. Genet Med. 2014;16(11):810–9. https://doi.org/10.1038/gim.2014.41.
153. Climent E, Benaiges D, Pedro-Botet J. Hydrophilic or lipophilic statins? Front Cardiovasc Med. 2021;8:687585. https://doi.org/10.3389/fcvm.2021.687585.
154. Thompson PD, Panza G, Zaleski A, Taylor B. Statin-associated side effects. J Am Coll Cardiol. 2016;67(20):2395–410. https://doi.org/10.1016/j.jacc.2016.02.071.
155. Rosenson RS, Baker SK, Jacobson TA, Kopecky SL, Parker BA. An assessment by the statin muscle safety task force: 2014 update. J Clin Lipidol. 2014;8(3, Supplement):S58-S71. https://doi.org/10.1016/j.jacl.2014.03.004.
156. Wilke RA, Lin DW, Roden DM, Watkins PB, Flockhart D, Zineh I, et al. Identifying genetic risk factors for serious adverse drug reactions: current progress and challenges. Nature Rev Drug Discov. 2007;6(11):904–16. https://doi.org/10.1038/nrd2423.
157. Buettner C, Rippberger MJ, Smith JK, Leveille SG, Davis RB, Mittleman MA. Statin use and musculoskeletal pain among adults with and without arthritis. Am J Med. 2012;125(2):176–82. https://doi.org/10.1016/j.amjmed.2011.08.007.
158. de Lemos JA, Blazing MA, Wiviott SD, Lewis EF, Fox KAA, White HD, et al. Early intensive vs a delayed conservative simvastatin strategy in patients with acute coronary syndromes phase Z of the A to Z trial. JAMA. 2004;292(11):1307–16. https://doi.org/10.1001/jama.292.11.1307.
159. Study of the Effectiveness of Additional Reductions in C, Homocysteine Collaborative G. Intensive lowering of LDL cholesterol with 80 mg versus 20 mg simvastatin daily in 12,064 survivors of myocardial infarction: a double-blind randomised trial. Lancet. 2010;376(9753):1658–69. https://doi.org/10.1016/S0140-6736(10)60310-8.
160. Food and Drug Administration. Drug safety communication: new restrictions, contraindications, and dose limitations for Zocor (simvastatin) to reduce the risk of muscle injury. Available at: https://www.fda.gov/drugs/postmarket-drug-safety-information-patients-and-providers/fda-drug-safety-communication-ongoing-safety-review-high-dose-zocor-simvastatin-and-increased-risk. Accessed 13 Nov 2022.
161. Niemi M, Pasanen MK, Neuvonen PJ. Organic anion transporting polypeptide 1B1: a genetically polymorphic transporter of major importance for hepatic drug uptake. Pharmacol Rev. 2011;63(1):157–81. https://doi.org/10.1124/pr.110.002857.
162. Shitara Y. Clinical importance of OATP1B1 and OATP1B3 in drug-drug interactions. Drug Metab Pharmacokin. 2011;26(3):220–7. https://doi.org/10.2133/dmpk.DMPK-10-RV-094.

163. Ramsey LB, Johnson SG, Caudle KE, Haidar CE, Voora D, Wilke RA, et al. The clinical pharmacogenetics implementation consortium guideline for SLCO1B1 and simvastatin-induced myopathy: 2014 update. Clin Pharmacol Ther. 2014;96(4):423–8. https://doi.org/10.1038/clpt.2014.125.

164. Voora D, Shah SH, Reed CR, Zhai J, Crosslin DR, Messer C, et al. Pharmacogenetic predictors of statin-mediated low-density lipoprotein cholesterol reduction and dose response. Circ Cardiovasc Genet. 2008;1(2):100–6. https://doi.org/10.1161/CIRCGENETICS.108.795013.

165. Hou Q, Li S, Li L, Li Y, Sun X, Tian H. Association between SLCO1B1 gene T521C polymorphism and statin-related myopathy risk: a meta-analysis of case-control studies. Medicine. 2015;94(37):e1268. https://doi.org/10.1097/MD.0000000000001268.

166. Xiang Q, Chen SQ, Ma LY, Hu K, Zhang Z, Mu GY, et al. Association between SLCO1B1 T521C polymorphism and risk of statin-induced myopathy: a meta-analysis. Pharmacogenomics J. 2018;18(6):721–9. https://doi.org/10.1038/s41397-018-0054-0.

167. Turner RM, Fontana V, Zhang JE, Carr D, Yin P, FitzGerald R, et al. A genome-wide Association Study of Circulating Levels of Atorvastatin and Its Major Metabolites. Clin Pharmacol Ther. 2020;108(2):287–97. https://doi.org/10.1002/cpt.1820.

168. Vrkić Kirhmajer M, Macolić Šarinić V, Šimičević L, Ladić I, Putarek K, Banfić L, et al. Rosuvastatin-induced rhabdomyolysis—possible role of ticagrelor and patients' pharmacogenetic profile. Basic Clin Pharmacol Toxicol. 2018;123(4):509–18. https://doi.org/10.1111/bcpt.13035.

169. Calderon-Ospina CA, Hernández-Sómerson M, García AM, Mejia A, Tamayo-Agudelo C, Laissue P, et al. A pharmacogenomic dissection of a rosuvastatin-induced rhabdomyolysis case evokes the polygenic nature of adverse drug reactions. Pharmgenomics Pers Med. 2020;13:59–70. https://doi.org/10.2147/PGPM.S228709.

170. Dagli Hernandez C, Freitas R, Marçal E, Goncalves R, Faludi A, Bassani J, et al. Late response to rosuvastatin and statin-related myalgia due to SLCO1B1, SLCO1B3, ABCB11, and CYP3A5 variants in a patient with Familial Hypercholesterolemia: a case report. Ann Transl Med. 2021;9:76. https://doi.org/10.21037/atm-20-5540.

171. Ruiz-Iruela C, Padró-Miquel A, Pintó-Sala X, Baena-Díez N, Caixàs-Pedragós A, Güell-Miró R, et al. KIF6 gene as a pharmacogenetic marker for lipid-lowering effect in statin treatment. PloS One. 2018;13(10):e0205430-e. https://doi.org/10.1371/journal.pone.0205430.

172. Ho RH, Choi L, Lee W, Mayo G, Schwarz UI, Tirona RG, et al. Effect of drug transporter genotypes on pravastatin disposition in European- and African-American participants. Pharmacogenet Genom. 2007;17(8). https://doi.org/10.1097/FPC.0b013e3280ef698f.

173. Niemi M, Pasanen MK, Neuvonen PJ. SLCO1B1 polymorphism and sex affect the pharmacokinetics of pravastatin but not fluvastatin. Clin Pharmacol Ther. 2006;80(4):356–66. https://doi.org/10.1016/j.clpt.2006.06.010.

174. Cooper-DeHoff RM, Niemi M, Ramsey LB, Luzum JA, Tarkiainen EK, Straka RJ, et al. The clinical pharmacogenetics implementation consortium guideline for SLCO1B1, ABCG2, and CYP2C9 genotypes and statin-associated musculoskeletal symptoms. Clin Pharmacol Ther. 2022;111(5):1007–21. https://doi.org/10.1002/cpt.2557.

175. Lim KS, Jang IJ, Kim BH, Kim J, Jeon JY, Tae YM, et al. Changes in the QTc interval after administration of flecainide acetate, with and without coadministered paroxetine, in relation to cytochrome P450 2D6 genotype: data from an open-label, two-period, single-sequence crossover study in healthy korean male subjects. Clin Ther. 2010;32(4):659–66. https://doi.org/10.1016/j.clinthera.2010.04.002.

176. Doki K, Homma M, Kuga K, Kusano K, Watanabe S, Yamaguchi I, et al. Effect of CYP2D6 genotype on flecainide pharmacokinetics in Japanese patients with supraventricular tachyarrhythmia. Eur J Clin Pharmacol. 2006;62(11):919–26. https://doi.org/10.1007/s00228-006-0188-x.

177. Group TDPW. The Dutch Pharmacogenomic Working Group (2020). Phamacogenomic recommendations, farmacogenetica-update. Available at: www.knmp.nl/. Accessed 12 July 2020.

178. Meloche M, Khazaka M, Kassem I, Barhdadi A, Dubé MP, de Denus S. CYP2D6 polymorphism and its impact on the clinical response to metoprolol: a systematic review and meta-analysis. Br J Clin Pharmacol. 2020;86(6):1015–33. https://doi.org/10.1111/bcp.14247.

179. Yoon DY, Lee S, Ban MS, Jang IJ, Lee S. Pharmacogenomic information from CPIC and DPWG guidelines and its application on drug labels. Transl Clin Pharmacol. 2020;28(4):189–98. https://doi.org/10.12793/tcp.2020.28.e18.

180. Hjalmarson Å, Goldstein S, Fagerberg B, Wedel H, Waagstein F, Kjekshus J, et al. Effects of controlled-release metoprolol on total mortality, hospitalizations, and well-being in patients with heart failure the metoprolol CR/XL randomized intervention trial in congestive heart failure (MERIT-HF). JAMA. 2000;283(10):1295 302. https://doi.org/10.1001/jama.283.10.1295.

181. White HL, de Boer RA, Maqbool A, Greenwood D, van Veldhuisen DJ, Cuthbert R, et al. An evaluation of the beta-1 adrenergic receptor Arg389Gly polymorphism in individuals with heart failure: a MERIT-HF sub-study. Eur J Heart Fail. 2003;5(4):463–8. https://doi.org/10.1016/s1388-9842(03)00044-8.

182. Savva J, Maqbool A, White HL, Galloway SL, Yuldasheva NY, Ball SG, et al. Polymorphisms of adrenoceptors are not associated with an increased risk of adverse event in heart failure: a MERIT-HF substudy. J Card Fail. 2009;15(5):435–41. https://doi.org/10.1016/j.cardfail.2008.12.005.

183. Thomas CD, Johnson JA. Pharmacogenetic factors affecting beta-blocker metabolism and response. Exp Opin Drug Metab Toxicol. 2020;16(10):953–64. https://doi.org/10.1080/17425255.2020.1803279.

184. Liggett SB, Mialet-Perez J, Thaneemit-Chen S, Weber SA, Greene SM, Hodne D, et al. A polymorphism within a conserved beta(1)-adrenergic receptor motif alters cardiac function and beta-blocker response in human heart failure. Proc Natl Acad Sci USA. 2006;103(30):11288–93. https://doi.org/10.1073/pnas.0509937103.

185. Pacanowski MA, Gong Y, Cooper-DeHoff RM, Schork NJ, Shriver MD, Langaee TY, et al. Beta-adrenergic receptor gene polymorphisms and beta-blocker treatment outcomes in hypertension. Clin Pharmacol Ther. 2008;84(6):715–21. https://doi.org/10.1038/clpt.2008.139.

186. Kao DP, Davis G, Aleong R, O'Connor CM, Fiuzat M, Carson PE, et al. Effect of bucindolol on heart failure outcomes and heart rate response in patients with reduced ejection fraction heart failure and atrial fibrillation. Eur J Heart Fail. 2013;15(3):324–33. https://doi.org/10.1093/eurjhf/hfs181.

187. Liggett SB, Cresci S, Kelly RJ, Syed FM, Matkovich SJ, Hahn HS, et al. A GRK5 polymorphism that inhibits beta-adrenergic receptor signaling is protective in heart failure. Nat Med. 2008;14(5):510–7. https://doi.org/10.1038/nm1750.

188. Lobmeyer MT, Wang LW, Zineh I, Turner ST, Gums JG, Chapman AB, et al. Polymorphisms in genes coding for GRK2 and GRK5 and response differences in antihypertensive-treated patients. Pharmacogenet Genom. 2011;21(1):42–9. https://doi.org/10.1097/FPC.0b013e328341e911.

189. Bradford LD. CYP2D6 allele frequency in European Caucasians, Asians, Africans and their descendants. Pharmacogenomics. 2002;3(2):229–43. https://doi.org/10.1517/14622416.3.2.229.

190. Zanger UM, Raimundo S, Eichelbaum M. Cytochrome P450 2D6: overview and update on pharmacology, genetics, biochemistry. Naunyn-Schmiedeberg's Arch Pharmacol. 2004;369(1):23–37. https://doi.org/10.1007/s00210-003-0832-2.

191. Luzum JA, Sweet KM, Binkley PF, Schmidlen TJ, Jarvis JP, Christman MF, et al. CYP2D6 genetic variation and beta-blocker maintenance dose in patients with heart failure. Pharmaceut Res. 2017;34(8):1615–25. https://doi.org/10.1007/s11095-017-2104-8.

Pharmacogenomics in Gastroenterology

Dragan Primorac and Lidija Bach-Rojecky

Abstract

Several classes of drugs are used in the treatment of wide spectra of gastrointestinal tract disorders. Some, like proton pump inhibitors, are widely used for self-medication of mild stomach disorders and are available without a prescription, while the use of others, like immunomodulators, is guided by medical doctors and specialists. Drugs' efficacy and safety are under influence of various endogenous and exogenous factors, where variations in genes encoding drug's

D. Primorac (✉)
St. Catherine Specialty Hospital, 10000 Zagreb, Croatia
e-mail: dragan.primorac@svkatarina.hr; draganprimorac2@gmail.com

University of Split School of Medicine, 21000 Split, Croatia

Josip Juraj Strossmayer University of Osijek Faculty of Medicine, 31000 Osijek, Croatia

University of Rijeka School of Medicine, 51000 Rijeka, Croatia

Josip Juraj Strossmayer University of Osijek Faculty of Dental Medicine and Health,
31000 Osijek, Croatia

Eberly College of Science, Pennsylvania State University, 517 Thomas St, State College,
University Park, PA 16803, USA

The Henry C. Lee College of Criminal Justice and Forensic Sciences, University of New Haven,
West Haven, CT, USA

National Forensic Science University, Gandhinagar, Gujarat, India

College of Medicine and Forensics, Xi'an Jiaotong University, Xi'an, China

Medical School REGIOMED, 96450 Coburg, Germany

L. Bach-Rojecky
University of Zagreb Faculty of Pharmacy and Biochemistry, 10000 Zagreb, Croatia

D. Primorac
International Center For Applied Biological Sciences, 10000, Zagreb, Croatia

protein targets, metabolic enzymes, and other proteins connected to drugs safety play a significant role. In this chapter, we review the clinical pharmacogenomics (PGx) of drugs used in the treatment of non-malignant disorders of the gastrointestinal tract. PGx information reduces the likelihood of adverse drug reactions and optimizes therapeutic efficacy. While for some drugs evidence-based guidelines recommend dosage adjustment according to a patient genotype, for others the role of PGx is still a matter of investigation.

Keywords

Pharmacogenomics • Gastrointestinal disorders • Proton pump inhibitors • Antiemetics • Thiopurines

1   Introduction

Functional gastrointestinal disorders represent the most common diagnoses in gastroenterology and are characterized by motility disturbances and visceral hypersensitivity. Among those, functional dyspepsia and irritable bowel syndrome are the most widely present and affect up to 20% of the general population around the world [1]. The most difficult to treat because of the complex immunopathophysiology are inflammatory bowel diseases (IBD), like ulcerative colitis and Crohn's disease. Because of the immunological background, the current treatment strategies are mostly oriented to modulation of the excessive intestinal immune response and reduction of mucosal inflammation [2].

Some of the medicines for mild acute gastrointestinal problems with well-known efficacy and safety profile, like antacids, blockers of histamine H2 receptors, some proton pump inhibitors, and laxatives, are available without the prescription. Others, like immunomodulators and biologicals, carry significant risk in long-term use, and patients should be monitored to prevent or treat adverse effects and toxicities. Efficacy and tolerability/toxicity for some of the drugs could be predicted based on some of the patient- and/or drug-related risk factors [3]. The influence of genetic variations as inherent risk factors for drug efficacy and safety is a matter of intensive investigation. For some drugs used to treat certain non-malignant disorders of the gastrointestinal tract, like proton pump inhibitors (PPI), 5-HT3 antagonists, and thiopurines, international expert consortium (The Clinical Pharmacogenetics Implementation Consortium, CPIC) has already published evidenced-based guidelines and recommend dosage adjustment according to patient genotype to optimize pharmacotherapy (Table 1).

2   Proton Pump Inhibitors

Proton pump inhibitors (PPIs) are the most potent and effective class of gastric acid-suppressing drugs, diminishing the basal and stimulated production of acid by around 70%. Their effect results from an irreversible inhibition of H^+/K^+—ATPase activity, due to the covalent binding to the protein. Because of their wide

Table 1 Drugs with available clinical guidelines linking the results of pharmacogenetic tests to specific therapeutic recommendations [4]

Drug class/drugs of interest	Gene/polymorphism	Phenotype	Clinical significance/recommendation	Refs.
Proton pump inhibitorsomeprazole, lansoprazole, pantoprazole	CYP2C19*17/*17 CYP2C19*1/*17 CPYC2C19*1/*1 CPYC2C19*1/*2, *1/*3, *2/*17, *3/*17 CPYC2C19*2/*2, *3/*3, 2/3	Ultrarapid metabolizers Rapid metabolizers Normal metabolizers Intermediate metabolizers Poor metabolizers	Increased metabolism to inactive compounds; increased risk of therapeutic failure CPIC recommends: — Increase in starting daily dose by 100% for ultrarapid metabolizers — Increase in dose by 50–100% for the treatment of Helicobacter pylori infection and erosive esophagitis for rapid and normal metabolizers — Reduction in daily dose by 50% for chronic therapy (> 12 weeks) in intermediate and poor metabolizers	[6]
Antiemetics 5-HT3 antagonists: ondansetron, tropisetron	CYP2D6*1/*1xN, *1/*2xN, *2/*2xNc	Ultrarapid metabolizers	Increased metabolism to less active compounds when compared to normal metabolizers and is associated with decreased response to ondansetron and tropisetron. CPIC recommends an alternative drug (granisetron)	[10]

(continued)

Table 1 (continued)

Drug class/drugs of interest	Gene/polymorphism	Phenotype	Clinical significance/recommendation	Refs.
Thiopurines: azathioprine, mercaptopurine, thioguanine	*TPMT* *1/*2, *1/*3A, *1/*3B, *1/*3C, *1/*4, *2/*8, *3A/*7 *3A/*3A, *2/*3A, *3A/ *3C, *3C/*4, *2/*3C, *3A/*4	Intermediate metabolizers Poor metabolizers	Increased risk of thiopurine-induced hematotoxicity in intermediate metabolizers. CPIC recommends start with reduced starting doses (30–80% of normal dose) Greatly increased risk of thiopurine-related myelosuppression in poor metabolizers. CPIC recommends alternative nonthiopurine immunosuppressant therapy.	[23]
	NUDT15 *1/*2, *1/*3 *2/*5, *3/*6 *2/*2, *2/*3, *3/*3	Intermediate metabolizers Poor metabolizers	Increased risk of thiopurine-related myelosuppression in intermediate metabolizers. CPIC recommends start with reduced starting doses (30–80% of normal dose). Greatly increased risk of thiopurine-related myelosuppression in poor metabolizers. CPIC recommends alternative nonthiopurine immunosuppressant therapy.	[23]

Legend CPIC—Clinical Pharmacogenetics Implementation Consortium therapeutic indications in adults and children, they are among the highest-selling drugs in the world. They are used in the therapy of chronic gastritis, gastroesophageal reflux disease, gastric and peptic ulcers, Zollinger-Ellison syndrome, as well as for treatment and prevention of gastrotoxic effects associated with chronic use of non-steroidal anti-inflammatory drugs. Furthermore, PPI are used in eradication therapy regimes for Helicobacter pylori infection because they increase the pH, thus providing optimal conditions for the antibacterial drugs' actions. Despite high safety-to-risk profile, higher exposure to the PPI and prolonged use have been associated with numerous adverse events and potential risks, including Clostridium difficile-associated infections, hypomagnesemia, kidney disease, osteoporosis, bone fractures, and dementia [5].

Six PPIs are available in clinical practice: the first-generation inhibitors omeprazole, lansoprazole pantoprazole, and the second-generation inhibitors esomeprazole (S-omeprazole), dexlansoprazole (R-lansoprazole), and rabeprazole. They share a common mechanism of action on H^+/K^+—ATPase but differ in pharmacokinetic properties which finally can impact their efficacy and safety. PPIs are rapidly absorbed from the small intestine and have a short plasma half-life, although their acid-suppressing effect lasts for 24–48 h. The first-generation PPIs are largely metabolized by hepatic CYP2C19 and to a lesser extent by CYP3A4, while the second-generation drugs esomeprazole and rabeprazole are less dependent on CYP2C19. In fact, rabeprazole mostly undergoes a non-enzymatic reduction in the liver, with only 10% of the parent compound being metabolized by CYP enzymes. Different factors may affect response to PPIs, like patient's age, other medications, as well as variations in the CYP2C19 gene, which is highly polymorphic [6].

The most common polymorphism, with allele frequencies of ~15% in Caucasians and Africans, 25–30% in Asians, and ~60% in Oceanians, is CYP2C19*2 (c.681G>A, rs4244285), which generates a non-functional protein. Poor (PM) and intermediate metabolizers (IM), which carry two copies or one copy of non-functional allele, respectively, share an impaired possibility to metabolize PPIs and therefore have increased PPIs plasma concentrations compared to normal metabolizers, with a potential higher risk of adverse events [6].

On the other hand, the CYP2C19*17 allele (c.−806C>T; rs12248560) results in increased activity, with allele frequencies of ~3–21% in different ethnic groups. Individuals with one or two increased function alleles (*1/*17, *17/*17) are categorized as rapid (RM) and ultrarapid metabolizers (UM) and are at increased risk of therapy failure due to increased PPIs clearance [6]. This is especially important when the strongest PPI antisecretory activity is needed, like in erosive esophagitis and the eradication of Helicobacter pylori infection. Royal Dutch Pharmacogenetics Working Group provided dose recommendations for four PPIs: omeprazole, esomeprazole, pantoprazole, and lansoprazole. They recommend a dose increase of 400%, 200%, 100–200%, and 50–100% for pantoprazole, lansoprazole, omeprazole, and esomeprazole, respectively, in the case of UM/RM phenotypes in Helicobacter pylori eradication therapy [5]. In 2021, Clinical Pharmacogenetics Implementation Consortium (CPIC) summarized the evidence from the literature and provided therapeutic recommendations for omeprazole, pantoprazole, lansoprazole, and dexlansoprazole prescribing, based on CYP2C19 phenotype (Table 1). Also, there is emerging evidence that *CYP2C19* genetic variation in children older than one year of age influences PPI pharmacokinetics and response [6].

Although more evidence is needed, the genotype-based corrections in the starting or maintaining PPI doses could, with other important factors taking into consideration, help in providing effective and safe therapy for a wide range of gastrointestinal disorders, in adults, as well as in the pediatric population.

3   Antiemetic Drugs

Antagonists of serotonin 5-HT3 receptors are used in the prevention of chemotherapy-induced, radiation-induced, as well as postoperative nausea and vomiting. They suppress nausea and vomiting by selectively blocking 5-HT3 receptors centrally and peripherally, thereby preventing serotonin-mediated emetogenic signaling. Drugs can be divided into two generations—the first is represented by dolasetron, granisetron, ondansetron, tropisetron, azasetron, and ramosetron (the last two being licensed in Southeast Asia only), while palonosetron is representative of the second generation. In comparison with the first-generation 5-HT3 receptor antagonists, palonosetron has a higher potency, a significantly longer half-life, and a different molecular interaction with 5-HT3 receptor. All drugs are well tolerated, with a headache, occasional diarrhea, and constipation being the most reported [7]. Ondansetron has been associated with dose-dependent cardiac adverse events such as QT prolongation [8].

Despite their shared mechanism of action, 5-HT3 receptor antagonists have different pharmacological characteristics, including differences in receptor binding affinity, biotransformation pathways, plasma half-lives, and duration of the effect. 5-HT3 antagonists are metabolized via multiple cytochrome P450 enzymes (CYP3A4, CYP1A2, CYP2D6), followed by glucuronidation to inactive metabolites. For ondansetron, CYP2D6 mediates approximately 30% of total metabolism, while around 91% of tropisetron metabolism is carried out by CYP2D6. On the contrary, metabolism of granisetron is not dependent on CYP2D6 [7]. Variation in CYP2D6 activity can impact on the pharmacokinetics of ondansetron and tropisetron, ultimately affecting their efficacy, as well as safety.

Gene *CYP2D6* is highly polymorphic with over 100 known allelic variants and subvariants identified. *CYP2D6* allele frequencies have been shown to vary substantially among world populations, with some allelic variants been detected only in a certain ethnic group. The most reported *CYP2D6* alleles are categorized into several functional groups: from reduced or complete lack of function *(CYP2D6*3, *4, *5, *6),* to normal function (e.g., *CYP2D6*1* and **2)* and increase in function *(CYP2D6*1/*1xN, *1/*2xN, *2/*2xN,* where xN represents the copy number of the *CYP2D6* gene) [9].

Individuals carrying duplications of functional alleles (around 1–2% of the world population) have the phenotype of ultrarapid metabolizers. Those patients have decreased exposure and a reduced response to ondansetron and tropisetron, as measured by an increased number of vomiting episodes compared to CYP2D6 normal metabolizers. For those patients, granisetron is a drug of choice since it is metabolized via CYP3A4 and CYP1A2 [10].

For individuals with poor CYP2D6 phenotype (carrying only no functional allele, 5–10%), potentially elevated blood levels of ondansetron might suggest a greater risk for torsade's de pointes; however, there are no clinical data to support this. It was also suggested, but without clear clinical relevance, that the synonymous variant rs1045642 in the *ABCB1* gene (encoding ATP-dependent drug efflux pump for xenobiotics) may affect ondansetron efficacy, where the G allele is associated with a reduced response to ondansetron [11]. Other genetic polymorphisms with potential impact on 5-HT3 receptor antagonists are still a matter of investigation.

4   Drugs Used for Inflammatory Bowel Diseases

Ulcerative colitis and Crohn disease represent inflammatory bowel diseases (IBDs)— chronic inflammatory intestinal conditions with increasing incidence and prevalence around the world. It is estimated that over 1 million residents in the USA and 2.5 million in Europe suffer from IBDs [2]. The pathogenesis of both conditions is multifactorial, involving genetic predisposition, intestinal epithelial barrier defects, dysregulated immune responses, and environmental factors. Pharmacological therapy for IBD mainly focuses on the reduction of inflammation, with specific goals of controlling acute exacerbations, maintaining remission, treating specific complications, and reducing the risk of colorectal cancer. Treatments, depending on the disease type and severity and therapy goals, include 5-aminosalicylic acid and derivatives, corticosteroids, immunosuppressants (thiopurines and methotrexate), and biologicals [12, 13].

4.1   5-Aminosalicylic Acid and Derivatives

First-line therapy for mild-to-moderate ulcerative colitis generally involves sulfasalazine and mesalazine (5-aminosalicylic acid, 5-ASA). This class of drugs reduces inflammation of colonic mucosa through a variety of anti-inflammatory mechanisms, like the activation of peroxisome proliferator-activated receptors-γ, inhibition of eicosanoid synthesis, reduction of NF-κB activation, etc. [14].

Sulfasalazine is a combination of 5-ASA and sulfapyridine linked together by an azo bond which is reduced by gut bacteria in the colon, thus releasing active 5-ASA and sulfapyridine. 5-ASA is primarily responsible for the efficacy, while sulfapyridine is the main cause of adverse effects. Sulfapyridine undergoes fast absorption from colon and transformation to N-acetyl-sulfapyridine by N-acetyltransferase 2 (NAT2) [15]. The enzyme is encoded by the *NAT2* gene, which has a high frequency of functional variations and has high levels of haplotype diversity. *NAT2* genotypes can be grouped into three different phenotypes: "slow acetylator" (two slow alleles), "intermediate acetylator" (1 slow and 1 rapid allele), and "rapid" acetylator (2 rapid alleles) [16]. The sulfapyridine biotransformation is significantly reduced in slow acetylators (carriers of two variant alleles *NAT2*5B*, **6A*, **7B* or **5, *6,* and **7*) compared to both normal and rapid acetylators (*NAT2*4/*4*), thus possibly increasing the risk of dose-related sulfapyridine-induced side effects, like headache, nausea, fatigue, and allergic reactions [17]. However, the clinical significance of these findings for the safety of sulfasalazine is not confirmed, and therefore, there are no evidence-based recommendations about dosing adjustment in different phenotypes. One study suggested that in the Chinese Han population, *HLA-B*13:01* is associated with a sulfasalazine-induced rash with eosinophilia and systemic symptoms. *HLA-B*13:01* might serve as a potential genetic marker for predicting the risk of those serious adverse effects. More information is needed for other patient populations and related risks [18]. Additionally, patients with glucose-6-phosphate dehydrogenase (G6PD) deficiency should be observed closely for signs of hemolytic anemia. Although drug monographs include warnings regarding sulfasalazine use in G6PD-deficient patients, the evidence indicates that there is no hemolytic effect at therapeutic dosages [19].

4.2   Corticosteroids

Because of their pronounced anti-inflammatory and immunomodulatory effects, corticosteroids (CSs): budesonide, prednisone, methylprednisolone, hydrocortisone, and beclomethasone dipropionate are used for the induction of remission of ulcerative colitis if 5-ASA induction therapy fails, or is not tolerated. Systemic CSs are an effective initial therapy for moderate to severely active Crohn's disease, regardless of disease location. They can be administered by oral, intravenous, or rectal route. CSs should be avoided as maintenance therapy due to toxicity and inability to induce symptomatic remission (steroid-resistant disease). Prolonging treatment with high-dose oral corticosteroids has a diminishing chance of achieving remission, and between responders, many will become corticosteroid-dependent [20].

It was postulated that the mechanisms of CSs resistance in IBDs may be associated with SNPs in the *NR3C1* gene (rs6189, rs6190, rs6195, and rs41423247) resulting in changed receptor structure and signal transduction. Additionally, genes encoding for enzymes involved in the proteasomal degradation of the GCs receptor, like steroid sulfatase and *MDM2* oncogene E3 ubiquitin-protein ligase, can be also involved in CSs resistance, but more studies are needed to further investigate possible connections [21].

4.3   Thiopurines

Immunosuppressant drugs azathioprine (AZA) and its metabolite mercaptopurine (6-MP) are used in the maintenance of remission in severe forms of IBD. Azathioprine is converted to the purine anti-metabolite 6-mercaptopurine by glutathione S-transferase, which inhibits purine synthesis as well as DNA and RNA synthesis and thus blocks the propagation of immune cells. 20–30% of IBD patients stop thiopurine treatment because of various side effects, like nausea, vomiting, anorexia, weight loss, headache, fatigue, stomatitis, alopecia, arthralgia, muscular weakness, rash, or pancreatitis. Other more serious adverse effects are dose-dependent, like hepatotoxicity, myelosuppression, and the risk for opportunistic infections [22]. To predict the risk for toxicities, the concentration of 6-MP's active metabolites (6-thioguanine nucleotides, TGN) can be measured in the cells (erythrocytes) and dosage adjusted accordingly. Furthermore, by understanding the complex thiopurines biotransformation pathways, it became evident that change in the activity of thiopurine-s-methyltransferase (TPMT) contributes to the risks for myelotoxicity. TPMT catalyzes the conversion of 6-MP to an inactive methylmercaptopurine base, leaving less 6-MP available for eventual conversion to active thioguanine nucleotides. TPMT is also involved in the generation of immunosuppressive methylmercaptopurine nucleotides (contribute to hepatotoxicity) from the thioinosine monophosphate. Another important enzyme in thiopurine metabolism is a nucleoside diphosphatase, nudix hydrolase 15 (NUDT15) which catalyzes the conversion of cytotoxic metabolites thioguanine triphosphates (TGTP) to the less toxic thioguanine monophosphates. Activities of both enzymes seem to be an important factor in the prediction of the risk of thioguanine-induced myelosuppression (TIM). While TPMT deficiency due to genetic polymorphisms is the main cause for thiopurine intolerance in Europeans and Africans, *NUDT15 gene polymorphisms* can explain the risks for TIM in Asian and Hispanic populations that carry variants with high allele frequencies [23]. However, based on increasing functional rare variants that have been identified in the *NUDT15* gene in Caucasians, analyzing this gene in conjunction with *TPMT* not only for Asians and Hispanics seems logical.

Individuals who inherit two loss-of-function *TPMT* alleles (*3A/*3A, *2/*3A, *3A/*3C, *3C/*4, *2/*3C, *3A/*4 dyplotypes) have the phenotype of poor metabolizers and have very high concentrations of TGN metabolites. In those individuals, fatal toxicity because of myelosuppression is possible, and thiopurines should be avoided. Additionally, intermediate metabolizers, carriers of *TPMT*1/*2, *1/*3A, *1/*3B, *1/*3C, *1/*4 dyplotypes, have one normal function allele and one no function allele, are also at increased risk of TIM. The guidelines suggest reduced starting dose (30–80% of the normal dose) and regular hematological monitoring of patients [24]. However, *TPMT* variants are only found in 25% of patients of European ancestry affected by TIM, suggesting the contribution of other genetic and environmental factors.

Individuals carrying two loss-of-function *NUDT15* alleles (*2/*2, *2/*3, *3/*3 dyplotypes), characterized as poor metabolizers, are also at increased risk of thiopurine-related leukopenia, neutropenia, and myelosuppression and should avoid the use of thiopurines, while NUDT15 intermediate metabolizers (*1/*2, *1/*3) should start the therapy with 30–80% lower than normal dose [23, 24].

Thiopurine-induced pancreatitis (TIP) is a dose-independent idiosyncratic drug reaction with unknown pathophysiology which affects 2–7% of patients with IBD treated with AZA. A genome-wide association study identified a strong association between the Class II *HLA* gene region polymorphism (rs2647087) and TIP. Recent studies showed a higher prevalence of TIP in individuals with the *HLA-DQA1*02:01-HLA-DRB1*07:01* haplotypes. Patients heterozygous carriers of the C allele have a 4.25% risk, whereas patients homozygous CC for rs2647087 has the estimated risk of developing pancreatitis 14.6% [25]. While waiting for more clinical evidence from well-designed studies in larger cohorts, routine screening of the respective polymorphism is not considered cost-effective at present.

4.4 Methotrexate

Methotrexate (MTX) in a single weekly low dose (15–25 mg intramuscularly or subcutaneously) is an effective immunosuppressive treatment for the induction and maintenance of remission of Crohn's disease if thiopurines are not tolerated or are contraindicated [20]. Methotrexate is an analog of reduced folate that targets endogenous cellular folate metabolism. At the high doses given in the treatment of neoplasms, its primary mechanism of action is disruption of purine and pyrimidine synthesis. At doses used for inflammatory disease treatment, its action likely occurs via accumulation of adenosine and through effects on cellular proliferation and cytokine expression [20]. Methotrexate in higher doses can cause bone marrow suppression, pulmonary fibrosis, hepatotoxicity, nausea, and vomiting. Pharmacogenetic studies were mostly performed on high-dose MTX in oncological patients. The most promising results came for *SLCO1B1* polymorphisms, which play a role in the pharmacokinetics of MTX and the risk of toxicity. Although a specific pharmacogenetic marker in routine clinical practice is not available for MTX therapy, the French National Network of Pharmacogenetics states that MTX pharmacogenetic tests can be potentially useful in cancer patients, but further evidence is needed, especially for the lower doses applied in IBD [26].

4.5 Biologicals

Biological therapy targets specific inflammatory pathways after binding to specific receptors or soluble molecules that play a significant role in mediating immune response ad inflammation. Biologicals significantly improved the treatment outcomes of IBD, because of a better quality of patients' life, reduced number of hospitalizations, improved mucosal healing, and reduced risks of drugs' side effects. The first-line biological drugs are the anti-TNF agents (like infliximab and adalimumab), which inhibit the pro-inflammatory activity of the cytokine

TNFα. Vedolizumab, on the contrary, exerts gut-selective anti-inflammatory activity because it prevents the migration of T-cells to inflamed gastrointestinal tissue. Ustekinumab, a biological drug first approved for the treatment of psoriasis, targets cytokines IL-12 and IL-23 involved in inflammatory and immune response [27].

Anti-TNF- Monoclonal antibodies to TNF-α are used to treat moderate-to-severe IBDs, usually refractory to immunomodulatory therapy despite dose optimization. Around 30% of patients do not respond to the treatment, and the ability to predict anti-TNF non-responders, by evaluating potential genetic markers, could improve therapeutic outcomes. One of the mechanisms accounting for diminished or lack of response is the formation of anti-drug antibodies, with the rates of anti-antibody formation varying greatly between studies and between the biologicals.

Recent studies on patients with IBDs taking infliximab and adalimumab with the *HLA-DQA1*05* (rs2097432) variant showed an increased risk to lose response to the drug and a higher incidence of discontinuation of the treatment. If proven significant in larger patients cohorts, this gene–drug interaction could lead to personalized approach to therapy detecting patients prone to auto-antibody development [28].

The *TNF-α* gene contains several SNPs, which have been found relevant to the response of anti-TNF treatment. One meta-analysis showed that *TNF-α gene polymorphisms* in the promoter region at the −308 and −857 positions could predict therapeutic response because in individuals with the −308 G/G genotype and −857 C/C genotype better anti-TNF response was observed [29].

One study suggested that variants in toll-like receptor 4 (*TLR*, rs55030728), FC fragment of IgG receptor IIIa (*FCGR3A*, rs396991), TNF receptor superfamily 1A (*TNFRS1A*, rs4149570), interferon-gamma (*IFNγ*, rs2439561), interleukin-6 (*IL-6*, rs10499563), and interleukin-1B (*IL-1B*, rs4848306) could be related to improved treatment response to anti-TNF, whereas *TLR2* rs3804099 and *TLR9* rs352139 SNPs might be associated with a weaker response [30].

However, despite some promising results, the level of evidence is not high enough to apply specific genetic markers in clinical practice, at least not before testing in larger cohorts over longer time periods is performed [27].

Other drugs—Monoclonal antibodies vedolizumab (specifically binds to α4β7 integrin expressed by gut-homing lymphocytes), ustekinumab (blocks interleukin IL-12 and IL-23), and small molecule tofacetinib (Janus kinase inhibitor) are used for the treatment of moderate-to-severe ulcerative colitis as well as Crohn's disease in case of a failure of TNF-antagonists [27]. Ustekinumab and tofacetinib are also employed in the treatment of other autoimmune inflammatory diseases, like psoriasis and rheumatoid arthritis. For these drugs, there is no clear evidence that any specific gene polymorphism could interfere with their efficacy and safety. Nevertheless, potential role of pharmacogenetics in guiding their use is a matter of investigation.

5   Conclusion

While we are waiting for more evidence about the influence of respective *gene polymorphisms* on the efficacy and safety profile of a broader range of drugs used in the treatment of non-malignant gastrointestinal diseases, it is without a doubt that pharmacogenomics can improve the therapeutic outcomes and decrease costs, especially in the therapy of complex diseases, such as IBDs. Choosing the best treatment and drug dose can prevent new disease episodes and increase patient adherence to the therapy, because of the lower incidence of adverse drug reactions [31].

References

1. Oshima T, Miwa H. Epidemiology of functional gastrointestinal disorders in japan and in the world. J Neurogastroenterol Motil. 2015;21(3):320–9. https://doi.org/10.5056/jnm14165.
2. Kaplan GG. The global burden of IBD: from 2015 to 2025. Nat Rev Gastroenterol Hepatol. 2015;12(12):720–7. https://doi.org/10.1038/nrgastro.2015.150.
3. Primorac D, Bach-Rojecky L, Vađunec D, Juginović A, Žunić K, Matišić V, et al. Pharmacogenomics at the center of precision medicine: challenges and perspective in an era of big data. Pharmacogenomics. 2020;21(2):141–56. https://doi.org/10.2217/pgs-2019-0134.
4. CPIC Guidelines. Available at https://cpicpgx.org/guidelines/. Accessed August 4, 2021.
5. El Rouby N, Lima JJ, Johnson JA. Proton pump inhibitors: from CYP2C19 pharmacogenetics to precision medicine. Expert Opin Drug Metab Toxicol. 2018;14(4):447–60. https://doi.org/10.1080/17425255.2018.1461835.
6. Lima JJ, Thomas CD, Barbarino J, Desta Z, Van Driest SL, El Rouby N, et al. Clinical pharmacogenetics implementation consortium (CPIC) Guideline for CYP2C19 and proton pump inhibitor dosing. Clin Pharmacol Ther. 2021;109(6):1417–23. https://doi.org/10.1002/cpt.2015.
7. Huddart R, Altman RB, Klein TE. PharmGKB summary: ondansetron and tropisetron pathways, pharmacokinetics and pharmacodynamics. Pharmacogenet Genom. 2019;29(4):91–7. https://doi.org/10.1097/FPC.0000000000000369.
8. Navari RM. 5-HT3 receptors as important mediators of nausea and vomiting due to chemotherapy. Biochim Biophys Acta. 2015;1848:2738–46. https://doi.org/10.1016/j.bbamem.2015.03.020.
9. Gaedigk A, Sangkuhl K, Whirl-Carrillo M. Prediction of CYP2D6 phenotype from genotype across world populations. Genet Med. 2017;19(1):69–76. https://doi.org/10.1038/gim.2016.80.
10. Bell GC, Caudle KE, Whirl-Carrillo M, Gordon RJ, Hikino K, Prows CA, et al. Clinical pharmacogenetics implementation consortium (CPIC) guideline for CYP2D6 genotype and use of ondansetron and tropisetron. Clin Pharmacol Ther. 2017;102(2):213–8. https://doi.org/10.1002/cpt.598.
11. He H, Yin JY, Xu YJ, Li X, Zhang Y, Liu ZG, et al. Association of ABCB1 polymorphisms with the efficacy of ondansetron in chemotherapy-induced nausea and vomiting. Clin Ther. 2014;36(8):1242-52.e2. https://doi.org/10.1016/j.clinthera.2014.06.016.
12. Ungaro R, Mehandru S, Allen PB, Peyrin-Biroulet L, Colombel JF. Ulcerative colitis. Lancet. 2017;389(10080):1756–70. https://doi.org/10.1016/S0140-6736(16)32126-2.

13. Torres J, Mehandru S, Colombel JF, Peyrin-Biroulet L. Crohn's disease. Lancet. 2017;389(10080):1741–55. https://doi.org/10.1016/S0140-6736(16)31711-1.
14. Perrotta C, Pellegrino P, Moroni E, De Palma C, Cervia D, Danelli P, Clementi E. Five-aminosalicylic acid: an update for the reappraisal of an old drug. Gastroentl Res Practice. 2015;2015:456895. https://doi.org/10.1155/2015/456895.
15. Kuhn UD, Anschütz M, Schmücker K, et al. Phenotyping with sulfasalazine—time dependence and relation to NAT2 pharmacogenetics. Int J Clin Pharmacol Ther. 2010;48(1):1–10. https://doi.org/10.5414/cpp48001.
16. Stanley LA, Sim E. Update on the pharmacogenetics of NATs: structural considerations. Pharmacogenomics. 2008;9(11):1673–93. https://doi.org/10.2217/14622416.9.11.1673.
17. McDonagh EM, Boukouvala S, Aklillu E. PharmGKB summary: very important pharmacogene information for N-acetyltransferase 2. Pharmacogenet Genom. 2014;24(8):409–25. https://doi.org/10.1097/FPC.0000000000000062.
18. Yang F, Gu B, Zhang L, Xuan J, Luo H, Zhou P, et al. HLA-B*13:01 is associated with salazosulfapyridine-induced drug rash with eosinophilia and systemic symptoms in Chinese Han population. Pharmacogenomics. 2014;15(11):1461–9. https://doi.org/10.2217/pgs.14.69.
19. Youngster I, Arcavi L, Schechmaster R, Akayzen Y, Popliski H, Shimonov J, et al. Medications and glucose-6-phosphate dehydrogenase deficiency: an evidence-based review. Drug Saf. 2010;33(9):713–26. https://doi.org/10.2165/11536520-000000000-00000.
20. Lamb CA, Kennedy NA, Raine T, Hendy PA, Smith PJ, Limdi JK, et al. British Society of Gastroenterology consensus guidelines on the management of inflammatory bowel disease in adults. Gut. 2019;68(Suppl 3):s1–106. https://doi.org/10.1136/gutjnl-2019-318484.
21. Chen HL, Li LR. Glucocorticoid receptor gene polymorphisms and glucocorticoid resistance in inflammatory bowel disease: a meta-analysis. Dig Dis Sci. 2012;57(12):3065–75. https://doi.org/10.1007/s10620-012-2293-2.
22. Frei P, Biedermann L, Nielsen OH, Rogler G. Use of thiopurines in inflammatory bowel disease. World J Gastroenterol. 2013;19(7):1040–8. https://doi.org/10.3748/wjg.v19.i7.1040.
23. Relling MV, Schwab M, Whirl-Carrillo M, Suarez-Kurtz G, Pui CH, Stein CM, et al. Clinical pharmacogenetics implementation consortium guideline for thiopurine dosing based on TPMT and NUDT15 genotypes: 2018 update. Clin Pharmacol Ther. 2019;105(5):1095–105. https://doi.org/10.1002/cpt.1304.
24. Luber RP, Honap S, Cunningham G, Irving PM. Can we predict the toxicity and response to thiopurines in inflammatory bowel diseases? Front Med. 2019;6:279. https://doi.org/10.3389/fmed.2019.00279.eCollection2019.
25. Wilson A, Jansen LE, Rose RV, Gregor JC, Ponich T, Chande N, et al. HLA-DQA1-HLA-DRB1 polymorphism is a major predictor of azathioprine-induced pancreatitis in patients with inflammatory bowel disease. Aliment Pharmacol Ther. 2018;47(5):615–20.
26. Quaranta S, Thomas F. Pharmacogenetics of anti-cancer drugs: State of the art and implementation—recommendations of the French national network of pharmacogenetics. Therapie. 2017;72(2):205–15. https://doi.org/10.1016/j.therap.2017.01.005.
27. Wang C, Baer HM, Gaya DR, Nibbs RJB, Milling S. Can molecular stratification improve the treatment of inflammatory bowel disease? Pharmacol Res. 2019;148:104442. https://doi.org/10.1016/j.phrs.2019.104442.
28. Sazonovs A, Kennedy NA, Moutsianas L, Heap GA, Rice DL, Reppell M, et al. HLA-DQA1*05 carriage associated with development of anti-drug antibodies to infliximab and adalimumab in patients with Crohn's disease. Gastroenterology. 2020;158(1):189–99. doi: 10.1053/j.gastro.2019.09.041
29. Tong Q, Zhao L, Qian X-D. Association of TNF-α polymorphism with the prediction of response to TNF blockers in spondyloarthritis and inflammatory bowel disease: a meta-analysis. Pharmacogenomics. 2013;14(14):1691–700. https://doi.org/10.2217/pgs.13.146.

30. Bek S, Nielsen JV, Bojesen AB. Systematic review: genetic biomarkers associated with anti-TNF treatment response in inflammatory bowel diseases. Aliment Pharmacol Ther. 2016;44(6):554–67. https://doi.org/10.1111/apt.13736.
31. Primorac D, Höppner W, editors. Pharmacogenetics in clinical practice: experience with 55 commonly used drugs. Zagreb, Hamburg, Philadelphia: St. Catherine Specialty Hospital, Bioglobe GmbH, ISABS; 2022. Available from: https://www.stcatherine.com/centre-of-excell ence/10/individualized-and-preventive-medicine/pharmacogenomics/69.

Pharmacogenomics in Cancer Therapeutics

Ron H. N. van Schaik

Abstract

The clinical application of pharmacogenomics/pharmacogenetics in cancer therapy holds significant potential due to the severe consequences of both over- and underdosing. Presently, genotyping for *DPYD* related to capecitabine/5-FU is employed in clinical practice, accompanied by dosing recommendations based on a Clinical Pharmacogenetics Implementation Consortium (CPIC) guideline. Regarding irinotecan/*UGT1A1*, a growing acceptance of genotyping for clinical use is observed after the publication of a recent prospective study demonstrating the benefits of reduced dosing in *UGT1A1* PMs. Although a CPIC guideline is not currently available, the European Medicine Agency (EMA) recognizes the elevated risk of toxicity in *UGT1A1* poor metabolizers (PMs) treated with the full dose of irinotecan and suggests dose reduction. As for tamoxifen/*CYP2D6*, there exists a current controversy surrounding its clinical utility. While a CPIC guideline with dose recommendations has been published, the European Society of Medical Oncology (ESMO) still advises against the use of *CYP2D6* genotyping to guide tamoxifen therapy due to insufficient evidence.

Keywords

Cancer · Genetic polymorphisms · Pharmacogenomics · Pharmacogenetics · DPD · DPYD · Capecitabine · 5-FU · UGT1A1 · Irinotecan · SN-38 · Tamoxifen · CYP2D6 · CPIC

R. H. N. van Schaik (✉)
Erasmus MC University Medical Hospital, Dr. Molewaterplein 40, 3015 GD Rotterdam, The Netherlands
e-mail: r.vanschaik@erasmusmc.nl

1   Introduction

In the field of cancer treatment, drug therapy plays a crucial role in managing disease progression. However, the therapeutic range of most anticancer drugs, which differentiates between toxicity and suboptimal treatment, is typically narrow. Most treatment regimens involve drug dosing slightly below the toxicity threshold, leaving little room for individual variations in drug metabolism, which can have severe consequences. In cases where drugs require activation by liver enzymes, a decreased enzymatic activity may lead to suboptimal treatment, potentially resulting in therapy failure. In other cases, decreased enzymatic activity may result in elevated blood concentration of anticancer drugs, thus resulting in increased toxicities. Therefore, interindividual differences in drug-metabolizing capacity and drug response between patients pose challenges in providing uniform treatment, even among individuals diagnosed with the same disease. Consequently, factors that can predict drug-metabolizing capacity are of utmost importance in cancer treatment.

Several potential targets for cancer treatment have been proposed (as discussed in [1]), with current attention in terms of clinical implementation on the gene/drug pairs *DPYD*/5-Fluorouracil (5-FU)/capecitabine, *UGT1A1*/irinotecan and *CYP2D6*/tamoxifen.

2   Capecitabine/5-FU and *DPYD*

Fluoropyrimidines, such as 5-FU and its precursor capecitabine, are commonly used in the treatment of various cancers, including colon and breast cancer. However, the administration of fluoropyrimidines can lead to significant treatment-related toxicities in approximately 30% of patients. These toxicities encompass adverse effects such as diarrhea, mucositis, myelosuppression and hand-foot syndrome. In rare cases, they can even result in treatment-related fatalities, occurring in up to 1% of patients [2–6].

The underlying cause of such toxicities often lies in the reduced activity of the critical metabolic enzyme dihydropyrimidine dehydrogenase (DPD). This enzyme is responsible for inactivating 5-FU and capecitabine [7]. Approximately 3–5% of the North American and European populations exhibit partial DPD deficiency, characterized by around 50% reduction in DPD enzymatic activity compared to normal individuals. Complete DPD deficiency is less common, estimated to occur in 0.01–0.1% of individuals [8–10].

The decreased enzymatic activity is primarily attributed to genetic variants within the *DPYD* gene, which encodes the DPD enzyme. Among these genetic variants, *DPYD*2A (rs3918290, c.1905+1G>A, IVS14 +1G>A), c.*2846A>T* (rs67376798, D949V), *DPYD*13 (rs55886062, c.1679T>G, I560S) and c.*1236G>A* (rs56038477, E412E, in haplotype B3) are considered the most significant clinically [11]. The frequency of the heterozygous *DPYD*2A genotype in Caucasian patients is approximately 1%, while for the c.*2846A>T* SNP, it is

1.1%. The frequency for c.*1236G>A*/HapB3 is 6.3%, and for *DPYD*13* it ranges from 0.07 to 0.1% (Xeloda EPAR).

In a study conducted by van Deenen et al. [12], it was demonstrated that reducing the capecitabine dose to 50% of the standard amount significantly decreased toxicity levels in individuals carrying the *DPYD*2A* variant allele, bringing them to a similar level as patients without this variant. The prospective study by Henricks et al. [13] in 2008 took into account dose reductions for all four DNA variants mentioned earlier (*DPYD*2A*, *DPYD*13*, *2846A>T* and *1236G>A*): carriers of the *DPYD*2A* and *13* variant alleles received a 50% dose reduction, while for carriers of the *DPYD 2846A>T* and *1236G>A* SNPs, an initial dose reduction of 25% was prescribed. After this initial dose reduction, doses were allowed to be uptitrated, as much as toxicity allowed. This study showed a significant reduction in toxicity when following this dosing protocol for the *2A* and *2846A>T* variants. As for the *1679T>G* variant, only one patient was identified, leading to lack of a statistical analysis. In the case of the *1236G>A* variant, a reduction in toxicity was not observed, suggesting that a larger dose reduction might be necessary. Importantly, the reduced dosing did not result in decreased drug exposure in patients, indicating that no loss in effectiveness should be expected [13]. With respect to economics, genotyping for the four *DPYD* variants was found to be cost-saving [14], and it is in fact nowadays performed as a routine practice in the Netherlands before initiating capecitabine therapy.

The European Medicine Agency provides the following annotation in the drug label of Xeloda (capecitabine):

*Patients with low or absence of DPD activity, an enzyme involved in fluorouracil degradation, are at increased risk of severe, life-threatening, or fatal adverse reactions caused by fluorouracil. Although DPD deficiency cannot be precisely defined, it is known that patients with certain homozygous or certain compound heterozygous mutations in the DPYD gene locus (e.g. DPYD*2A, c.1679T>G, c.2846A>T and c.1236G >A/HapB3 variants), which can cause complete or near complete absence of DPD enzymatic activity (as determined from laboratory assays), have the highest risk of life-threatening or fatal toxicity and should not be treated with Xeloda. No dose has been proven safe for patients with complete absence of DPD activity.*

For patients with complete absence of DPD activity, capecitabine and 5-FU are contraindicated.

Clinical guidelines for *DPYD* genotyping for capecitabine/5-FU therapy have been published by the Clinical Pharmacogenetics Implementation Consortium (CPIC) in 2013 [15] with an update in 2017 [16], as well as by the Dutch Pharmacogenetics Working Group (DPWG) [17].

Since then, the distinction into "normal", "intermediate" and "poor metabolizers" has been abandoned for *DPYD*. Instead, activity scores (AS) are used, in which the *DPYD*2A* and *13* alleles have a score of 0, and the c.*2846G>A* and c.*1236G>A* alleles have a score of 0.5 [18]. When the combined activity score of both alleles is 1.0–1.5, a reduced dose of 25-50% is recommended by CPIC, as stated in their November 2018 update:

The current DPYD guideline recommends to reduce the dose of fluoropyrimidines by 25–50% (from the full standard dose) in DPYD Intermediate Metabolizers with an activity score of 1.5. At the time of the guideline publication, this dose range was recommended due to limited evidence for genotype-guided dosing of decreased function alleles/variants. However, a recent prospective study (PMID: 30348537) provides evidence to support a recommendation for a 50% dose reduction in heterozygous carriers of the decreased function variants c.2846A>T (rs67376798) or c.1129–5923C>G (rs75017182; HapB3 or its tagging SNP c.1236G>A; rs56038477). These data suggest that all Intermediate Metabolizers with an activity score of 1.5 should receive a 50% dose reduction. Therefore, CPIC revises its recommendation such that all DPYD Intermediate Metabolizers should receive a 50% dose reduction from the full standard starting dose, whether the activity score is 1 or 1.5 followed by dose titration, based on clinical judgement and ideally therapeutic drug monitoring.

In addition, recent case reports from patients who are homozygous for c.2846A>T (activity score of 1) indicate that a dose reduction of more than 50% may be required in some carriers of this genotype. Therefore, in patients with an activity score of 1 due to a homozygous c.[2846A>T];[2846A>T] genotype, clinicians should be aware that a > 50% reduction in starting dose might be warranted.

(https://cpicpgx.org/guidelines/guideline-for-fluoropyrimidines-and-dpyd/)

3   Irinotecan and UGT1A1

Irinotecan (CPT-11) is a derivative of camptothecin and has demonstrated effective anticancer activity against various solid tumors. It is commonly used in the treatment of colorectal, pancreatic and lung cancer. Irinotecan serves as a pro-drug that is converted into its active form, SN-38, which acts by inhibiting topoisomerase-I, an enzyme involved in DNA replication [19, 20]. The conversion of irinotecan to SN-38 is mediated by carboxylesterases (CES1 and CES2) and butyrylcholinesterase (BChE) [21, 22].

Once converted, SN-38 is actively transported into the liver by the organic anion transporter polypeptide (OATP) 1B1 [23]. SN-38 is significantly more cytotoxic, with 100- to 1000-fold greater potency as compared to irinotecan. SN-38 is subsequently inactivated through enzymatic conversion into SN-38 glucuronide (SN-38G) by the enzyme UGT1A1. However, the exposure to SN-38 exhibits considerable variability [24]. Multiple UGT subtypes participate in the hepatic (UGT1A1, UGT1A9) and extrahepatic (UGT1A1, UGT1A7, UGT1A10) conversion of SN-38, with UGT1A1 being the primary isoform involved, along with contributions from UGT1A7 and UGT1A9 [23]. UGT1A1 is also responsible for the conjugation of bilirubin, and a notable correlation between SN-38 levels and bilirubin glucuronidation has been observed [25].

UGT1A1 exhibits significant genetic variability with over 100 reported genetic variants [26]. Among these, *UGT1A1*6* and *UGT1A1*28* have been extensively studied in relation to irinotecan-induced toxicities, particularly neutropenia and diarrhea [27]. The wild-type *UGT1A1* allele is characterized by six thymine adenine (TA) repeats in the promoter region, whereas *UGT1A1*28* (rs8175347) involves an additional TA repeat that impairs *UGT1A1* transcription, resulting in approximately 70% reduced enzyme expression [28, 29]. *UGT1A1*28* is relatively common in Caucasians, with a minor allele frequency (MAF) of 26–39%; in Africans/African-Americans, it has a MAF of 30–56%. In Asian populations, the prevalence of *UGT1A1*28* is lower, with a MAF of 9–20% [30, 31]. Another variant, *UGT1A1*6* (rs4148323, 211G>A), is more prevalent in Asian populations, with a MAF of up to 47%, and may therefore be a better predictor for irinotecan-related toxicities for this population than *UGT1A1*28* [32]. *UGT1A1*6* leads to a 70% reduction in UGT1A1 enzymatic activity in individuals homozygous for the *UGT1A1*6/*6* genotype [33]. Both *UGT1A1*6* and *UGT1A1*28* variants result in homozygous carriers in increased systemic exposure to SN-38, the active metabolite of irinotecan, thereby increasing the risk of irinotecan-related adverse events [34, 35].

Adjusting the dosing of irinotecan, based on the *UGT1A1* genotype, has been demonstrated to be effective in a recent prospective multicenter randomized controlled trial. This study evaluated *UGT1A1*28* and *UGT1A1*93*. Patients with poor metabolizer status (homozygous for *UGT1A1*28* and/or *UGT1A1*93*) received an initial 30% dose reduction[36]. The incidence of febrile neutropenia in the poor metabolizer group treated with the adjusted dose was 6.5% compared to the historically higher rate of 24%. Moreover, the incidence was comparable to that of normal metabolizers treated with the full dose of irinotecan. Importantly, the systemic exposure to SN-38 was not reduced in patients receiving adjusted dosing, indicating no compromise in therapeutic efficacy [36]. Subsequent cost analysis demonstrated that the genotyping approach was not only safer for patients but also cost-saving, with a reduction of €183 per patient [36].

Both the FDA and EMA regard *UGT1A1* genotyping for irinotecan as "Actionable PGx" (www.pharmgkb.org, accessed 23-04-2022), based on the *UGT1A1*28* polymorphism:

Individuals who are 7/7 homozygous for the UGT1A1*28 allele are at increased risk for neutropenia from nonliposomal irinotecan. In the clinical study evaluating ONIVYDE + 5-FU/LV, the frequency of = Grade 3 neutropenia in these patients (2 of 7 (28.6%)) was similar to the frequency in patients not homozygous for the UGT1A1*28 allele who received a starting dose of ONIVYDE of 70 mg/m² (30 of 110 (27.3%)).

A reduced starting dose of ONIVYDE (liposomal irinotecan) of 50 mg/m² should be considered for patients known to be homozygous for the UGT1A1*28 allele. A dose increase of ONIVYDE to 70 mg/m² should be considered if tolerated in subsequent cycles.

At this moment, there is no CPIC guideline on irinotecan and *UGT1A1*.

4   Tamoxifen and CYP2D6

Tamoxifen is widely used for prevention and treatment of hormone receptor-positive breast cancer and is considered a crucial adjuvant endocrine therapy for Estrogen Receptor (ER)-positive breast cancer [37, 38]. As a Selective Estrogen Receptor Modulator (SERM), tamoxifen inhibits tumor growth, promotes apoptosis in ER-positive tumors [39] and reduces the risk of breast cancer recurrence and mortality [40]. However, its use in the preventive setting is approached cautiously due to reported side effects, such as an increased risk of deep vein thrombosis, pulmonary embolism and endometrial cancer [41].

Tamoxifen is a prodrug that undergoes conversion into multiple derivatives by phase-I enzymes. Among these, 4-hydroxytamoxifen (4OH-TAM) and endoxifen (4OH-N-desmethyl tamoxifen) exhibit the highest affinity for the ER [37, 42]. Endoxifen, with plasma concentrations 6–12 times higher than 4OH-TAM, is considered the major active metabolite of tamoxifen. The conversion of tamoxifen into inactive N-desmethyltamoxifen (NDM-TAM) is primarily mediated by CYP3A4 and CYP3A5 enzymes, accounting for 90% of tamoxifen metabolism, while only 10% is metabolized to 4OH-TAM. Subsequent hydroxylation of NDM-TAM, predominantly catalyzed by CYP2D6, leads to the formation of endoxifen [37, 42].

In a 2005 study, involving 200 breast cancer patients receiving tamoxifen as adjuvant therapy, it was observed that CYP2D6 poor metabolizers had worse relapse-free ($p = 0.023$) and disease-free ($p = 0.012$) survival compared to other patients. This finding suggested a lack of effectiveness of tamoxifen treatment due to reduced activation to endoxifen [43]. Since then, the clinical and predictive value of *CYP2D6* genotyping for tamoxifen therapy has been extensively discussed, with conflicting results reported in various studies (reviewed in [44]). Notably, conflicting studies by Schroth et al. in [45], showing worse disease-free survival for breast cancer patients on adjuvant tamoxifen, and studies by Rae et al. [46] and Regan et al. [47], failing to demonstrate such an effect, created controversy. The negative studies used DNA derived from tumor tissue and were not in Hardy–Weinberg equilibrium, thus deemed scientifically invalid by several researchers [48]. A meta-analysis conducted on all published studies, confirmed the correlation between CYP2D6 poor metabolizer status and worse outcomes on adjuvant tamoxifen treatment [49]. However, this conclusion has not been universally adopted, leading to ongoing controversy regarding the clinical value of *CYP2D6* genotyping in tamoxifen therapy.

In 2018, CPIC released a tamoxifen/*CYP2D6* guideline [50] recommending using an alternative drug (aromatase inhibitor) or considering a doubling of the dose to 40 mg/day for CYP2D6 poor metabolizers (but noting this would not fully compensate the CYP2D6PM status), as compared to the standard dose of 20 mg/day. Conversely, the European Society for Medical Oncology (ESMO) guideline, published in 2019, stated that routine *CYP2D6* genotyping should not be performed outside a clinical trial [51]. However, the same ESMO guideline cautioned against combining tamoxifen with strong CYP2D6 inhibitors, such as paroxetine, as it could affect therapy efficacy because of inhibiting the CYP2D6 enzyme, thereby in fact acknowledging the importance of CYP2D6 enzymatic activity in tamoxifen therapy [51].

5 CPIC Guidelines

For pharmacogenomics in cancer treatment, two CPIC guidelines have been published. A. For capecitabine/5-FU and *DPYD* originally in 2013 [15] and updated in 2017 [16], with an online update in November 2018 (www.pharmgkb.org), based on *DPYD* genotyping for (*2A*, *13*, 2846A>T and 1236G>A):

DPYD IM (as 1.0–1.5)

All DPYD Intermediate Metabolizers should receive a 50% dose reduction from the full standard starting dose, whether the activity score is 1 or 1.5 followed by dose titration, based on clinical judgement and ideally therapeutic drug monitoring.
In patients with an activity score of 1 due to a homozygous c.[2846A>T];[2846A>T] genotype, clinicians should be aware that a > 50% reduction in starting dose might be warranted.

*DPYD*2A/*2A*
For patients with complete absence of DPD activity, capecitabine and 5-FU are contraindicated.

B. For tamoxifen/*CYP2D6*, the 2018 CPIC guideline [50] states:

CYP2D6 IM (AS 0.25–1.0)

This patient is predicted to be a CYP2D6 poor metabolizer and may be at an increased risk of a poor tamoxifen response due to low endoxifen (active component of tamoxifen) concentrations. Recommend alternative hormonal therapy such as an aromatase inhibitor for postmenopausal women or aromatase inhibitor along with ovarian function suppression in premenopausal women. If aromatase inhibitor use is contraindicated, consideration should be given to use a higher but FDA approved tamoxifen dose (40 mg/day). Avoid CYP2D6 inhibitors. Please consult a clinical pharmacist for more information.

(http://cpicpgx.org/guidelines/)

CYP2D6 PM (AS 0)

This patient is predicted to be a CYP2D6 poor metabolizer and may be at an increased risk of a poor tamoxifen response due to low endoxifen (active component of tamoxifen) concentrations. Recommend alternative hormonal therapy such as an aromatase inhibitor for postmenopausal women or aromatase inhibitor along with ovarian function suppression in premenopausal women. Note, higher dose tamoxifen (40 mg/day) increases, but does not normalize endoxifen concentrations in CYP2D6 poor metabolizers.

(http://cpicpgx.org/guidelines/)

6   Conclusion

For the clinical use of pharmacogenomics/pharmacogenetics in cancer therapy, genotyping for *DPYD* for capecitabine/5-FU apparently has sufficient support and is used in clinical practice. CPIC guideline with dose recommendations are available. For irinotecan and *UGT1A1*, there is a recent uptake due to the publication of a prospective study, showing the benefits of reduced dosing in *UGT1A1* PMs. A CPIC guideline is not (yet) available. For tamoxifen/*CYP2D6*, there is a current controversy about the clinical value. A CPIC guideline has been published with dose recommendations, the ESMO discourages the use of *CYP2D6* genotyping to guide tamoxifen therapy.

References

1. van Schaik RH. CYP450 pharmacogenetics for personalizing cancer therapy. Drug Resist Updat. 2008;11(3):77–98.
2. Froehlich TK, et al. Clinical importance of risk variants in the dihydropyrimidine dehydrogenase gene for the prediction of early-onset fluoropyrimidine toxicity. Int J Cancer. 2015;136(3):730–9.
3. Hoff PM, et al. Comparison of oral capecitabine versus intravenous fluorouracil plus leucovorin as first-line treatment in 605 patients with metastatic colorectal cancer: results of a randomized phase III study. J Clin Oncol. 2001;19(8):2282–92.
4. Meta-Analysis Group In, C, et al. Toxicity of fluorouracil in patients with advanced colorectal cancer: effect of administration schedule and prognostic factors. J Clin Oncol. 1998;16(11):3537–41.
5. Mikhail SE, Sun JF, Marshall JL. Safety of capecitabine: a review. Expert Opin Drug Saf. 2010;9(5):831–41.
6. Van Cutsem E, et al. Oral capecitabine compared with intravenous fluorouracil plus leucovorin in patients with metastatic colorectal cancer: results of a large phase III study. J Clin Oncol. 2001;19(21):4097–106.

7. Longley DB, Harkin DP, Johnston PG. 5-fluorouracil: mechanisms of action and clinical strategies. Nat Rev Cancer. 2003;3(5):330–8.
8. Etienne MC, et al. Population study of dihydropyrimidine dehydrogenase in cancer patients. J Clin Oncol. 1994;12(11):2248–53.
9. Mattison LK, et al. Increased prevalence of dihydropyrimidine dehydrogenase deficiency in African-Americans compared with Caucasians. Clin Cancer Res. 2006;12(18):5491–5.
10. Ogura K, et al. Dihydropyrimidine dehydrogenase activity in 150 healthy Japanese volunteers and identification of novel mutations. Clin Cancer Res. 2005;11(14):5104–11.
11. Meulendijks D, et al. Clinical relevance of DPYD variants c.1679T>G, c.1236G>A/HapB3, and c.1601G>A as predictors of severe fluoropyrimidine-associated toxicity: a systematic review and meta-analysis of individual patient data. Lancet Oncol. 2015;16(16):1639–50.
12. Deenen MJ, et al. Upfront genotyping of DPYD*2A to individualize fluoropyrimidine therapy: a safety and cost analysis. J Clin Oncol. 2016;34(3):227–34.
13. Henricks LM, et al. DPYD genotype-guided dose individualisation of fluoropyrimidine therapy in patients with cancer: a prospective safety analysis. Lancet Oncol. 2018;19(11):1459–67.
14. Henricks LM, et al. A cost analysis of upfront DPYD genotype-guided dose individualisation in fluoropyrimidine-based anticancer therapy. Eur J Cancer. 2019;107:60–7.
15. Caudle KE, et al. Clinical pharmacogenetics implementation consortium guidelines for dihydropyrimidine dehydrogenase genotype and fluoropyrimidine dosing. Clin Pharmacol Ther. 2013;94(6):640–5.
16. Amstutz U, et al. Clinical pharmacogenetics implementation consortium (CPIC) guideline for dihydropyrimidine dehydrogenase genotype and fluoropyrimidine dosing: 2017 update. Clin Pharmacol Ther. 2018;103(2):210–6.
17. Lunenburg C, et al. Dutch pharmacogenetics working group (DPWG) guideline for the gene-drug interaction of DPYD and fluoropyrimidines. Eur J Hum Genet. 2020;28(4):508–17.
18. Henricks LM, et al. Translating DPYD genotype into DPD phenotype: using the DPYD gene activity score. Pharmacogenomics. 2015;16(11):1277–86.
19. Hsiang YH, Liu LF. Identification of mammalian DNA topoisomerase I as an intracellular target of the anticancer drug camptothecin. Cancer Res. 1988;48(7):1722–6.
20. Shao RG, et al. Replication-mediated DNA damage by camptothecin induces phosphorylation of RPA by DNA-dependent protein kinase and dissociates RPA:DNA-PK complexes. EMBO J. 1999;18(5):1397–406.
21. Morton CL, et al. The anticancer prodrug CPT-11 is a potent inhibitor of acetylcholinesterase but is rapidly catalyzed to SN-38 by butyrylcholinesterase. Cancer Res. 1999;59(7):1458–63.
22. Slatter JG, et al. Bioactivation of the anticancer agent CPT-11 to SN-38 by human hepatic microsomal carboxylesterases and the in vitro assessment of potential drug interactions. Drug Metab Dispos. 1997;25(10):1157–64.
23. de Man FM, et al. Individualization of irinotecan treatment: a review of pharmacokinetics, pharmacodynamics, and pharmacogenetics. Clin Pharmacokinet. 2018;57(10):1229–54.
24. Rivory LP, Robert J. Identification and kinetics of a beta-glucuronide metabolite of SN-38 in human plasma after administration of the camptothecin derivative irinotecan. Cancer Chemother Pharmacol. 1995;36(2):176–9.
25. Iyer L, et al. Genetic predisposition to the metabolism of irinotecan (CPT-11). Role of uridine diphosphate glucuronosyltransferase isoform 1A1 in the glucuronidation of its active metabolite (SN-38) in human liver microsomes. J Clin Invest. 1998;101(4):847–54.
26. Barbarino JM, et al. PharmGKB summary: very important pharmacogene information for UGT1A1. Pharmacogenet Genom. 2014;24(3):177–83.
27. Douillard JY, et al. Irinotecan combined with fluorouracil compared with fluorouracil alone as first-line treatment for metastatic colorectal cancer: a multicentre randomised trial. Lancet. 2000;355(9209):1041–7.
28. Bosma P, Chowdhury JR, Jansen PH. Genetic inheritance of Gilbert's syndrome. Lancet. 1995;346(8970):314–5.
29. Bosma PJ, et al. The genetic basis of the reduced expression of bilirubin UDP-glucuronosyltransferase 1 in Gilbert's syndrome. N Engl J Med. 1995;333(18):1171–5.

30. Beutler E, Gelbart T, Demina A. Racial variability in the UDP-glucuronosyltransferase 1 (UGT1A1) promoter: a balanced polymorphism for regulation of bilirubin metabolism? Proc Natl Acad Sci USA. 1998;95(14):8170–4.
31. Hall D, et al. Variability at the uridine diphosphate glucuronosyltransferase 1A1 promoter in human populations and primates. Pharmacogenetics. 1999;9(5):591–9.
32. Akaba K, et al. Neonatal hyperbilirubinemia and mutation of the bilirubin uridine diphosphate-glucuronosyltransferase gene: a common missense mutation among Japanese, Koreans and Chinese. Biochem Mol Biol Int. 1998;46(1):21–6.
33. Sugatani J, et al. Identification of a defect in the UGT1A1 gene promoter and its association with hyperbilirubinemia. Biochem Biophys Res Commun. 2002;292(2):492–7.
34. Iyer L, et al. Phenotype-genotype correlation of in vitro SN-38 (active metabolite of irinotecan) and bilirubin glucuronidation in human liver tissue with UGT1A1 promoter polymorphism. Clin Pharmacol Ther. 1999;65(5):576–82.
35. Wang Y, et al. UGT1A1 predicts outcome in colorectal cancer treated with irinotecan and fluorouracil. World J Gastroenterol. 2012;18(45):6635–44.
36. Hulshof EC, et al. UGT1A1 genotype-guided dosing of irinotecan: a prospective safety and cost analysis in poor metaboliser patients. Eur J Cancer. 2022;162:148–57.
37. Briest S, Stearns V. Tamoxifen metabolism and its effect on endocrine treatment of breast cancer. Clin Adv Hematol Oncol. 2009;7(3):185–92.
38. Jordan VC. Tamoxifen as the first targeted long-term adjuvant therapy for breast cancer. Endocr Relat Cancer. 2014;21(3):R235–46.
39. Jordan VC. Fourteenth Gaddum memorial lecture. A current view of tamoxifen for the treatment and prevention of breast cancer. Br J Pharmacol 1993;110(2):507–17.
40. Osborne CK. Tamoxifen in the treatment of breast cancer. N Engl J Med. 1998;339(22):1609–18.
41. White IN. Tamoxifen: is it safe? Comparison of activation and detoxication mechanisms in rodents and in humans. Curr Drug Metab. 2003;4(3):223–39.
42. Saladores PH, et al. Impact of metabolizing enzymes on drug response of endocrine therapy in breast cancer. Expert Rev Mol Diagn. 2013;13(4):349–65.
43. Goetz MP, et al. Pharmacogenetics of tamoxifen biotransformation is associated with clinical outcomes of efficacy and hot flashes. J Clin Oncol. 2005;23(36):9312–8.
44. Mulder TAM, et al. Clinical CYP2D6 genotyping to personalize adjuvant tamoxifen treatment in ER-positive breast cancer patients: current status of a controversy. Cancers. 2021;13(4).
45. Schroth W, et al. Association between CYP2D6 polymorphisms and outcomes among women with early stage breast cancer treated with tamoxifen. JAMA. 2009;302(13):1429–36.
46. Rae JM, et al. CYP2D6 and UGT2B7 genotype and risk of recurrence in tamoxifen-treated breast cancer patients. J Natl Cancer Inst. 2012;104(6):452–60.
47. Regan MM, et al. CYP2D6 genotype and tamoxifen response in postmenopausal women with endocrine-responsive breast cancer: the breast international group 1–98 trial. J Natl Cancer Inst. 2012;104(6):441–51.
48. Ratain MJ, Nakamura Y, Cox NJ. CYP2D6 genotype and tamoxifen activity: understanding interstudy variability in methodological quality. Clin Pharmacol Ther. 2013;94(2):185–7.
49. Province MA, et al. CYP2D6 genotype and adjuvant tamoxifen: meta-analysis of heterogeneous study populations. Clin Pharmacol Ther. 2014;95(2):216–27.
50. Goetz MP, et al. Clinical pharmacogenetics implementation consortium (CPIC) guideline for CYP2D6 and tamoxifen therapy. Clin Pharmacol Ther. 2018;103(5):770–7.
51. Cardoso F, et al. Early breast cancer: ESMO clinical practice guidelines for diagnosis, treatment and follow-up. Ann Oncol. 2019;30(10):1674.

Pharmacogenomics on Immunosuppressive Drugs in Solid Organ Transplantation

Ron H. N. van Schaik

Abstract

Tacrolimus, a calcineurin inhibitor, plays a significant role in immunosuppressive drug therapy following solid organ transplantation. It is commonly prescribed alongside mycophenol mofetil (MMF) and a glucocorticosteroid. While tacrolimus effectively prevents acute rejection, it carries notable toxicity and exhibits considerable variability in its pharmacokinetics and pharmacodynamics among individuals. One particular genetic variation, a single nucleotide polymorphism (SNP) known as 6986A>G in *cytochrome P450 (CYP) 3A5*, has consistently shown an association with the required dose of tacrolimus. Patients expressing CYP3A5 (*CYP3A5*1* carriers, referred to as CYP3A5 expressers) typically require 50% higher doses compared to non-expressers (such as *CYP3A5*3/*3* individuals). Non-expressers of CYP3A5 constitute a significant proportion of different populations, including 80–90% of Caucasians, 70% of Asians and 30% of Africans. While there have been effects reported of *CYP3A4*22* and *POR*28* on tacrolimus metabolism, the Clinical Pharmacogenetic Implementation Consortium (CPIC) has currently only published guidelines for *CYP3A5* and tacrolimus, and not for other genes. As for MMF, a combined promotor polymorphism in *UGT1A9* has been associated with an increased risk on biopsy-proven acute rejection (BPAR) due to a higher UGT1A9 enzymatic activity.

Keywords

Solid organ transplantation · Genetic polymorphisms · CYP3A4 · CYP3A5 · POR*28 · UGT1A9 · MMF · Pharmacogenetics · Pharmacogenomics · Drug-gene interactions · Tacrolimus · CPIC · Drug-metabolizing enzymes

R. H. N. van Schaik (✉)
Erasmus MC University Medical Hospital, Dr. Molewaterplein 40, 3015 GD Rotterdam, The Netherlands
e-mail: r.vanschaik@erasmusmc.nl

1   Introduction

The mid-1950s marked a significant milestone in the history of kidney transplantation with the first successful procedure, introducing a highly effective therapy for end-stage renal disease. Since then, kidney transplantations have been showing improved outcomes, such as a reduction in early acute rejection (AR) and enhanced patient survival. This can be primarily attributed to improvements in immunosuppressive therapy [1]. Immunosuppressive drugs play a crucial role in solid organ transplantation, with transplant physicians usually prescribing a combination of mycophenol mofetyl (MMF), a calcineurin inhibitor (CNI) such as tacrolimus or cyclosporin, and a glucocorticoid, to prevent graft rejection. Among CNIs, tacrolimus has emerged as the preferred choice, serving as the cornerstone of current immunosuppressive therapy after solid organ transplantation [2]. Despite its effectiveness in preventing acute rejection, tacrolimus therapy is hindered by significant toxicity that may lead to loss of kidney function. Due to substantial inter-individual variability in its pharmacokinetics [3], therapeutic drug monitoring (TDM) is essential for tacrolimus. Striking a delicate balance between therapeutic efficacy and adverse events becomes crucial as the margin between beneficial and harmful concentration levels is narrow [4]. The individualization of drug therapy to optimize the trade-off between effectiveness and side effects has become a paramount objective for transplant physicians. Consequently, there is a growing need to explore additional factors beyond TDM that can contribute to this goal.

2   Pharmacokinetics of Tacrolimus

Tacrolimus, originally known as FK506 during its research phase, undergoes biotransformation through the polymorphic cytochrome P450 (CYP) 3A4 and 3A5 enzymes, resulting in the formation of at least 15 different metabolites. Tacrolimus is mainly excreted through the bile (> 90%); approximately, 5% is directly eliminated by the kidneys, whereas < 1% is excreted renally without alteration [7]. Among the cytochromes involved, CYP3A5 plays the most prominent role, showing a 1.6-fold higher catalytic activity in vitro as compared to CYP3A4 [8]. Tacrolimus demonstrates a clearance rate of approximately 0.06 L/h/kg, with a corresponding terminal elimination half-life of around 12 h, ranging from 4 to 41 h [4, 6, 7]. Additionally, tacrolimus acts as a substrate for the drug-efflux pump P-glycoprotein, which is encoded by the *ABCB1* gene. *ABCB1* expression in the brush border of proximal tubular epithelial cells and in the renal tubules may contribute to renal elimination, while *ABCB1* expression at the canalicular surface of hepatocytes ensures excretion into the bile [9].

3   Pharmacogenetics of CYP3A5

In 2011, Kuehl et al. [10] and Hustert et al. [11] made a significant discovery regarding the expression of CYP3A5 protein in the liver. They identified two groups of individuals: CYP3A5 expressers, who showed the presence of CYP3A5 protein, and CYP3A5 non-expressers, who lacked its expression. The underlying genetic cause for this polymorphic expression was identified as a single nucleotide polymorphism (SNP) within the CYP3A5 gene at position 6986 in intron 3 (rs776746). The A nucleotide at position 6986 was associated with expression of CYP3A5 protein, and thus referred to as the CYP3A5*1 allele, despite not being the most prevalent allele in the (Caucasian) population. The inactive 6986G allele (CYP3A5*3) had a minor allele frequency (MAF) as high as 90% in the Caucasian population, resulting in approximately 80% of Caucasians being classified as CYP3A5 non-expressers [12] since the CYP3A5*3 allele leads to alternative splicing, causing protein truncation [10]. Individuals carrying at least one CYP3A5*1 allele (CYP3A5*1/*1 and CYP3A5*1/*3 individuals) were found to express substantial levels of CYP3A5 protein [10]. Therefore, both intermediate and normal metabolizers are usually grouped together in the CYP3A5 expresser category [13]. Notably, the prevalence of CYP3A5 expresser status varies considerably among different ethnicities, reflecting the differences in MAFs, with 5–15% of Caucasians, 30% of Asians, and 70% of Africans being CYP3A5 expressers [10–13]. While several other variants of CYP3A5 exist, they have limited clinical relevance due to their low frequency compared to the CYP3A5*3 allele [13].

The significance of CYP3A5 in tacrolimus metabolism became evident when it was established that kidney transplant recipients carrying at least one CYP3A5*1 allele (CYP3A5 expressers) required a substantially higher tacrolimus dose to achieve the desired therapeutic blood concentration as compared to CYP3A5 non-expressers [14–18]. This observation has been consistently replicated in various studies involving patients of different ethnic backgrounds, both in adult and pediatric kidney transplant recipients, as well as in recipients of other organs like heart, liver or lung [19]. Two meta-analyses, involving 1443 and 2028 renal transplant recipients, respectively, confirmed that CYP3A5 expressers need a higher tacrolimus dosage in comparison to CYP3A5 non-expressers [20, 21]. However, no consistent evidence demonstrating a direct association between CYP3A5 variant alleles and an individual's risk of acute rejection has been demonstrated [19].

4   CYP3A4*22, ABCB1 3435C >T and POR*28

While the CYP3A5 genotype is the most influential genetic predictor of tacrolimus dose requirements today, it does not account for all of observed variability. The TacTic study demonstrated that only 43.2% (95% CI 36.0–51.2) of patients in the CYP3A5 genotype-based dosing group achieved the target blood concentration at the first steady state time point [22], leaving the possibility that other genetic variants may contribute to the additional variation in tacrolimus dose requirements.

Because CYP3A4 also plays a role in tacrolimus metabolism, the identification of the clinically relevant *CYP3A4*22* allele (rs35599367; C>T SNP in intron 6) in 2011 by Wang et al. [23] enabled the investigation of the pharmacogenetic effect of CYP3A4 on tacrolimus metabolism. Indeed, the T-variant (identifying the *CYP3A4*22* allele) was associated with reduced CYP3A4 mRNA expression and lower in vitro CYP3A4 enzymatic activity, demonstrated using the CYP3A4 gold standard phenotyping probes midazolam and erythromycin [23]. The *CYP3A4*22* allele has a minor allele frequency of approximately 5% in Caucasians and significantly impacts CYP3A4 expression in vivo [24]. Notably, *CYP3A4*22* has also demonstrated a significant effect on tacrolimus metabolism on top of the influence of *CYP3A5* genetic polymorphisms [25]. Patients with a combined CYP3A4/ 5 poor metabolizer status showed the highest risk on supra-therapeutic tacrolimus concentrations following standard, body weight-based tacrolimus dosing shortly after transplantation [25].

The drug transporter P-glycoprotein, encoded by the *ABCB1* gene, plays a role in the transport of tacrolimus over cell membranes. More than 50 single nucleotide polymorphisms (SNPs) have been identified in this gene. Due to the significance of P-glycoprotein in the absorption, distribution, and elimination of tacrolimus, several SNPs have been investigated in relation to tacrolimus pharmacokinetics, including *ABCB1* 3435C>T (rs1045642), 1236C>T (rs1128503) and 2677G>T/A (rs2032582; Ala893Ser/Thr) SNPs. These three SNPs are in linkage disequilibrium, although the *ABCB1* 3435C>T polymorphism is considered the most important pharmacogenetic variant as it affects *ABCB1* mRNA levels and P-glycoprotein protein expression. However, these finding have not always been consistently confirmed [26–28]. Most association studies have reported negative results regarding the impact of *ABCB1* genetic variations on tacrolimus pharmacokinetics. As a result, the clinical relevance of *ABCB1* pharmacogenetic analysis for tacrolimus metabolism is likely to be minor and therefore not clinically significant.

Nicotinamide adenine dinucleotide phosphate (NADPH)-CYP oxidoreductase (POR) plays a crucial role as an electron donor for CYP monooxygenase enzymes, including CYP3A [29]. More than 100 SNPs have been found in the *POR* gene, and these genetic variations can influence the interaction between POR and CYP enzymes. This, in its turn, then leads to alterations in CYP activity [29, 30]. One specific variant allele, *POR*28* (rs1057868; C>T; Ala503Val), has a relative high minor allelic frequency of 28% [29, 30].

In a study by de Jonge et al. [31], involving 298 de novo renal transplant recipients, it was observed that patients who expressed CYP3A5 and carried the *POR*28* T-variant allele, required a 25% higher tacrolimus dose compared to CYP3A5 expressers with the *POR*28* CC genotype. Additionally, individuals carrying the *POR*28* T-variant allele took significantly longer to reach the target tacrolimus concentration (C_0) and were more likely to be underexposed during the early phase after transplantation. Notably, the *POR*28* SNP did not affect tacrolimus C_0 in CYP3A5 non-expressers [31]. These findings were confirmed by

Elens et al. [32], who demonstrated an increased tacrolimus dose requirement in CYP3A5-expressing kidney transplant recipients carrying the *POR*28* T-variant allele.

---

5 Mycophenolic acid and *UGT1A9*

Mycophenolate mofetil (MMF), an essential component of immunosuppressive therapy in renal transplantation, undergoes hydrolysis by esterases to form mycophenolic acid (MPA), its active metabolite. The primary metabolic pathway of MPA involves glucuronidation by uridine diphosphate-glucuronosyltransferases (UGTs), primarily UGT1A9, leading to the formation of the inactive metabolite MPA-glucuronide (MPAG) [33]. Significant correlations have been observed between MPA plasma concentrations and therapeutic efficacy. Studies have demonstrated that MPA exposure on day 3 is associated with the risk of BPAR within both the first month ($P = 0.009$) and the first year ($P = 0.006$) after transplantation [34]. These findings indicate that monitoring MPA plasma concentrations early after transplantation can provide valuable information about the risk of rejection and help optimize the immunosuppressive regimen.

Patients carrying the increased-expression promoter polymorphisms −275T>A and/or −2152C>T in the UGT1A9 gene have been shown to exhibit lower mycophenolic acid (MPA) AUC_{0-12} values when treated with tacrolimus. This suggests increased metabolism of MPA by UGT1A9. These findings were consistent with a study by Sanchez-Fructuosa et al. in 2009 [36]. On the other hand, patients carrying the inactivating 98T>C SNP (*UGT1A9*3*) consistently displayed higher MPA AUC_{0-12} values, indicating reduced metabolism of MPA [35].

Using a mixed-model analysis, it was observed that carriers of *UGT1A9* −275T>A and/or −2152C>T polymorphism had a 20% lower MPA AUC_{0-12} compared to patients with the wild-type *UGT1A9* genotype ($p = 0.012$). Furthermore, these *UGT1A9* polymorphisms were found to be significant predictors of BPAR within the first year after transplantation, showing an odds ratio of 13.3 (95% confidence interval 1.1–162.3; $p = 0.042$) [35]. These results suggest that genetic variations in *UGT1A9* can influence MPA metabolism and thus may impact the risk of BPAR in renal transplant recipients.

---

6 CPIC Guidelines

In 2015, the Clinical Pharmacogenetics Implementation Consortium (CPIC) published a guideline for tacrolimus and *CYP3A5* [13]. CPIC recommendations for tacrolimus dosing are:

Extensive Metabolizer (CYP3A5 Expresser)
Increase starting dose 1.5–2.0 times. Total starting dose should not exceed 0.3 mg/ kg/day. Use TDM to guide dose adjustments.

Intermediate Metabolizer (CYP3A5 Expresser)
Increase starting dose 1.5–2.0 times. Total starting dose should not exceed 0.3 mg/ kg/day. Use TDM to guide dose adjustments.

Poor Metabolizer (CYP3A5 Non-expresser)
Initiate therapy with standard recommended dose. Use TDM to guide dose adjustments.

7   Conclusion

Indeed, in the field of immunosuppressive therapy involving medications like tacrolimus, *CYP3A5* genotyping is currently the most relevant factor to consider. The presence of at least one *CYP3A5*1* allele (CYP3A5 expressers) or homozygously *CYP3A5*3* alleles (CYP3A5 non-expressers) has been consistently associated with differences in tacrolimus dose requirements and blood concentrations. While the *CYP3A4*22* variant allele has shown additional value, there are currently no specific guidelines from the CPIC published yet regarding *CYP3A4*22* and tacrolimus dosing.

When it comes to the risk of undertreatment in solid organ transplantation with a tacrolimus/MMF/corticosteroid regimen, *UGT1A9* genotyping may be relevant. SNPs in *UGT1A9* have been associated with differences in MPA metabolism, and have been correlated with BPAR. However, there are no CPIC guidelines published so far specifically addressing *UGT1A9* genotyping and its impact on immunosuppressive therapy. Therefore, at present, *CYP3A5* genotyping for tacrolimus and its interaction remains the main actionable pharmacogenetic gene-drug interaction in the field of immunosuppressant therapy for solid organ transplantation.

References

1. Hariharan S, et al. Improved graft survival after renal transplantation in the United States, 1988 to 1996. N Engl J Med. 2000;342(9):605–12.
2. Kaufman DB, et al. Immunosuppression: practice and trends. Am J Transplant. 2004;4(Suppl 9):38–53.
3. Bouamar R, et al. Tacrolimus predose concentrations do not predict the risk of acute rejection after renal transplantation: a pooled analysis from three randomized-controlled clinical trials(dagger). Am J Transplant. 2013;13(5):1253–61.
4. Venkataramanan R, et al. Clinical pharmacokinetics of tacrolimus. Clin Pharmacokinet. 1995;29(6):404–30.
5. Kamdem LK, et al. Contribution of CYP3A5 to the in vitro hepatic clearance of tacrolimus. Clin Chem. 2005;51(8):1374–81.
6. Staatz CE, Tett SE. Clinical pharmacokinetics and pharmacodynamics of tacrolimus in solid organ transplantation. Clin Pharmacokinet. 2004;43(10):623–53.
7. Moller A, et al. The disposition of 14C-labeled tacrolimus after intravenous and oral administration in healthy human subjects. Drug Metab Dispos. 1999;27(6):633–6.
8. Lamba J, et al. PharmGKB summary: very important pharmacogene information for CYP3A5. Pharmacogenet Genom. 2012;22(7):555–8.

9. Thiebaut F, et al. Cellular localization of the multidrug-resistance gene product P-glycoprotein in normal human tissues. Proc Natl Acad Sci USA. 1987;84(21):7735–8.
10. Kuehl P, et al. Sequence diversity in CYP3A promoters and characterization of the genetic basis of polymorphic CYP3A5 expression. Nat Genet. 2001;27(4):383–91.
11. Hustert E, et al. The genetic determinants of the CYP3A5 polymorphism. Pharmacogenetics. 2001;11(9):773–9.
12. van Schaik RH, et al. CYP3A5 variant allele frequencies in Dutch Caucasians. Clin Chem. 2002;48(10):1668–71.
13. Birdwell KA, et al. Clinical pharmacogenetics implementation consortium (CPIC) guidelines for CYP3A5 genotype and tacrolimus dosing. Clin Pharmacol Ther. 2015;98(1):19–24.
14. Haufroid V, et al. The effect of CYP3A5 and MDR1 (ABCB1) polymorphisms on cyclosporine and tacrolimus dose requirements and trough blood levels in stable renal transplant patients. Pharmacogenetics. 2004;14(3):147–54.
15. Hesselink DA, et al. Genetic polymorphisms of the CYP3A4, CYP3A5, and MDR-1 genes and pharmacokinetics of the calcineurin inhibitors cyclosporine and tacrolimus. Clin Pharmacol Ther. 2003;74(3):245–54.
16. Macphee IA, et al. Tacrolimus pharmacogenetics: the CYP3A5*1 allele predicts low dose-normalized tacrolimus blood concentrations in whites and South Asians. Transplantation. 2005;79(4):499–502.
17. Thervet E, et al. Impact of cytochrome p450 3A5 genetic polymorphism on tacrolimus doses and concentration-to-dose ratio in renal transplant recipients. Transplantation. 2003;76(8):1233–5.
18. Tsuchiya N, et al. Influence of CYP3A5 and MDR1 (ABCB1) polymorphisms on the pharmacokinetics of tacrolimus in renal transplant recipients. Transplantation. 2004;78(8):1182–7.
19. Hesselink DA, et al. The role of pharmacogenetics in the disposition of and response to tacrolimus in solid organ transplantation. Clin Pharmacokinet. 2014;53(2):123–39.
20. Tang HL, et al. Lower tacrolimus daily dose requirements and acute rejection rates in the CYP3A5 nonexpressers than expressers. Pharmacogenet Genom. 2011;21(11):713–20.
21. Terrazzino S, et al. The effect of CYP3A5 6986A>G and ABCB1 3435C>T on tacrolimus dose-adjusted trough levels and acute rejection rates in renal transplant patients: a systematic review and meta-analysis. Pharmacogenet Genomics. 2012;22(8):642–5.
22. Thervet E, et al. Optimization of initial tacrolimus dose using pharmacogenetic testing. Clin Pharmacol Ther. 2010;87(6):721–6.
23. Wang D, et al. Intronic polymorphism in CYP3A4 affects hepatic expression and response to statin drugs. Pharmacogenomics J. 2011;11(4):274–86.
24. Elens L, et al. CYP3A4 intron 6 C>T SNP (CYP3A4*22) encodes lower CYP3A4 activity in cancer patients, as measured with probes midazolam and erythromycin. Pharmacogenomics. 2013;14(2):137–49.
25. Elens L, et al. A new functional CYP3A4 intron 6 polymorphism significantly affects tacrolimus pharmacokinetics in kidney transplant recipients. Clin Chem. 2011;57(11):1574–83.
26. Hoffmeyer S, et al. Functional polymorphisms of the human multidrug-resistance gene: multiple sequence variations and correlation of one allele with P-glycoprotein expression and activity in vivo. Proc Natl Acad Sci USA. 2000;97(7):3473–8.
27. Kimchi-Sarfaty C, et al. A "silent" polymorphism in the MDR1 gene changes substrate specificity. Science. 2007;315(5811):525–8.
28. Wang D, et al. Multidrug resistance polypeptide 1 (MDR1, ABCB1) variant 3435C>T affects mRNA stability. Pharmacogenet Genomics. 2005;15(10):693–704.
29. Hart SN, Zhong XB. P450 oxidoreductase: genetic polymorphisms and implications for drug metabolism and toxicity. Expert Opin Drug Metab Toxicol. 2008;4(4):439–52.
30. Huang N, et al. Genetics of P450 oxidoreductase: sequence variation in 842 individuals of four ethnicities and activities of 15 missense mutations. Proc Natl Acad Sci USA. 2008;105(5):1733–8.

31. de Jonge H, et al. The P450 oxidoreductase *28 SNP is associated with low initial tacrolimus exposure and increased dose requirements in CYP3A5-expressing renal recipients. Pharmacogenomics. 2011;12(9):1281–91.
32. Elens L, et al. Impact of POR*28 on the clinical pharmacokinetics of CYP3A phenotyping probes midazolam and erythromycin. Pharmacogenet Genom. 2013;23(3):148–55.
33. Bernard O, Guillemette C. The main role of UGT1A9 in the hepatic metabolism of mycophenolic acid and the effects of naturally occurring variants. Drug Metab Dispos. 2004;32(8):775–8.
34. van Gelder T, et al. A randomized double-blind, multicenter plasma concentration controlled study of the safety and efficacy of oral mycophenolate mofetil for the prevention of acute rejection after kidney transplantation. Transplantation. 1999;68(2):261–6.
35. van Schaik RH, et al. UGT1A9-275T>A/-2152C>T polymorphisms correlate with low MPA exposure and acute rejection in MMF/tacrolimus-treated kidney transplant patients. Clin Pharmacol Ther. 2009;86(3):319–27.
36. Sanchez-Fructuoso AI, et al. The prevalence of uridine diphosphate-glucuronosyltransferase 1A9 (UGT1A9) gene promoter region single-nucleotide polymorphisms T-275A and C-2152T and its influence on mycophenolic acid pharmacokinetics in stable renal transplant patients. Transplant Proc. 2009;41(6):2313–6.

The Application of Pharmacogenomics to Infectious Disease

Bernard Esquivel

Abstract

One of the most disruptive and game-changer events in the history of medicine, thus humankind, was the discovery of penicillin by Alexander Fleming in the twentieth century. Fleming's work paved the way for modern antimicrobial therapies that have dramatically impacted the human lifespan. Nevertheless, as with almost any other medication, unexpected adverse drug reactions and other related factors affect the efficacy and overall patients' outcome. Since the "genomic revolution" started, it is well known that both the host and the pathogen's genetic information plays a crucial role in treatment response, thus, outcome. In this chapter, using a clinical utility lens, the implications of pharmacogenomics in infectious diseases in an evidence-based approach will be discussed.

Keywords

Pharmacogenomics · Pharmacogenetics · Infectious diseases · HIV · HCV · Aminoglycosides

1 Introduction

One of the most disruptive and game-changer events in the history of medicine, thus humankind, was the discovery of penicillin by Alexander Fleming in the twentieth century. Since then, the human lifespan was positively impacted due to the direct benefits that penicillin brought and because it preceded a broad range of antibiotics that made several life-threatening bacterial infections treatable [1].

B. Esquivel (✉)
Personalized Medicine Latin American Association, GenXys Health Care Systems Inc., Vancouver, BC, Canada
e-mail: ber.doc@gmail.com

Also called "communicable diseases," infectious diseases are caused by pathogens that are transmitted either directly between persons or indirectly via a vector or the environment. The spread of an infectious disease through populations is determined by the characteristics of the infectious agent, the host, and the environment [2]. It has been widely documented that each individual may respond differently to an anti-infectious treatment, primarily due to the complex and dynamic interaction between the environment, the host, and the agent. In terms of the host, the response (effectivity) to the treatment and tolerability play a crucial role thus; pharmacogenetics starts making much sense. In order to bring the full potential of precision medicine into infectious diseases, the application of pharmacogenomics to infectious diseases requires consideration of the genomes of both the pathogen and the host. The pathogen's genome may be used for antigen identification, identifying infecting organisms, and determining antimicrobial resistance [3]. However, the scientific efforts, hence, the scientific evidence, have been mainly focusing on the host, probably due to the pathogens' underlying complexity and constant rapid mutating capabilities. Specifically, the most robust evidence behind the clinical applicability of pharmacogenomics in infectious diseases relies on genetic polymorphisms related to the immune system and its responses to pathogens, as well as genetic variants associated with metabolic pathways that impact drugs' tolerability and toxicity.

There have been described hundreds of possible gene–drug interactions in the infectious disease space; however, the Clinical Pharmacogenetics Implementation Consortium (CPIC) has narrowed it down based on scientific evidence and provided specific recommendations and guidelines:

2   *HLA-B* and Abacavir

According to the World Health Organization (WHO) and published via the Summary of the global HIV epidemic (2019), about 38 million people are currently living with Human Immunodeficiency Virus (HIV). That number represents a 24% increase if compared with 2010 figures.

HIV is a lent virus that causes infection and acquired immunodeficiency syndrome (AIDS). AIDS is a condition in humans in which progressive failure of the immune system allows life-threatening infections and cancers to thrive. Infection with HIV occurs by transferring blood, semen, vaginal fluid, breast milk. HIV is present as both free virus particles and virus within infected immune cells within these bodily fluids. HIV infects vital cells in the human immune system, such as helper CD4+ T cells, macrophages. HIV infection leads to low levels of T cells through several mechanisms, including pyroptosis of infected T cells. The symptoms of AIDS are primarily the result of conditions that do not usually develop in individuals with healthy immune systems. Most of these conditions are opportunistic infections caused by bacteria, viruses, fungi, and parasites usually controlled by the immune system elements that HIV damages [4].

Abacavir is a nucleoside reverse-transcriptase inhibitor with activity against the HIV, available for once-daily use in combination with other antiretroviral agents, that has shown efficacy, few drug interactions, and a favorable long-term safety profile. The most important adverse effect of abacavir that limits its use in therapy and mandates a high degree of clinical vigilance is an immunologically mediated hypersensitivity reaction affecting 5–8% of patients during the first six weeks of treatment [5]. Since 2002, an association between a diagnosis of hypersensitivity reaction to abacavir and carriage of the major histocompatibility complex class I allele *HLA-B*5701* was reported independently by two research groups and was subsequently corroborated by several independent studies [5–7].

Excerpt from the CPIC abacavir dosing guidelines:

HLA-B*57:01 screening should be performed in all abacavir-naive individuals before initiation of abacavir-containing therapy; this is consistent with the recommendations of the FDA, the US Department of Health and Human Services, and the European Medicines Agency (EMA). In abacavir-naive individuals who are *HLA-B*57:01*-positive, abacavir is not recommended and should be considered only under exceptional circumstances when the potential benefit, based on resistance patterns and treatment history, outweighs the risk [5, 8].

Nowadays, the correlation between hypersensibility and *HLA-B*5701*, in fact, several global regulatory agencies state that HLA-B*5701 testing prior to prescribing abacavir is required. Some of them are the US Food and Drug Administration, the EMA, the Swiss Agency of Therapeutic Products, and Health Canada (Canada).

3   *UGT1A1* and Atazanavir

Atazanavir is an antiretroviral protease inhibitor used to treat and prevent HIV-1 infection and AIDS. Atazanavir is a substrate and inhibitor of cytochrome P450 isozyme 3A and an inhibitor and inducer of P-glycoprotein. It has similar virologic efficacy as efavirenz and ritonavir-boosted lopinavir in antiretroviral-naive individuals [9–11]. It has been described that atazanavir may cause unconjugated bilirubinemia in over 40% of the patients. Atazanavir has a mean elimination half-life of 7–8 h, and it is eliminated 7% in urine and 20% in feces. The explanation for the dose-related hyperbilirubinemia has been associated with the nonprotein-bound atazanavir direct inhibition of bilirubin glucuronidation via UGT1A1 [10, 12].

The Uridine Diphosphate (UDP) Glucuronosyltransferases (UGT) enzymes family mediate glucuronic acid conjugate with lipophilic drugs, xenobiotics, and endogenous substances, which enable their efficient elimination in bile and urine by increasing their water solubility [13].

Three UGT subfamilies have been identified based on gene sequence similarity: UGT1A, UGT2A, and UGT2B. The UGT1A subfamily of enzymes encoded by a single-gene locus through differential splicing of unique first exons (exon 1) to shared exons 2–5 [14].

The primary UGT1A subfamily enzyme, UGT1A1, is expressed predominantly in the liver and gastrointestinal tract and is crucial for eliminating bilirubin. Reduced UGT1A1 activity either through developmental delay in neonates, genetic variation, or catalytic inhibition by drugs results in the accumulation of unconjugated bilirubin in blood and tissues [10].

The most frequent genetic variant that affects UGT1A1 the enzyme function is a dinucleotide TAn repeat polymorphism (rs8175347) located in a TATAA consensus element in the *UGT1A1* promoter at –53 relative to the translation start site. This varies from five to eight TA repeats. TA6 (*UGT1A1*1*) and TA7 (*UGT1A1*28*) are most frequent, while TA5 (*UGT1A1*36*) and TA8 (*UGT1A1*37*) repeats are infrequent or absent depending on the geographic region of ancestry [10]. Clinically, *UGT1A1* variant *28 has been correlated with Gilbert syndrome: a genetic disorder of bilirubin metabolism in the liver with the phenotypic expression of recurrent episodes of jaundice due to a decreased glucuronidation, thus bilirubin excretion [12].

Studies using promoter-reporter constructs have shown that the TA7 (*UGT1A1*28*) allele causes a moderate reduction in gene transcription as compared with the reference TA6 (*UGT1A1*1*) allele, perhaps due to reduced binding affinity for transcription factors including TATA-binding protein. The TA8 repeat (*UGT1A1*37*) appears to drive lower transcription levels than TA7, while TA5 (*UGT1A1*36*) appears to cause higher transcription levels than TA6. Studies of human liver microsomes show that UGT1A1 protein is ~twofold less in *UGT1A1*28/*28* donors than in *UGT1A1*1/*1* donors [12, 15].

According to PharmGKB, a Very Important Pharmacogene (VIP) summary provides an overview of a significant gene involved in the metabolism of, or response to, one or several drugs. VIP summaries typically include background information on the gene, including any disease associations, as well as in-depth information on the gene's pharmacogenetics. PharmGKB has categorized the correlation between UGT1A1 and atazanavir in terms of the level of evidence as a Level-1 Tier-1 VIP. CPIC Guideline for UGT1A1 and atazanavir prescribing [10] has established prescribing recommendations based on the assignment of likely UGT1A1 phenotypes based on genotypes:

- *Extensive metabolizer:* An individual carrying two reference function *1 (Reference function refers to the *UGT1A1* alleles to which other alleles are compared. The reference function *1 allele is fully functional and refers to the rs8175347 TA6 allele) and or increased function alleles (*36). Alternatively identified by homozygosity for rs887829 C/C. Diplotypes included in this phenotypic classification are *1/*1; *1/*36; *36/*36; rs887829 C/C.
- *Intermediate metabolizer:* An individual carrying one reference function (*1) or increased function allele (*36) plus one decreased function allele (*6, *28, *37). Alternatively identified by heterozygosity for rs887829 C/T. The correlated haplotypes are *1/*28; *1/*37; *36/*28; *36/*37; rs887829 C/T, *1/ *6.

- *Poor metabolizer:* An individual carrying two decreased function alleles (*6, *28, *37). Alternatively identified by homozygosity for rs887829 T/T (*80/*80). Diplotypes examples are **28/*28; *28/*37; *37/*37*; rs887829 T/T (**80/*80*), **6/*6*.

Based on the high level of quality evidence, CPIC has also provided clinical recommendations on how to use atazanavir, boosted with either ritonavir or cobicistat (Table 1):

Table 1 Clinical recommendations for atazanavir [10]

Phenotype	Implications for phenotypic measures	Dosing recommendations	Classification of recommendations
Extensive metabolizer	Reference UGT1A1 activity; very low likelihood of bilirubin-related discontinuation of atazanavir	There is no need to avoid prescribing of atazanavir based on *UGT1A1* genetic test result. Inform the patient that some patients stop atazanavir because of jaundice (yellow eyes and skin), but that this patient's genotype makes this unlikely (less than about a 1 in 20 chance of stopping atazanavir because of jaundice)	Strong
Intermediate metabolizer	Somewhat decreased UGT1A1 activity; low likelihood of bilirubin-related discontinuation of atazanavir	There is no need to avoid prescribing of atazanavir based on *UGT1A1* genetic test result. Inform the patient that some patients stop atazanavir because of jaundice (yellow eyes and skin), but that this patient's genotype makes this unlikely (less than about a 1 in 20 chance of stopping atazanavir because of jaundice)	Strong
Poor metabolizer	Markedly decreased UGT1A1 activity; high likelihood of bilirubin-related discontinuation of atazanavir	Consider an alternative agent particularly where jaundice would be of concern to the patient If atazanavir is to be prescribed, there is a high likelihood of developing jaundice that will result in atazanavir discontinuation (at least 20% and as high as 60%)	Strong

*All studies correlating *UGT1A1* genotypes with atazanavir adverse events have involved ritonavir boosting. However, concentration-time profiles are equivalent when boosted with either cobicistat or ritonavir and bilirubin-related adverse events including discontinuation of atazanavir occur in a similar percentage of patients prescribed atazanavir with cobicistat or ritonavir. Associations between UGT1A1 genotype, bilirubin elevations, and atazanavir/r discontinuation therefore almost certainly translate to atazanavir/cobicistat

4   *CYP2B6* and Efavirenz

Efavirenz is a non-nucleoside reverse transcriptase inhibitor (NNRTI) and is used as part of highly active antiretroviral therapy (HAART) for the treatment of HIV type 1 [16].

For HIV infection that has not previously been treated, efavirenz and lamivudine in combination with zidovudine or tenofovir is the preferred NNRTI-based regimen. Efavirenz is also used in combination with other antiretroviral agents as part of an expanded postexposure prophylaxis regimen to prevent HIV transmission for those exposed to materials associated with a high risk for HIV transmission. Efavirenz is highly bound (approximately 99.5–99.75%) to human plasma proteins, predominantly albumin. In HIV-1-infected patients (n = 9) who received Sustiva® 200–600 mg once daily for at least one month, cerebrospinal fluid concentrations ranged from 0.26 to 1.19% (mean 0.69%) of the corresponding plasma concentration. This proportion is approximately threefold higher than the plasma's non-protein-bound (free) fraction of efavirenz. Studies in humans and in vitro studies using human liver microsomes have demonstrated that the cytochrome P450 system principally metabolizes efavirenz to hydroxylated metabolites with subsequent glucuronidation of these hydroxylated metabolites (Fig. 1). These metabolites are essentially inactive against HIV-1. The in vitro studies suggest that CYP3A4 and CYP2B6 are the major isozymes responsible for efavirenz metabolism. Efavirenz has been shown to induce P450 enzymes, resulting in the induction of its own metabolism. Multiple doses of 200–400 mg per day for 10 days resulted in a lower than predicted extent of accumulation (22–42% lower) and a shorter terminal half-life of 40–55 h (single dose half-life 52–76 h). Efavirenz has a terminal half-life of 52–76 h after single doses and 40–55 h after multiple doses. A one-month mass balance/excretion study was conducted using 400 mg per day with a 14C-labeled dose administered on Day 8. Approximately 14–34% of the radiolabel was recovered in the urine and 16–61% was recovered in the feces. Nearly, all of the urinary excretion of the radiolabeled drug was in the form of metabolites. Efavirenz accounted for the majority of the total radioactivity measured in feces [16, 17].

CYP2B6 is highly polymorphic with 38 known variant alleles and multiple sub-alleles. Substantial differences in allele frequencies occur across ancestrally diverse groups. Alleles are categorized into functional groups as follows: normal function, decreased function, no function, and increased function. *CYP2B6*6* (p.Q172H, p.K262R) is the most frequently decreased function allele (15–60% minor allele frequency depending on ancestry). Even though reduced protein expression due to aberrant splicing caused by the c.516G>T (rs3745274, p.Q172H) Single-Nucleotide Polymorphism (SNP) contributes to reduced function of *CYP2B6*6*, two in vitro studies also suggest complex substrate-dependent catalytic effects. Thus, giving function to *CYP2B6* alleles is reasonably challenging, as function may be substrate specific [17].

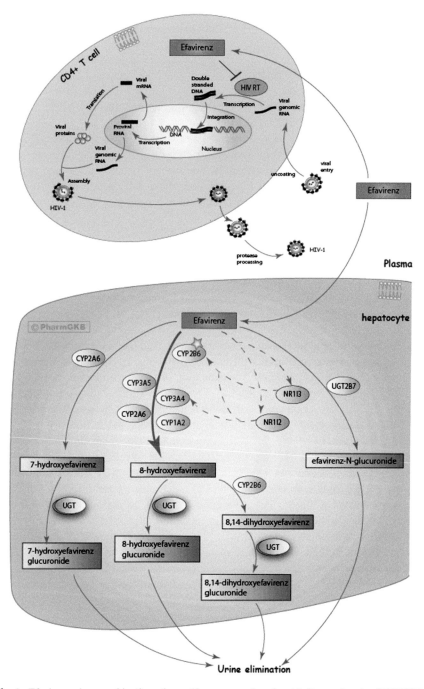

Fig. 1 Efavirenz pharmacokinetic pathway *Image reproduced and is licensed under CC BY-SA 4.0 from PharmGKB

CPIC via their Guideline for CYP2B6 and Efavirenz-Containing Antiretroviral Therapy has proposed the following assessment of likely CYP2B6 phenotypes based on genotypes:

- Ultrarapid metabolizer; an individual carrying two increased function alleles (*4/*4, *22/*22, *4/*22).
- Rapid metabolizer; an individual carrying one normal function allele and one increased function allele (*1/*4, *1/*22).
- Normal metabolizer; an individual carrying two normal function alleles (*1/*1).
- Intermediate metabolizer; an individual carrying one normal function allele and one decreased function allele OR one normal function allele and one no-function allele OR one increased function allele and one decreased function allele OR one increased function allele and one no-function allele (*1/*6, *1/*18, *4/*6, *4/*18, *6/*22, *18/*22).
- Poor metabolize; an individual carrying two decreased function alleles OR two no-function alleles OR one decreased function allele and one no-function allele (*6/*6, *18/*18, *6/*18).

In the guideline mentioned above, CPIC also provides efavirenz dosing recommendations for children >40 kg and adult patients [17]:

- CYP2B6 ultrarapid metabolizer: Slightly lower dose-adjusted trough concentrations of efavirenz compared with normal metabolizers. Initiate efavirenz with standard dosing (600 mg/day). Classification of recommendation-strong
- CYP2B6 rapid metabolizer: Slightly lower dose-adjusted through concentrations of efavirenz compared with normal metabolizers. Initiate efavirenz with standard dosing (600 mg/day). Classification of recommendation-strong
- CYP2B6 normal metabolizer: Normal efavirenz metabolism. Initiate efavirenz with standard dosing (600 mg/day). Classification of recommendation-strong
- CYP2B6 intermediate metabolizer: Higher dose-adjusted trough concentrations of efavirenz compared with normal metabolizers; increased risk of CNS adverse events. Consider initiating efavirenz with decreased dose of 400 mg/day. Classification of recommendation-moderate
- CYP2B6 poor metabolizer: Higher dose-adjusted trough concentrations of efavirenz compared with normal metabolizers; significantly increased risk of CNS adverse events and treatment discontinuation. Consider initiating efavirenz with decreased dose of 400 or 200 mg/day. Classification of recommendation-moderate.

5   *MT-RNR1* and Aminoglycosides

Aminoglycosides are powerful, broad-spectrum antibiotics that act through the inhibition of protein synthesis. Aminoglycosides are active against various Gram-positive and Gram-negative organisms. Aminoglycosides are particularly potent against members of the *Enterobacteriaceae* family, including *Escherichia coli, Klebsiella pneumoniae* and *K. oxytoca, Enterobacter cloacae* and *E. aerogenes, Providencia spp., Proteus spp., Morganella spp.*, and *Serratia spp.* Aminoglycosides have good activity against *Staphylococcus aureus*, including methicillin-resistant and vancomycin-intermediate and -resistant isolates, *P. aeruginosa* and to a lesser extent *Acinetobacter baumannii*. Recent large-scale surveillance programs explain aminoglycoside susceptibility among essential pathogens associated with common infection types. A recent surveillance study of Gram-negative organisms isolated from patients hospitalized in Intensive Care Units (ICUs) in the United States and the EU found that amikacin and gentamicin showed good activity against key Gram-negative pathogens. In the United States, 99.5% and 87.9% of *E. coli* isolates were susceptible to amikacin and gentamicin, respectively, according to the Clinical and Laboratory Standards Institute (CLSI) criteria. Likewise, 97.3% and 87.2% of *E. coli* isolates from the EU samples were susceptible to amikacin and gentamicin, respectively, according to the European Committee on Antimicrobial Susceptibility Testing (EUCAST) criteria [18].

The human mitochondrial genome contains 37 genes; 13 encode the mitochondrial respiratory chain components, whereas the other 24 encode a mature RNA product. Mature RNA products are mitochondrial tRNA molecules, a 16s rRNA subunit, and a 12s rRNA subunit. These sub-units are necessary for the translation of mRNAs into mitochondrial proteins (Fig. 2). Variants in *MT-RNR1*, which predispose to aminoglycosides-induced hearing loss (AIHL), appear to drive the 12s rRNA subunit to resemble the bacterial 16s rRNA subunit more closely, thus permitting aminoglycosides to bind better. The variant m.1555A>G has been extensively correlated with AIHL. Early family studies recognized that the predisposition toward AIHL seemed to be inherited down the maternal lineage in an extra-nuclear inheritance pattern [18, 19].

CPIC guidelines recognized the risk of developing AIHL when certain *MT-RNR1* variants are present. CPIC 2021 guideline provides recommendations for both adult and pediatric patients. Excerpts from the guideline [19]:

- "The critical pharmacogenetics recommendation for a person with an *MT-RNR1* variant which predisposes to AIHL is that aminoglycoside antibiotics are relatively contraindicated, meaning that aminoglycosides should be avoided unless the increased risk of hearing loss is outweighed by the severity of infection and lack of safe or effective alternative therapies."
- "There is insufficient evidence to suggest that the adverse drug reaction may be more profound with some members of the aminoglycoside class than others. As such, this guidance covers all aminoglycoside antibiotics irrespective of class. We provide a strong recommendation that carriers of *MT-RNR1* variants that

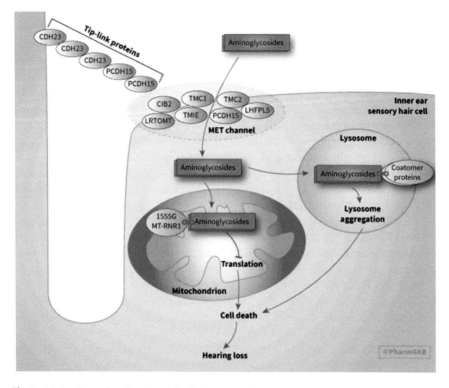

Fig. 2 Mechanism of aminoglycosides-induced hearing loss. Image reproduced and is licensed under CC BY-SA 4.0 from PharmGKB

predispose to AIHL should avoid aminoglycosides unless the increased risk of permanent hearing loss is outweighed by the risk of infection without safe or effective alternative therapies."

- "If no effective alternative to an aminoglycoside is thought to be available, we advise use for the shortest possible time, consultation with an infectious disease expert for alternative approaches, therapeutic drug monitoring and frequent assessment for hearing loss, both during and after therapy, in consultation with an audiovestibular physician."
- "An individual with no detectable *MT-RNR1* variant or carrying *MT-RNR1* variants not considered to be predisposing to AIHL (normal risk), including the m.827A>G variant, should still be considered at risk of AIHL."

AIHL is caused by the death of hair cells in the inner ear following exposure to aminoglycosides. Aminoglycosides cross the blood-labyrinth barrier in the inner ear and enter the endolymph. They then selectively enter sensory hair cells through Mechanoelectrical Transduction (MET) channels in a calcium-dependent manner. The exact composition of the MET channel has not been definitively ascertained but is known to contain the TMC1 protein le. This pathway displays the MET channel components.

Tip-link protein chains consisting of cadherin 23 and protocadherin 15 (PCDH15) regulate MET channel gating. Gentamicin uptake and subsequent cell death was found to be prevented in hair cells derived from CDH23 knockout mice [7].

6   *CYP2C9* and Voriconazole

Invasive fungal diseases are associated with significant morbidity and mortality in immunocompromised patients. Voriconazole is the first-line treatment of invasive aspergillosis and has been successfully used in other invasive fungal infections, such as candidiasis, fusariosis or scedosporidiosis. It is a second-generation triazole and a derivate of fluconazole. Voriconazole has nonlinear pharmacokinetics and undergoes extensive hepatic metabolism by the cytochrome P450 system that depends on age, genetic factors, and interactions with other drugs [20]. The cytochrome P450 2C19 (CYP2C19) enzyme seems to play a significant role in the metabolism of voriconazole, and polymorphisms in CYP2C19 are linked with slow voriconazole metabolism. As many as 20% of non-Indian Asians have low CYP2C19 activity and develop voriconazole levels as much as fourfold higher than those in homozygous subjects, leading to potentially augmented toxicity [20].

CYP2C19 is highly polymorphic with 35 defined variant star (*) alleles. *CYP2C19*1* allele encodes a normal function CYP2C19 enzyme, and the most common no function allele is *2* (c.681G>A; rs4244285). Other *CYP2C19* alleles with decreased or no function have been identified; nevertheless, they are commonly rare in the general population with the exception of *CYP2C19*3* (c.636G>A; rs4986893) in Asians. In contrast, the increased function *CYP2C19*17* allele (c.-806C>T; rs12248560) enhances transcription and increases enzyme activity for some substrates [21]. CPIC guidelines for CYP2C19 and Voriconazole Therapy proposed the following assignment of likely CYP2C19 phenotypes based on genotypes [21]:

- CYP2C19 ultrarapid metabolizer (2–5% of patients): An individual carrying two increased function alleles;
- CYP2C19 rapid metabolizer (2–30% of patients): An individual carrying one normal function allele and one increased function allele.
- CYP2C19 normal metabolizer (35–50% of patients): An individual carrying two normal function alleles.
- CYP2C19 intermediate metabolizer (18–45% of patients): An individual carrying one normal function allele and one no function allele or one no function allele and one increased function allele
- CYP2C19 poor metabolizer (2–15% of patients): An individual carrying two no-function alleles.

Also, within the same guideline mentioned above, CPIC has published dosing recommendations for voriconazole treatment based on the CYP2C19 phenotype for adults, children and pediatric patients. The recommendations for adult patients are:

- Ultrarapid metabolizer (*17/*17): the probability of attainment of therapeutic voriconazole concentrations is small with standard dosing. Choose an alternative agent that is not dependent on CYP2C19 metabolism as primary therapy in lieu of voriconazole. Such agents include isavuconazole, liposomal amphotericin B, and posaconazole. Classification of the recommendations: moderate
- Rapid metabolizer (*1/*17): the probability of attainment of therapeutic concentrations is modest with standard dosing. Choose an alternative agent that is not dependent on CYP2C19 metabolism as primary therapy in lieu of voriconazole. Such agents include isavuconazole, liposomal amphotericin B, and posaconazole. Classification of the recommendations: moderate
- Normal metabolizer: Normal voriconazole metabolism. Initiate therapy with the recommended standard of care dosing. Classification of the recommendations: strong
- Intermediate metabolizer: Higher dose-adjusted trough concentrations of voriconazole compared with normal metabolizers. Initiate therapy with the recommended standard of care dosing. Classification of the recommendations: moderate
- Poor metabolizer: Higher dose-adjusted trough concentrations of voriconazole and may increase the probability of adverse events. Choose an alternative agent that is not dependent on CYP2C19 metabolism as primary therapy in lieu of voriconazole. Such agents include isavuconazole, liposomal amphotericin B, and posaconazole. In the event that voriconazole is considered to be the most appropriate agent, based on clinical advice, for a patient with poor metabolizer genotype, voriconazole should be administered at a preferably lower than standard dosage with careful therapeutic drug monitoring. Classification of the recommendations: moderate.

The dosing recommendations for voriconazole based on CYP2C19 phenotype for pediatric patients (children and adolescents < 18 years old) are [21]:

- Ultrarapid metabolizer (*17/*17): the probability of attainment of therapeutic concentrations is small. Choose an alternative agent that is not dependent on CYP2C19 metabolism as primary therapy in lieu of voriconazole. Such agents include liposomal amphotericin B, and posaconazole. Classifications of recommendations: moderate.
- Rapid metabolizer (*1/*17): the probability of attainment of therapeutic concentrations is variable. Initiate therapy with the recommended standard of care dosing. Use therapeutic drug monitoring to titrate dose to therapeutic trough concentrations. Classifications of recommendations: moderate.

- Normal metabolizer: Normal voriconazole metabolism. Initiate therapy with the recommended standard of care dosing. Classifications of recommendations: strong.
- Intermediate metabolizer: Higher dose-adjusted trough concentrations of voriconazole compared with normal metabolizers. Initiate therapy with the recommended standard of care dosing. Classifications of recommendations: moderate.
- Poor metabolizer: Higher dose-adjusted trough concentrations of voriconazole and may increase the probability of adverse events. Choose an alternative agent that is not dependent on CYP2C19 metabolism as primary therapy in lieu of voriconazole. Such agents include liposomal amphotericin B and posaconazole. In the event that voriconazole is considered to be the most appropriate agent, based on clinical advice, for a patient with poor metabolizer genotype, voriconazole should be administered at a preferably lower than standard dosage with careful therapeutic drug monitoring. Classifications of recommendations: moderate.

From the regulatory standpoint, the FDA has also provided a safety recommendation on the Tables of Pharmacogenetic Associations: "intermediate or poor metabolizers: results in higher systemic concentrations and may result in higher adverse reaction risk."

Other possible gene–drug interactions still need additional scientific and clinical evidence to bring them closer to the point of care. Some of them are G6PD-chloramphenicol, G6PD-ciprofloxacin, G6PD-dapsone, G6PD-moxifloxacin, G6PD-nalidixic acid, G6PD-nitrofurantoin, G6PD-norfloxacin, G6PD-primaquine, G6PD-quinine, G6PD-sulfadiazine, G6PD-sulfamethoxazole/trimethoprim, NAT2-sulfamethoxazole/trimethoprim, NAT2-sulfasalazine, HLA(B)-dapsone, VDR-ribavirin, among others.

7 *IFNL3/IFNL4* and Pegylated Interferon Alpha-Based Regimens

Pegylated interferon alpha-2a and 2b are conjugates of recombinant interferon attached to a polyethylene glycol (PEG) chain, which improves its pharmacokinetic and pharmacodynamic performance [22]. The interferon moiety of PEG-interferon alpha binds membrane receptors, triggering a cellular response that inhibit virus-replication in infected cells. Until 2011, a PEG-interferon alpha and ribavirin combination was used as the main form of hepatitis C virus treatment. With the approval of new direct-acting antiviral medicines, medical guidelines no longer suggest the use of PEG-interferon alpha as a first-line therapy [23]. However, it is still used in specific situations [24, 25].

Worldwide, approximately 58 million people have chronic hepatitis C virus infection [26]. In order to treat chronic hepatitis C virus infection, the virus levels must be eradicated. This is monitored through Sustained Virological Response

(SVR), defined as the absence of hepatitis C virus levels for 24 weeks after the end of treatment [27]. The use of PEG-interferon alpha and ribavirin for the treatment of hepatitis C virus infection leads to different SVR rates depending on the hepatitis C virus genotype. For instance, patients with genotype 2 and 3 infections treated with PEG-interferon alpha and ribavirin have SVR rates of 80%, but for those with genotype 1, this SVR rate decreases to 40% [28, 29].

Several studies have shown that *IFNL3* genetic variations affect PEG-interferon alpha clinical response [30]. The *IFNL3* gene, also known as IL28B, encodes interferon-lambda 3, a protein capable of inducing antiviral immunity [31].

Single-Nucleotide Polymorphism (SNP) rs12979860 is located upstream of IFNL3, and homozygous carriers of the C allele have a higher probability of PEG-interferon alpha therapeutic success, compared to those carrying the T allele [32]. It was later discovered that rs12979860 is located in *IFNL4*, a gene that produces a protein that shares less than 30% amino-acid identity with interferon-lambda 3 [33]. Another SNP, rs8099917, has also been associated to PEG-interferon alpha treatment response [34]. Both rs12979860 and rs8099917 are in strong linkage disequilibrium, however the frequency of rs8099917 differs across different populations [35].

The CPIC guideline for PEG interferon-alpha-based regimens has assigned two observed phenotypes depending on the rs12979860 genotype that is detected. People carrying two favorable response alleles (rs12979860 CC), have a favorable response genotype, and an "increased likelihood of response (higher SVR rate) to PEG-interferon alpha and ribavirin therapy as compared with patients with unfavorable response genotype". People carrying at least one unfavorable response allele (rs12979860 CT and TT), have an unfavorable response genotype, and a "decreased likelihood of response (lower SVR rate) to PEG-interferon alpha and ribavirin therapy as compared with patients with favorable response genotype" [34].

The CPIC guideline includes the following recommendations for PEG-interferon alpha and ribavirin therapy [34]:

- Favorable response genotype: Approximately 70% chance for SVR after 48 weeks of treatment. Consider implications before initiating PEG-interferon alpha and ribavirin-containing regimens.
- Unfavorable response genotype: Approximately 30% chance of SVR after 48 weeks of treatment. Consider implications before initiating PEG-interferon alpha and ribavirin-containing regimens.

If protease inhibitors are combined with PEG-interferon alpha and ribavirin therapy, the CPIC recommendations for each genotype are [34]:

- Favorable response genotype: Approximately 90% chance for SVR after 24–48 weeks of treatment. Approximately 80–90% of patients are eligible for shortened therapy (24–28 weeks vs. 48 weeks). Weighs in favor of using PEG-interferon alpha and ribavirin-containing regimens.

– Unfavorable response genotype: Approximately 60% chance of SVR after 24–48 weeks of treatment. Approximately 50% of patients are eligible for shortened therapy regimens (24–28 weeks). Consider implications before initiating PEG-interferon alpha and ribavirin-containing regimens.

8   Conclusion

Pharmacogenomics has evolved exponentially within the last five years. Robust scientific evidence has boosted its clinical actionability, thus bringing it closer to the point of care, and the infectious disease space is not the exception. CPIC has led the effort by bringing closer together global field experts fostering scientific collaboration. The pharmacogenetic advances in the infectious disease space exponentially increase the safety and efficacy of treatments; 5–8% of patients will present a hypersensitivity reaction to abacavir; a broad standardization of pharmacogenetic testing could avoid it. In order to continue increasing the effectiveness and utility of pharmacogenetics in infectious diseases, scientific research needs to be more inclusive with different ethnic sub-group/populations. Also, it will be instrumental in including the genomic information of the pathogen and its implications. Ideally, in order to make this information fit into the clinical workflow smoothly, the pharmacogenetic components from both the host and the pathogen should be funneled into a precision prescribing solution: a comprehensive solution powered by artificial intelligence that takes into account the relevant data points that impact the patient treatment response hence outcome such as pharmacogenetic information from both the host and the pathogen, possible drug-drug interaction, other diagnoses and relevant comorbidities, kidney function, liver function, allergies, and social determinants of health.

References

1. Ganguly NK, Saha GK. Pharmacogenomics and personalized medicine for infectious diseases. Omics Personalized Med. 2013:603–635. https://doi.org/10.1007/978-81-322-1184-6_27
2. Krämer A, Akmatov M, Kretzschmar M. Principles of infectious disease epidemiology. Mod Infect Dis Epidemiol. 2009;28:85–99. https://doi.org/10.1007/978-0-387-93835-6_5.
3. Hayney MS. Pharmacogenomics and infectious diseases: impact on drug response and applications to disease management. Am J Health Syst Pharm. 2002;59(17):1626–31. https://doi.org/10.1093/ajhp/59.17.1626.
4. Kapila A, Chaudhary S, Sharma R, Vashist H, Sisodia S, Gupta A. A review on: HIV AIDS. Indian J Pharm Biol Res. 2016;4(3):69–73. https://doi.org/10.30750/ijpbr.4.3.9.
5. Mallal S, Phillips E, Carosi G, Molina JM, Workman C, Tomazic J, et al. HLA-B*5701 screening for hypersensitivity to abacavir. N Engl J Med. 2008;358(6):568–79. https://doi.org/10.1056/NEJMoa0706135.

6. Ren J, Bird LE, Chamberlain PP, Stewart-Jones GB, Stuart DI, Stammers DK. Structure of HIV-2 reverse transcriptase at 2.35-A resolution and the mechanism of resistance to non-nucleoside inhibitors. Proc Natl Acad Sci U S A. 2002;99(22):14410–14415. https://doi.org/10.1073/pnas.222366699

7. Whirl-Carrillo M, Huddart R, Gong L, Sangkuhl K, Thorn CF, Whaley R, et al. An evidence-based framework for evaluating pharmacogenomics knowledge for personalized medicine. Clin Pharmacol Ther. 2021;110(3):563–72. https://doi.org/10.1002/cpt.2350.

8. Whirl-Carrillo M, McDonagh EM, Hebert JM, Gong L, Sangkuhl K, Thorn CF, et al. Pharma-cogenomics knowledge for personalized medicine. Clin Pharmacol Ther. 2012;92(4):414–7. https://doi.org/10.1038/clpt.2012.96.

9. Wood R. Atazanavir: its role in HIV treatment. Expert Rev Anti Infect Ther. 2008;6(6):785–96. https://doi.org/10.1586/14787210.6.6.785.

10. Gammal RS, Court MH, Haidar CE, Iwuchukwu OF, Gaur AH, Alvarellos M, et al. Clinical pharmacogenetics implementation consortium (CPIC) guideline for UGT1A1 and atazanavir prescribing. Clin Pharmacol Ther. 2016;99(4):363–9. https://doi.org/10.1002/cpt.269.

11. National Center for Biotechnology Information. PubChem Compound Summary for CID 148192, Atazanavir PubChem2021. Available from: https://pubchem.ncbi.nlm.nih.gov/compound/Atazanavir. Accessed 11 Oct 2022.

12. Thoguluva Chandrasekar V, John S. Gilbert syndrome. Treasure Island, FL: StatPearls Pub-lishing; 2021. Available from: https://www.ncbi.nlm.nih.gov/books/NBK470200/. Accessed 11 Oct 2022.

13. Johnson AD, Kavousi M, Smith AV, Chen MH, Dehghan A, Aspelund T, et al. Genome-wide association meta-analysis for total serum bilirubin levels. Hum Mol Genet. 2009;18(14):2700–10. https://doi.org/10.1093/hmg/ddp202.

14. Bartlett MG, Gourley GR. Assessment of UGT polymorphisms and neonatal jaundice. Semin Perinatol. 2011;35(3):127–33. https://doi.org/10.1053/j.semperi.2011.02.006.

15. Sugatani J, Yamakawa K, Yoshinari K, Machida T, Takagi H, Mori M, et al. Identification of a defect in the UGT1A1 gene promoter and its association with hyperbilirubinemia. Biochem Biophys Res Commun. 2002;292(2):492–7. https://doi.org/10.1006/bbrc.2002.6683.

16. Michaud V, Ogburn E, Thong N, Aregbe AO, Quigg TC, Flockhart DA, et al. Induction of CYP2C19 and CYP3A activity following repeated administration of efavirenz in healthy volunteers. Clin Pharmacol Ther. 2012;91(3):475–82. https://doi.org/10.1038/clpt.2011.249.

17. Desta Z, Gammal RS, Gong L, Whirl-Carrillo M, Gaur AH, Sukasem C, et al. Clinical pharmacogenetics implementation consortium (CPIC) guideline for CYP2B6 and efavirenz-containing antiretroviral therapy. Clin Pharmacol Ther. 2019;106(4):726–33. https://doi.org/10.1002/cpt.1477.

18. Krause KM, Serio AW, Kane TR, Connolly LE. Aminoglycosides: an overview. Cold Spring Harb Perspect Med. 2016;6(6): a027029. https://doi.org/10.1101/cshperspect.a027029.

19. McDermott JH, Wolf J, Hoshitsuki K, Huddart R, Caudle KE, Whirl-Carrillo M, et al. Clinical pharmacogenetics implementation consortium guideline for the use of aminoglycosides based on MT-RNR1 genotype. Clin Pharmacol Ther. 2022;111(2):366–72. https://doi.org/10.1002/cpt.2309.

20. Mikulska M, Novelli A, Aversa F, Cesaro S, de Rosa FG, Girmenia C, et al. Voriconazole in clinical practice. J Chemother. 2012;24(6):311–27. https://doi.org/10.1179/1973947812Y.0000000051.

21. Moriyama B, Obeng AO, Barbarino J, Penzak SR, Henning SA, Scott SA, et al. Clinical phar-macogenetics implementation consortium (CPIC) guidelines for CYP2C19 and voriconazole therapy. Clin Pharmacol Ther. 2017;102(1):45–51. https://doi.org/10.1002/cpt.583.

22. Palumbo E. PEG-interferon in acute and chronic hepatitis C: a review. Am J Ther. 2009;16(6):573–8. https://doi.org/10.1097/MJT.0b013e3181960819.

23. Shah H, Bilodeau M, Burak KW, Cooper C, Klein M, Ramji A, et al. The management of chronic hepatitis C: 2018 guideline update from the Canadian Association for the study of the liver. CMAJ. 2018;190(22):E677–87. https://doi.org/10.1503/cmaj.170453.

24. Gonzalez-Grande R, Jimenez-Perez M, Gonzalez Arjona C, Mostazo TJ. New approaches in the treatment of hepatitis C. World J Gastroenterol. 2016;22(4):1421–32. https://doi.org/10. 3748/wjg.v22.i4.1421.
25. Lawitz E, Poordad F, Brainard DM, Hyland RH, An D, Dvory-Sobol H, et al. Sofosbuvir with peginterferon-ribavirin for 12 weeks in previously treated patients with hepatitis C genotype 2 or 3 and cirrhosis. Hepatology. 2015;61(3):769–75. https://doi.org/10.1002/hep.27567.
26. World Health Organization. Hepatitis C 2021. Available from: https://www.who.int/news-room/fact-sheets/detail/hepatitis-c. Accessed 11 Oct 2022.
27. van der Meer AJ, Veldt BJ, Feld JJ, Wedemeyer H, Dufour JF, Lammert F, et al. Association between sustained virological response and all-cause mortality among patients with chronic hepatitis C and advanced hepatic fibrosis. JAMA. 2012;308(24):2584–93. https://doi.org/10. 1001/jama.2012.144878.
28. Manns MP, McHutchison JG, Gordon SC, Rustgi VK, Shiffman M, Reindollar R, et al. Peginterferon alfa-2b plus ribavirin compared with interferon alfa-2b plus ribavirin for initial treatment of chronic hepatitis C: a randomised trial. Lancet. 2001;358(9286):958–65. https://doi.org/10.1016/s0140-6736(01)06102-5.
29. Hadziyannis SJ, Sette H Jr, Morgan TR, Balan V, Diago M, Marcellin P, et al. Peginterferon-alpha2a and ribavirin combination therapy in chronic hepatitis C: a randomized study of treatment duration and ribavirin dose. Ann Intern Med. 2004;140(5):346–55. https://doi.org/10.7326/0003-4819-140-5-200403020-00010.
30. Suppiah V, Moldovan M, Ahlenstiel G, Berg T, Weltman M, Abate ML, et al. IL28B is associated with response to chronic hepatitis C interferon-alpha and ribavirin therapy. Nat Genet. 2009;41(10):1100–4. https://doi.org/10.1038/ng.447.
31. Kotenko SV. IFN-lambdas. Curr Opin Immunol. 2011;23(5):583–90. https://doi.org/10.1016/j.coi.2011.07.007.
32. Stattermayer AF, Ferenci P. Effect of IL28B genotype on hepatitis B and C virus infection. Curr Opin Virol. 2015;14:50–5. https://doi.org/10.1016/j.coviro.2015.07.011.
33. Zhou H, Mohlenberg M, Terczynska-Dyla E, Winther KG, Hansen NH, Vad-Nielsen J, et al. The IFNL4 gene is a noncanonical interferon gene with a unique but evolutionarily conserved regulation. J Virol. 2020;94(5):e01535-e1619. https://doi.org/10.1128/JVI.01535-19.
34. Muir AJ, Gong L, Johnson SG, Lee MT, Williams MS, Klein TE, et al. Clinical Pharmacogenetics Implementation Consortium (CPIC) guidelines for IFNL3 (IL28B) genotype and PEG interferon-alpha-based regimens. Clin Pharmacol Ther. 2014;95(2):141–6. https://doi.org/10. 1038/clpt.2013.203.
35. Fischer J, Bohm S, Scholz M, Muller T, Witt H, George J, et al. Combined effects of different interleukin-28B gene variants on the outcome of dual combination therapy in chronic hepatitis C virus type 1 infection. Hepatology. 2012;55(6):1700–10. https://doi.org/10.1002/hep.25582.

Pharmacogenomics in Primary Care

Ghada Elnashar, Victor Tam, and Julie Ceno-England

Abstract

Primary care providers (PCP) are often the first healthcare professionals that patients will visit when they have a health concern or for routine preventative visits. The majority of primary care visits involve medication therapy, e.g., the initiation of a new prescription or the review and continuation of maintenance drug therapy. In prescribing medications, providers use many clinical factors such as age, weight, and renal function. PCP's can use pharmacogenomics (PGx) as another tool in their therapeutic decisions to help optimize patients' medications. The goals of PGx are to aid in the selection or dosing of drug therapy, reduce potential trial and error, help avoid possible adverse drug reactions (ADRs), and maximize potential drug efficacy. Germline PGx does not change over time. Thus, PCP's can use this valuable information over many visits for a multitude of conditions and medications. Obstacles that may exist to the use of PGx include lack of provider education, cost of the test, and the burden of additional workflow. Primary care physicians and clinical pharmacists can be collaborators which will help to overcome some of these obstacles and aid in the implementation and advancement of PGx. Clinical pharmacists can be PGx champions and partner with PCP's to bring the valuable knowledge of PGx into the clinic. Together, with these advancements in technology and available PGx resources, PCP's can make more informed decisions to help achieve optimal individualized patient care.

G. Elnashar · V. Tam · J. Ceno-England (✉)
OneOme LLC, Minneapolis, MN 55413, USA
e-mail: julieengland@oneome.com

G. Elnashar
e-mail: ghadaelnashar@oneome.com

V. Tam
e-mail: victortam@oneome.com

© The Author(s), under exclusive license to Springer Nature Switzerland AG 2023   289
D. Primorac et al. (eds.), *Pharmacogenomics in Clinical Practice*,
https://doi.org/10.1007/978-3-031-45903-0_16

Keywords

PGx in primary care • Germline PGx • PGx in comprehensive medication management • Resources for PGx • Precision medicine

1   Introduction

1.1   Why PGx is Valuable in Primary Care

Primary care clinicians can use this chapter as a starting point and reference for their education and to aid in the implementation of PGx into their practice. The goal of this chapter is to provide a quick reference to primary care providers who would like to get started using PGx and have a basic understanding. Learning objectives of this chapter are the following:

– provide the value behind PGx in primary care
– explain the basic molecular biology of PGx
– explain the benefits and limitations of PGx
– bring awareness to the freely available PGx educational resources
– describe lab considerations
– explain the benefits of collaborating with a clinical pharmacist
– describe what patients need to know.

The number of overall healthcare office visits involving a prescription are approximately 70% (1). The percentage of ambulatory office visits made to a primary care physician in the USA is over 50% and often much higher in other countries (2). The percent of drug mentions in primary care office visits is over 50% (3). Primary care providers prescribe a broad range of medications to their patients, and many patients are taking multiple medications. Although no consensus definition exists for polypharmacy, a widely accepted definition is the regular use of five or more medications (4). Polypharmacy increases a patient's risk of adverse drug events, drug–drug interactions, and may result in increased healthcare costs (5). Medication initiation and management is a large portion of what primary care providers oversee.

Pharmacogenomics (PGx) is the study of pharmacology and genetics/genomics, to aid in the selection of drug and drug doses that are likely to work for an individual patient (6). PGx has an emerging role to assist providers in their therapeutic strategies to help improve the safety and efficacy of medication use by their patients with the goal of an individualized approach. Evidence is present that PGx can help improve the safety and efficacy of medications commonly prescribed in primary care (7). Given these facts and that much prescribing takes place in primary care offices, it reasons that PGx is an important tool for primary care clinicians. In addition, genetic variants that may lead to an increased risk of ADRs and or failure of therapy are also common. The Mayo Clinic RIGHT study (8) and Vanderbilt Predict study (9) have shown over 90% of people carry at least one pharmacogene variant for a common medication. Therefore, there is opportunity for the utilization and implementation of PGx in the primacy care environment.

Primary care providers often treat their patients for multiple comorbidities over a long period of time. Thus, PGx results have longitudinal value in primary care as the germline DNA does not change. An important consideration to keep in mind for patients who have had hematopoietic or liver transplants is that results may be inconsistent or not applicable. If a patient fits one of these criteria, the clinical laboratory should be consulted prior to testing as the patient may be ineligible for PGx testing.

PGx testing may be utilized at the time the medication is considered or proactively when testing is completed ahead of any known future treatment. For example, a PGx test may be ordered to help in therapeutic strategy to select an antidepressant for a patient at the time the patient is diagnosed with major depression disorder. Furthermore, if that patient developed a cardiac or neurological condition, for example, PGx may also help in other therapeutic areas (refer to the "When and Who to Test" section of this chapter for further information). As mentioned above, many patients are on more than one medication and PGx can provide further insights on drug–gene interactions as well. A clinical pharmacist may help the team through a comprehensive medication management (CMM) review (please refer to the CMM section for further information). Physicians and pharmacists can be great collaborators in the implementation of PGx in the clinic. Pharmacists can provide great value to the provider regarding the addition of PGx to medication management. The clinical pharmacist is an expert in the therapeutic use of medications, and is qualified to advise the provider in the role of drug therapy (10). In addition, there exists a plethora of PGx resources and professional guidelines/guidance (e.g., FDA (5), CPIC (6), DPWG (7), PharmGKB (8)) that are easily accessible.

1.2   How Does PGx Work?

Pharmacogenomics, looks at genes that produce proteins that are involved in a drug's pharmacological action or metabolism. These are known as pharmacogenes. Pharmacogenes can be classified as pharmacokinetic (PK) or pharmacodynamic (PD). A PK gene is associated with the absorption, distribution, metabolism, and excretion of the drug. A PD pharmacogene influences how the target cells respond to the drug. These PD targets can be receptors, ion channels, or immune system components, among others (12).

Foundational Pharmacogenomic Definitions:

– Allele: One of two or more alternative forms in a gene
    Wild type: Refers to the natural form or reference form of the gene occurring in the majority of the population. Often referred to as "normal" due to the normal functional gene product that is predicted (13).

- Genetic variant: An individual change found in a person's genetic code. Also referred to as polymorphism (14).
- Germline: Refers to the DNA that is inheritable and derived from the reproductive cells. A germline variation may be passed from parent to offspring (15).
- Ultrarapid metabolizer: Increased enzyme activity compared to normal metabolizers (16).
- Rapid metabolizer: Increased enzyme activity compared to normal metabolizers but less than ultrarapid (16).
- Normal metabolizer: Fully functional enzyme activity, also known as an extensive metabolizer in some literature (16).
- Intermediate metabolizer: Decreased enzyme activity (activity between normal and poor metabolizer) (16).
- Poor metabolizer: Little to no enzyme activity (16).
- Prodrug: Is a medication that is inactive of its intended action until it undergoes transformation by the body via metabolism or chemical transformation into its pharmacologically active form (17). Example is codeine. Codeine is inactive when it enters the body and it depends on CYP2D6 to activate it into its analgesic form (18).
- Active ingredient: Is the ingredient that provides pharmacological activity (19).

Genetic variants can cause individuals to react differently to medications. Variants in pharmacogenes can cause an increase or decrease in the gene product. A pharmacogene known as *CYP2C19* produces a metabolizing enzyme. If patient A inherits a wild-type "normal" allele and patient B inherits a variant, the variant can lead to a change in the gene product. In this case example, the variant may cause an increase or decrease in the function of the metabolizing enzyme. If the variant in patient B causes an increased function of the CYP2C19 metabolizing enzyme, it has the potential to metabolize active medications faster for drugs that utilize this CYP2C19 enzyme pathway. Figure 16.1 shows a representation of such an example with the different serum concentration levels. Through advanced technology, these variants are now able to be genotyped in a relatively short period of time and relatively low cost via a saliva, buccal, or blood sample.

The clinical outcome of this is that patient B may have a decreased serum concentration of the drug potentially limiting their therapeutic response (20, 21).

1.3   Benefits and Limitations of PGx

Pharmacogenomics is an important tool that clinicians can use in their practice to make more informed decisions in their medication decisions. PGx can help to minimize harmful effects of medications and optimize medication response (22). It may also help decrease trial and error and contain medical costs (23, 6). Furthermore, PGx is helpful in complex medication problems and polypharmacy interactions.

Serum Concentrations

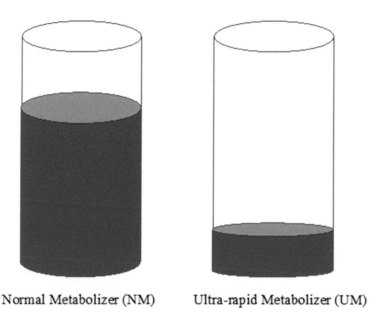

Normal Metabolizer (NM)   Ultra-rapid Metabolizer (UM)

Fig. 16.1 Representation of an example with the different serum concentration levels described above

Not all gene–drug interactions have the same level of evidence. Depending on the gene, allele and the medication, there are different degrees of severity and importance of information that PGx can provide. Since germline PGx results do not change over time, a broad panel germline PGx test can be ordered once and used repeatedly. Incorporating PGx information into an electronic health record (EHR) will help to ensure the results stay with the patient despite the fact that they may see multiple healthcare providers.

It is important to note that PGx alone is not a solution for all medication difficulties. Some medications are not clinically impacted by PGx, while others may have varying levels of evidence (LOE). PGx alone cannot explain lack of medication response or ADRs in all circumstances. Clinicians must also consider other clinical factors such as age, sex, renal function, and adherence. There are also laboratory considerations that will be addressed in the lab section of this chapter.

Adding PGx as another tool in therapeutic decision making helps to personalize treatment for patients. As the sciences advance, transcriptomics (mRNA), proteomics, epigenetics, and artificial intelligence and machine learning will be additional layers clinicians or scientists can build upon.

PGx should not be used in isolation and all other appropriate clinical factors (e.g., renal function, comorbidities, drug–drug interactions, drug–drug–gene interactions) should be taken into consideration.

The science of PGx continues to grow it is important to stay current as new information becomes available.

2 When and Who to Test

2.1 Pre-Emptive Versus Reactive

When should a patient get a PGx test? There are many factors to consider in this question. Clinical factors such as age, existing medical conditions, current medications, and family history are just a few examples of the complete picture the clinician must consider. The type of practice (concierge, community health, government run, etc.) and the cost of the test also needs to be considered as some insurance companies/government funding will not cover genetic testing. Single gene versus panel testing, medical necessity versus prevention are all considerations that must be made at the time of testing.

The difference between pre-emptive and reactive testing is as follows:

– Pre-emptive pharmacogenomic testing refers to having the patient's results available, at point of care, before the need/indication for the medication therapy is identified.
– Reactive pharmacogenomic testing indicates that the testing is performed when the need for the medication is realized.

Pre-emptive PGx testing is emerging as best practice as it helps to avoid delays in medication decisions (24). It guides decision making in real time, at point of care using a patient's genomic data. Many providers are asking how they can utilize this in their workflow and what clinical decision support tools exist. It is ideal to have PGx information loaded into the EHR so that the information can be utilized at the point of care and travel with the patient when the decision is made to initiate medication therapy. Clinical decision support (CDS) tools that alert providers when gene–drug interactions exist and give professional guidelines to support the provider in their clinical decisions and actionability are ideal but not without obstacles including significant information technology (IT) time and cost.

A case example of how PGx can be used reactively at the time of introducing a new medication and proactively in the future.

2.2 Behavioral/Mental Health Case Example

This case study will cover an example of reactive PGx testing in behavioral health while still being able to use the results prospectively for the future.

James is a 45-year-old male with a history of major depressive disorder (MDD) and generalized anxiety disorder (GAD). James is also a pack per day smoker. He has had a long history with MDD, spanning over the course of the last 10 years. James has tried a number of antidepressant treatments over these years. He had initially found some success at the start with fluoxetine, but found that it was becoming less effective. He has tried and failed a few different medications including bupropion, paroxetine, fluvoxamine, and venlafaxine—finding intermittent success but ultimately losing effectiveness with each one.

Chief Complaint (CC): Feeling down and hopeless.

Past Medical History (PMH):

Major depressive disorder

Generalized anxiety disorder

Tobacco abuse

Current Medications: venlafaxine

Background

The primary care provider recently learned about PGx and recalled that there is strong evidence for utilizing PGx testing in depression, as well as professional PGx guidelines for selective serotonin reuptake inhibitors (SSRIs). With James' current depression therapy not achieving efficacy and a long history of failing different antidepressants, the provider orders PGx testing as an additional tool to help with antidepressant selection and dosing.

At this time, the PCP orders a PGx consult to be co-managed by the clinical pharmacist on the care team. A broad-panel PGx test is ordered to aid in antidepressant selection and provide support for future conditions and medication selection. PGx testing is obtained and follow-up is scheduled in 2 weeks.

At the follow-up visit, PGx results are available for his providers to view. The clinical pharmacist notes that the strongest evidence from available data bases such as CPIC and DPWG for PGx in antidepressant use revolve around two genes: *CYP2C19* and *CYP2D6*. The results for these genes are presented in Table 16.1.

Table 16.1 Genotype and predicted phenotype

Gene/genotype	Phenotype	Expected activity/function of protein
CYP2C19 *1/*1	Normal Metabolizer	Normal enzyme activity
CYP2D6 *1 × 2/*2	Ultrarapid Metabolizer	Increased enzyme activity

Considerations

Professional PGx guidelines exist for this class of medications. Since the patient is an ultrarapid metabolizer, he may not be able to achieve therapeutic efficacy with a CYP2D6-associated antidepressant due to inadequate serum concentrations of the active medication. CYP2D6-associated antidepressants may be metabolized and inactivated too quickly. Many of the past antidepressant (fluoxetine, paroxetine, fluvoxamine, and venlafaxine) were all CYP2D6-associated medications. It is not a definitive conclusion that this was the reason for their failure, but it may have played a role.

Additionally, the results do not mean that the provider cannot or should not use a medication metabolized by an affected enzyme—the provider may have to adjust the dosage and/or monitor more closely. This can be referenced with appropriate information from drug labels and professional guidelines.

Action Plan

The provider decides to go with a CYP2C19 (normal metabolizer) metabolized medication—sertraline. Choosing an unaffected medication from the tested panel makes clinical sense. The provider is seeking to use genomics to individualize the medication choice due to the multiple failures the patient experienced.

Conclusion

PGx is one factor among many that assists prescribers in their therapeutic decision making. The patient does not have any known genetic variants at CYP2C19 (normal metabolizer) that may cause the medication to be metabolized at a faster or slower rate than expected. Standard dosing will be used in this case.

James Case Continued

Reason for visit: Follow-up on antidepressant therapy and hyperlipidemia

PMH:

Major depressive disorder

Generalized anxiety disorder

Tobacco abuse

Current Medications:

Sertraline

Table 16.2 Genotype and predicted phenotype

Gene/genotype	Phenotype	Expected activity/ function of protein
*SLCO1B1 *1/*5*	Decreased Function	Decreased transporter function

At the follow-up visit, the patient is feeling better and continues to stay on his treatment plan as directed. The patient is more confident with the treatment plan because of the reassurance from the PGx testing, and this also improves the confidence of the clinical team.

James is now willing to address health concerns from previous lab testing. Lab results show total cholesterol and low-density lipoprotein (LDL) were elevated. Based on his elevated cardiovascular risk score, the provider chooses to start a statin—using the appropriate treatment/PGx guidelines and algorithm.

Using the appropriate resources, the clinical pharmacist finds that the gene *SLCO1B1* encodes for a relevant transporter used in statin function. Depending on the function of this transporter, a patient may be at a higher risk for developing statin-related toxicities such as myalgias and myopathies when given a statin. The risk of statin-associated toxicity related to *SLCO1B1* varies by statin. The SLCO1B1 gene was also tested in the broad panel and is available in Table 16.2.

Considerations

James' SLCO1B1 has a phenotype of decreased function, which results in an increased risk of side effects. Referencing the clinical PGx guidelines, the clinical pharmacist chooses pravastatin as it has a smaller risk for statin-related toxicities than other statins such as simvastatin. There are other genes with emerging evidence for statin-associated toxicities that are currently being investigated.

Action Plan

The patient has decreased function of SLCO1B1. The provider decides to go with a SLCO1B1 transported medication with lower risk of toxicity—pravastatin.

Choosing a less PGx-affected statin medication makes clinical sense as the provider is seeking to use genomics in their clinical decision making to individualize the medication choice and reduce risk for toxicity.

Conclusion

This is an example of a PGx use case where the testing was initially done reactively—for antidepressant selection, but then also able to be used preemptively—for statin selection. The PCP and clinical pharmacist were able to utilize PGx knowledge. The patients' success resulted in more confidence of the treatment plan.

2.3   Pain Case Study

Jeff is a 60-year-old male and presents to the clinic for follow-up on chronic back pain. Decompression and lumbar fusion of L3-L5 six months ago and leg pain is gone but the low back pain is still present. The patient is requesting a new pain medication due to failed response to codeine. The provider suggests ordering PGx testing to help optimize pain management. A 1-week follow-up appointment is made to discuss the PGx results (Table 16.3).

CC: Low back pain

PMH: Chronic back pain secondary to spinal stenosis, former smoker

Current Medications: codeine

Considerations
There are various PGx guidelines as outlined in this chapter. For example, CPIC, DPWG, the FDA package label insert and so forth. In addition, there are CPIC guidelines for pain medications such as certain opioids and NSAIDs. Using the appropriate resources, the team discusses with the patient that being a poor metabolizer at CYP2D6 may result in an increased risk for lack of codeine efficacy. The patient is a normal metabolizer at CYP2C9, and according to the CPIC guidelines for NSAIDs, normal metabolism is predicted.

Key Points
The patient is a CYP2D6 poor metabolizer, which puts him at increased risk for lack of drug efficacy as this enzyme is required to activate codeine.

Also, due to this poor metabolizer status at CYP2D6, other medications that could be needed in the future are impacted.

Jeff agrees to a non-opioid pain medication so celecoxib is introduced.

Table 16.3 Genotype and predicted phenotype

Gene	Genotype	Predicted phenotype	Medication examples
CYP2D6	*3/*4	Poor metabolizer	Tramadol, codeine
CYP2C9	*1/*1	Normal metabolizer	Ibuprofen, celecoxib, meloxicam

3   Comprehensive Medication Management and Complex PGx Cases

3.1   Comprehensive Medication Management and PGx

Comprehensive medication management (CMM) is utilized by clinical pharmacists with the end goal of reviewing all medications (including supplements, non-prescriptions, etc.) to evaluate its indication, effectiveness, safety, and convenience for the patient (26). This is an interdisciplinary team effort, where clinical pharmacists work with the provider, patient, and other appropriate clinical team members. In the United States, the clinical pharmacist usually performs CMM under a collaborative practice agreement (CPA), which varies depending on the institution and state (28). For example, a clinical pharmacist may be permitted to initiate, change, and/or discontinue a medication within the scope of the CPA (26, 27).

CMM is a well-defined process that includes assessment tools to be utilized on all patients. Furthermore, incorporating CMM into practice may help achieve what is known as the quadruple aim: improved clinical outcomes, patient satisfaction, reduced total cost of care, provider well-being (26, 29).

PGx is an integral part of the clinical picture. It provides a more personalized approach as opposed to a "one size fits all," which may help provide additional insight into the overall CMM process.

Utilization of PGx testing through the CMM process is an important factor. Creatinine clearance (CrCl), one clinical factor, is used for many reasons, including determining appropriate dosing of a particular medication. Similarly, knowing if one is a potential poor metabolizer at CYP2D6 may help in understanding the associated risks and implications of the gene–drug interaction. Furthermore, knowledge of being a normal metabolizer at CYP2D6, for example, is equally as important. A phenomenon known as phenoconversion may convert a genotypic normal metabolizer into a phenotypic poor metabolizer of a drug (30). Hence, the predicted drug metabolism based on the genotype does not match with the clinically observed phenotypic metabolizer status (31, 32). There are various reasons this could happen, including drug–drug–gene interactions. The following are some examples illustrating this phenomenon:

Example 1

Fluoxetine is a strong CYP2D6 inhibitor. Per the FDA package insert for fluoxetine: "Fluoxetine inhibits the activity of CYP2D6, and may make individuals with normal CYP2D6 metabolic activity resemble a poor metabolizer." Please refer to the appropriate drug package insert accordingly for more information (33).

Example 2 (34, 35)

clopidogrel + omeprazole (Avoid X)

The following is similar to an example referenced above (34).

Patient is *CYP2C19 *1/*2* genotypically, which may have a predicted phenotype of Intermediate Metabolizer. If taking clopidogrel (a prodrug), this may result in a drug–gene interaction (clopidogrel—CYP2C19), which may have a reduced clopidogrel efficacy (see Boxed Warning on the FDA label for more information). However, if considering omeprazole (a CYP2C19 inhibitor), this may result in a drug–drug–gene interaction and result in a phenoconversion (a clinical observed phenotype of a poor metabolizer). It is important to note that the FDA label for clopidogrel warns against the concomitant use of clopidogrel and omeprazole together (refer to the FDA package label for more information) (36).

By combining both CMM and PGx, it provides an opportunity for finding potential drug–drug–gene interactions. Collaborating and working together as a team is essential. An interprofessional collaboration together with the patient helps capture potential polypharmacy risks (e.g., drug–drug–gene interactions, phenoconversion). In addition to working as a team, stakeholder acceptance is crucial for the implementation of PGx into a CMM care model.

An alternative approach is to start the combined PGx–CMM strategy in specific populations. For example, clinicians may want to start in the oncology field or mental health field depending on what aligns with their clinical goals (27).

Education is an additional key component. Sometimes, lack of education or knowledge of PGx may hinder the implementation of PGx into practice. Thus, it is important to provide the appropriate and necessary education to increase clinician engagement. There are a variety of resources available that can help one start, e.g., PharmGKB, CPIC, DPWG, etc.

The field is moving toward a pre-emptive testing approach versus a reactive testing approach. More specifically, shifting from a reactive (meaning one has tried and failed certain medication(s) and now trying PGx testing) to pre-emptive (testing before giving a medication). It is crucial to remember that pharmacogenomics is one part of the clinical picture and it should not be used in isolation. Furthermore, utilization of advanced clinical decision support systems (CDSS) may be helpful to clinicians, especially when each institution may have its own standard policies and procedures (37).

3.2   Polypharmacy PGx Case Study

A 52-year-old female presents to the clinic with muscle pain and also states that she is not receiving adequate pain control for her leg and back. Her clinic visit today is with a CMM clinical pharmacist, who is working under a CPA with the PCP.

CC: Muscle pain and not receiving adequate pain control for leg and back pain

PMH: MDD, pain, diabetes, hypertension (HTN), hypercholesterolemia, gastroesophageal reflux disease (GERD)

Table 16.4 Genotype and predicted phenotype

Gene	Genotype	Predicted phenotype	Medication examples
CYP2D6	*3/*4	Poor metabolizer	Tramadol, codeine
CYP2C9	*1/*1	Normal metabolizer	Ibuprofen, celecoxib
CYP2C19	*1/*1	Normal metabolizer	Sertraline, citalopram, escitalopram
SLCO1B1	*5/*5	Poor function, Homozygous variant	Simvastatin

Current Medications:

Sertraline

Tramadol

Metformin

Insulin glargine

Insulin aspart

Simvastatin (40 mg)

Lisinopril

Considerations
The team review's the PGx results (Table 16.4) and references the appropriate PGx guidelines. Further, they take all other clinical factors, including appropriate revision of medical charts. They note the appropriate PGx-related information. CPIC is used below as an example:

Current Relevant Medications

Tramadol
CPIC Example PGx Guidelines (38)

- CYP2D6 Poor Metabolizer—Greatly reduced O-desmethyltramadol (active metabolite) formation leading to diminished analgesia. Avoid tramadol use because of possibility of diminished analgesia. If opioid use is warranted, consider a non-codeine opioid.

Sertraline
CPIC Example PGx Guidelines (39)

- CYP2C19 Normal Metabolizer—"Initiate therapy with recommended starting dose."

Simvastatin
CPIC Example PGx Guidelines (40)

- SLCO1B1 Poor function—High myopathy risk. Prescribe a lower dose or consider an alternative statin (e.g., pravastatin or rosuvastatin); consider routine creatine kinase (CK) surveillance.

Future Medications
Ibuprofen Example PGx Guidelines (41)

- CYP2C9 NM—Normal metabolism. Initiate therapy with recommended starting dose. In accordance with the prescribing information, use the lowest effective dosage for shortest duration consistent with individual patient treatment goals.

Action Plan/Key Points
The clinical team decides that based on the historical and current data the following would be next steps:

- Patient is a CYP2D6 poor metabolizer. Knowing she is a poor metabolizer at CYP2D6 puts her at increased risk for lack of drug efficacy as this enzyme is required to activate tramadol. STOP tramadol due to potential lack of efficacy.
- Patient has a predicted normal metabolism at CYP2C9 and it is associated with certain NSAIDs like ibuprofen. START ibuprofen PRN
- Patient reports experiencing muscle pain. SLCO1B1 poor function is predicted, which may potentially increase risk of muscle myopathy. PCP also wanted to provide an alternative that is equivalent to a moderate intensity statin per the AHA/ACC guidelines. STOP simvastatin 40 mg duo to muscle pain. START pravastatin 40 mg (Note: Since new evidence continues to emerge, the most up to date information must be referenced).

Screening for drug–drug interactions the team plans to monitor therapy. PCP follows up in 2 weeks with the patient. Patient reports no muscle pain and back pain has significantly reduced.

3.3   Oncology/Supportive Care Case Study

Many patients in primary care may go through cancer treatment and will likely have a team of specialists including an oncologist. Patients will rely on their PCP for support throughout the process. The medical oncologist can use germline PGx to help them in their selection of certain chemotherapy medications to help avoid toxicity. A PCP can add value to the care of an oncology patient by helping in other areas that oncology patients are affected by. With the long-term relationship that many patients have with their PCP's, they may turn to them for help with the anxiety or depression they are suffering or from or the unrelenting nausea that they are experiencing. Germline PGx can be valuable to both the oncologist and PCP when these problems arise for a patient during their cancer journey.

Introduction
Chloe is a 19-year-old female.

Diagnosis: Acute lymphoblastic leukemia (ALL), pre-bone marrow transplant (BMT), and presents to the emergency room (ER) with fever and cough. Patient admitted to hospital; workup reveals fungal pneumonia.

The team is consulted and they treat her with IV voriconazole. She also has severe nausea and vomiting (N&V) and ondansetron was given. The patient is not responding to ondansetron.

CC: Severe N&V (Not responding to ondansetron)

PMH: ALL, depression, anxiety

Current medications:

voriconazole iv

ondansetron

The CMM clinical pharmacist on the team recalled she had a PGx testing (Table 16.5) completed as part of her pre-transplant workup.

Considerations
The team review's Chloe's PGx results and references the appropriate PGx guidelines. As per CPIC, an ultrarapid metabolizer at CYP2D6 may result in increased

Table 16.5 Genotype and predicted phenotype

Gene	Genotype	Predicted phenotype	Medication examples
CYP2D6	*1/*1 × 2	Ultrarapid Metabolizer	Ondansetron
CYP2C19	*1/*1	Normal Metabolizer	Voriconazole

metabolism and therefore a potential decreased response to ondansetron. Hence, CPIC suggests an alternative drug not predominantly metabolized by CYP2D6 (e.g., granisetron). Of course, drug–drug interactions and other patient characteristics (e.g., age, renal function, and liver function) should be considered when selecting alternative therapy. CPIC is illustrated below as an example:

Ondansetron
CPIC Example PGx Guidelines (43)

- CYP2D6 Ultrarapid Metabolizer—Increased metabolism to less active compounds when compared to normal metabolizers and is associated with decreased response to ondansetron and tropisetron (i.e., vomiting). Select an alternative drug not predominantly metabolized by CYP2D6 (i.e., granisetron). Consideration for alternative 5-HT3 receptor antagonists antiemetics: Dolasetron, palonosetron, and ramosetron are also metabolized by CYP2D6. Limited evidence is available regarding the utilization of CYP2D6 genetic variation to guide use of these drugs. Drug–drug interactions and other patient characteristics (e.g., age, renal function, and liver function) should be considered when selecting alternative therapy.

Voriconazole
CPIC Example PGx Guidelines (44)

- CYP2C19 Normal Metabolizer—Normal voriconazole metabolism. For pediatric or adult patients: initiate therapy with recommended standard of care dosing. Further dose adjustments or selection of alternative therapy may be necessary due to other clinical factors, such as drug interactions, hepatic function, renal function, species, site of infection, TDM, and comorbidities.

Key Points
The team decides that based on the patient's historical and current data the following would be next steps:

- Voriconazole: Initiate therapy with recommended standard of care dosing.
- Ondansetron: Select an alternative drug not predominantly metabolized by CYP2D6; decided to use granisetron.

All other patient and clinical characteristics were taken into consideration prior to selecting an alternative.

With the granisetron Chloe's N/V symptoms improved. Within 48–72 h the fever and cough improved.

PGx results can be utilized in a variety of settings, such as with a PCP who can utilize it from a PGx perspective for depression/anxiety considerations.

4   PGx Considerations, Education, and Resources

4.1   Lab Considerations

One of the most important factors to consider is lab credentials. In the United States, laboratories that are doing high complexity molecular testing should be CAP accredited (College of American Pathologists) and CLIA (Clinical Laboratory Improvement Amendments) certified by the Center for Medicare and Medicaid Services (CMS) to ensure the highest quality of standards and quality review (45). Equivalent recognition with proper lab credentials and certification may differ in each country.

A second factor to consider is the genes and alleles that the PGx lab tests. The genes and variants included would optimally have high levels of evidence and clinical actionability. Understanding the gene and allele coverage is important for the treating team. If a patient has a variant that is not tested for this will not be captured on the report. In such a scenario, it may default as the wild type (example: *1) or the nomenclature that is most often seen in the population. The Association for Molecular Pathology (AMP) has released several guidelines (46) for commonly tested for PGx genes that guide in the identification of the minimum set of alleles that should be included on a test panel.

Important questions, especially from the patient perspective are as follows:

– How will the test be obtained?
– Does it require a blood draw or sample through saliva or buccal swab can be performed?
– What is the cost of the test?
– Does the patient's insurance or government health system cover the cost of the test or does the patient have to pay out of pocket?
– What is the turnaround time for the test?

Other factors to consider from the primary care providers perspective include delivery of the report and turnaround time.

– Will a PCP utilize a website outside of the clinic or health system?
– Will a PCP access a PDF or does EHR have integration capabilities to order and see the report through the EHR?
– With current workflow will the turnaround time be feasible?

These answers will depend on the clinical reason for testing the patient and the accepted time frame of treatment.

Lastly, additional questions to ask are what type of support does the lab offer? Do they offer live customer service, educational or clinical support? Do other support tools exist?

Secondary Findings

Genetic test results provide information about changes (variants) in a gene unrelated to the primary purpose for the testing but may be medically actionable (47).

4.2   Pharmacogenomics Education and Resources

Clinician Education

This section covers examples of available PGx resources. These resources may be used to help guide and facilitate treatment strategy when using PGx. They can offer insight into how to interpret patient's PGx test into an actionable clinical plan. Available resources for guidelines and education in PGx will be covered and how to stay on top of relevant developments in the PGx field.

PharmGKB, FDA label, FDA Table of Pharmacogenetic Associations, CPIC, DPWG, PGx Certification Courses

When looking at available resources, focus on guidelines gives clinically actionable decisions that are supported by strong evidence. A starting point may be to look for PGx information or guidelines for a medication of interest. For that given medication, start by looking into the drug label or package insert for that medication. Similar to how providers may use the label for indication, dosage, warnings, and contraindications—relevant PGx information may be found here. The label may offer recommendations or insight into whether testing may be required, how dosing might be changed with different genetic results, or any findings from the manufacturer about relevant gene–drug interactions or drug–drug–gene interactions. Depending on nation's governing body in drug usage, these recommendations may be different. However, it is still important to keep in mind regulatory and governing body recommendations in addition to utilizing clinical judgment.

Another resource is clinical guidelines which are prepared by workgroups of distinguished and practicing providers in the field of interest. Similar to other areas of medicine, these guidelines provide recommendations on clinical actionability and how to develop treatment plans utilizing the testing. In PGx, there are a number of different professional organizations that work to provide guidance utilizing results from PGx testing (Table 16.6). Most in the PGx field will be familiar with Clinical Pharmacogenetics Implementation Consortium (CPIC) and Dutch Pharmacogenetics Working Group (DPWG). CPIC is a working group of clinicians based out of St. Jude Hospital in the USA and DPWG is based out of the Netherlands. Depending on the location, one of these groups may carry more weight than the other. Nonetheless, providers should consider all appropriate factors and guidelines.

Table 16.6 PGx resources

Resource name	Resource description	Resource URL
FDA Label	Manufacturer information submitted to the FDA	https://labels.fda.gov/
FDA Table of Pharmacogenetic Associations	FDA Recognized PGx associations	https://www.fda.gov/medical-devices/precision-medicine/table-pharmacogeneticPharma cogenetics-associations
EMA European Public Assessment Report	Medication info provided by the EMA	https://www.ema.europa.cu/en/medicines
Health Canada Label	Medication info provided by Health Canada	https://www.canada.ca/en/health-canada/services/drugs-health-products.html
CPIC	Professional PGx guidelines and info	https://cpicpgx.org/
DPWG	Professional PGx guidelines and info	https://upgx.eu/guidelines/
PharmGKB	PGx resource collection of guidelines, labels, and more	https://www.pharmgkb.org/

The Pharmacogenomics Knowledge Base (PharmGKB) is a great resource that houses and summarizes much of the available literature surrounding pharmacogenomics. It is funded by the National Institutes of Health in the United States and managed at Stanford University. On their website (PharmGKB.org), medication specific PGx information such as drug labels annotated for PGx information, clinical PGx guidelines for gene–drug associations, PGx literature with annotations for gene-specific results, and metabolism pathways can be found. They also provide some gene-specific information such as allele definitions, allele functionalities, population-based allele frequencies, and diplotype-phenotype conversions.

As noted above, different PGx resource organizations may define their levels of evidence (LOE) differently, so be sure to check their definitions and criteria for evidence.

Some academic institutions and pharmacy schools/organizations offer PGx courses to become certified. These often are allowed to be taken at the attendee's own pace and offer continuing medical education credits. In recent years, many webinars and conferences are also available to advance clinician knowledge of pharmacogenomics and address many topics such as evidence review, clinical actionability, and implementation. Interested clinicians can also join organizations such as CPIC, and Standardizing Laboratory Practices in Pharmacogenomics (STRIPE) where they have regular scheduled meetings and bring key stakeholders together.

4.3   Patient Education

Educating and obtaining a patient's informed consent prior to PGx testing is the ethical obligation of the ordering provider. It is the role of the clinician to explain to the patient why the test is ordered and how the information will be used. Demystifying genetic testing is very important when it comes to educating a patient. Without setting the correct expectations, patients can mistakenly believe that PGx is the sole factor when it comes to what medications are best for them. Level setting the patient with proper expectations from the beginning will help establish trust and avoid frustrations. There are some patient friendly resources that may help with expectations (6). It is important for patient to understand that PGx is one piece of the medication response equation. In addition, the information will not be used in isolation, but all clinical factors must be considered. It is important that providers consider secondary findings or variants of uncertain significance when performing genetic testing. Clinicians must be prepared to answer questions of how this may impact patients' family members. Utilizing a genetic counselor is an appropriate solution in this situation.

5   Final Discussion on PGx Adoption in Primary Care

Genetics rules and regulations

Laws and regulations around genetic testing vary from country to country (and even state to state) is beyond the scope of this chapter. It is important to be familiar with the governing rules around genetic testing and data privacy of the country or state in which the clinician practices. It is critical to know how the lab is handling the patient samples. Do they biobank the samples; do they sell data to third parties; are they compliant in the data protection laws of your country?

Lastly, it is important to also keep in mind that cultural attitudes may play a role in whether patients will opt in or out of genetic testing. Certain cultures were more likely to believe that genetic test results could lead to discrimination or to interfere with the natural order of things (48).

How to implement PGx into practice

Primary care clinicians have a great opportunity to adopt and utilize PGx into their practice. It has the potential to optimize medication dosing and selection through individuals' genomic data to improve the efficacy of medications as well as avoiding potential ADRs. Depending on practice, clinicians can start with a single therapeutic area such as behavioral/mental health or pain management, for example. The PCP together with a clinical pharmacist can begin by collaborating through a comprehensive medication management process that addresses polypharmacy. With resources available such as CPIC, DPWG, and PharmGKB, it brings freely available evidence-based knowledge with clinical actionability. PGx can benefit patients in primary care and many other specialties with the potential to have more precise prescribing and reduced overall healthcare costs.

References

1. Centers for Disease Control and Prevention. National Center for Health Statistics. Health Care and Insurance. Therapeutic Drug Use. Available from: https://www.cdc.gov/nchs/fastats/drug-use-therapeutic.htm. Accessed 07 Oct 2021.
2. Centers for Disease Control and Prevention. National Center for Health Statistics. Ambulatory and Hospital Care. Ambulatory Care Use and Physician office visits. Available from: https://www.cdc.gov/nchs/fastats/physician-visits.htm. Accessed 07 Oct 2021.
3. Rui P, Okeyode T. National ambulatory medical care survey: 2016 national summary tables. Available from: https://www.cdc.gov/nchs/data/ahcd/namcs_summary/2016_namcs_web tab les.pdf. Accessed 07 Oct 2021.
4. Halli-Tierney AD, Scarbrough C, Carroll D. Polypharmacy: evaluating risks and deprescribing. Am Fam Phys. 2019;100(1):32–8.
5. Maher RL, Hanlon J, Hajjar ER. Clinical consequences of polypharmacy in elderly. Expert Opin Drug Saf. 2014;13(1):57–65. https://doi.org/10.1517/14740338.2013.827660.
6. National Human Genome Research Institute. Pharmacogenomics FAQ. Available from: https://www.genome.gov/FAQ/Pharmacogenomics. Accessed 18 Nov 2021.
7. Krebs K, Milani L. Translating pharmacogenomics into clinical decisions: do not let the perfect be the enemy of the good. Hum Genomics. 2019;13(1):39. https://doi.org/10.1186/s40246-019-0229-z.
8. Ji Y, Skierka JM, Blommel JH, Moore BE, VanCuyk DL, Bruflat JK, et al. Preemptive pharmacogenomic testing for precision medicine: a comprehensive analysis of five actionable pharmacogenomic genes using next-generation DNA sequencing and a customized CYP2D6 genotyping cascade. Mol Diagn. 2016;18(3):438–45. https://doi.org/10.1016/j.jmoldx.2016.01.003.
9. Van Driest SL, Shi Y, Bowton EA, Schildcrout JS, Peterson JF, Pulley J, et al. Clinically actionable genotypes among 10,000 patients with preemptive pharmacogenomic testing. Clin Pharmacol Ther. 2014;95(4):423–31. https://doi.org/10.1038/clpt.2013.229.
10. American College of Clinical Pharmacy. The definition of clinical pharmacy. Pharmacotherapy. 2008;28(6):816–7. https://doi.org/10.1592/phco.28.6.816.
11. Clancy S, Brown W. Translation: DNA to mRNA to protein. Nat Educ. 2008;1(1):101.
12. Adams J. Pharmacogenomics and personalized medicine. Nat Educ. 2008;1(1):194.
13. Kalman LV, Agúndez JA, Appell ML, Black JL, Bell GC, Boukouvala S, et al. Pharmacogenetic allele nomenclature: international workgroup recommendations for test result reporting. Clin Pharmacol Ther. 2016;99(2):172–85. https://doi.org/10.1002/cpt.280.
14. PharmGKB. Pharmacogenomics glossary. Available from: https://www.pharmgkb.org/page/glossary. Accessed 18 Nov 2021.
15. National Human Genome Research Institute. Talking glossary of genetic terms. Germ Line. Available from: https://www.genome.gov/genetics-glossary/germ-line. Accessed 18 Nov 2021.
16. Caudle KE, Dunnenberger HM, Freimuth RR, Peterson JF, Burlison JD, Whirl-Carrillo M, et al. Standardizing terms for clinical pharmacogenetic test results: consensus terms from the Clinical Pharmacogenetics Implementation Consortium (CPIC). Genet Med. 2017;19(2):215–23. https://doi.org/10.1038/gim.2016.87.
17. Wu KM. A new classification of prodrugs: regulatory perspectives. Pharmaceuticals (Basel). 2009;2(3):77–81. https://doi.org/10.3390/ph2030077.
18. Smith HS. Opioid metabolism. Mayo Clin Proc. 2009;84(7):613–24. https://doi.org/10.1016/S0025-6196(11)60750-7.
19. U.S. Food & Drug Administration. Drugs@FDA Glossary of Terms. Available from: https://www.fda.gov/drugs/drug-approvals-and-databases/drugsfda-glossary-terms. Accessed 18 Nov 2021.

20. Sim SC, Ingelman-Sundberg M. The Human Cytochrome P450 (CYP) Allele Nomenclature website: a peer-reviewed database of CYP variants and their associated effects. Hum Genomics. 2010;4(4):278–81. https://doi.org/10.1186/1479-7364-4-4-278.
21. Belle DJ, Singh H. Genetic factors in drug metabolism. Am Fam Phys. 2008;77(11):1553–60.
22. Weinshilboum RM, Wang L. Pharmacogenomics: precision medicine and drug response. Mayo Clin Proc. 2017;92(11):1711–22. https://doi.org/10.1016/j.mayocp.2017.09.001.
23. Verbelen M, Weale ME, Lewis CM. Cost-effectiveness of pharmacogenetic-guided treatment: are we there yet? Pharmacogenomics J. 2017;17(5):395–402. https://doi.org/10.1038/tpj.2017.21.
24. Nicholson WT, Formea CM, Matey ET, Wright JA, Giri J, Moyer AM. Considerations when applying pharmacogenomics to your practice. Mayo Clin Proc. 2021;96(1):218–30. https://doi.org/10.1016/j.mayocp.2020.03.011.
25. Weitzel KW, Cavallari LH, Lesko LJ. Preemptive panel-based pharmacogenetic testing: the time is now. Pharm Res. 2017;34(8):1551–5. https://doi.org/10.1007/s11095-017-2163-x.
26. McFarland MS, Finks SW, Smith L, Buck ML, Ourth H, Brummel A. Am Health Drug Benefits. 2021;14(3):111–4.
27. Bingham JM, Michaud V, Wiisanen K, Bates J, Morreale AP, Empey PE, et al. Outcomes through the integration of pharmacogenomic testing into comprehensive medication management care models. J Precis Med. 2021;7(3):28–37.
28. McInnis T, et al., editors. The patient-centered medical home: integrating comprehensive medication management to optimize patient outcomes. 2nd ed. PCPCC Medication Management Task Force collaborative document.
29. Funk KA, Pestka DL, McClurg MT, Carroll JK, Sorensen TD. Primary care providers believe that comprehensive medication management improves their work-life. Am Board Fam Med. 2019;32(4):462–73. https://doi.org/10.3122/jabfm.2019.04.180376.
30. Shah RR, Smith RL. Addressing phenoconversion: the Achilles' heel of personalized medicine. Br J Clin Pharmacol. 2015;79(2):222–40. https://doi.org/10.1111/bcp.12441.
31. Klomp SD, Manson ML, Guchelaar HJ, Swen JJ. Phenoconversion of cytochrome P450 metabolism: a systematic review. J Clin Med. 2020;9(9):2890. https://doi.org/10.3390/jcm9092890.
32. Abubakar A, Bentley O. Precision medicine and pharmacogenomics in community and primary care settings. Pharm Today. 2018;24(2):55–68.
33. U.S. Food & Drug Administration. Drugs @FDA: FDA-Approved Drugs. fluoxetine drug label. Accessed Oct 2021. Available from: https://www.accessdata.fda.gov/drugsatfda_docs/label/2021/018936s111lbl.pdf
34. Westervelt P, Cho K, Bright DR, Kisor DF. Drug–gene interactions: inherent variability in drug maintenance dose requirements. P T. 2014;39(9):630–7.
35. Malki MA, Pearson ER. Drug–drug–gene interactions and adverse drug reactions. Pharmacogenomics J. 2020;20(3):355–66. https://doi.org/10.1038/s41397-019-0122-0.
36. U.S. Food & Drug Administration. Drugs @FDA: FDA-Approved Drugs. clopidogrel bisulfate drug label. Available from: https://www.accessdata.fda.gov/drugsatfda_docs/label/2021/020839s074lbl.pdf. Accessed Oct 2021.
37. Turgeon J, Michaud V. Clinical decision support systems: great promises for better management of patients' drug therapy [published correction appears in Expert Opin Drug Metab Toxicol. 2016;12(9):iii]. Expert Opin Drug Metab Toxicol. 2016;12(9):993–995. https://doi.org/10.1517/17425255.2016.1171317
38. Crews KR, Monte AA, Huddart R, Caudle KE, Kharasch ED, Gaedigk A, et al. Clinical Pharmacogenetics Implementation Consortium guideline for CYP2D6, OPRM1, and COMT genotypes and select opioid therapy. Clin Pharmacol Ther. 2021;110(4):888–96. https://doi.org/10.1002/cpt.2149.
39. Hicks JK, Bishop JR, Sangkuhl K, Müller DJ, Ji Y, Leckband SG, et al. Clinical Pharmacogenetics Implementation Consortium (CPIC) guideline for CYP2D6 and CYP2C19 genotypes and dosing of selective serotonin reuptake inhibitors. Clin Pharmacol Ther. 2015;98(2):127–34. https://doi.org/10.1002/cpt.147.

40. Ramsey LB, Johnson SG, Caudle KE, Haidar CE, Voora D, Wilke RA, Maxwell WD, McLeod HL, Krauss RM, Roden DM, Feng Q. The clinical pharmacogenetics implementation consortium guideline for SLCO1B1 and simvastatin-induced myopathy: 2014 update. Clin Pharmacol Ther. 2014;96(4):423–8. https://doi.org/10.1038/clpt.2014.125.
41. Theken KN, Lee CR, Gong L, Caudle KE, Formea CM, Gaedigk A, Klein TE, Agúndez JA, Grosser T. Clinical Pharmacogenetics Implementation Consortium Guideline (CPIC) for CYP2C9 and nonsteroidal anti-inflammatory drugs. Clin Pharmacol Ther. 2020;108(2):191–200. https://doi.org/10.1002/cpt.1830.
42. Grundy SM, Stone NJ, Bailey AL, Beam C, Birtcher KK, Blumenthal RS, et al. AHA/ACC/AACVPR/AAPA/ABC/ACPM/ADA/AGS/APhA/ASPC/NLA/PCNA guideline on the management of blood cholesterol: a report of the American College of Cardiology/American Heart Association Task Force on Clinical Practice Guidelines. J Am Coll Cardiol. 2019;73(24):3168–209. https://doi.org/10.1016/j.jacc.2018.11.002.
43. Hicks JK, Bishop JR, Sangkuhl K, Müller DJ, Ji Y, Leckband SG, Leeder JS, Graham RL, Chiulli DL, LLerena A, Skaar TC. Clinical Pharmacogenetics Implementation Consortium (CPIC) guideline for CYP2D6 and CYP2C19 genotypes and dosing of selective serotonin reuptake inhibitors. Clin Pharmacol Ther. 2015;98(2):127–134. https://doi.org/10.1002/cpt.147
44. Moriyama B, Obeng AO, Barbarino J, Penzak SR, Henning SA, Scott SA, Agúndez JA, Wingard JR, McLeod HL, Klein TE, Cross SJ. Clinical Pharmacogenetics Implementation Consortium (CPIC) guidelines for CYP2C19 and voriconazole therapy. Clin Pharmacol Ther. 2017;102(1):45–51. https://doi.org/10.1002/cpt.583.
45. College of American Pathologists. Laboratory Accreditation. Available from: https://www.cap.org/laboratory-improvement/accreditation/laboratory-accreditation-program. Accessed 18 Nov 2021.
46. Association for Molecular Pathology. Available from: https://www.amp.org/clinical-practice/practice-guidelines/. Accessed 22 Nov 2021.
47. Kalia SS, Adelman K, Bale SJ, Chung WK, Eng C, Evans JP, et al. Recommendations for reporting of secondary findings in clinical exome and genome sequencing, 2016 update (ACMG SF v2.0): a policy statement of the American College of Medical Genetics and Genomics. Genet Med. 2017;19(2):249–255. https://doi.org/10.1038/gim.2016.190
48. Hann KE, Freeman M, Fraser L, Waller J, Sanderson SC, Rahman B, et al. Awareness, knowledge, perceptions, and attitudes towards genetic testing for cancer risk among ethnic minority groups: a systematic review. BMC Public Health. 2017;17(1):503. https://doi.org/10.1186/s12889-017-4375-8.

Pharmacogenomics and Big Data

Dragan Primorac, Lidija Bach-Rojecky, Petar Brlek, and Vedrana Škaro

Abstract

The advancement of new technologies has been one of the crucial drivers for precision medicine implementation in practice. Pharmacogenomics (PGx) can improve patient outcomes by using a patient's genetic profile to optimize the selection and efficacy of drug therapy and reduce the likelihood of adverse drug reactions. When linked to electronic health record data, genomic approaches provide valuable information needed for more detailed understandings of diseases, discovering and prioritizing potential drug targets, predicting side effects, data mining for unknown drug effects, repurposing medications, and accelerating PGx. However, PGx studies generate a large amount of information ("big data") and are associated with some challenges. They include data collection and processing, data storage, and results interpretation and their clinical implementation, which includes search, sharing, transfer, visualization, querying, updating information privacy, and data source. Artificial intelligence (AI) is

D. Primorac (✉) · P. Brlek
St. Catherine Specialty Hospital, Zagreb, Croatia
e-mail: dragan.primorac@svkatarina.hr; draganprimorac2@gmail.com

P. Brlek
e-mail: petar.brlek@svkatarina.hr

D. Primorac
University of Split School of Medicine, Split, Croatia

Josip Juraj Strossmayer University of Osijek Faculty of Medicine, Osijek, Croatia

University of Rijeka School of Medicine, Rijeka, Croatia

Josip Juraj Strossmayer University of Osijek Faculty of Dental Medicine and Health, Osijek, Croatia

Eberly College of Science, Penn State University, University Park, PA, USA

© The Author(s), under exclusive license to Springer Nature Switzerland AG 2023
D. Primorac et al. (eds.), *Pharmacogenomics in Clinical Practice*,
https://doi.org/10.1007/978-3-031-45903-0_17

a potent tool for "big data" analysis because it helps understand the heterogeneity in processes that contribute to the individualized genetic-tailored therapeutics approach, leading to better quality and more cost-effective healthcare.

Keywords

Artificial intelligence • Electronic health records • Big data • Personalized medicine • Pharmacogenomics • Therapy optimization

1   Introduction

Contemporary drug management has a positive impact on many medical conditions. However, predicting the efficacy and safety of a given medication for an individual patient is still greatly limited, primarily due to insufficient comprehensive gene–drug reports on which current prescribing practices rely.

There are some challenges associated with reducing medication errors and achieving the maximum desired efficacy of medication administration. In addition, new drugs are approved each year, with new mechanisms of action and limited clinical experience, which demand continuous education of healthcare providers [1].

It is widely accepted that treatment outcomes are strongly associated with an individual's genotype, among others, thus apostrophizing the potential of precision medicine to improve the current healthcare model.

Implementation of precision medicine in everyday clinical practice relies on the advancements of new technologies [2–4]. Pharmacogenomics (PGx) can improve therapy outcomes because it uses a patient's genetic profile to optimize drug therapy selection. Therefore, PGx is considered one of precision medicine's core elements. Unlike pharmacogenetics which studies variations of a single gene on drug disposition and response, PGx focuses on the genome-wide examination of

The Henry C. Lee College of Criminal Justice and Forensic Sciences, University of New Haven, West Haven, CT, USA

Medical School REGIOMED, Gustav-Hirschfeld-Ring 3, Coburg, Germany

National Forensic Science University, Gandhinagar, Gujarat, India

L. Bach-Rojecky
University of Zagreb Faculty of Pharmacy and Biochemistry, Zagreb, Croatia
e-mail: lbach@pharma.hr

V. Škaro
Greyledge Europe Ltd, Zagreb, Croatia
e-mail: vedranaskaro@greyledgebiotech.com; vskaro@genos.hr

Genos Ltd, DNA Laboratory Zagreb, Zagreb, Croatia

D. Primorac
International Center For Applied Biological Sciences, 10000, Zagreb, Croatia

genetic factors influencing drug effects. Continuous development of new technologies enables the identification of genetic and genomic factors of importance for drug treatment response. These findings are crucial for genetic-tailored therapeutics, thus optimizing therapeutic efficacy and minimizing adverse effects. Genetic and genomic information can integrate into comprehensive electronic health record (EHR) data. This approach provides valuable information that is necessary for a more precise understanding of diseases, discovering and prioritizing potential drug targets, predicting side effects, data mining for unknown drug effects, repurposing medications, and accelerating PGx.

A systematic evaluation of the impact of common individual genetic variants, known as Single-Nucleotide Polymorphisms (SNPs), for a given trait has been provided by Genome-Wide Association Studies (GWAS). The identification of complex phenotypes and subpopulations of the patient is enabled by new biomedical informatics and machine-learning approaches that advance the ability to interpret clinical information [5].

However, since PGx studies generate a considerable amount of information, commonly referred to as "big data," there are also some challenges. These challenges are mostly related to big data issues, including data collection, processing, and storage, then interpretation and clinical implementation of obtained results, which include search, sharing, transfer, visualization, querying, updating, information privacy, and data source [6, 7]. To make decision-making easier, collected information assets must rely on cost-effective, accessible, and advanced forms of information processing [8].

Data collection, processing, and analysis are all critical points that can influence the production of reliable results for clinical interpretation. The type of study (genomic, transcriptomic, or epigenomic) and the type of data studied generate information that can be analyzed and processed based on biological knowledge (using annotation only or adding functional prediction or pathways), statistics, or a combination of both [9].

2   Big Data in Biomedicine

Due to its versatility, the power of big data depends on gathered datasets and the ability of algorithms to make the most of them. The integration of big data into clinical care has raised expectations. Three key big data concepts are characterized as high volume, velocity, and variety. In the healthcare system, variability and value are often included as added qualities [10].

Volume refers to the clinical information associated with laboratory tests, physician visits, and administrative load. Associated with the greater use of precision medicine, these data grow and will expand as genomic and environmental information become more ubiquitous.

Velocity refers to the rapidly increasing speed at which new data are created by technological advances and the corresponding need for faster analysis, interpretation, and clinical implementation.

Variety refers to the tremendous diversity of data types that healthcare organizations encounter on daily basis. With increasing volume and velocity, variety increases as well. Variety is caused by the collection of different kinds of traditional, clinical, and administrative data combined with socioeconomic data, unstructured notes, and even social media data. In turn, these data might be interpreted differently by different clinicians. With the increasing adoption of population health and big data analytics, the variety of data becomes greater.

Variability refers to the many factors that may impact data access and the adequate care provided to a patient. For example, information retrieved from a patient during the initial exam and the clinician's specialty (the source of the clinician's knowledge and training affecting the professional opinion) may impact the decision on further medical intervention. Such data variability can have meaningful interpretation when the care setting and delivery process are taken into context.

Value refers to the cost–benefit of investment in the infrastructure required to collect and interpret data on a large scale. Acquired information must be based on accurate data with measurable improvements as its final result. However, handling big data is challenging and variable. It affects delivering of high-quality patient care by different healthcare systems. The same tools and technologies for gathering and analyzing the data used by organizations and clinicians might result in different ways to put that data to work.

With the rapid development and increasing prevalence of high-throughput multidimensional genomics data, the PGx field is facing extraordinary challenges to develop and use appropriate analytical approaches to keep up with the continuous growth of the data volume, the increasing number of independent variables, and the increasing variety of data types—all accompanied with the increase of biases and noise in the data. More attention is needed to cope with the data veracity as well [7, 9].

3   Emerging Role of Artificial Intelligence

It is challenging to analyze and handle huge amounts of data collected over time just by using common database management tools. Therefore, big data need integration with artificial intelligence (AI) to provide a powerful tool for data analysis and handling. The implementation of AI is growing. Its importance is already recognized to various degrees in the healthcare system (i.e., risk management, remote patient monitoring, and hospital management), but also in drug research and discovery, clinical trials, diagnostics, imaging, etc. [11]. Furthermore, nowadays IT companies such as Google, Amazon, or IBM apply AI principles to almost everything, from medical devices to lifestyle management solutions. It is, therefore, expected to witness their significant impact on healthcare as well [12]. Machine learning (ML) is an application of AI that uses intelligent software that enables machines to perform their work skillfully.

If successfully used, the ML technique relying on high-performance computing methodologies can help to predict the clinical response of drugs. Sources and ways of big data employment are numerous. The process of extracting knowledge from a data set is called data mining, and it involves several steps [13]. ML techniques can be supervised or unsupervised. When under supervision, the algorithm learns on a labeled data set, providing an answer key that the algorithm can use to evaluate its accuracy on training data. When unsupervised, the algorithm is extracting features and patterns on its own, trying to make sense of unlabeled data [14]. Semi-supervised and reinforcement learning methods are used as well.

ML techniques are often used to analyze raw data in "omics". Because a relationship between particular "omics" is very complex, identification and understanding underlying relationships in a set of data in order to interpret the results is a great challenge.

As a subclass of ML, Deep Learning (DL) algorithms called Artificial Neural Networks (ANN), specifically Deep Neural Networks (DNN), can continually evaluate data with a logic structure equivalent to how a human would make conclusions. In contrast to ML algorithms which can make mistakes in outcome prediction and require adjustment of the basic formula by humans, ANN/DNN is more advanced because of their own rule-association and pattern discovery capacity [11, 15, 16]. ML can also be of value in developing systems for automated analysis of images in routine clinical practice [17]. Despite the many advantages of big data-AI tools, current applications to healthcare systems are still limited. Some methodologic issues, such as deficiencies in model calibration and the lack of or insufficient data sharing, unrepresentative or selected populations, data inaccuracy, and missing information, with measurement and data-collecting issues, need to be addressed before the big data analytics routine employment in clinical practice [18].

One of the obstacles to a broader-scale implementation of PGx into clinical practice will be using AI methods for patient categorization into subpopulations. This requires analysis of high-complexity data, which along with heterogeneous biomedical, also includes sociometric and demographic information [19]. There is a significant risk of bias in predictive analytics, as shown in some studies. For example, genetic risk prediction models based on genome-wide association studies are less accurate in non-European populations because most such studies were conducted in populations of European descent [20]. Furthermore, an ML risk assessment tool, widely used in U.S. healthcare organizations, has incorrectly assigned a proportion of Black patients to the same level of a health risk as White patients [21]. There are also other important issues, such as preserving privacy and confidentiality and continuous evaluation of ethical, legal, and social implications of big data [22].

In their excellent review article, Kalinin et al. [19] suggest the importance of DL algorithms in overcoming the challenges of PGx data implementation in the electronic health record (EHR). Deep learning (DL) already has a significant role in medication selection and dosing, as well as in individual drug response prediction, all based on information analyzed from "big data"databases [19]. The main strengths, weaknesses, opportunities, and threats of AI implementation in clinical practice, especially in the context of PGx, are shown in Fig. 1 [23].

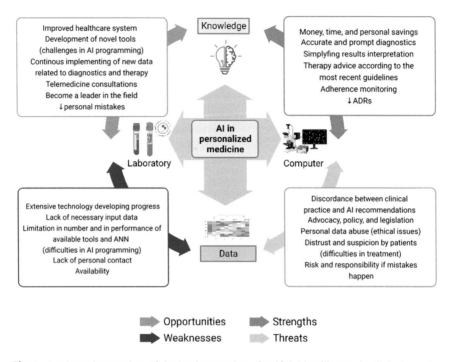

Fig. 1 A schematic overview of the implementation of artificial intelligence in clinical practice and patient care, specifically in the field of pharmacogenomics, is presented through a SWOT analysis. This analysis includes an evaluation of the strengths, weaknesses, opportunities, and threats associated with the introduction of Artificial Intelligence (AI) and Artificial Neural Networks (ANNs) in personalized medicine. Legend: ADRs—adverse drug reactions

4   Implementing Pharmacogenomics in Clinical Practice

Although the "trial and error" approach leads to positive clinical outcomes for most of treated patients, some may suffer from either a partial or complete lack of therapeutic response or serious adverse reactions. Despite various barriers to implementation, the powerful merge between big data analytics and PGx provides a tool for integrating pharmacogenomics into routine clinical settings, intending to guide the optimal drug selection and dosing. However, since PGx knowledge is relatively new, complex, and continuously developing, relying on the clinicians' comprehension alone is insufficient for clinical implementation. Therefore, all relevant clinical recommendations relating to gene–drug pairs need to be summarized and presented to clinicians in a manner that allows understandable and effortless translation of PGx into the clinical practice.

Evidence-based guidelines for developing and using pharmacogenomic Clinical Decision Support (CDS) are provided by relevant institutions and associations such as the Clinical Pharmacogenetics Implementation Consortium and the U.S.

National Academy of Medicine. Also, the Food and Drug Administration continually updates information on potential interactions between drugs and genomic biomarkers [24]. Additionally, some considerations for a pharmacogenomic CDS successful implementation into the EHR include clinical workflows, identification of alert triggers, and tools to guide the interpretation of results. In some circumstances, additional systems and applications outside the EHR may be integrated to enhance its potential [25, 26].

Several international organizations and research networks are evaluating different aspects of PGx implementation in clinical practice [27, 28]. The initiatives with the greatest emphasis on the integration of PGx data into EHR and translation of PGx guidelines into clinical workflows are:

1. The Electronic Medical Records and Genomics Network (eMERGE) [29, 30],
2. The Implementing Genomics in Practice (IGNITE) [31],
3. Displaying and Integrating Genetic Information Through the EHR (DIGITizE) [32].

There is a growing number of medical institutions with programs related to the integration of PGx into their clinical workflows and among the first ones were:

1. Pharmacogenomic Program, Mayo Clinic, Center for Individualized Medicine [33, 34],
2. 1200 Patients Project, University of Chicago [35],
3. Personalized Medicine Program, University of Florida [36],
4. CLIPMERGE PGx program, Mount Sinai Medical Center [37],
5. PG4KDS program, St. Jude Children's Research Hospital [38],
6. Pharmacogenomic Resource for Enhanced Decisions in Care and Treatment (PREDICT) project, Vanderbilt University Medical Center [39, 40],
7. Personalized Medication Program and Pharmacogenomic Service, Cleveland Clinic [25, 26],
8. Personalized Anti-Platelet Pharmacogenetics Program, University of Maryland [41],
9. eMERGE project, Northwestern University [42].

In addition, the US National Institutes of Health (NIH)-funded resource, the "Pharmacogenomics Knowledgebase" (PharmGKB), is dedicated to the curation and dissemination of pharmacogenomic (PGx) information [43]. Drug labels containing PGx information are approved by regulatory agencies worldwide, including the US Food and Drug Administration, the European Medicine Agency, and the Pharmaceuticals and Medical Devices Agency of Japan.

One of the useful clinician-oriented tools is the RightMed® panel, developed by OneOme in collaboration with Mayo Clinic that is used in clinical practice by St. Catherine Specialty Hospital, Zagreb, Croatia [23] as well as the book "Pharmacogenetics in clinical practice, Experience with 55 commonly used drugs" which contains information obtained from authentic and highly regarded sources [44].

An example of successive PGx implementation in clinical decision-making to provide optimal treatment to their patients in St. Catherine Specialty Hospital in Zagreb is described by Primorac et al. [23] and briefly summarized in the following text. This approach to PGx testing determines SNPs using a TaqMan real-time PCR method and copy number variations (CNV) analysis. Results of the DNA analysis are generated in individual test reports available in OneOme's HIPAA-secure portal. OneOme's data curation and clinical annotations are performed by a team of clinical pharmacists and scientists, supported by scientific evidence that meets OneOme's rigorous inclusion criteria and professional guidelines (e.g., Clinical Pharmacogenetics Implementation Consortium (CPIC), Dutch Pharmacogenomics Working Group, French National Pharmacogenetics Network/Group of Clinical Onco-Pharmacology and Canadian Pharmacogenomics Network for Drug Safety). The PGx testing results are then interpreted by a genetic counseling team. The CDS tool used for drug–gene interactions interpretation and possible drug-drug/food/supplements interactions is RightMed Advisor. The interpreted results and clinical recommendations are then presented to the patient by the attending clinician, who advises on the best pharmacological option based on the main principles of individualized medicine: the right drug for the right patient at the right time (Fig. 2) [23].

The use of PGx in the clinic workflow showed that implementation is a complex process that depends on clinical evidence and structured pharmacogenomics data, information technology, CDS systems, clinician access to PGx knowledge, and continuous maintenance of CDS interventions [45, 46]. The help of AI for PGx is needed so that large quantities of data from patients who do PGx tests are analyzed altogether and not on a case-by-case basis. It will help in understanding the heterogeneity in processes that contribute to how a patient reacts to a specific drug and dose, thus allowing prescribers to tailor or "personalize" medicines to the individual patient [47]. Additionally, new data on genomic variations, drug–gene, drug–drug interactions, and more could emerge, which lead to better quality and more cost-effective healthcare.

To enhance the application of PGx in clinical practice, PGx CDS must become more integrated into the infrastructure of commercial EHR systems. Also, healthcare institutions have to adopt EHRs to enable more interaction and information sharing. Since this is an evolutionary process, current and future challenges should be embraced, and all available tools applied to pioneer the application of AI principles to PGx-guided treatment. These efforts will make future treatments safer, more efficient, and cost-effective, which, in turn, will benefit all.

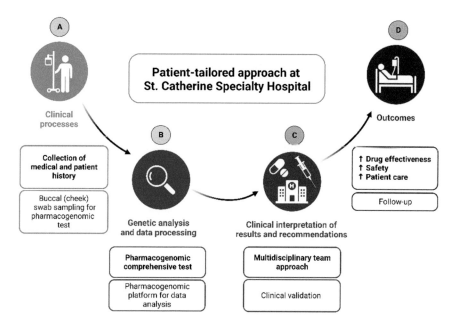

Fig. 2 The personalized pharmacogenomic-based treatment and healthcare system is presented in a diagrammatic format. The first step (A) involves completing a specific form to gather medical and patient history, followed by collecting a sample for DNA analysis through RT-PCR or next generation sequencing (NGS). The results are then processed using a pharmacogenomic platform for data analysis to generate pharmacogenomic reports (e.g., RightMed Advisor report) (B). Next, a multidisciplinary clinical team interprets the results, which include checks for drug–gene interactions, drug–drug interactions, and drug-other xenobiotic (food, dietary supplement, alcohol, smoking) interactions (C). The outcome of this process leads to improved patient care, superior therapy outcomes, increased drug effectiveness, and a reduction in the incidence of adverse drug reactions (D)

References

1. Kinch MS, Haynesworth A, Kinch SL, Hoyer D. An overview of FDA-approved new molecular entities: 1827–2013. Drug Discov Today. 2014;19(8):1033–9. https://doi.org/10.1016/j.drudis.2014.03.018.
2. Agyeman AA, Ofori-Asenso R. Perspective: does personalized medicine hold the future for medicine? J Pharm Bioallied Sci. 2015;7(3):239–44. https://doi.org/10.4103/0975-7406.160040.
3. Hong KW, Oh B. Overview of personalized medicine in the disease genomic era. BMB Rep. 2010;43(10):643–8. https://doi.org/10.5483/BMBRep.2010.43.10.643.
4. Tian Q, Price ND, Hood L. Systems cancer medicine: towards realization of predictive, preventive, personalized and participatory (P4) medicine. J Int Med. 2012;271(2):111–21. https://doi.org/10.1111/j.1365-2796.2011.02498.x.
5. Denny JC, Van Driest SL, Wei WQ, Roden DM. The influence of big (clinical) data and genomics on precision medicine and drug development. Clin Pharmacol Ther. 2018;103(3):409–18. https://doi.org/10.1002/cpt.951.

6. Chenoweth MJ, Giacomini KM, Pirmohamed M, Hill SL, van Schaik RHN, Schwab M, et al. Global pharmacogenomics within precision medicine: challenges and opportunities. Clin Pharmacol Ther. 2020;107(1):57–61. https://doi.org/10.1002/cpt.1664.
7. Li R, Kim D, Ritchie MD. Methods to analyze big data in pharmacogenomics research. Pharmacogenomics. 2017;18(8):807–20. https://doi.org/10.2217/pgs-2016-0152.
8. Glossary G. Big data. www.gartner.com/en/information-technology/glossary/big-data. Accessed 17 Nov 2021.
9. Barrot CC, Woillard JB, Picard N. Big data in pharmacogenomics: current applications, perspectives and pitfalls. Pharmacogenomics. 2019;20(8):609–20. https://doi.org/10.2217/pgs-2018-0184.
10. Jain A. The 5 V's of big data: IBM Watson Health. 2016. https://www.ibm.com/blogs/watson-health/the-5-vs-of-big-data/. Accessed 17 Nov 2021.
11. Topol EJ. High-performance medicine: the convergence of human and artificial intelligence. Nat Med. 2019;25(1):44–56. https://doi.org/10.1038/s41591-018-0300-7.
12. He J, Baxter SL, Xu J, Xu J, Zhou X, Zhang K. The practical implementation of artificial intelligence technologies in medicine. Nat Med. 2019;25(1):30–6. https://doi.org/10.1038/s41591-018-0307-0.
13. Mohammed M, Khan MB, Bashier EBM. Machine learning: algorithms and applications, 1st ed. CRC Press; 2016.
14. Rumbold JMM, O'Kane M, Philip N, Pierscionek BK. Big data and diabetes: the applications of big data for diabetes care now and in the future. Diabet Med. 2020;37(2):187–93. https://doi.org/10.1111/dme.14044.
15. Hessler G, Baringhaus KH. Artificial intelligence in drug design. Molecules. 2018;23(10):2520. https://doi.org/10.3390/molecules23102520.
16. Esteva A, Robicquet A, Ramsundar B, Kuleshov V, DePristo M, Chou K, et al. A guide to deep learning in healthcare. Nat Med. 2019;25(1):24–9. https://doi.org/10.1038/s41591-018-0316-z.
17. Hosny A, Parmar C, Quackenbush J, Schwartz LH, Aerts H. Artificial intelligence in radiology. Nat Rev Cancer. 2018;18(8):500–10. https://doi.org/10.1038/s41568-018-0016-5.
18. Khoury MJ, Armstrong GL, Bunnell RE, Cyril J, Iademarco MF. The intersection of genomics and big data with public health: opportunities for precision public health. PLoS Med. 2020;17(10):e1003373. https://doi.org/10.1371/journal.pmed.1003373.
19. Kalinin AA, Higgins GA, Reamaroon N, Soroushmehr S, Allyn-Feuer A, Dinov ID, et al. Deep learning in pharmacogenomics: from gene regulation to patient stratification. Pharmacogenomics. 2018;19(7):629–50. https://doi.org/10.2217/pgs-2018-0008.
20. Roberts MC, Khoury MJ, Mensah GA. Perspective: the clinical use of polygenic risk scores: race, ethnicity, and health disparities. Ethn Dis. 2019;29(3):513–6. https://doi.org/10.18865/ed.29.3.513.
21. Obermeyer Z, Powers B, Vogeli C, Mullainathan S. Dissecting racial bias in an algorithm used to manage the health of populations. Science. 2019;366(6464):447–53. https://doi.org/10.1126/science.aax2.
22. Flaxman AD, Vos T. Machine learning in population health: opportunities and threats. PLoS Med. 2018;15(11):e1002702. https://doi.org/10.1371/journal.pmed.1002702.
23. Primorac D, Bach-Rojecky L, Vađunec D, Juginović A, Žunić K, Matišić V, et al. Pharmacogenomics at the center of precision medicine: challenges and perspective in an era of Big Data. Pharmacogenomics. 2020;21(2):141–56. https://doi.org/10.2217/pgs-2019-0134.
24. U.S. Food and Drug Administration. Table of pharmacogenomic biomarkers in drug labeling with labeling text. https://www.fda.gov/drugs/science-and-research-drugs/table-pharmacogenomic-biomarkers-drug-labeling. Accessed 19 Nov 2021.
25. Hicks JK, Stowe D, Willner MA, Wai M, Daly T, Gordon SM, et al. Implementation of clinical pharmacogenomics within a large health system: from electronic health record decision support to consultation services. Pharmacotherapy. 2016;36(8):940–8. https://doi.org/10.1002/phar.1786.

26. Hicks JK, Dunnenberger HM, Gumpper KF, Haidar CE, Hoffman JM. Integrating pharmacogenomics into electronic health records with clinical decision support. Am J Health Syst Pharm. 2016;73(23):1967–76. https://doi.org/10.2146/ajhp160030.

27. Manolio TA, Chisholm RL, Ozenberger B, Roden DM, Williams MS, Wilson R, et al. Implementing genomic medicine in the clinic: the future is here. Genet Med. 2013;15(4):258–67. https://doi.org/10.1038/gim.2012.157.

28. Manolio TA, Abramowicz M, Al-Mulla F, Anderson W, Balling R, Berger AC, et al. Global implementation of genomic medicine: we are not alone. Sci Transl Med. 2015;7(290):290ps13. https://doi.org/10.1126/scitranslmed.aab0194.

29. Rasmussen-Torvik LJ, Stallings SC, Gordon AS, Almoguera B, Basford MA, Bielinski SJ, et al. Design and anticipated outcomes of the eMERGE-PGx project: a multicenter pilot for preemptive pharmacogenomics in electronic health record systems. Clin Pharmacol Ther. 2014;96(4):482–9. https://doi.org/10.1038/clpt.2014.137.

30. eMERGE Network. 2021. https://emerge-network.org/. Accessed 19 Nov 2021.

31. Weitzel KW, Alexander M, Bernhardt BA, Calman N, Carey DJ, Cavallari LH, et al. The IGNITE network: a model for genomic medicine implementation and research. BMC Med Genom. 2016;9:1. https://doi.org/10.1186/s12920-015-0162-5.

32. DIGITizE. Displaying and Integrating Genetic Information Through the EHR: National Academies of Sciences, Engineering, and Medicine. https://www.nationalacademies.org/our-work/digitize-displaying-and-integrating-genetic-information-through-the-ehr-action-collaborative. Accessed 19 Nov 2021.

33. Bielinski SJ, Olson JE, Pathak J, Weinshilboum RM, Wang L, Lyke KJ, et al. Preemptive genotyping for personalized medicine: design of the right drug, right dose, right time-using genomic data to individualize treatment protocol. Mayo Clin Proc. 2014;89(1):25–33. https://doi.org/10.1016/j.mayocp.2013.10.021.

34. Caraballo PJ, Bielinski SJ, St Sauver JL, Weinshilboum RM. Electronic medical record-integrated pharmacogenomics and related clinical decision support concepts. Clin Pharmacol Ther. 2017;102(2):254–64. https://doi.org/10.1002/cpt.707.

35. O'Donnell PH, Bush A, Spitz J, Danahey K, Saner D, Das S, et al. The 1200 patients project: creating a new medical model system for clinical implementation of pharmacogenomics. Clin Pharmacol Ther. 2012;92(4):446–9. https://doi.org/10.1038/clpt.2012.117.

36. Johnson JA, Elsey AR, Clare-Salzler MJ, Nessl D, Conlon M, Nelson DR. Institutional profile: University of Florida and Shands Hospital Personalized Medicine Program: clinical implementation of pharmacogenetics. Pharmacogenomics. 2013;14(7):723–6. https://doi.org/10.2217/pgs.13.59.

37. Gottesman O, Scott SA, Ellis SB, Overby CL, Ludtke A, Hulot JS, et al. The CLIPMERGE PGx Program: clinical implementation of personalized medicine through electronic health records and genomics-pharmacogenomics. Clin Pharmacol Ther. 2013;94(2):214–7. https://doi.org/10.1038/clpt.2013.72.

38. Hoffman JM, Haidar CE, Wilkinson MR, Crews KR, Baker DK, Kornegay NM, et al. PG4KDS: a model for the clinical implementation of pre-emptive pharmacogenetics. Am J Med Genet C Semin Med Genet. 2014;166c(1):45–55. https://doi.org/10.1002/ajmg.c.31391.

39. Westbrook MJ, Wright MF, Van Driest SL, McGregor TL, Denny JC, Zuvich RL, et al. Mapping the incidentalome: estimating incidental findings generated through clinical pharmacogenomics testing. Genet Med. 2013;15(5):325–31. https://doi.org/10.1038/gim.2012.147.

40. Snyder B. PREDICT program expands, opens new Genomics Clinic: Vanderbilt University Medical Center. 2020. https://news.vumc.org/2020/04/30/predict%E2%80%88program-expands-opens-new-genomics-clinic/. Accessed 19 Nov 2021.

41. Shuldiner AR, Palmer K, Pakyz RE, Alestock TD, Maloney KA, O'Neill C, et al. Implementation of pharmacogenetics: the University of Maryland Personalized Anti-platelet Pharmacogenetics Program. Am J Med Genet C Semin Med Genet. 2014;166c(1):76–84. https://doi.org/10.1002/ajmg.c.31396.

42. Center for Genetic Medicine FSoM, Northwestern University. Electronic Medical Records and Genomics (eMERGE) Network. https://www.cgm.northwestern.edu/research/emerge-net work/index.html. Accessed 19 Nov 2021.
43. Thorn CF, Klein TE, Altman RB. PharmGKB: the pharmacogenomics knowledge base. Methods Mol Biol. 2013;1015:311–20. https://doi.org/10.1007/978-1-62703-435-7_20.
44. Primorac D, Höppner W, editors. Pharmacogenetics in clinical practice: Experience with 55 commonly used drugs. Zagreb, Hamburg, Philadelphia: St. Catherine Specialty Hospital, Bioglobe GmbH, ISABS; 2022. Available from: https://www.stcatherine.com/centre-of-exc ellence/10/individualized-and-preventive-medicine/pharmacogenomics/69. Accessed: 2 April, 2022
45. Glicksberg BS, Li L, Chen R, Dudley J, Chen B. Leveraging big data to transform drug discovery. Methods Mol Biol. 2019;1939:91–118. https://doi.org/10.1007/978-1-4939-9089-4_ 6.
46. Arwood MJ, Chumnumwat S, Cavallari LH, Nutescu EA, Duarte JD. Implementing pharmacogenomics at your institution: establishment and overcoming implementation challenges. Clin Transl Sci. 2016;9(5):233–45. https://doi.org/10.1111/cts.12404.
47. Schork NJ. Artificial intelligence and personalized medicine. Cancer Treat Res. 2019;178:265–83. https://doi.org/10.1007/978-3-030-16391-4_11.

Public Health Issues in Pharmacogenomics

Marius Geanta, Bianca Cucos, and Angela Brand

Abstract

COVID-19 is the first pandemic in the post-genomic era, showcasing how advancements in fundamental research can be translated for real-time, global monitoring of viral variants, identifying the viral origin, understanding the host responses and differences in outcomes, as well as for drug repurposing and drug discovery. Genomic epidemiology and precision public health are some of the interdisciplinary fields which have come of age during this pandemic. Genomics will likely become an essential component of public health strategies for communicable and non-communicable diseases. Genomic medicine leads to disruption in terms of clinical management of the individual patient (precision medicine) or population health (precision public health).

M. Geanta (✉) · B. Cucos
Centre for Innovation in Medicine, Bucharest, Romania
e-mail: marius.geanta@ino-med.ro

M. Geanta
Kol Medical Media, Bucharest, Romania

United Nations University-Maastricht Economic and Social Research Institute on Innovation and Technology, Maastricht, The Netherlands

B. Cucos
Genomed Consulting, Bucharest, Romania

A. Brand
Department of Public Health Genomics, Manipal School of Life Sciences, Manipal Academy of Higher Education, Manipal, India

Faculty of Health, Medicine and Life Sciences, Maastricht University, Maastricht, Netherlands

Manipal School of Life Sciences, Dr. TMA Pai Endowment Chair in Public Health Genomics, Manipal Academy of Higher Education, Manipal, India

© The Author(s), under exclusive license to Springer Nature Switzerland AG 2023   325
D. Primorac et al. (eds.), *Pharmacogenomics in Clinical Practice*,
https://doi.org/10.1007/978-3-031-45903-0_18

Keywords

Precision public health • Personalized prevention • Preemptive
pharmacogenomic testing • Personalized medicine • Population health •
Genomics

1   Introduction

Understanding how genomic variation affects drug metabolism and response is an
essential part of implementing precision medicine. Due to advances in sequencing
technologies and molecular sciences, there is a transition from small studies on
candidate genes to genome-wide studies, from pharmacogenetics to pharmacogenomics and ultimately toward a multiomic approach to pharmacological responses
and profiles. All these popular research areas have clinical and public health implications. Such as genomic medicine is changing clinical standards across disciplines
(e.g., oncology, cardiology, and psychiatry), public health is predicted to undertake
an increasing role in prevention, aiming to maintain health and define medical risks
using new tools, including the use of knowledge related to the variation associated
with pharmacogenes.

Since whole genome sequencing is becoming more accessible, the perspective for preemptive pharmacogenomic testing will likely impact routine care in the
years to come. Results of comprehensive pharmacogenomic screening can become
part of the patient's electronic health record (EHR), providing lifelong value for
the individual and the healthcare system. Making this information available will
be key to support clinicians in day-to-day decision making, but also for informing
health policies and programs as well as for citizen empowerment and health liter-
acy. EHR will become an indispensable tool to understand risk distribution across
populations.

2   The Rise of Precision Public Health
in the Pharmacogenomics Era

All human diseases are the result of complex interactions between genes, the environment, and social determinants [1, 2]. Multiple risk factors and mechanisms can
be described nowadays to explain the variety of phenotypes encountered in real
life. Genomic variation describes naturally occurring differences among individuals of the same species and is a result of diverse phenomena such as genetic drift,
natural selection, and migration [3, 4].

Advances in sequencing technologies led to significant improvements to the
human reference genome [5, 6]. In March 2022, the Telomere-to-Telomere (T2T)
Consortium announced the final sequence of a complete human genome, gathering
a detailed description of each human chromosome from end to end [6, 7]. Building
on this achievement, a new ambitious international project aims to provide a better
representation of human genomic diversity, The Human Pangenome Project. The

development of long-read sequencing technologies and data analytic tools have led to new methods for detecting global genomic variation. The Human Pangenome Reference Consortium intends to create a more comprehensive human reference that illustrates global genomic diversity, enabling more accurate research and the implementation of true precision medicine approaches [5]. To make large-scale genomic analyses more accessible, Siren et al. report a new bioinformatic tool, *Giraffe*, which will allow researchers to compare natural variations in human genes against genome sequences collected from diverse group of subjects [8].

Other international projects such as All of US or the UK's 100.000 Genomes also contribute to a deeper characterization of diverse human genomic profiles. Understanding population diversity at the molecular level complements efforts to define other types of health determinants, resulting in better strategies for health promotion, prevention, screening, surveillance, and treatment decisions.

Genetic variations in populations living in different geographical areas have profound effects on infectious disease susceptibility. It has been long known that having *the sickle cell trait* (certain sickle cell allele of hemoglobin), for example, offers protection against severe forms of malaria in people living in Sub-Saharian Africa [9]. The *CCR5* deletion allele protects against HIV infection in homozygotes and leads to slower progression of disease in heterozygotes [10]. Even though nicotine displays ethnic differences in its metabolism, studies show that the disease risk cannot be explained solely by behavioral factors involving smoking [11].

In the field of non-communicable diseases, the most successful human genomic application in public health was traditionally newborn screening [12]. These applications expanded with the emergence of tumor biomarkers, testing for rare disorders, and discovering pharmacogenes. The COVID-19 pandemic built the foundation for the broad use of the genomics in public health, with applications ranging from fast identification of the virus to the use of genomics for viral surveillance, variants identification, and as well for the stratification of high risk for COVID-19 individuals. The influence is likely to be major in other medical disciplines [13, 14].

"Public health genomics" was defined in 2005 as *"the responsible and effective translation of genome-based knowledge and technologies for the benefit of the population"* [15]. Precision public health is evolving around new methods enabling integration of all determinants of health (biological, social, behavioral, or environmental). Increased access to genomic data can offer new ways of identifying and defining a target population, beyond the classical association of parameters such as gender, age, or socio-economic status. The field of personalized medicine is expanding to include more possibilities for better population health management, moving further from the narrow applications that impact so far only clinical medicine [16]. Genomics reveals a new mechanism that proves populations are not homogeneous. Genomic technologies could be applied using a precision public health approach to identify the impact of genomic variants in different population subgroups. Each subgroup could then be targeted with tailored interventions that are more relevant to their level of risk, resulting in more efficient and effective disease prevention, screening, and surveillance strategies [14].

Based on the advances in pharmacogenomics, in the post-genomics era, public health is moving toward preventive, precision, and participatory healthcare. Reducing medical costs in various human diseases requires the broad implementation of pharmacogenomic at the health system level, enabling a new understanding of medical risks and avoiding drug indications that can trigger adverse reactions. Data from more than 7.7 million US veterans show that almost 99% of people carry at least one actionable pharmacogene variant [17]. A report published by the British Pharmacological Society and the Royal College of Physicians confirms that almost 99% of people carry at least one genetic variation that affects their response to certain drugs, including commonly prescribed painkillers, heart disease drugs and antidepressants, and that by the time they reach the age of 70, about 90% of people are taking at least one therapeutic agent from these classes [18].

Population-based information about the distribution of genotypes in different populations is not uniform at the global level, which poses limitations to increase access to early interventions. Currently, the development of public health programs and policies do not reflect progress in the field of genomics. As science progresses, the role of public health in translating data related to new genes for applications to prevent disease is increasing [19]. There is a major need for expanding the use EHR as a valuable way to understand risk distribution in a population and maximize the advantages of novel therapies [20].

The ways, in which public health interventions and activities may become more *"precise"* because of technological innovations and the data they produce, are evident in a number of areas including epidemiology, knowledge of the determinants of health, targeting of healthcare disparities, screening and prevention, diagnosis, surveillance, and response to communicable diseases.

Decades of studying pharmacogenes and searching for new variants involved in drug metabolism prove that it is difficult to easily translate genotypes to accurate phenotypes. Pharmacogene tests that use RT-PCR, DNA microarrays, Sanger sequencing have been replaced over the years with panel sequencing, whole exome, or whole genome sequencing, taking into account the fact that drug response can be influenced by multiple genes. Long-read sequencing data offers promising opportunities in elucidating complex pharmacogenes. For instance, CYP2D6 is one of the genes being associated with guideline recommendations for clinical management. However, it is a very complex gene with over 100 variants described to date [21]. The gene is also involved in large-scale gene rearrangements, forming hybrid genes with neighboring partners. Using long-read sequencing allows for full-gene characterization, discovering new alleles, characterizing large structural variants which will improve phenotype prediction and screening prior to administration of drugs [22].

Over 200 genome-wide association studies (GWAS) of pharmacotherapy responses have been reported to date, becoming popular tools for searching susceptibility genes [23]. For example, GWAS studies offer insights into treatment response to hepatitis C virus (HCV) infection, which led to changes in clinical practice [24]. Initially, patients were treated with combinations of pegylated inter-ferons and ribavirin that failed to clear the infection in over half of cases [25]. Direct-acting antivirals improved treatment success rate, especially in patients with unfavorable *IFNL3* genotype [26].

Mendelian randomization (MR) is another epidemiological method that is gain-ing ground; using genetic variants follow an exposure and predicts its causal association with an outcome. MR applications include disease risk evaluation and pointing to causal relationships, supporting evidence of prior observational data, identifying new drug targets, and drug repurposing, providing evidence for PGx implementation [27]. With all these new technologies, population genomic-based screening across the lifespan is becoming feasible.

The impact of public health programs based on genomics will increase in the years to come, based on the development in the field of pharmacogenomics and as well in the field of polygenic risk scores (PRS), in addition to the current use of genomic information in public health interventions (e.g., early identification of Lynch syndrome, hereditary breast and ovarian cancer or familial hyperc-holesterolemia). Brigham and Women's Hospital, Veterans Affairs (VA) Boston Healthcare System, and Harvard Medical School published polygenic risk scores (PRS) for six common diseases as part of the Genomic Medicine at VA (GenoVA) Study providing the lab report and informational resources that succinctly told the doctor and patient what they need to know to decide about using PRS results in their health care [28].

In a report published in the early 2000s, aiming to set a framework for the integration of human genetics into public health practice, the US Centers for Dis-ease Control (CDC), called for more public health leadership as many complex issues related to deciphering the human genome, with public health relevance are emerging.

Public health genomics is a transversal field, requiring the contribution of a wide variety of academic domains from medical sciences, population sciences, epidemiology, social sciences, law, and strategies for improved health outcomes should be based on multistakeholder engagement. In this context, public health professionals must take an active role in promoting the use of genomic knowledge and services when there are cost-effective interventions to prevent disease or dis-ability, which has also been described as the *commitment for change management* to deliver improved health [29, 30].

3   The COVID-19 Pandemic and the Rebirth of Public Health: The Pivotal Role of Genomics

COVID-19 is the first pandemic in the post-genomic era, representing an important opportunity to showcase how advancements in genomics can enhance understand-ing of the viral evolution, host response, and influence the public health response, but also other medical fields [31, 32]. The costs of massive parallel sequencing have dropped significantly, as have the time to return results and data analysis.

Technologies that allow high throughput sequencing, second or third generation, can now inform the world about the emergence of a new virus or variants of the virus, allowing for diagnostic tests and vaccines to be developed in record time [33].

SARS-CoV-2 is one of the most tested viruses in human history, with many technologies available to enable real-time tracking on a global scale. Within six months from the start of the pandemic (by May 2020), GISAID (Global Initiative on Sharing Avian Influenza Data) already had 110,000 full-length SARS-CoV-2 genome sequences. As of February 2022, the UK is the world leader in sequencing capacity, uploading over 2 million genome sequences to the international GISAID database, accounting for a quarter of all SARS-CoV-2 genomes shared globally to date [34]. SARS-CoV-2 sequencing data collected all over the world and rapidly shared in online databases allowed public health officials and governments to make better-informed decisions.

The cornerstone technology for nanopore sequencing, developed in 2014, allows sequencing to happen remotely during a disease outbreak. Validated during the Ebola outbreak and then during the Zika epidemic, it enabled scientists to identify where each outbreak originated [35]. Sequencing technologies which proved their value during COVID-19 will allow researchers to identify new pathogens, paving an early start on understanding and tracking the next outbreak as well as providing frameworks for developing new testing and screening programs for other diseases. The unprecedented volume of SARS-CoV-2 genomic data coupled with available bioinformatics tools accelerated the prompt and effective characterization of SARS-CoV-2 genomes and provided tools enabling epidemiologists and public health officials to respond to the COVID-19 pandemic more effectively [36]. Genomic epidemiology and precision public health are two key fields which have come of age during this pandemic [37].

Targeted genomic surveillance of SARS-CoV-2 in immunocompromised patients has been shown useful in understanding the mechanisms of appearance of newly emerging variants of concern [38].

The role of genomics in infectious diseases ranges from early assessing vaccine antigens to inform vaccine composition, diagnosis, understanding antimicrobial resistance determinants to inform treatment but as well understanding the host-related factors.

Although some well-known risk factors (such as older age, obesity, gender) have been associated with increased disease severity of COVID-19, these risk factors alone do not explain all the variability encountered in disease severity [39]. Young, otherwise healthy individuals still develop severe forms of COVID-19 leading to hospitalizations or even deaths. Identifying host-specific genetic factors may reveal biological mechanisms of therapeutic relevance and clarify causal relationships of modifiable environmental risk factors for SARS-CoV-2 infection and outcomes [40].

Some individuals are more or less likely to become infected or their risk for developing severe disease manifestations is higher. This has also been observed with previous outbreaks. According to WHO, in 2009 during the H1N1 influenza pandemic, pregnant women and infants and young children (< 2 years of age) were at an increased risk for severe complications in the context of infection [41].

ACE2 gene polymorphisms were shown to be correlated with pulmonary and cardiovascular conditions by modifying the angiotensinogen-ACE2 system [42]. The viral entry to the host cell by binding to the cell membrane through S protein can be blocked by transmembrane serine protease 2 (TMPRSS2) [43]. Early studies showed that missense polymorphisms and stop-gains of *TMPRSS2* polymorphisms may be sensitive to treatment with hydroxychloroquine [44].

An international, open-science collaboration, the COVID-19 Host Genetics Initiative has been established to map the host genetic determinants of SARS-CoV-2 infection and the severity of the resulting COVID-19 disease [45]. COVID Human Genetic Effort is another project focused on identifying monogenic cases with rare, highly penetrant mutations through the analysis of young patients (<50 years of age) who were previously well and developed life-threatening disease, as well as those naturally resistant despite repeated exposure [46].

The application of pharmacogenomics to infectious diseases requires consideration of the genomes of both the pathogen and the host. Variation in genes related to the control of the innate or adaptive immune response against infectious diseases impacts pathogen escape from the specific immune response, disease pathogenesis, and disease morbidity. Variants in genes encoding drug-metabolizing enzymes, transporters, or receptors could also provide the insights to implement personalized therapy strategies leading to a better outcome in the context of infectious diseases [47].

COVID-19 treatment standards vary in different countries and since the beginning of the pandemic included multiple classes of drugs: antivirals, antibiotics, antiparasitics, anti-inflammatory drugs previously used for other infectious and non-infectious diseases [48]. All these classes have been intensively studied and are associated with well-established pharmacogenomic biomarkers. The RECOVERY trial has demonstrated the therapeutic utility of existing drugs such as dexamethasone for treatment of severe disease [49]. However, many drugs were being administered in COVID-19 patients without establishing clinical effectiveness or safety, across age groups, ethnic backgrounds, and comorbidities [48].

Drugs like hydroxychloroquine, azithromycin, and lopinavir, frequently used in the beginning of the pandemic, can cause patients to develop *long QT syndrome and torsades de pointes* [50]. Moreover, studies point to the importance of testing for *G6PD* (glucose-6-phosphate dehydrogenase) gene for patients taking antimalarial medication. G6PD deficiency, caused by a genetic mutation in the red blood cell enzyme G6PD, should be considered in every patient who develops hemolysis after taking new medication. COVID-19 has turned the attention once again on hydroxychloroquine use and G6PD deficiency [51].

Certain variants in *ITPA gene* are reported to have protective effects against hemolytic anemia, a well-known adverse effect of ribavirin, RNA polymerase inhibitor drug used for severe COVID-19 cases, originally prescribed for hepatitis C infection [52, 53]. More recently, *GYPC* variation affecting erythrocyte membrane strength is important in predicting risk for developing ribavirin-induced anemia [54].

Shana et al. evaluated drug–gene, drug–drug, and drug–drug–gene interactions associated with COVID-19 therapy in the Indian population and showed that COVID-19-associated pharmacogenes were substantially overlapped with those of metabolic disorder therapeutics [55]. Aschenbrenner et al. [56] evaluated transcriptomes of COVID-19 patients, showing differences in the immune response of patients with severe versus mild disease. RNA-seq of whole blood cell transcriptomes capture important information related to granulocytes which are major drivers of disease severity and points to patient subgroup-specific drug candidates targeting the dysregulated systemic immune response of the host [56].

Ongoing clinical trials on COVID-19 medicines can benefit more from incorporation of pharmacogenomic information as an enrollment criterion [57]. A repurposing strategy might be more effective and successful if pharmacogenetic interventions are being considered in future clinical trials [58].

Populations at risk for severe COVID-19 such as the elderly are also in many instances populations with multiple comorbidities, being prescribed with multiple drugs. In this context, they are also susceptible to drug–drug interactions and toxicities associated COVID-19 therapeutics [59]. Therefore, is critical to understand the pharmacogenomics of COVID-19 therapies and develop population-specific PGx maps for the widely used drugs [55].

The identification of pharmacogenetic biomarkers of relevance in drugs used for COVID-19 treatment and integrating information about nongenetic factors could inform dosage adjustments or the selection of the optimal treatment. Achieving a personalized therapy would assure drug plasma concentrations within the therapeutic range, leading to several advantages in the disease's clinical outcome. If institutions used pre-emptive PGx testing or extracted PGx information from research biorepositories, these results would be highly relevant during COVID-19 hospitalization. PGx results would be relevant for nearly all individuals hospitalized with COVID-19 and would provide the opportunity to improve clinical care [17].

Understanding the substantial differences between populations in terms of genetic variation will be crucial to improve current strategies to tackle the burden of communicable diseases. Global trends are correlating with an increased risk of infectious disease outbreaks. Climate change and rapid urbanization will only contribute to the risk of disease emergence in the coming decades [60]. New infectious diseases will continue to emerge at a global level and others will become more difficult to tackle if we also consider the issue of antimicrobial resistance which is becoming an increasing public health threat [61]. Understanding genomic mechanisms with impact on infectious disease susceptibility offers the opportunity for new insights into finding drug targets, ensuring better risk stratification of populations and prediction of response to therapy. Data obtained from large-scale genomic sequencing projects based on innovative molecular technologies confirm the complexity of the host biology on disease susceptibility and outcomes. The implementation of planetary health genomics for the prevention of future pandemics could be considered as well, a step further in addition to the implementation of the one health approach [62].

4 Increase the Efficacy of Public Health Interventions Using Pharmacogenomics in Primary, Secondary, Tertiary Non-communicable Diseases Prevention

Adverse drug reactions (ADRs) are a major public health problem globally in relation to non-communicable diseases (NCD). Up to 200,000 people lose their lives in Europe every year due to ADRs and the total cost to society of ADRs in the EU is €79 billion [63]. Data from the WHO pharmacovigilance database, VigiBase, show that in 2010–2019, fatal ADRs correspond to over 1% of the total number of ADRs. They occurred more in males, over 65 years and with antineoplastic/immunomodulating drugs, followed by central nervous system and cardiac drugs [64].

Insani et al. [65] published the first systematic review providing a comprehensive evaluation of the overall burden of ADRs in primary care. The most frequent drug class involved in the ADRs among adults were cardiovascular drugs (antihypertensive, lipid-modifying, antithrombotic drugs), followed by psychiatric drugs. Data also showed that one-fifth of ADRs in primary care were preventable. Patients with ADRs were reported to take almost three times the number of drugs compared to those without ADRs [65].

A study assessing the burden of ADR on the National Health Service (NHS) showed that they accounted for 6.5% of all admissions to 2 major medical centers in England and the majority were because of cardiovascular severe adverse reactions. The drugs most implicated were diuretics, warfarin, and nonsteroidal anti-inflammatory drugs, including aspirin. Most reactions were either definitely or possibly avoidable [66].

There has been an upward trend in the inclusion of PGx labeling in new drug approvals in the USA and Europe over the last two decades. More than half of PGx information in new drug approvals are clinically actionable [67]. Inclusion of PGx information in drug labels has increased for all clinical areas between 2000 and 2020, especially for oncology, which comprise the largest proportion—over 75% of biomarker—drug pairs for which PGx testing is required. FDA defines genomic biomarkers as a measurable DNA and/or RNA characteristic that can be used as an indicator of either normal biologic processes, pathogenic phenomena, and/or response to therapeutic or other interventions [68].

An ongoing CDC project will measure the prevalence of PGx variation in 150 pharmacogenes in a diverse US population, using 5,000 DNA samples from the population based NHANES (The National Health and Nutrition Examination Survey) project. These data will be used as population reference to evaluate clinical validity and associations of PGx variants with health outcomes in various populations (African American, Asian, Hispanic) [69].

PGx may be particularly beneficial in medically underserved populations, helping to allocate resources more effectively, reducing the number of appointments needed for establishing drug doses. Dalton et al. analyzed EHRs from over 60.000 cases in Florida showing that improved geographic access to PGx testing may allow prescribers to make more efficient use of limited opportunities to optimize therapy for drugs with PGx testing guidelines [70]. Another study conducted in Columbia confirms that population-centered approaches to pharmacogenomics can help realize the promise of precision medicine in resource-limited settings [19].

4.1 Improving Cardiovascular Disease Prevention with Pharmacogenomics

Cardiovascular diseases (CVD) impact the lives of 60 million people in the EU and account for 36% of all deaths across the EU [69]. Around 20% of all premature deaths (below the age of 65) in the EU are caused by CVD [72]. Genomics offers the potential to improve cardiovascular disease primary, secondary, and tertiary prevention, including by optimizing cardiovascular pharmacotherapy.

An important milestone in the field of cardiovascular pharmacogenomics was the publishing of a position paper by the European Society of Cardiology (ESC) in 2021 that brings together the scientific evidence accumulated over the years on the value that pharmacogenomics can bring to the management of CVD [73].

For example, statins are the most common lipid-lowering drugs used in practice. However, about 50% of patients stop treatment with statins because of side effects. In heterozygous carriers, and especially homozygous, for the *SLCO1B1*5* variant with loss of function, an increase in the risk of myopathy has been identified by increasing the plasma concentration of most statins [74].

Given the large number of patients receiving antiplatelet therapy, the use of pharmacogenomics to personalize treatment could have a significant impact at the population level. Clopidogrel is an antiplatelet drug used since 1997 for patients with acute coronary syndromes. However, up to 30% of patients do not respond adequately to therapy with this antiplatelet due to genetic variability in the population, which induces differences in the metabolism of the drug [75].

Metoprolol should be avoided in people with ultra-rapid or weak metabolism profile, and an alternative (e.g., bisoprol) should be chosen. Drugs that prolong the QT interval should also be avoided in those with genetic variants associated with long QT syndrome. Before initiating warfarin treatment, it is recommended to genotype all relevant alleles (*CYP2C9, VKORC1, CYP4F*), regardless of the ethnic group to which the patient belongs to.

ESC recognizes there is a need for professional bodies and health systems to support prescribers in understanding, interpreting, and implementing evidence-based PGx in cardiovascular medicine [73].

According to a recent study by Murdock et al. [76], routine genetic testing in cardiology outpatients can lead to a significant number of actionable results. About 700 patients were enrolled in Baylor College of Medicine's cardiology clinics and tested multigenic panel for cardiovascular diseases as part of routine care. The results showed that genetic testing influenced the course of treatment in a third of patients. Of the doctors surveyed, 84% said they had changed the course of patient care based on test results, including sending patients to another specialist, performing additional cardiac tests, and changing medications [76].

4.2   Familial Hypercholesterolemia: A Model for the Primary Prevention of CVDs

The world's most common and non-modifiable CVD risk factor is Familial Hypercholesterolemia (FH). Less than 10% of those born with FH are diagnosed and adequately treated, leading to heart attacks, strokes, heart disease, and deaths, early in life, even as early as 4 years of age [77, 78].

A genetically confirmed diagnosis of FH is essential both for treatment of the affected individual and for finding and treating other affected family members. Multiple observational studies indicate that raised LDL during childhood is associated with carotid thickening and coronary calcifications. More recent data from Mendelian randomization studies point to the fact that exposure to lower LDL-C beginning early in life is associated with a greater cardiovascular risk reduction versus lowering LDL-C later in life. One of the main goals of primary and secondary cardiovascular prevention is to reach and sustain recommended LDL-C goals. HMG-CoA reductase inhibitors (statins) at the highest tolerable dose are recommended in all international guidelines to be initiated immediately at diagnosis in all FH adults. However, statin efficacy is lower in FH patients because of genetic variation as well as lack of adherence related to toxicities (myopathy, hepatotoxicity) [79, 80].

The increasing options for cholesterol-lowering therapies in recent years led to challenges in clinical practice related to assessing the right medication for the right patients, understanding the therapeutic response and potential adverse effects. Race, gender, age along with genetic variations involving *LDLR, APOB, PCSK9*, which are the main genes involved in monogenic FH, can lead to variable responses to available therapeutic options. For example, the *HMGCR* polymorphism, rs3846662, modulates women's sensitivity to statin treatments and several GWAS studies show an association between *PCSK9* polymorphisms and statin efficacy [81, 82].

The FH genetic defects are modulated by various genetic and epigenetic factors leading to a variety of genotypes which can influence the circulating levels of LDL-C, drug response and outcomes. For example, studies show the essential role for the LDLR mutation type in predicting response to statins. Moreover, people with certain *HMGCR* haplotypes also have difficulties in achieving guideline-recommended LDL-C [83].

Recent studies using non-statin lipid-lowering drugs demonstrate that LDL-C can be significantly reduced, even below 70, or even beyond 55 mg/dl, which is associated with an incremental risk reduction. For example, adding the new generation monoclonal antibody evinacumab (targeted against angiopoietin-like 3) to standard of care lipid-lowering therapy in patients with homozygous familial hypercholesterolaemia and refractory hypercholesterolemia may facilitate more patients attaining guideline-defined LDL-C goals and potentially reduce risk of cardiovascular disease events and overall mortality [84, 85].

A new generation of therapies, which are completely different from conventional approaches, are gene silencing therapies, such as those based on small interfering RNA or antisense oligonucleotides. Both approaches lead to temporary reductions in the expression of various genes. RNA-based approaches are convenient ways, with an infrequent dosing interval, to provide sustained reductions in LDL-C because of the mode of action and how it is delivered. This is already used for secondary CVD prevention in the UK population and studies are undergoing to validate the role in primary prevention [86, 87]. In the EU, inclisiran–siRNA directed against proprotein convertase subtilisin/kexin type 9 protein (PCSK9), has been approved in 2020 for the treatment of adults with primary hypercholesterolemia or mixed dyslipidemia.

Isgut et al. [88] show that PRS improves cardiovascular risk stratification early in life when later-life risk factors are unknown. By middle age, when many risk factors are known, improvement attributed to PRS is marginal for the general population. In the case of PCSK9 inhibitors treatment for familial hypercholesterolemia, a reduction in relative and absolute risk among people at high genetic risk has been demonstrated, which suggests an important role for PRS in identifying subgroups of people for whom these therapies would be cost-effective [88].

Despite the growing burden of CVD, drug development has faced multiple challenges. Compared to other therapeutic areas, the development of drugs for cardiovascular diseases is more expensive [89]. Pharmacogenomics represents an opportunity to revolutionize the design of drugs and clinical trials and make them cost-effective. Randomized clinical trials (RCTs) require a large number of patients to demonstrate a clinical effect. The interest of the scientific world is focused on selecting the patients who would have the greatest benefits from a particular treatment and thus reducing the need for very large cohorts [90].

Population differences in ADR susceptibility also have an impact on the drug development process. Performing clinical trials in a population that is different from the intended target market, especially when the drug is intended for use by individuals of diverse ethnicities can lead to challenges in real life. Pereira et al. demonstrated the importance of genotype-based RCTs in cardiovascular disease, showing that by identifying population groups that are likely to be more susceptible to a potential ADR, drug development companies can eliminate the huge cost and length of clinical trials [91].

5 Cancer, Pharmacogenomics, and the Public Health Impact

Although many efforts in cancer control have routinely focused on behavioral risk factor, advances in genetic testing have created new opportunities for cancer prevention through the evaluation of family history and identification of cancer-causing inherited mutations. The identification of *BRCA* or *HNPCC* gene mutation carriers has already impacted public health programs dedicated to breast and colorectal cancer, informing screening strategies for early detection and prophylactic surgery or preventive medicines (CDC tier 1 genomic applications) [92]. As sequencing costs are dropping, more application in cancer genomics are feasible in practice, including pharmacogenomic testing which can identify populations who might be susceptible to developing toxicity or severe adverse reactions, allowing a paradigm shift from the trial and error approach.

The proportion of drugs with genomic biomarker labeling has increased nearly threefold in the last two decades [67]. Oncology indications represent 39% of all FDA drug label warnings related to pharmacogenomic markers [93].

Pharmacogenomics can help chose dosage regimens and optimization of a therapeutic window of anticancer drugs. Genetic polymorphisms can be found in the genes that code for the metabolic enzymes, transporters, receptors. For example, dihydropyramidine dehydrogenase (*DPD*) gene shows great variability with different effects from treatment with 5-fluorouracil (5-FU) drugs being observed in terms of efficacy, resistance, or toxicity [94].

Different types of cancer immunotherapies, ranging from monoclonal antibodies, cancer vaccines to cell therapies, are currently revolutionizing clinical practice, working by activating the host immune response to eliminate cancer cells.

Microsatellite instability (MSI)/mismatch repair deficiency (dMMR) and tumor mutational burden (TMB) have been approved to guide treatment with PD-1 inhibitors (checkpoint inhibitors) such as pembrolizumab. Patients with MSI-high/dMMR or high TMB generally have higher overall response rates and longer progression-free survival in various solid tumors treated with PD-1 inhibitors. However, some NSCLC patients who show primary resistance are unresponsive to immune checkpoint inhibitors (ICIs), while others develop secondary resistance during/after the treatment. Other patients experience immune-related adverse events, which also limits the use of ICIs. Immunopharmacogenomics can explain such mechanisms that restrict the population which can benefit from immunotherapies [95].

To predict responses to oncology drugs, germline testing is important to explain inherited genomic characteristics which can influence systemic drug pharmacokinetics and pharmacodynamics. Testing the somatic mutations at the tumor level helps to assess the mutations which may be acquired in time and influence the way cancer cells respond to drugs. Germline genetic profile can also influence somatic change; therefore, somatic mutations have been used as endophenotypes to test for germline genetic variants that confer risk for obtaining specific somatic mutations.

Hutchcraft et al. [96] showed that germline whole exome data originally obtained for quality control purposes may be used to report pharmacogenomic variants. More than 90% of cancer patients carried at least one clinically action-able pharmacogenetic variant. One-quarter carried at least one pharmacogenomic variant for at least one therapeutic option indicated in their disease type. The data indicated that universal pharmacogenomic screening are feasible and may be an effective germline pharmacogenomic screening strategy for patients who are candidates for irinotecan, 5-fluorouracil, capecitabine, or 6-mercaptopurine [96].

Germline PGx and management of drug–drug interactions are likely to benefit advanced cancer patients who are frequently prescribed multiple concomitant med-ications to treat cancer and other associated conditions. Shugg et al. demonstrate important clinical utility of PGx germline testing and drug to drug interaction eval-uation on a cohort of 481 patients with advanced cancers. About 60% of subjects were prescribed at least one medication with CPIC recommendations, and around 14% of subjects had opportunities for actionable PGx [97].

Tamoxifen is a selective estrogen receptor modulator commonly used to both treat and prevent breast cancer [93]. Its pharmacological activity depends to some extent on the hepatic enzyme cytochrome P450 2D6 (CYP2D6), which converts tamoxifen to its active metabolite endoxifen. Over 100 *CYP2D6* variant alleles have been found so far. *CYP2D6* is a highly polymorphic gene and 5–10% of the population carry 2 nonfunctional alleles, and are referred to as CYP2D6 poor metabolizers, who have worse relapse-free breast cancer survival and increased risk for recurrence. Guidelines state that these categories should receive an alternative therapy such as aromatase inhibitors or an increase in tamoxifen dose [98].

Although individual genes with a major influence on the therapeutic response have been described so far, there is an increasing number of studies that show the genome-wide polygenic contribution. The UK Biobank includes data on the preva-lence of pharmacogenes in the population, on drug response profiles and disease information for over 500,000 individuals. Recent results, published by Marden-stein et al., point to corticosteroids as modulators of breast cancer genetic risk (by triggering cancer growth or modifying the immune response). The *IGSF23* rs62119267 genotype can stratify breast cancer risk among corticosteroid users [99].

Such data prove that there is a complex interaction between risk factors and that new tools such as GWAS and multiomic approaches are needed to point for new mechanisms and capture the contribution of polygenic variations. Moreover, biobanks are essential to advance future studies on gene–drug interactions and contribute to personalized recommendation in specific populations.

For example, incorporating a single cell technique with drug screening may help analyze the effects of intra-tumor heterogeneity and offer a better description of tumors as they evolve. It is known that sensitive clones are killed during treatment, and resistant clones keep growing. In some instances, prediction based on the molecular characteristics of a tumor before treatment may not reflect the evolution in time nor is suitable to assess the tumor evolution [100].

A less known area is pharmacoepitranscriptomics, studying the influence of RNA modifications on drug effects. Over two-thirds of pharmacogenes' RNAs have chemical modifications, with m6A being the most frequent. Several m6A regulators have been shown to affect drug sensitivity, especially for cancer chemotherapy and immunotherapy. A recent study shows that m6A modifications can become drug-effect biomarkers for treatment of TNBC, ovarian cancer, and acute myeloid leukemia (AML) [101].

6   Opportunities for Preemptive Pharmacogenomic Testing in Clinical Practice

Most economic evaluations of PGx-guided treatment indicate favorable cost-effectiveness; however, there are still gaps related to assessing the feasibility of preemptive PGx testing in routine care. In a review of 44 economic evaluations of pharmacogenetics, 30% were found to be cost-effective and 27% even cost saving [102].

There is a clear opportunity for concrete healthcare savings from improving prescription drug management. The pharmacogenetic information that is currently available to guide therapy selection and adjust dose requirements can significantly enhance the utility of prescription drugs, especially in patients with polytherapy [103].

PGx is useful not only in its ability to identify individual susceptibility to drug side effects when multiple therapeutic options have failed, but also in terms of pre-treatment assessment of the patient's individual response to a particular drugs combination.

Preemptive genetic testing is cost-effective in most situations, virtually benefits all, given that 95% of individuals present at least one clinically actionable PGx variant and could improve drug dosage while reducing ADRs [17]. At the level of the healthcare system, it could be more efficient to test once as the data have lifelong value in most cases. This involves the creation of a framework for storing the information, making it accessible, creating alerts to support clinicians in decision making, and returning results to patients that may be clinically impacted. Any healthcare professional within the health system can see PGx results and use them in making drug therapy decisions.

The Mayo-Baylor RIGHT 10K Study enabled preemptive, sequence-based pharmacogenomics (PGx)-driven drug prescribing practices in routine clinical care within a large cohort. In 10,077 individuals, 79% carried clinically actionable variants in ≥ 3 genes. Implementation of preemptive revealed nearly universal patient applicability, as opposed to the reactive, sequence-based traditional approach [104]. This requires integrated institution-wide resources to fully realize individualized drug therapy and to show more efficient use of healthcare resources.

A study conducted at the University of Colorado shows the feasibility of clinical implementation of pharmacogenomics via a health system-wide research biobank.

Some of the key factors for success are strong institutional support, a multidisciplinary team working on implementation, the use automated clinical decision support tools, developing strategies to engage stakeholders early in the clinical decision support tool development process [105].

Lanillos et al. [106] performed a comprehensive analysis on diagnostic exome data showing the untapped potential of pharmacogenomic information contained in this data which could be used preemptively in clinical practice. About 95% of the cohort of almost 5000 participants from Spain and Latin American countries could be informed of at least one actionable pharmacogenetic phenotype. Data that could be easily retrieved from exome data could prevent severe even fatal drug adverse reactions and guide drug dosing adjustments, according to international guidelines [106].

7   Future Perspectives for Pharmacogenomics and Public Health: Personalized Prevention

The developments in omics disciplines, the rise of polygenic risk scores, considering the citizen behavior and other health determinants, already built the foundation for a new era in public health: personalized prevention. Compared to one-size-fits-all preventive interventions that failed to reach the targets in both non-communicable (e.g., cancer, cardiovascular diseases, diabetes) and communicable diseases, the personalized prevention refers to a transversal discipline which aims to intersect the classical prevention types: primary, secondary, and tertiary. Personalized prevention is only possible if data on as many as possible health determinants are available, collected, and analyzed, with the pharmacogenomics data as an immediate to be implemented and essential pillar.

References

1. Jackson M, Marks L, May GHW, Wilson JB. The genetic basis of disease. Essays Biochem. 2018;62:643–723. https://doi.org/10.1042/EBC20170053.
2. Chakravarti A, Little P. Nature, nurture and human disease. Nature. 2013;421:412–4. https://doi.org/10.1038/nature01401.
3. The Genetic Variation in a Population Is Caused by Multiple Factors | Learn Science at Scitable. https://www.nature.com/scitable/topicpage/the-genetic-variation-in-a-population-is-6526354/. Accessed 25 Apr 2022
4. Fuselli S. Beyond drugs: the evolution of genes involved in human response to medications. Proc R Soc B Biol Sci. 2019;286:20191716. https://doi.org/10.1098/rspb.2019.1716.
5. Wang T, Antonacci-Fulton L, Howe K, et al. The Human Pangenome Project: a global resource to map genomic diversity. Nature. 2022;604:437–46. https://doi.org/10.1038/s41586-022-04601-8.
6. Nurk S, Koren S, Rhie A, Rautiainen M, Bzikadze AV, Mikheenko A, et al. The complete sequence of a human genome. Science. 2022;376(6588):44–53. https://doi.org/10.1126/science.abj6987.

7. Researchers generate the first complete, gapless sequence of a human genome. https://www.genome.gov/news/news-release/researchers-generate-the-first-complete-gapless-sequence-of-a-human-genome. Accessed 25 Apr 2022

8. Sirén J, Monlong J, Chang X, et al. Pangenomics enables genotyping of known structural variants in 5202 diverse genomes. Science. 2021;374(6574):abg8871. https://doi.org/10.1126/science.abg8871.

9. Grosse SD, Odame I, Atrash HK, Amendah DD, Piel FB, Williams TN. Sickle cell disease in Africa. Am J Prev Med. 2011;41:S398–405. https://doi.org/10.1016/j.amepre.2011.09.013.

10. Al-Jabri, Hasson SS. Genetic Diversity within Chemokine Receptor 5 (CCR5) for Better Understanding of AIDS. In: Bitz, L., editor. Genetic Diversity. London: IntechOpen; 2017. https://www.intechopen.com/chapters/53953. https://doi.org/10.5772/67256

11. Bachtiar M, Lee CGL. Genetics of population differences in drug response. Curr Genet Med Rep. 2013;1:162–70. https://doi.org/10.1007/s40142-013-0017-3.

12. Bowen MS, Kolor K, Dotson WD, Ned RM, Khoury MJ. Public health action in genomics is now needed beyond newborn screening. Public Health Genomics. 2012;15:327–34.

13. Molster CM, Bowman FL, Bilkey GA, Cho AS, Burns BL, Nowak KJ, Dawkins HJS. The evolution of public health genomics: exploring its past, present, and future. Front Public Health. 2018;6:247. https://doi.org/10.1159/000341889.

14. Khoury MJ, Holt KE. The impact of genomics on precision public health: beyond the pandemic. Genome Med. 2021;13:67. https://doi.org/10.1159/000341889.

15. Genome-based research and population health. Report of an Expert Workshop Held at the Rockefeller Foundation Study and Conference Center. Bellagio. 2005. http://www.phgfoundation.org/documents/74_1138619841.pdf. Accessed 17 Oct 2022.

16. The Path from Genome-based Research to Population Health: Development of an International Public Health Genomics Network. CDC. 2021. https://www.cdc.gov/genomics/hugenet/publications/populationhealth.htm. Accessed 25 Apr 2022

17. Stevenson JM, Alexander GC, Palamuttam N, Mehta HB. Projected utility of pharmacogenomic testing among individuals hospitalized with COVID-19: a retrospective multicenter study in the United States. Clin Transl Sci. 2021;14:153–62. https://doi.org/10.1111/cts.1291.

18. Personalised prescribing: using pharmacogenomics to improve patient outcomes. 2022. https://www.rcp.ac.uk/projects/outputs/personalised-prescribing-using-pharmacogenomics-improve-patient-outcomes. Accessed 26 Apr 2022

19. Nagar SD, Moreno AM, Norris ET, et al. Population pharmacogenomics for precision public health in Colombia. Front Genet (eCollection 2019). 2019;10:241. https://doi.org/10.3389/fgene.2019.00241.

20. Auwerx C, Sadler MC, Reymond A, Kutalik Z. From pharmacogenetics to pharmaco-omics: milestones and future directions. Hum Genet Genomics Adv. 2022;3: 100100. https://doi.org/10.1016/j.xhgg.2022.10010.

21. Pratt VM, Cavallari LH, Del Tredici AL, et al. Recommendations for clinical CYP2D6 genotyping allele selection: a joint consensus recommendation of the association for molecular pathology, College of American Pathologists, Dutch Pharmacogenetics Working Group of the Royal Dutch Pharmacists Association, and the European Society for Pharmacogenomics and Personalized Therapy. J Mol Diagn. 2021;23:1047–64. https://doi.org/10.1016/j.jmoldx.2021.05.013.

22. Charnaud S, Munro JE, Semenec L, et al. PacBio long-read amplicon sequencing enables scalable high-resolution population allele typing of the complex CYP2D6 locus. Commun Biol. 2022;5:1–10. https://doi.org/10.1038/s42003-022-03102-8.

23. Ko DC, Urban TJ. Understanding human variation in infectious disease susceptibility through clinical and cellular GWAS. PLoS Pathog. 2013;9: e1003424. https://doi.org/10.1371/journal.ppat.1003424.

24. Eslam M, George J. Genome-wide association studies and hepatitis C: harvesting the benefits of the genomic revolution. Semin Liver Dis. 2015;35:402–20. https://doi.org/10.1055/s-0035-1567830.

25. Davis GL, Wong JB, McHutchison JG, Manns MP, Harvey J, Albrecht J. Early virologic response to treatment with peginterferon alfa-2b plus ribavirin in patients with chronic hepatitis C. Hepatology. 2003;38:645–52. https://doi.org/10.1053/jhep.2003.50364.

26. McFarland AP, Horner SM, Jarret A, et al. IFNL3 (IL28B) favorable genotype escapes hepatitis C virus-induced microRNAs and mRNA decay. Nat Immunol. 2014;15:72–9. https://doi.org/10.1038/ni.2758.

27. Khasawneh LQ, Al-Mahayri ZN, Ali BR. Mendelian randomization in pharmacogenomics: the unforeseen potentials. Biomed Pharmacother. 2022;150: 112952. https://doi.org/10.1016/j.biopha.2022.112952.

28. Hao L, Kraft P, Berriz GF, et al. Development of a clinical polygenic risk score assay and reporting workflow. Nat Med. 2022;28(5):1006–13. https://doi.org/10.1038/s41591-022-017 67-6.

29. Part I: Genetics and public health: an overview Chapter 1. CDC. 2019. https://www.cdc.gov/genomics/resources/books/21stcent/chap01.htm. Accessed 25 Apr 2022

30. Özdemir V, Fisher E, Dove ES, Burton H, Wright GEB, Masellis M, Warnich L. End of the beginning and public health pharmacogenomics: knowledge in 'Mode 2' and P5 medicine. Curr Pharmacogenomics Pers Med. 2012;10:1–6. https://doi.org/10.2174/187569211120101 0001.

31. Saravanan KA, Panigrahi M, Kumar H, Rajawat D, Nayak SS, Bhushan B, Dutt T. Role of genomics in combating COVID-19 pandemic. Gene. 2022;823: 146387. https://doi.org/10.1016/j.gene.2022.146387.

32. van Dorp L, Houldcroft CJ, Richard D, Balloux F. COVID-19, the first pandemic in the post-genomic era. Curr Opin Virol. 2021;50:40–8. https://doi.org/10.1016/j.coviro.2021.07.002.

33. Chiara M, D'Erchia AM, Gissi C, et al. Next generation sequencing of SARS-CoV-2 genomes: challenges, applications and opportunities. Brief Bioinform. 2021;22:616–30. https://doi.org/10.1093/bib/bbaa297.

34. UK completes over 2 million SARS-CoV-2 whole genome sequences. https://www.gov.uk/government/news/uk-completes-over-2-million-sars-cov-2-whole-genome-sequences. Accessed 25 Apr 2022.

35. Bull RA, Adikari TN, Ferguson JM, et al. Analytical validity of nanopore sequencing for rapid SARS-CoV-2 genome analysis. Nat Commun. 2020;11:6272. https://doi.org/10.1038/s41467-020-20075-6.

36. Knyazev S, Chhugani K, Sarwal V, et al. Unlocking capacities of genomics for the COVID-19 response and future pandemics. Nat Methods. 2022;19:374–80.

37. Cyranoski D. Alarming COVID variants show vital role of genomic surveillance. Nature. 2021;589:337–8. https://doi.org/10.1038/d41586-021-00065-4.

38. Corey L, Beyrer C, Cohen MS, Michael NL, Bedford T, Rolland M. SARS-CoV-2 variants in patients with immunosuppression. N Engl J Med. 2021;385(6):562–6. https://doi.org/10.1056/NEJMsb2104756.

39. Velavan TP, Pallerla SR, Rüter J, Augustin Y, Kremsner PG, Krishna S, Meyer CG. Host genetic factors determining COVID-19 susceptibility and severity. EBioMedicine. 2021;72: 103629. https://doi.org/10.1016/j.ebiom.2021.103629.

40. Kwok AJ, Mentzer A, Knight JC. Host genetics and infectious disease: new tools, insights and translational opportunities. Nat Rev Genet. 2021;22:137–53. https://doi.org/10.1038/s41576-020-00297-6.

41. Rasmussen SA, Jamieson DJ, Uyeki TM. Effects of influenza on pregnant women and infants. Am J Obstet Gynecol. 2012;207:S3-8. https://doi.org/10.1016/j.ajog.2012.06.068.

42. Al-Azzawi MA, Sakr MA. Co-evolution between new coronavirus (SARS-CoV-2) and genetic diversity: insights on population susceptibility and potential therapeutic innovations. In: Maia RT, de Araújo Campos M, editors. Genetic variation. London: IntechOpen. 2020. https://www.intechopen.com/chapters/73379. https://doi.org/10.5772/intechopen.93676

43. Li J, Wang Y, Liu Y, Zhang Z, Zhai Y, Dai Y, Wu Z, Nie X, Du L. Polymorphisms and mutations of ACE2 and TMPRSS2 genes are associated with COVID-19: a systematic review. Eur J Med Res. 2022;27:26. https://doi.org/10.1186/s40001-022-00647-6.

44. Hou Y, Zhao J, Martin W, Kallianpur A, Chung MK, Jehi L, Sharifi N, Erzurum S, Eng C, Cheng F. New insights into genetic susceptibility of COVID-19: an ACE2 and TMPRSS2 polymorphism analysis. BMC Med. 2020;18:216. https://doi.org/10.1186/s12916-020-016 73-z.

45. COVID-19 Host Genetics Initiative. https://www.covid19hg.org/. Accessed 25 Apr 2022

46. COVID human genetic effort. https://www.covidhge.com. Accessed 25 Apr 2022

47. Malheiro A, Ramasawmy R, Courtin D, Donadi EA. Editorial: The role of gene polymorphisms in modulating the immune responses against tropical infectious diseases. Front Immunol. 2021;12: 714237. https://doi.org/10.3389/fimmu.2021.714237.

48. Zarkesh K, Entezar-Almahdi E, Ghasemiyeh P, et al. Drug-based therapeutic strategies for COVID-19-infected patients and their challenges. Future Microbiol. 2021;16:1415–51. https://doi.org/10.2217/fmb-2021-0116.

49. Taboada M, Rodríguez N, Varela PM, et al. Effect of high versus low dose of dexamethasone on clinical worsening in patients hospitalised with moderate or severe COVID-19 Pneumonia: An Open-label, randomised clinical trial. Eur Respir J. 2022;60(2):2102518. https://doi.org/10.1183/13993003.02518-2021.

50. Jankelson L, Karam G, Becker ML, Chinitz LA, Tsai M-C. QT prolongation, torsades de pointes, and sudden death with short courses of chloroquine or hydroxychloroquine as used in COVID-19: a systematic review. Heart Rhythm. 2020;17:1472–9. https://doi.org/10.1016/j.hrthm.2020.05.008.

51. Onori ME, Ricciardi Tenore C, Urbani A, Minucci A. Glucose-6-phosphate dehydrogenase deficiency and hydroxychloroquine in the COVID-19 era: a mini review. Mol Biol Rep. 2021;48:2973–8. https://doi.org/10.1007/s11033-021-06234-y.

52. Pineda-Tenor D, García-Álvarez M, Jiménez-Sousa MA, Vázquez-Morón S, Resino S. Relationship between ITPA polymorphisms and hemolytic anemia in HCV-infected patients after ribavirin-based therapy: a meta-analysis. J Transl Med. 2015;13:320. https://doi.org/10.1186/s12967-015-0682-y.

53. Xu Y, Li M, Zhou L, Liu D, He W, Liang W, Sun Q, Sun H, Li Y, Liu X. Ribavirin treatment for critically Ill COVID-19 patients: an observational study. Infect Drug Resist. 2021;14:5287–91. https://doi.org/10.2147/IDR.S330743.

54. Lin JJ, Loucks CM, Trueman JN, et al. Novel variant in glycophorin c gene protects against ribavirin-induced anemia during chronic hepatitis C treatment. Biomed Pharmacother. 2021;143: 112195. https://doi.org/10.1016/j.biopha.2021.112195.

55. Sahana S, Sivadas A, Mangla M, et al. Pharmacogenomic landscape of COVID-19 therapies from Indian population genomes. Pharmacogenomics. 2021;22:603–18. https://doi.org/10.2217/pgs-2021-0028.

56. Aschenbrenner AC, Mouktaroudi M, Krämer B, et al. Disease severity-specific neutrophil signatures in blood transcriptomes stratify COVID-19 patients. Genome Med. 2021;13:7. https://doi.org/10.1186/s13073-020-00823-5.

57. Şardaş S, Özdemir V. Pharmacogenomics for clinical trials of COVID-19 medicines: why is this important now? OMICS J Integr Biol. 2021;25:679–80. https://doi.org/10.1089/omi.2021.0176.

58. Biswas M, Sawajan N, Rungrotmongkol T, Sanachai K, Ershadian M, Sukasem C. Pharmacogenetics and precision medicine approaches for the improvement of COVID-19 therapies. Front Pharmacol. 2022;13: 835136. https://doi.org/10.3389/fphar.2022.835136.

59. O'Shea J, Ledwidge M, Gallagher J, Keenan C, Ryan C. Pharmacogenetic interventions to improve outcomes in patients with multimorbidity or prescribed polypharmacy: a systematic review. Pharmacogenomics J. 2022;22:89–99. https://doi.org/10.1038/s41397-021-00260-6.

60. Baker RE, Mahmud AS, Miller IF, et al. Infectious disease in an era of global change. Nat Rev Microbiol. 2022;20:193–205. https://doi.org/10.1038/s41579-021-00639-z.

61. Dandekar T, Dandekar G. Pharmacogenomic strategies against microbial resistance: from bright to bleak to innovative. Pharmacogenomics. 2010;11:1193–6. https://doi.org/10.2217/pgs.10.18.

62. Geanta M, Tanwar AS, Lehrach H, Satyamoorthy K, Brand A. Horizon scanning: rise of planetary health genomics and digital twins for pandemic preparedness. OMICS. 2022;26(2):93–100. https://doi.org/10.1089/omi.2021.0062.
63. Pharmacovigilance legislation (2018). Available at: https://www.ema.europa.eu/en/pharma covigilance-legislation. Accessed 25 Apr 2022
64. Montastruc J-L, Lafaurie M, de Canecaude C, Durrieu G, Sommet A, Montastruc F, Bagheri H. Fatal adverse drug reactions: a worldwide perspective in the World Health Organization pharmacovigilance database. Br J Clin Pharmacol. 2021;87:4334–40. https://doi.org/10.1111/bcp.14851.
65. Insani WN, Whittlesea C, Alwafi H, Man KKC, Chapman S, Wei L. Prevalence of adverse drug reactions in the primary care setting: a systematic review and meta-analysis. PLoS One. 2021;16: e0252161. https://doi.org/10.1371/journal.pone.0252161.
66. Pirmohamed M, James S, Meakin S, Green C, Scott AK, Walley TJ, Farrar K, Park BK, Breckenridge AM. Adverse drug reactions as cause of admission to hospital: prospective analysis of 18 820 patients. BMJ. 2004;329:15–9. https://doi.org/10.1136/bmj.329.7456.15.
67. Kim JA, Ceccarelli R, Lu CY. Pharmacogenomic biomarkers in US FDA-approved drug labels (2000–2020). J Pers Med. 2021;11:179. https://doi.org/10.3390/jpm11030179.
68. Guidance for Industry: E15 definitions for genomic biomarkers, pharmacogenomics, pharmacogenetics, genomic data and sample coding. https://www.fda.gov/media/71389/download. Accessed 17 Oct 2022
69. Abrishamcar S, Dotson WD, Khoury MJ. Tracking the scientific literature on the impact of pharmacogenomics on clinical practice and public health. https://blogs.cdc.gov/genomics/2022/04/04/tracking-the-scientific/. Accessed 18 Oct 2022
70. Dalton R, Brown JD, Duarte JD. Patients with geographic barriers to health care access are prescribed a higher proportion of drugs with pharmacogenetic testing guidelines. Clin Transl Sci. 2021;14:1841–52. https://doi.org/10.1111/cts.13032.
71. An EU cardiovascular action plan. https://www.europarl.europa.eu/doceo/document/E-9-2021-003111_EN.html. Accessed 26 Apr 2022
72. European organisations join forces to shine spotlight on cardiovascular health. https://www.escardio.org/The-ESC/Press-Office/Press-releases/European-organisations-join-forces-to-shine-spotlight-on-cardiovascular-health. Accessed 26 Apr 2022
73. Magavern EF, Kaski JC, Turner RM, et al. The role of pharmacogenomics in contemporary cardiovascular therapy: a position statement from the European Society of Cardiology Working Group on Cardiovascular Pharmacotherapy. Eur Heart J Cardiovasc Pharmacother. 2022;8:85–99. https://doi.org/10.1093/ehjcvp/pvab018.
74. CPIC® guideline for statins and SLCO1B1, ABCG2, and CYP2C9. https://cpicpgx.org/gui delines/cpic-guideline-for-statins/. Accessed 26 Apr 2022
75. Pereira NL, Rihal CS, So D, et al. Clopidogrel pharmacogenetics: state of the art review and the TAILOR-PCI study. Circ Cardiovasc Interv. 2019;12: e007811. https://doi.org/10.1161/CIRCINTERVENTIONS.119.007811.
76. Murdock DR, Venner E, Muzny DM, et al. Genetic testing in ambulatory cardiology clinics reveals high rate of findings with clinical management implications. Genet Med Off J Am Coll Med Genet. 2021;23:2404–14. https://doi.org/10.1038/s41436-021-01294-8.
77. Cuchel M, McGowan MP. Familial hypercholesterolaemia: too many lost opportunities. Lancet. 2021;398:1667–8. https://doi.org/10.1016/S0140-6736(21)01372-6.
78. Wiegman A, Gidding SS, Watts GF, et al. Familial hypercholesterolaemia in children and adolescents: gaining decades of life by optimizing detection and treatment. Eur Heart J. 2015;36:2425–37. https://doi.org/10.1093/eurheartj/ehv157.
79. Schaefer JR, Kurt B, Sattler A, Klaus G. Soufi M (2012) Pharmacogenetic aspects in familial hypercholesterolemia with the special focus on FHMarburg (FH p.W556R). Clin Res Cardiol Suppl. 2012;7:2–6. https://doi.org/10.1007/s11789-012-0041-y.
80. Kim H, Lee CJ, Pak H, et al. GENetic characteristics and REsponse to lipid-lowering therapy in familial hypercholesterolemia: GENRE-FH study. Sci Rep. 2020;10(1):19336. https://doi.org/10.1038/s41598-020-75901-0.

81. Hindi NN, Alenbawi J, Nemer G. Pharmacogenomics variability of lipid-lowering therapies in familial hypercholesterolemia. J Pers Med. 2021;11:877. https://doi.org/10.3390/jpm110 90877.

82. Chuan J, Qian Z, Zhang Y, Tong R, Peng M. The association of the PCSK9 rs562556 polymorphism with serum lipids level: a meta-analysis. Lipids Health Dis. 2019;18:105. https://doi.org/10.1186/s12944-019-1036-1.

83. Mangravite LM, Medina MW, Cui J, Pressman S, Smith JD, Rieder MJ, et al. Combined influence of LDLR and HMGCR sequence variation on lipid-lowering response to simvastatin. Arterioscler Thromb Vasc Biol. 2010;30:1485–92. https://doi.org/10.1161/ATVBAHA.110. 203273.

84. Park K, Vishnevetskaya K, Vaidyanathan J, Burckart GJ, Green DJ. Pediatric drug development studies for familial hypercholesterolemia submitted to the US Food and Drug Administration between 2007 and 2020. J Clin Pharmacol. 2022;62:397–408. https://doi.org/10.1002/ jcph.1973.

85. Three-part, single-arm, open-label study to evaluate the efficacy, safety, and pharmacokinetics of evinacumab in pediatric patients with homozygous familial hypercholesterolemia. https:// clinicaltrials.gov/ct2/show/NCT04233918. Accessed 18 Oct 2022

86. A placebo-controlled, double-blind, randomized trial to evaluate the effect of 300 mg of inclisiran sodium given as subcutaneous injections in subjects with atherosclerotic cardiovascular disease (ASCVD) or ACSVD risk-equivalents and elevated low-density lipoprotein cholesterol (LDL-C). https://clinicaltrials.gov/ct2/show/NCT03400800. Accessed 18 Oct 2022

87. Overview. Inclisiran for treating primary hypercholesterolaemia or mixed dyslipidaemia. https://www.nice.org.uk/guidance/TA733. Accessed 25 Apr 2022

88. Isgut M, Sun J, Quyyumi AA, Gibson G. Highly elevated polygenic risk scores are better predictors of myocardial infarction risk early in life than later. Genome Med. 2021;13:13. https:// doi.org/10.1186/s13073-021-00828-8.

89. Fordyce CB, Roe MT, Ahmad T, et al. Cardiovascular drug development: is it dead or just hibernating? J Am Coll Cardiol. 2015;65(15):1567–82. https://doi.org/10.1016/j.jacc.2015. 03.016.

90. Hockings JK, Pasternak AL, Erwin AL, Mason NT, Eng C, Hicks JK. Pharmacogenomics: an evolving clinical tool for precision medicine. Cleve Clin J Med. 2020;87:91–9. https://doi. org/10.3949/ccjm.87a.19073.

91. Pereira NL, Sargent DJ, Farkouh ME, Rihal CS. Genotype-based clinical trials in cardiovascular disease. Nat Rev Cardiol. 2015;12:475–87. https://doi.org/10.1038/nrcardio.2015.64.

92. Rodriguez JL, Thomas CC, Massetti GM, et al. CDC grand rounds: family history and genomics as tools for cancer prevention and control. MMWR Morb Mortal Wkly Rep. 2016;65(46):1291–4. https://doi.org/10.15585/mmwr.mm6546a3.

93. Carr DF, Turner RM, Pirmohamed M. Pharmacogenomics of anticancer drugs: personalising the choice and dose to manage drug response. Br J Clin Pharmacol. 2021;87:237–55. https:// doi.org/10.1111/bcp.14407.

94. Donadio MDS, Carraro DM, Torrezan GT, de Mello CAL. Dihydropyrimidine dehydrogenase (DPD) polymorphisms knocking on the door. Ecancermedicalscience. 2022;16:1344. https://doi.org/10.3332/ecancer.2022.1344.

95. Calibasi-Kocal G, Baskin Y. Immunopharmacogenomics in Cancer Management. In: Liu Y, editor. Genetic Diversity and Disease Susceptibility. London: IntechOpen; 2018. https:// www.intechopen.com/chapters/61177. https://doi.org/10.5772/intechopen.76934

96. Hutchcraft ML, Lin N, Zhang S, et al. Real-world evaluation of universal germline screening for cancer treatment-relevant pharmacogenes. Cancers. 2021;13:4524. https://doi.org/10. 3390/cancers13184524.

97. Shugg T, Ly RC, Rowe EJ, et al. Clinical opportunities for germline pharmacogenetics and management of drug-drug interactions in patients with advanced solid cancers. JCO Precis Oncol. 2022;6: e2100312. https://doi.org/10.1200/PO.21.00312.

98. Yang Y, Botton MR, Scott ER, Scott SA. Sequencing the CYP2D6 gene: from variant allele discovery to clinical pharmacogenetic testing. Pharmacogenomics. 2017;18:673–85. https://doi.org/10.2217/pgs-2017-0033.

99. Marderstein AR, Kulm S, Peng C, Tamimi R, Clark AG, Elemento O. A polygenic-score-based approach for identification of gene-drug interactions stratifying breast cancer risk. Am J Hum Genet. 2021;108:1752–64. https://doi.org/10.1016/j.ajhg.2021.07.008.

100. Feng F, Shen B, Mou X, Li Y, Li H. Large-scale pharmacogenomic studies and drug response prediction for personalized cancer medicine. J Genet Genomics. 2021;48:540–51. https://doi.org/10.1016/j.jgg.2021.03.007.

101. Liu K, Ouyang QY, Zhan Y, et al. Pharmacoepitranscriptomic landscape revealing m6A modification could be a drug-effect biomarker for cancer treatment. Mol Ther Nucleic Acids. 2022;28:464–76. https://doi.org/10.1016/j.omtn.2022.04.001.

102. Verbelen M, Weale ME, Lewis CM. Cost-effectiveness of pharmacogenetic-guided treatment: are we there yet? Pharmacogenomics J. 2017;17(5):395–402. https://doi.org/10.1038/tpj.2017.21.

103. Saldivar J-S, Taylor D, Sugarman EA, Cullors A, Garces JA, Oades K, Centeno J. Initial assessment of the benefits of implementing pharmacogenetics into the medical management of patients in a long-term care facility. Pharmacogenomics Pers Med. 2016;9:1–6. https://doi.org/10.2147/PGPM.S93480.

104. Wang L, Scherer SE, Bielinski SJ, et al. Implementation of preemptive DNA sequence–based pharmacogenomics testing across a large academic medical center: The Mayo-Baylor RIGHT 10K Study. Genet Med. https://doi.org/10.1016/j.gim.2022.01.022

105. Aquilante CL, Kao DP, Trinkley KE, et al. Clinical implementation of pharmacogenomics via a health system-wide research biobank: the University of Colorado experience. Pharmacogenomics. 2020;21:375–86. https://doi.org/10.2217/pgs-2020-0007.

106. Lanillos J, Carcajona M, Maietta P, Alvarez S, Rodriguez-Antona C. Clinical pharmacogenetic analysis in 5,001 individuals with diagnostic exome sequencing data. NPJ Genomic Med. 2022;7:1–9. https://doi.org/10.1038/s41525-022-00283-3.

Ethical Issues in Pharmacogenomics

Erin D. Williams and Michele M. Schoonmaker

Abstract

The ethical issues raised by clinical pharmacogenomics fall broadly into three interrelated categories: ownership, access, and use. Ownership issues relate to who controls and may profit from genomic data and biological samples. Access issues relate to who may leverage genomic data and biological samples, and who benefits from the fruits of pharmacogenomics in medicine. Use issues relate to the purposes for which genomic information, biological specimens, and pharmacogenomic findings may be harnessed. Associated key ethical concepts include justice and equity; autonomy and informed consent; nonmaleficence, beneficence, and utility; and privacy and confidentiality. This chapter defines the key ethical concepts involved in clinical pharmacogenomics, applies the ethical concepts to pharmacogenomic issues of ownership, access, and use, and presents the most common rules and guidelines designed to protect and direct those involved in pharmacogenomics.

Keywords

Pharmacogenomics · Ethics · Biobank · Human subjects research · Informed consent

E. D. Williams (✉)
The MITRE Corporation, McLean, VA, USA
e-mail: erinw@mitre.org

M. M. Schoonmaker
Michele Schoonmaker, LLC, Annapolis, MD, USA
e-mail: michele@mmschoo.com

© The Author(s), under exclusive license to Springer Nature Switzerland AG 2023
D. Primorac et al. (eds.), *Pharmacogenomics in Clinical Practice*,
https://doi.org/10.1007/978-3-031-45903-0_19

1   Introduction

Pharmacogenomics is a powerful tool that, in different circumstances, can produce life-saving or life-threatening discriminatory effects. Understanding and addressing ethical issues related to pharmacogenomics enables practitioners to realize its benefits while mitigating its risks.

The issues raised by pharmacogenomics fall broadly into three interrelated categories: ownership, access, and use. Ownership issues relate to who controls and may profit from genomic data and biological samples. Access issues relate to who may leverage genomic data and biological samples, and who benefits from the fruits of pharmacogenomics in medicine. Use issues relate to the purposes for which genomic information, biological specimens, and pharmacogenomic findings may be harnessed.

Ethics can help those involved with the practice of pharmacogenomics recognize and resolve issues. The key ethical concepts raised by pharmacogenomics are justice and equity; autonomy and informed consent; nonmaleficence, beneficence, and utility; and privacy and confidentiality. These concepts are useful for practitioners not only in raising and evaluating issues, but also because the concepts form the foundation of many rules and guidelines that govern pharmacogenomics research and clinical practice.

This chapter defines the key ethical concepts in pharmacogenomics. Next, it applies the ethical concepts to pharmacogenomic issues of ownership, access, and use. Finally, it presents the most common rules and guidelines designed to protect and direct those involved in pharmacogenomics.

2   Key Ethical Concepts in Pharmacogenomics

For purposes of this chapter, ethics refers to well-established standards of right and wrong. It is worth noting that this definition is not universal. In fact, many definitions and types of ethics have evolved over the centuries—virtue-based, deontological, utilitarian, feminist, normative, applied, subjective, hedonist, contractual, liberation, and religious, just to name a few—sometimes sparking spirited debate among their proponents.

Like the definition of ethics itself, there are many ethical concepts that have been explored over time—honesty, integrity, professionalism, responsibility, caring, citizenship, avoiding deception, human solidarity, the common good, and many more. This section introduces a set of ethical concepts that lend themselves to evaluating issues in the practice of pharmacogenomics: justice and equity; autonomy and informed consent; nonmaleficence, beneficence, and utility; and privacy and confidentiality.

The definition of ethics and concepts presented are well established, underscore many practice guidelines, illuminate potential issues in the practice of pharmacogenomics, and lead to guidance for those involved.

2.1   Justice and Equity

Justice refers to the allocation of burdens and benefits in a society. There are several types of justice, and the one most pertinent to pharmacogenomics is distributive justice. Distributive justice means fair, equitable, and appropriate distribution and includes policies that allot diverse benefits and burdens, like property, resources, taxation, privileges, or opportunities [1]. Equity is a related concept. The Institute of Medicine defines equitable health care provided in a way that does not vary in quality because of personal characteristics such as gender, ethnicity, geographic location, and socioeconomic status [2].

Pharmacogenomics has the potential to raise issues of distributive justice and exacerbate inequities—some along racial lines. Populations may become (further) disadvantaged if their diseases or conditions are not in pharmacogenomic research, or if pharmacogenomic testing is not available to them due to a lack of healthcare infrastructure, insurance coverage, or provider training [3]. They may also be disadvantaged by the use of race as the basis for research or clinical decision-making, which is being scrutinized due to a growing recognition that race-based diagnosis and treatment reflect flawed biological, social, and genetic assumptions [4].

2.2   Autonomy and Informed Consent

Autonomy refers to respecting people and their choices. In health care, it is associated generally with enabling patients to make their own decisions about treatment and what happens to their own body [5]. Autonomy emphasizes privacy and self-determination [6]. Informed consent is a process that supports autonomy in health care and research. It involves ensuring a person is made aware of pertinent risks and benefits so they can make an autonomous choice consistent with their personal beliefs. Informed consent is based on respect for the individual and his or her right both to define personal goals and make choices designed to achieve those goals [7].

In pharmacogenomic research, protecting autonomy with informed consent requires that participants be told about and understand the risks of the study, have the right to decline or withdraw at any point, and explicitly agree to participate [8]. In clinical practice, patients should be made aware of the services that they are agreeing to undergo, the risks and benefits of the test/treatment itself, the risks and benefits of how information from a test could affect their lifestyle, whether the information would impact a risk (or benefit) for responding to other treatments; information needs to be accurate [9]. Patients and research participants both should have the option to receive only certain information, such as the main result of a pharmacogenetic test, and opt-out of receiving any secondary information [9, 10].

Informed consent for research or clinical testing may be a challenging process for a number of reasons. For example, the sheer volume of information that may be revealed can create a barrier to truly informed consent. There may be an overwhelming amount to consider. Patients or consumers may be given the opportunity to decide what kinds of information they do and do not want to receive [11].

Another challenge can be created by the evolving nature of our knowledge. It is possible for a person to have their genome sequenced now and only learn the range of possible implications of that choice in the future as research turns data into knowledge. Even if they have consented to diagnostic testing, patients may provide specimens for research in clinical trials. In this case, hospital laboratories have often not provided consent for additional testing for research purposes [12]. Consent is generally specific to a given purpose rather than being broad based to cover any potential purpose; it is impractical to recontact individuals for every future study. Open consent is a relatively new practice that may allow an individual to grant unrestricted consent to future use of specimens or genomic information, which can help to enable future research [13].

2.3   Nonmaleficence and Beneficence and Utilitarianism

Nonmaleficence refers to the duty to do no harm. Beneficence refers to the duty to benefit others. Utilitarianism generally refers to a duty to do the greatest good for the greatest number of people. Beneficence is an underpinning of utilitarianism (the duty to do good for the most people). There are differences of opinion about what constitutes good [1].

In pharmacogenomics and healthcare generally, nonmaleficence and beneficence have long been staples underpinning the rules that govern doctor patient relationships. Physicians are commonly bound to benefit and not to harm their patients. These are reflected in UNESCO's Declaration on Bioethics and Human Rights, which calls for benefits to research participants and other affected individuals to be maximized and harm to be minimized [14]. In pharmacogenomic research, nonmaleficence requires that potential harm from the development and use of pharmacogenomics, such as stigmatization, be reduced [15]. Participation in research can also have elements of beneficence, because it can benefit the participant, and may also benefit others [16]. Wide-scale pharmacogenomic research can be supported by utilitarianism to the extent that it aims to benefit most people in society.

2.4   Privacy and Confidentiality

Privacy generally means a state of being free from intrusion or observation. Confidentiality, by contrast, refers to a state in which information is shared in a protected relationship, such as that between a doctor and patient. Both may involve control over how and when information is revealed, but confidentiality typically arises in a relationship of trust. In medicine and biomedical research, both are governed by a complex set of rules, governing when health information, including genetic information, may be disclosed. For example, when required for law enforcement purposes confidentiality of health information may be waived.

Pharmacogenomics creates some challenges to protecting both privacy and confidentiality. Genomes are both unique and shared with families and subpopulations. As a result, the emergence of whole genome sequencing has implications not just for the individuals who elect to have sequencing done, but also for their family members. Once samples or genomics data are collected and stored, abridgements of privacy and confidentiality may lead to risks of discrimination, stigmatization, loss of insurance coverage, raised premiums, or even criminal prosecution.

With this overview of general ethical concepts and principles that should influence practice, we turn to a set of ethical issues raised in pharmacogenomics.

3 Ethical Issues Raised by Pharmacogenomics

Pharmacogenomics can produce many benefits. It is a key to unlocking the potential of precision medicine: delivering the right drug at the right dose at the right time to the right patient [17]. Pharmacogenomic research and development can result in drugs to treat heritable or somatic diseases. It can enable risk assessments to determine the safety and efficacy of drugs in certain individuals with cancer or other conditions. It can identify fast and slow metabolizers of common medicines, so clinicians can design drug regimens based on a patients' metabolic enzyme activity. It can prevent prescribing drugs that would not benefit—or could even harm—specific patients [18]. Adverse drug reactions may harm patients and be expensive—costing up to $30.1 billion annually in the US health system alone [19]. Pharmacogenomic testing can be a significant tool for reducing some adverse drug reactions, which are estimated to be responsible for 3%–12% of hospital admissions and 5% of deaths of those patients in US hospitals [20].

Pharmacogenomics also raises issues, which if not properly managed can lead to undesirable consequences. This section explores the issues raised by pharmacogenomics, breaking them into three interrelated categories: ownership, access, and use. Each subsection reviews one category, describing the relevant issues and evaluating them using the ethical principles.

3.1 Ownership Issues

Most ethical, legal, social issues related to non-targeted (whole genome) testing have to do with information, starting with who owns that information [11]. Ownership issues in pharmacogenomics relate to who controls and may profit from genomic data and biological samples. There is a need to balance risk to individual with the benefit to society as fear of repercussions or negative impact from inappropriate use of the information may make patients reluctant to undergo tests.

This section focuses on ownership by individuals, corporations, and biobanks. It explores issues of justice, equity, beneficence, utility, confidentiality, autonomy, and informed consent.

Individual ownership

There are presumptions, which are reflected in law, that each individual owns his or her DNA, and that genomic information derived from testing that DNA should be kept confidential in the health system. The presumption that individuals own their own DNA is based on respect for individuals' autonomy. It enables one's ability to choose what is done with one's own genomic information.

Corporate ownership

Corporations or other organizations may acquire rights to an individual's genomic information legally and ethically through an agreement with the individual. This typically occurs in exchange for a service, or in the course of research or treatment. Rights to genomic information are valuable for a number of reasons. Pharmacogenomic variants are often the subject for diagnostic tests that could predict the likelihood of a drug response or adverse reaction. Intellectual property rights to genomic information enable companies to develop commercial diagnostic tests for profit.

When individuals undergo testing either from private ancestry companies or provide samples for use in clinical studies, they may give rights to that information to the company. For example, 23andMe is a US-based company that collects consumer saliva, isolates DNA, and provides interpretative information regarding the health and ancestry of that individual. Individuals who send samples to 23andMe may opt-in to agree that their data may be shared with third parties. With individuals' consent, 23andMe has collected and catalogued thousands of individuals' DNA. About 80% of 23andMe customers agree to share their data. 23andMe has a contractual relationship with Genentech, a pharmaceutical company, to share data as part of the company's research on Parkinson's disease [21].

When individuals agree that 23andMe may provide their genetic information to a biotech company for research to develop tests and treatments for diseases, the biotech company also helps to subsidize the cost of testing. Some of this research has benefitted society. For example, user data has recently been leveraged to investigate the genetics of attention deficit/hyperactivity disorder (ADHD), neuroticism, and depression [21].

Corporate rights to genomic information may support utilitarian objectives to the extent that they create societal benefits with new medical tests and treatments. Such rights—if acquired through meaningful informed consent—also reflect respect for data donors' autonomy. People's ability to transfer of intellectual property rights is premised on the notion that they have a right to decide whether and how their body, body parts, and associated data will be used [22]. An individual may make an autonomous choice to, reflected in informed consent, share his or her genomic information in exchange for a service and/or to enable a benefit to society.

Issues of equity and justice may arise if the risks flow to one group (e.g., data donors facing discrimination or higher life insurance premiums), while benefits flow to another (for example, those who commercialize the data receive profits). While corporations, not the people who contribute their genomic data, typically do the work to develop and commercialize products and take on associated financial risks, they also reap the rewards. Possible inequities or injustices may be mitigated by ensuring that data donation is truly informed and voluntary, that research occurs to benefit all participants, including those in historically underrepresented groups, and that testing and treatment are widely available.

Genomic data that are donated are often anonymized before they are shared. In the case of whole genome sequencing, because genomes are unique, there are questions about whether true anonymization is possible, or whether re-identification may occur. In order to protect donor's privacy and enable those handling the data to maintain the confidentiality of the data and related health information, good practice guidelines and security measures should be followed (e.g., [23]).

Biobank Ownership

Biobanks are public or private entities that collect and store specimens and associated information for future studies. Specimens are typically remnants from clinical pharmaceutical trials, (e.g., tumor sections from a prospective study of patients who did and did not receive a drug). Biobanked specimens are useful to enable retrospective analyses leading to rapid evaluations of the analytical or clinical validity of a new pharmacogenomic biomarker. Just as corporations may acquire rights to genomic information, biobanks may acquire rights to specimens and their corresponding annotated information. Like genomic data, acquiring rights to biospecimens typically occurs in exchange for a service, or in the course of research or treatment.

One famous case that highlights ownership issues was that of Henrietta Lacks. She was a young African American mother who was diagnosed with an aggressive form of cervical cancer. Before she succumbed to the disease, tissue samples were taken by her physician. Cells from the tumor grew extremely well in vitro and are viable today. HeLa cells as they became known have contributed significantly to both discovery and the development of medicines [24].

While originally HeLa cells were freely available, they later were commercialized in a way that was extremely lucrative for companies that sold them. The Lacks family received no renumeration and remained poor, with little access to health care. In 2013, researchers sequenced the HeLa cell genome, providing publicly available health information about Henrietta Lacks and her family. As a result of intense scrutiny that followed, the Director of the National Institutes of Health removed the sequence information from the public domain. Now, any researcher seeking to use HeLa cells or the information must go through committee review that includes members of the Lacks family [24].

The case of Henrietta Lacks raises significant issues of equity and justice. The valuable tissue was taken from one woman's body and not amassed from the aggregated genomic information from many donors. And it was companies that used her cells who profited, while her family remained uncompensated. The benefits were not equitably distributed. The inclusion of her family members on a research committee supports autonomy and justice, but not financial equity.

As with genomic information, rights to biospecimens acquired through meaningful informed consent reflect respect donors' autonomy. Consent signifies individuals' decisions to share their specimens to enable a benefit to society. For biobanking, consent should include critical information about sample storage, usage, destruction, and anonymity and include an option for withdrawing samples and sharing results [25–27]. For biobanks operating in international networks, the informed consent should be amenable to universal models [28].

Biobanking may also spark utilitarian, privacy, and confidentiality issues. The fruits of biobanking arguably support utilitarian objectives, to the extent that they create societal benefits with new medical tests and treatments. However, they may raise issues of privacy and confidentiality, if anonymization is not possible, or if re-identification can occur. Protecting the privacy of donors and treating information that may be gleaned about as confidential is possible with sound guidelines and security measures that protect specimens and related information during sample collection, storage, use, and sharing [29, 30].

3.2   Access Issues

There are two broad categories of issues related to access in clinical pharmacogenomics explored in this section. One set of access issues relates to the question of who may obtain genomic data, such as donors or patients, health providers, recreational genetics companies, targeted advertisers, or law enforcement agents. The other set of access issues focus on who can obtain pharmacogenomic services, which may be based on research with limited populations, may be expensive, and may require specialized training, staff, and/or equipment. These two categories raise ethical issues related to access, including autonomy, consent, privacy, confidentiality, nonmaleficence, justice, and equity.

Access to genomic data

Health information, including genomic information, was traditionally solely accessible to health practitioners. The US Clinical Laboratory Improvement Amendments of 1988 gave laboratories rights to give patients direct access to their laboratory test reports, whereas in past only healthcare providers were authorized to receive results [31]. Now, in the form of personal health records, genomic and other health information can be accessed by individuals or even third parties [31]. Within the health system, genomic test results may be shared by not only the patient and the ordering provider, but with other authorized parties, such multiple providers within that institution, to facilitate coordinated medical care and improved outcomes.

Barriers to data sharing include resources, data ownership, assurance in data curation, and the belief in the accuracy and protection of sensitive information.

Despite the issues, the US Association of Molecular Pathology (AMP) supports widespread sharing of de-identified variant data and encourages inclusion of data from diverse populations [32]. Both AMP and the American College of Medical Genetics and Genomics (ACMG) agree that clinical laboratories should share data to advance the development and validation of tests and treatments. In 2017, the ACMG called for the extensive sharing of laboratory and clinical data from genetic testing in a position paper [33]. Both AMP and the College of American Pathologists (CAP) support insurance coverage of pharmacogenetic tests that are supported by clinical guidelines, such as the Clinical Pharmacogenetic Implementation Consortium (CPIC) guidelines in addition to the pharmacogenomic information included in FDA-labeling [34].

ACMG recommends that laboratories be fully transparent in all uses of patient data including when conducting quality assurance checks, in test development, and in sharing data with public databases. They have made the following recommendations, among others [23]: (1) clinicians should alert patients about their results when they order tests, and let patients know that data may be shared in de-identified form for research, ultimately giving patients the choice of whether to participate; (2) a Data Use Agreement should be in place to prevent consumers from being exploited, with the testing laboratory protecting the privacy of genetic information, particularly for sensitive uses, like for studies involving genetics and psychosocial traits; (3) resale or other transfer of genomic data should be prohibited unless de-identification can be assured with informed consent required by the patient should re-identification be necessary; and (4) it is ultimately the patient's decision whether to allow their data to be shared for any reason. In making this decision, patients should be able to choose to either opt-in or opt-out of participation following an informed discussion of how data would be used.

In another program, the Cancer Moonshot Public Access and Data Sharing (PADS) Program, the US National Cancer Institute sought to enhance data sharing and make evidence-based approaches to cancer therapy more broadly available to patients. As a result, the program required the submission of a PADS plan with each funding application, emphasizing that funding priority would be given to applicants that ensured maximal sharing of resulting publications and data. Despite the requirements, a study of 33 PADS plans submitted with funded FY18 Cancer Moonshot applications reveals that few fully addressed the requirements of the PADS Policy [35].

Within the US health system, patient data exchange is regulated by provisions of the Health Insurance Portability and Accountability Act of 1996 (HIPAA), which specifies how and when protected health information can be shared [36].

Under HIPAA, data can be accessed by regulatory agencies and insurance companies for defined business purposes. Non-healthcare agencies that provide rehabilitation, educational, or long-term care services for patients may have access to information in the electronic health record and fall outside the HIPAA.

Organizations that operate outside of the health system in the USA can obtain health information, including genomic information, directly from individuals. In these cases, the protections and restrictions in HIPAA typically do not attach.

Individuals may choose to give samples for genomic testing to non-health companies to learn about their ancestry, paternity, or to find relatives, for example. These organizations can share or sell the data, giving others' access, without having to adhere to HIPAA's requirements.

It has been suggested that complete protection of privacy is not realistic when direct-to-consumer genetic tests are sold on the Internet [37]. Though health care and research companies explicitly use informed consent processes to maintain data anonymity, public company Web sites may offer no such assurances, which may lead to unforeseen uses of the data. For example, GEDMatch is a service that allows individuals to upload their own information to find relatives. The information on GEDMatch has been accessed by law enforcement to solve crimes such as the case of the Golden State killer in California [21]. The act of sharing one's genomic information remains at the discretion of the individual. There are no protections for relatives who may or may not want to be found, or who may or may not want to know certain information.

Looking with an ethics lens, practitioners of clinical genomics should ensure their patients understand the risks and benefits of genomic testing before doing the analysis to obtain genomic data. Practitioners should also protect their patients' privacy by keeping the data confidential, limiting disclosures to those required or permitted by law. In this way, they can limit possible harm that could come from disclosures, supporting their non-maleficent obligation to do no harm.

Access to pharmacogenomic services

A complex set of issues arises when considering how to make the fruits of clinical pharmacogenomics available across society. Individual access to clinical pharmacogenomics varies due to research and resource limitations. If a population is underrepresented in research, products like diagnostics or therapeutics developed from the research ultimately may not work for them. Even if there are applicable products, the analysis and expertise needed to use pharmacogenomics in clinical settings is not yet widely or equitably available.

Access sparked from research
One type of interference with access to the fruits of pharmacogenomics can arise upstream, during research. Some have noted that drug companies might be discouraged from developing drugs that would benefit only a small number of patients, simply because the financial incentives are not present, particularly for individuals with rare genetic variants or rare conditions [38, 39]. A possible solution could be to use bioinformatic prediction of the effects of mutations on drug response/in silico prediction of drug response [39].

Research conducted in only certain groups leads to the development of products untested in others. If inequity continues in study enrollment, the benefits of the research will continue to be unevenly distributed among population groups [31]. This effectively makes the resulting products inaccessible, because they are of unproven utility among those underrepresented.

Historically, underrepresentation of certain groups in research was due in part to a bias in favor of white males as research subjects, which left products undertested in women and minorities. It can be difficult to gather the necessary genetic information from underrepresented populations (e.g., poor, developing countries) that may have limited access to health care generally or conditions that are not present in developed countries. Therefore, these groups may receive suboptimal benefits from the research [31].

The underrepresentation of some populations in research has also been caused by skepticism about participating in research. This skepticism is due in part to history: some research involving minorities has resulted in debacle [40]. Debacles undermine trust and lead some to be reluctant to participate in or trust biomedical research.

The Tuskegee Syphilis Study was a notable example of a study that undermined trust in the research enterprise. In 1932, the US Public Health Service started a 40-year study of the natural history of syphilis in African American men. Of 600 men enrolled, 399 had syphilis, and 201 did not. The men were not offered informed consent at the time they were enrolled in the study. Worse, although penicillin was available for treatment of syphilis in 1943, the men were not treated and were observed while they suffered the long-term effects of the disease, such as damage to the brain, eyes, heart, nerves, bones, liver, and joints. The government stopped the study in 1972, almost 30 years after treatment became available, following the publication of a news in article. In 1973, there was a class action lawsuit filed on behalf of the participants and their families. This resulted in an out-of-court settlement of $10 million in 1974 [41]. Knowledge of this study diminished the willingness of people, particularly African Americans, to participate in research [42].

Today, patients participating in clinical research in the USA are protected under Human Subjects Research Protection regulations (see 45 Code of Federal Regulation (CFR) part 46, and 21 CFR parts 50 and 56). Some note that if enthusiasm for research threatens those protections, human rights and scientific integrity come into question [43]. Even with strict compliance, however, there may still be room for improvement diversifying research participant populations. In a 2011 study of publications that included the National Human Genome Research Institute (NHGRI) Catalog of Genome-Wide Associations, nearly 75% of studies only involved populations of European descent, with fewer than 10% focused exclusively on non-Europeans (primarily China, Japan, and other Asian countries) [44].

Pharmacogenomics may be used to facilitate research if the underlying data and decisions are sound. Selecting clinical study participants based on pharmacogenomic biomarkers can result in smaller trials by limiting the number of patients to those that may receive the greatest benefit (fairness) at lower cost [45]. However, if the information regarding the association of the biomarker and the disease or condition is not valid, there is potential for stigmatization and discrimination among a group with that particular characteristic, some of which characteristics are visible, some are not.

Despite the obstacles, there have been significant efforts to ensure that historically underrepresented or hard to reach populations are included in genomic and other research [46]. For example, one study found that participation of medically underserved populations could be increased by improving research awareness and knowledge of clinical trials. In addition, reducing time needed for participation and compensating for travel also led to increased participation [47]. Others recommend conducting studies in developing countries whose populations tend to be underrepresented in medical research [48]. These types of efforts toward inclusion in turn enable the evaluation of the clinical and analytical validity of new pharmacogenetic biomarkers to prove that the markers will benefit underrepresented patients.

Once again looking through an ethics lens, issue of equity is quite important in research. The benefits of research should be distributed across society. Efforts need to persist to ensure that no participants are unjustly excluded from research because of race, location, or other incidental reason. In addition, ensuring adequate informed consent and balancing possible benefits with risks (beneficence and nonmaleficence) help build trust that ultimately enhances access to research its results.

Access to clinical pharmacogenomic expertise and services
Ensuring equity in access to pharmacogenomics in clinical medicine is challenging. It is also important, as groups that are underrepresented in research are likely to receive suboptimal benefits from existing healthcare services [49]. The ability of people to access clinical pharmacogenomic services will depend on the availability of payment, on trained providers to interpret tests and deliver services, and on having the appropriate associated infrastructure.

An ability to pay represents one essential component of access to clinical pharmacogenomic services. One's ability to pay is based in part on the cost of pharmacogenomic testing. Some have noted that, while such testing may have potential to decrease overall costs to healthcare system, it may raise direct costs of medications at individual level [50, 51]. Personalized medicines developed with pharmacogenomics may target smaller subpopulations and not be appropriate for all. Drug companies that produce personalized medicines may thus have smaller markets and charge more for those drugs.

The cost of custom drug development for rare variants is a barrier to accessibility of genomic technologies in drug development. It raises issues related to rationing and who will bear the costs of development of rare treatments for rare diseases [39]. If the cost of pharmacogenomic or personalized medicine services is too high, it will limit access and bring social justice challenges to personalized genomic medicine [52]. Because of these issues, there are special programs to fund and reduce the time to market for tests and treatments for rare diseases and conditions [53].

An individuals' ability to pay for and access services may also depend on whether a patient has health insurance coverage for the service or has the means to pay out-of-pocket. Some note a danger of creating orphan populations when patients are potentially stratified depending on their economic status, as personalized drugs are expensive. Access then becomes either prohibitive or, stratification occurs based on race or nationality as a proxy [9]. The uneven availability of "boutique style" health care—like personalized medicine—may create a disadvantage to less developed countries [48].

Many countries have developed guidelines to address the potential discrimination, bias, or disadvantages, favoring the widespread availability of the benefits or research. For example, the Iranian National Ethical Guideline for Genetic Research recommends that the results of research on human genome be broadly accessible for the society [45]. The Universal Declaration on Human Genome and Human Rights (1997) insists that the benefits from advances in biology, genetics, and medicine be widely available to all not just to patients who can afford them as most services are expensive and not covered by insurance [45].

Even for those with insurance, pharmacogenomic services may not be covered. In the USA, private insurers' coverage and payments for pharmacogenomic tests vary, and research demonstrating clinical utility of gene-drug pairs may remain suboptimal, according to a 2020 study [54]. National health insurance systems may not cover expensive tests, like pharmacogenomic ones, without proven efficacy [31].

Tests need to be analytically and clinically valid so that individuals make sound decisions regarding treatment options [55]. When payment is available for analytically and clinically valid pharmacogenomic tests, access may still be limited by clinicians' ability and willingness to use them. Emerging medical technologies makes medicine more complex, increasing the chance of medical error and adding to physician responsibility [31]. A 2008 survey of more than 100,000 physicians found that while most (98% of respondents) were aware that a patient's genetic profile could influence response to drug therapy, few (only 10%) were comfortable applying pharmacogenetic information to clinical decision-making [56]. Those who considered themselves to be well informed were twice as likely to order pharmacogenomic tests. In the survey, only a quarter (26%) reported that they had received pharmacogenomic training during medical school or postgraduate studies [56]. If pharmacogenomic services are clinically unreliable and clinicians are not equipped to interpret them, there is a risk to the welfare of patients and the public [57]. International Society of Pharmacogenomics has requested that deans at medical schools include pharmacogenomic training in the core medical curriculum [58]. Steps like these can help to improve patient access to reliable pharmacogenomic care.

Even with trained providers, the burden on them may interfere with patient access. There are a few ways that clinical pharmacogenomics creates additional requirements for providers. Healthcare providers may require additional time to be able to interpret the results of pharmacogenomic tests and communicate risks and benefits to patients [31]. Providers need to listen to and engage with patients when pharmacogenomic-oriented options are presented to ensure patients understand what their choices are. The required time for these conversations may not be reimbursable by insurers [31].

Further adding to the complexity and time pressure on providers, patients increasingly seek information about their conditions on the Internet [59]. They may arrive at their provider with complex questions or even demands about what treatment they want [60]. This level of involvement is in sharp contrast to the more traditional medical model where the physician was always considered more knowledgeable about medical conditions than the patient. Providers need to be equipped to address patient concerns when patient wants a treatment, but a pharmacogenetic biomarker indicates that the treatment may not be beneficial or could even be harmful [11].

In 2019, AMP convened a group of members with expertise in pharmacogenomics testing and determined that clinically meaningful pharmacogenomic tests can improve patient care and professional practice, provided the following conditions are met [61]: (1) all health-related pharmacogenomic claims require well-established clinical validity; (2) the provider of pharmacogenomic testing must comply with the CLIA statute and regulations, as for all other clinical laboratory tests, including having a robust quality management system, documented analytical validity, and appropriately licensed or credentialed laboratory personnel; (3) the pharmacogenomic test report should be comprehendible by healthcare providers without training in medical genetics or pharmacogenomics; it should include the significance of the results, interpretation of the findings, as well as the limitations of the test; and (4) AMP strongly recommends that patients talk to their healthcare provider before changing their treatment plan.

Adopting an ethics lens, training and payment policies may support the adoption of clinical pharmacogenomics in a way consistent with equity and distributive justice. Without such adoption, existing inequities facing underserved populations may be exacerbated. With them, clinicians can exercise beneficence, using clinical pharmacogenomics tools for the good of their patients.

3.3   Use Issues

Use issues relate to the purposes for which genomic information may be harnessed. Pharmacogenomic information and its relationship to race can potentially be used for a range of purposes, with implications for the individuals tested and their family members. Its use in clinical practice and research may reveal unexpected results, which raise ethical issues. The same pharmacogenomic information may be used beyond clinical care, such as for insurance, employment, ancestry, advertising, paternity, and law enforcement. Interplay among the possible uses sparks additional ethical issues.

Clinical and Research Use, Informed Consent, and Security Pharmacogenomic testing may be used to reveal sought-after information regarding drug response. It may be used to expose a risk for genetically transmitted disease. Large-scale pharmacogenomic data collection can generate in information that was not requested by the patient or the clinician and that may have current or future health implications [39].

Clinical practice and research require informed consent. As covered in earlier sections, consent is based upon individuals' autonomous decision to share data for their own benefit and enable some utilitarian benefits across society. Typically, individuals do not receive renumeration when their genomic information is used to generate profits for private companies, but services they receive may be subsidized.

Informed consent is important in the practice of clinical pharmacogenomics because it determines how data may be used. Consent should address patient preferences about how the results may be used and shared, even with the patients themselves. Patients may not want to receive unexpected information. For example, nondisclosure may be preferable and is standard practice in many places if testing reveals a child is likely to develop a condition in adulthood [62]. Providers should speak to patients about what to do if tests reveal of unintended information or variants of unknown significance. Doing so may help avoid issues such as possible liability for failing to warn a patient of possible adverse events based on the genetic predisposition [63].

In pharmacogenomic studies, the informed consent is also important and should contain special elements. It should account for the range of information that may be revealed by genomic testing. It should cover testing pertinent to the drug effect being studied and should address nonspecific testing needed for subsequent pharmacogenetics studies [64]. It may also include, if relevant, authorization to link personal and/or family information to the research. If the consent is associated with future studies, neither the study design, purpose, or risks or benefits are likely to be known. In all cases, participants should be fully informed about possible risks, including previously unanticipated information being revealed, or any potential personal risk for exploitation [64].

Informed consent is based on respect for autonomy. Its practice protects privacy and confidentiality, including physicians' duty not to disclose patient health info unless authorized by the patient or required by law. Both the USA and Europe place similar requirements on providers to protect their patients' privacy and confidentiality [31].

Some information generated by pharmacogenomic testing may be of unknown clinical significance, making consent more difficult. The ACMG recommends that disclosure of incidental findings taking into account autonomy, justice, beneficence, and nonmaleficence in their debates [65]. However, there are cases where the significance of the information may not be known at the time of testing but may become important at some time in the future [11]. This could possibly create a future duty to warn, which may be addressed in the informed consent process.

Once obtained with informed consent, protecting the confidentiality of pharmacogenomic information is important for several reasons. The disclosure of sensitive data can cause embarrassment, stigma, and discrimination. The fear of improper disclosure of sensitive information may compromise the quality of care an individual seeks. Also, peoples' fear of loss of privacy could result in delays in treatment that result in public health harms, for example, related to mental illness or infectious disease [31].

Protecting privacy and maintaining confidentiality requires sound security measures. This is increasingly so in a connected world, for example, featuring electronic health records (EHRs), which may include pharmacogenomic information and reduce barriers to sharing information. US law created financial incentives for institutions capable of demonstrating "meaningful use" of EHRs [31, 66]. In 2020, the ACMG urged specific types of inclusion of genomic information into EHRs [67]. Security measures are required to ensure the protection of patients' privacy. With specific regard to EHR, ACMG urges that the following be considered, among other things [67]: (1) that the patient should be able to access any genetic data contained in their medical record; (2) that any clinical diagnoses made are visible to the patient's healthcare providers; (3) that access to data only be available via a secure patient portal; and (4) that results be in a format easily understandable by reasonable persons with updates as necessary. In future EHRs, the ability to easily retrieve genomic information will be essential for targeted testing for family members, facilitating cost reduction, earlier diagnosis, and treatment. ACMG further recommends that access to genetic data by minors and adolescents should be treated as other medical information. Secondary findings like carrier status for autosomal recessive disorders and pathogenic variants for adult-onset disorders should not be disclosed to minors except in special circumstances [68].

Race-Based Prescribing

Pharmacogenomics may identify the genetic variants that contribute to recognized differences in drug responses among racial and ethnic groups [69]. It has also led to the use of race-based prescribing in certain cases. This use is the source of some controversy.

In one notable example of race-based prescribing, the US Food and Drug Administration (FDA) approved the drug under the trade name BiDil in 2005 as a race-specific drug to treat heart failure among African Americans. The application for race-based approval and related marketing has been critiqued by some as a misguided effort to race as a proxy for genotype for commercial and regulatory advantage [70]. BiDil remains approved as a race-based drug today.

BiDil is not the only example of a treatment with race-based prescribing guidelines. Hydrochlorothiazide is recommended as first line hypertension therapy for Black patients as an alternative the angiotensin convertase inhibitor therapy recommended for all other groups [71]. A drug used to treat thrombocytopenia (trade name Eltrombopag) has a lower recommended starting dose for East Asian patients than all other patients. Similarly, the FDA recommends a lower starting dose of a statin used to lower lipid levels (trade name Crestor) for Asian patients, based on a gene that confers metabolic variability, though this gene may be present in any population [72]. There has also been ongoing discussion around race-based dosing and the utility of race-based genetic screening for drugs such as warfarin for anticoagulation therapy [73]and abacavir for HIV treatment [74].

Viewpoints on race-based prescribing vary. For example, a study of American cardiologists found that many providers believe race-based drug labels in treatment of heart failure may help prescribe effective medications sooner [75]. Others expressed concerns that considering race could potentially harm patients by resulting in some patients not receiving the drug [75].

Some assert that race and ethnicity are good proxies for pharmacogenomics science and can be used to increase effectiveness and decrease side effects [76]. Others think race is imprecise proxy for genotype and the two should not be equated [40]. Still others posit that, if personalized medicine amounts to no more than patient-risk stratification along ethnic, racial, or socioeconomic lines, it will further exacerbate the social inequities that currently exist [77]. In all cases, a clinician should act for the benefit of patients (with beneficence), and to do no harm (nonmaleficence).

Other Uses

When the Human Genome Project began in 1990, concerns were raised that personalized medicine be used to amplify differential treatment, as slight genetic differences could have significant ethical, legal, and social implications. The use of clinical pharmacogenomics has the potential to alleviate health discrepancies, but also to exacerbate them if the results are used for non-clinical purposes [31]. Individuals labeled "non-responders" for a therapy could result in patients facing significant psychological costs, stigmatization, isolation, or discrimination [77]. Discrepancies could be exacerbated in an international context between developed and developing countries.

Raw pharmacogenetic data are unusable; they must be interpreted. The interpretation can affect an individual's personhood and global position [45]. It can result in discrimination, the practice of drawing a socially or legally unacceptable distinction among individuals [78]. Genomic information can be used non-clinical purposes, such as insurance, employment, law enforcement, paternity, ancestry, advertising, and others, which may result in discrimination.

In the USA, the Genetic Information Nondiscrimination Act (GINA) builds on HIPAA and places restrictions on the use of genetic information by employers and health insurers, and on its handling in the health system [79]. In many other countries, genetic discrimination legislation has also been enacted [80].

In the USA, GINA does not cover all uses of genetic information. Notably, restrictions under US law do not apply to life insurance companies and do not attach if the information is collected outside the health system. A life insurance company could use genomic information to create exclusions or set premiums [31, 81].

GINA and HIPAA restrictions also do not apply to companies not involved in health. For example, a company that collects DNA samples for ancestry testing is not bound to protect the information in the same way as health researcher or provider. Unless the company policies and contracts state otherwise, the information could be used for advertising or law enforcement purposes. Further, companies like DNA ancestry that collect genomic information from individuals can be mined for additional purposes, as it was to catch the Golden State Killer, noted earlier. Genomic information could also be linked to medical records, or testing could be done on leftover specimens, which could be especially problematic if it could identify a person from the data [39].

Restrictions on the use or handling of genomic information ensure confidentiality. They also promote justice by preventing individuals from suffering the harm of losing a job or health insurance based on what their genomic information reveals.

Use Related to Family Members

Pharmacogenomic testing has implications not only for the person being tested, but also for family members. When performing methods that evaluate either whole genome sequencing information or large panels of pharmacogenomic variants, information is likely to arise that is unanticipated [45]. For example, non-paternity could be identified in a family being treated for an inherited cancer, as family members may share pharmacogenomic variants as well as genetic markers of disease.

The discovery of information with disease susceptibility or diagnosis implications for family members raises issues about what, if anything should be done. Some suggest a possible duty to warn family members [82]. Others note that family members may not want to know [83]. In particular, this may be the case for children, and/or conditions such as mental illness, which may carry the potential for stigmatization within the family or society.

Providers in the USA are generally bound to keep individuals' pharmacogenomic information confidential, even from family members who may be affected. Attitudes toward the question of sharing the information can vary across cultures. For example, according to one study, public opinion in the USA supports the current requirements; however, in the United Kingdom there was public support for a legal duty to share patients' genetic information with their relatives [84].

Despite restrictions placed on providers, individuals who undergo testing are permitted to share the results of their tests with others, including family members. Many guidelines encourage directive counselling to encourage individuals to share relevant information with family members with the support of genetic health professionals [85]. Conversations between health professionals and patients support autonomy and can lead to a beneficent result without breaching privacy.

4 Pharmacogenomics Practice Guidelines

Clinicians have a range of easily accessible web resources available to help them find and interpret pharmacogenomics information. Some are federal or national regulators, and others are professional groups.

4.1   Federal Regulators (US)

Regulators play a significant role in translating pharmacogenomics into clinical practice [86]. For example, in the USA, the FDA and the Office of Human Research Protections (OHRP) each play a role, which are the focus of this subsection. Clinicians practicing outside of the USA should familiarize themselves with their domestic regulatory requirements.

The FDA requires companies that offer direct-to-consumer pharmacogenetic tests to put their tests through premarket review and clearance [87]. The FDA has not currently authorized any direct-to-consumer pharmacogenetic tests predicting whether an individual is likely to respond to or have adverse reactions from a specific therapeutic drug [88]. As of August 20, 2021, FDA had licensed 483 drugs with pharmacogenomic biomarker information included in their labels at the time of their initial or supplemental approval [89]. However, laboratories that are performing such testing are doing so as a laboratory service may not be subject to FDA review, leading many to question the validity of such testing.

The OHRP helps ensure protection of the rights, welfare, and well-being of participants in US government-supported research. ORHP provides clarification and guidance, develops educational programs and materials, maintains regulatory oversight, and provides advice on ethical and regulatory issues in protecting human subjects [90].

4.2   Professional Groups

Many professional groups make information available to assist clinicians. Some host data aggregation sites, some publish evidence-based clinical guidelines, and others compile regulatory data [91]. Two organizations that compile pharmacogenomics evidence to develop clinical guidelines are the Clinical Pharmacogenetics Implementation Consortium (CPIC; www.cpicpgx.org) and the Dutch Pharmacogenetics Working Group [92]. The CPIC was created support implementation with standardized clinical pharmacogenomics guidelines. Since 2012, CPIC has published more than 20 guidelines, and they are publicly available to help clinicians translate genetic laboratory test results into actionable prescribing decisions [93]. Pharmacogenomic Knowledge Base (PharmGKB) tracks approvals by various regulatory bodies. It reports how many drugs have pharmacogenomic biomarker information where testing is required, recommended, actionable, or informative [94].

The AMP has several position papers on pharmacogenetic testing [95]. Many AMP professionals, using their education, training, and clinical experience, work with medical teams to provide information about the role of a person's genetic makeup in predicting the likelihood of medication response and/or risk for adverse drug reactions. This information can be critical, and it is imperative that those receiving it understand the test result's implications and limitations [96].

The Personalized Medicine Coalition (PMC) consists of innovators, scientists, patients, providers, and payers. It promotes the understanding and adoption of personalized medicine concepts, services, and products. It also supports investment in and adoption of personalized medicine through education, advocacy, and evidence development to benefit patients. PMCs Pharmacogenomics Working Group includes members with interest or expertise in issues related to pharmacogenomic testing. The group guides PMCs efforts in pharmacogenomics and its related engagements with FDA, clinical guidelines developers, and other stakeholders. In August 2020, PMC published a set of guidelines for advancing patient centered personalized medicine [97].

Many professional organizations offer health practitioners, students, and researchers the opportunity to participate in working groups or committees that promulgate recommendations regarding current best practices given the state of knowledge and science. Interested persons can contact a national or local association or society in their country to enquire about membership and participation.

References

1. Beauchamp TL, Childress JF. Principles of biomedical ethics. 6th ed. Oxford: Oxford University Press; 2009.
2. Institute of Medicine (US) Committee on Quality of Health Care in America. Crossing the quality chasm: a new health system for the 21st century. Washington (DC): National Academies Press (US); 2001.
3. Rosen S, Buckles S. 8 steps to implementing pharmacogenomics into your clinical practice. Mayo Clinic. https://individualizedmedicineblog.mayoclinic.org/2017/01/10/8-steps-to-implementing-pharmacogenomics-into-your-clinical-practice/. Accessed 8 April 2022.
4. Goodman CW, Brett AS. Race and pharmacogenomics—personalized medicine or misguided practice? JAMA. 2021;325(7):625–6. https://doi.org/10.1001/jama.2020.25473.
5. Schloendorff V. Society of New York Hospital. 1914 (105 N.E. 92, 93). https://biotech.law.lsu.edu/cases/consent/schoendorff.htm. Accessed 22 Aug 2022.
6. Pellegrino E. The metamorphosis of medical ethics: a 30-year retrospective. JAMA. 1993;269:1158–62.
7. President's Commission for the Study of Ethical Problems in Medicine and Biomedical and Behavioral Research. Making Health Care Decisions: The ethical and legal implications of informed consent in the patient-practitioner relationship. Vol 1. Report. Washington: Government Printing Office; 1982.
8. Nuffield Council on Bioethics Pharmacogenetics. Ethical issues. London: Nuffield Council on Bioethics; 2005.
9. Butnariu A, Samsca G, Lupan I. Ethical implications in pharmacogenetics and pharmacogenomics. Med Con. 2015;10(4):41–4.
10. Netzer C, Biller-Andorno N. Pharmacogenetic testing, informed consent and the problem of secondary information. Bioethics. 2004;18(4):344–60. https://doi.org/10.1111/j.1467-8519.2004.00401.x.
11. Bunnik EM, Schermer MHN, Janssens ACJW. Personal genome testing: test characteristics to clarify the discourse on ethical, legal and societal issues. BMC Med Ethics. 2011;12:11.
12. Barash CI. Ethical issues in pharmacogenetics. Action Biosci. 2013;170:968–76.
13. Hallinan D, Friedewald M. Open consent, biobanking and data protection law: can open consent be 'informed' under the forthcoming data protection regulation? Life Sci Soc Policy. 2015;11:1–1.

14. United Nations Educational, Scientific and Cultural Organization. Universal Declaration on Bioethics and Human Rights. 2005. https://portal.unesco.org/en/ev.php-URL_ID=31058& URL_DO=DO_TOPIC&URL_SECTION=201.html. Accessed 18 Apr 2022.
15. World Health Organization. The ethical, legal, and social implications of pharmacogenomics in developing countries, report of an international group of experts. Geneva: WHO Press; 2007. https://apps.who.int/iris/bitstream/handle/10665/43669/9789241595469_eng.pdf;seq uence=1. Accessed 8 Apr 2022.
16. Richardson LD, Wilets I, Ragin DF, Holohan J, Smirnoff M, Rhodes R, et al. Research without consent: community perspectives from the community VOICES study. Acad Emerg Med. 2005;12(11):1082–90. https://doi.org/10.1197/j.acm.2005.06.008.
17. Pharmacogenomics. https://www.nih.gov/about-nih/what-we-do/nih-turning-discovery-into-health/pharmacogenomics. Accessed 11 Feb 2020.
18. Fulton CR, Swart M, De Luca T, Liu SN, Collins KS, Desta Z, Gufford BT, Eadon MT. Pharmacogenetics and practice: tailoring prescribing for safety and effectiveness. J Nurse Pract. 2018;14(10):697-704.e1. https://doi.org/10.1016/j.nurpra.2018.09.021.
19. Sultana J, Cutroneo P, Trifirò G. Clinical and economic burden of adverse drug reactions. J Pharmacol Pharmacother. 2013;4(1):S73–7. https://doi.org/10.4103/0976-500X.120957.
20. Cressey D. Adverse drug reactions a big killer. Nature. 2008. https://doi.org/10.1038/news.2008.676.
21. Segert J. Understanding ownership and privacy of genetic data. Harvard University Blog. 2018. https://sitn.hms.harvard.edu/flash/2018/understanding-ownership-privacy-genetic-data/. Accessed 27 Mar 2022.
22. Cambon-Thomsen A, Rial-Sebbag E, Knoppers BM. Trends in ethical and legal frameworks for the use of human biobanks. Eur Respir J. 2007;30:373–82. https://doi.org/10.1183/09031936.00165006.
23. Best RG, Khushf G, Rabin-Havt SS, Clayton EW, Grebe TA, Hagenkord J, et al. Electronic address: documents@acmg.net. Stewardship of patient genomic data: apolicy statement of the American College of Medical Genetics and Genomics (ACMG). Genet Med. 2022;24(3):509–11. https://doi.org/10.1016/j.gim.2021.11.001.
24. Beskow LM. Lessons from HeLa cells: the ethics and policy of biospecimens. Ann Rev Genom Hum Genet. 2016;17: 395–417.
25. Hansson MG, Dillner J, Bartram CR, Carlsson J, Helgesson G. Should donors be allowed to give broad consent to future biobank research? Lancet Oncol. 2006;7:266–9.
26. Stjernschantz Forsberg J, Hansson MG, Eriksson S. Changing perspectives in biobank research-from individual rights to concerns about public health regarding the return of results. Eur J Hum Genet. 2009;17:1544–9. https://doi.org/10.1038/ejhg.2009.87.
27. Wolf SM, Lawrenz FP, Nelson CA, Kahn JP, Cho MK, Clayton EW, et al. Managing incidental findings in human subjects research: analysis and recommendation. J Law Med Ethics. 2008;36:219–48. https://doi.org/10.1111/j.1748-720X.2008.00266.x.
28. Beskow LM, Friedman JY, Hardy NC, Lin L, Weinfurt KP. Developing a simplified consent form for biobanking. PLoS ONE. 2010;8:e2133. https://doi.org/10.1371/journal.pone.0013302.
29. Breckenridge A, Lindpaintner K, Lipton P, McLeod H, Rothstein M, Wallace H. Pharmacogenetics: ethical problems and solutions. Nat Rev Genet. 2004;5:676–80. https://doi.org/10.1038/nrg1431.
30. Haga SB, Beskow LM. Ethical, legal, and social implications of biobanks for genetics research. Adv Genet. 2008;60:505–44. https://doi.org/10.1016/S0065-2660(07)00418-X.
31. Brothers KB, Rothstein MA. Ethical, legal and social implications of incorporating personalized medicine into healthcare. Per Med. 2015;12:43–51. https://doi.org/10.2217/pme.14.65.
32. AMP Position Statement on Variant Sharing. https://www.amp.org/AMP/assets/File/advocacy/AMP_Position_Variant_Data_Sharing_7_29_2021.pdf?pass=46 Accessed 27 Mar 2022 (Published 7/29/21, updated 12/3/21).

33. ACMG Board of Directors. Laboratory and clinical genomic data sharing is crucial to improving genetic health care: a position statement of the American College of Medical Genetics and Genomics (ACMG). Genet Med. 2017;19:721–2. https://doi.org/10.1038/gim.2016.196.
34. AMP and CAP Comments on Pharmacogenomics Testing. Submitted to First Coast Service Options and Novitas, Medical Administrative Contractors for the Centers for Medicare and Medicaid Services. 2021. https://www.amp.org/AMP/assets/File/advocacy/AMP-CAP%20C omments%20on%20Pharmacogenomics%20Testing_7-23-2021.pdf?pass=58. Accessed 27 Mar 2022.
35. Frisby TM, Contreras JL. The national cancer institute cancer moonshot public access and data sharing policy—initial assessment and implications. Data Policy. 2020;2:e9. https://doi.org/10. 1017/dap.2020.9.
36. Health Insurance Portability and Accountability Act of 1996, Pub.L. 104-91; HIPAA Privacy Rule, 45 CFR Part 160. https://www.govinfo.gov/app/details/PLAW-104publ191. Accessed 22 Aug 2022.
37. Knoppers BM. Consent to 'personal' genomics and privacy. Direct-to-consumer genetic tests and population genome research challenge traditional notions of privacy and consent. EMBO Rep. 2010;11:416–19. https://doi.org/10.1038/embor.2010.69.
38. Singh D. Ethical issues in pharmacogenomics must be addressed, says Nuffield Council. BMJ. 2003;327(7417):701. https://doi.org/10.1136/bmj.327.7417.701-a.
39. Gershon ES, Alliey-Rodriguez N, Grennan K. Ethical and public policy challenges for pharmacogenomics. Dial Clin Neurosci. 2014;16(4):567–74. https://doi.org/10.31887/DCNS.2014. 16.4/egershon.
40. Peterson-Iyer K. Pharmacogenomics, ethics, and public policy. Kennedy Inst Ethics J. 2008;18(1):35–56. https://doi.org/10.1353/ken.0.0004.
41. The US Public Health Service Syphilis Study at Tuskegee: Timeline. https://www.cdc.gov/tus kegee/timeline.htm. Accessed 27 Mar 2022.
42. Shavers VL, Lynch CF, Burmeister LF. Knowledge of the Tuskegee study and its impact on the willingness to participate in medical research studies. J Natl Med Assoc. 2000;92(12):563–72.
43. Rhodes R. Rethinking research ethics. Am J Bioethics. 2005;5(1):7–28. https://doi.org/10. 1080/15265160590900678.
44. Rosenberg NA, Huang L, Jewett EM, Szpiech ZA, Jankovic I, Boehnke M. Genome-wide association studies in diverse populations. Nat Rev Genet. 2010;11(5):356–66. https://doi.org/ 10.1038/nrg2760.
45. Salari P, Larijani B. Ethical issues surrounding personalized medicine: a literature review. Acta Med Iran. 2017;55(3):209–17 (citing United Nations Educational, Scientific and Cultural Organization. Universal Declaration on the Human Genome and Human Rights. 1997)
46. All of Us Research Project, Core Values. National Institutes of Health. https://allofus.nih.gov/ about/core-values. Accessed 5 Apr 2022.
47. Shah-Williams E, Levy KD, Zang Y, Holmes AM, Stoughton C, Dexter P, Skaar TC. Enrollment of diverse populations in the INGENIOUS pharmacogenetics clinical trial. Front Genet. 2020;11:571. https://doi.org/10.3389/fgene.2020.00571.
48. Daar AS, Singer PA. Pharmacogenetics and geographical ancestry: implications for drug development and global health. Nat Rev Genet. 2005;6:241–6. https://doi.org/10.1038/nrg 1559.
49. McClellan KA, Avard D, Simard J, Knoppers BM. Personalized medicine and access to health care: potential for inequitable access? Eur J Hum Genet. 2013;21(2):143–7. https://doi.org/10. 1038/ejhg.2012.149.
50. Reese ES, Daniel Mullins C, Beitelshees AL, Onukwugha E. Cost–effectiveness of cytochrome P450 2C19 genotype screening for selection of antiplatelet therapy with clopidogrel or prasugrel. Pharmacotherapy. 2012;32(4):323–32. https://doi.org/10.1002/PHAR. 1048.
51. Nocera J. The $300,000 drug. The New York Times. 2014. https://www.nytimes.com/2014/07/ 19/opinion/joe-nocera-cystic-fibrosis-drug-price.html. Accessed 22 Aug 2022.

52. Hedgecoe A. The politics of personalised medicine—pharmacogenetics in the clinic. Cambridge, UK: Cambridge University Press; 2004.
53. Orphan Products Grants Program. https://www.fda.gov/industry/developing-products-rare-diseases-conditions/orphan-products-grants-program. Accessed 7 Apr 2022.
54. Park SK, Tgpen J, Lee IJ. Coverage of pharmacogenetic tests by private health insurance companies. J Am Pharm Assoc. 2020;60(2):352–356.e3. https://doi.org/10.1016/j.japh.2019.10.003.
55. Association for Molecular Pathology recommendations. https://www.amp.org/clinical-practice/practice-guidelines. Accessed 8 Apr 2022.
56. Prainsack B, Wolinsky H. Direct-to-consumer genome testing: opportunities for pharmacogenomics research. Pharmacogenomics. 2010;11(5):651–5. https://doi.org/10.2217/pgs.10.33.
57. Avard D, Knoppers B. Genomic medicine: considerations for health professionals and the public. Genome Med. 2009;1(2):25. https://doi.org/10.1186/gm25.
58. Squassina A, Manchia M, Manolopoulos VG, Artac M, Lappa-Manakou C, Karkabouna S, et al. Realities and expectations of pharmacogenomics and personalized medicine: impact of translating genetic knowledge into clinical practice. Pharmacogenomics. 2010;11(8):1149–67. https://doi.org/10.2217/pgs.10.97.
59. Neal-Gualtieri L. The doctor as the second opinion and the Internet as the first. In: Extended abstracts on human factors in computing systems. CHI EA'09. New York, NY: ACM; 2009. p. 2489–98.
60. Dilliway G, Maudsley G. Patients bringing information to primary care consultations: a cross-sectional (questionnaire) study of doctors' and nurses' views of its impact. J Eval Clin Pract. 2008;14(4):545–7. https://doi.org/10.1111/j.1365-2753.2007.00911.x.
61. AMP Position Statement: Best Practices for Pharmacogenomic Testing. 2019. https://www.amp.org/AMP/assets/File/advocacy/AMP_Response_to_PGx_Citizen_Petition_5-4-2020.pdf?pass=73. Accessed 27 Mar 2022.
62. Clarke A. The genetic testing of children. Working Party of the Clinical Genetics Society (UK). J Med Genet. 1994;31(10):785–97. https://doi.org/10.1136/jmg.31.10.785.
63. Morreale AP, McFarland MS. Legal and liability implications of pharmacogenomics for physicians and pharmacists. J Prec Med. 2021;7(4):20.
64. Corrigan OP. Pharmacogenetics, ethical issues: a review of the Nuffield Council on Bioethics Report. J Med Ethics. 2005;31:144–8. https://doi.org/10.1136/jme.2004.007229.
65. Green R, Berg J, Grody W, Kalia SS, Korf BR, Martin CL, et al. ACMG recommendation for reporting of incidental findings in clinical exome and genome sequencing. Genet Med. 2013;15:565–74. https://doi.org/10.1038/gim.2013.73.
66. Health Information Technology for Economic and Clinical Health (HITECH) Act. 2009. https://www.hhs.gov/hipaa/for-professionals/special-topics/hitech-act-enforcement-interim-final-rule/index.html. Accessed 22 Aug 2022.
67. Grebe TA, Khushf G, Chen M, Bailey D, Brenman LM, Williams MS, Seaver LH, ACMG Social, Ethical and Legal Issues Committee. The interface of genomic information with the electronic health record: a points to consider statement of the American College of Medical Genetics and Genomics (ACMG). Genet Med. 2020;22:1431–6. https://doi.org/10.1038/s41436-020-0841-2.
68. Ross LF, Saal HM, David KL, Anderson RR, American Academy of Pediatrics, American College of Medical Genetics and Genomics. Technical report: ethical and policy issues in genetic testing and screening of children. Genet Med. 2013;15:234–45. https://doi.org/10.1038/gim.2012.176.
69. Rahemtulla T, Bhopal R. Pharmacogenetics and ethnically targeted therapies. Br Med J. 2005;330(7499):1036–7. https://doi.org/10.1136/bmj.330.7499.1036.
70. Sankar P, Kahn J. BiDil: race medicine or race marketing? Health Aff. 2005;Suppl Web Exclusives:W5-455–63. https://doi.org/10.1377/hlthaff.w5.455.
71. Joint National Committee (JNC) 8 Hypertension Guideline Algorithm. The Philippine Academy of Family Physicians. https://thepafp.org/website/wp-content/uploads/2017/05/2014-JNC-8-Hypertension.pdf. Accessed 6 Apr 2022.

72. Wu HF, Hristeva N, Chang J, Liang X, Li R, Frassetto L, Benet LZ. Rosuvastatin pharmacokinetics in Asian and white subjects wild type for both OATP1B1 and BCRP under control and inhibited conditions. J Pharm Sci. 2017;106(9):2751–57. https://doi.org/10.1016/j.xphs.2017.03.027.

73. Limdi NA, Brown TM, Yan Q, Thigpen JL, Shendre A, Liu N, et al. Race influences warfarin dose changes associated with genetic factors. Blood. 2015;126(4):539–45. https://doi.org/10.1182/blood-2015-02-627042.

74. Wan BP, Pyoeng GC, Kyoung-Ho S, Shinwon L, Hee-Chang J, Jae Hyun J, et al. Should HLA-B*5701 screening be performed in every ethnic group before starting Abacavir? Clin Inf Dis. 2009;48(3):365–7. https://doi.org/10.1086/595890.

75. Callier SL, Cunningham BA, Powell J, McDonald MA, Royal CDM. Cardiologists' perspectives on race-based drug labels and prescribing within the context of treating heart failure. Health Equity. 2019;3(1): 246–53. https://doi.org/10.1089/heq.2018.0074

76. Joly Y, Ngueng Feze I, Simard J. Genetic discrimination and life insurance: a systematic review of the evidence. BMC Med. 2013;11:25.

77. Juengst ET, Settersten RA, Fishman JR, McGowan ML. After the revolution? Ethical and social challenges in personalized genomic medicine. Per Med. 2012;9:429–39. https://doi.org/10.2217/pme.12.37.

78. Rothstein MA, Anderlik MR. What is genetic discrimination, and when and how can it be prevented? Genet Med. 2001;3(5):354–8. https://doi.org/10.1097/00125817-200109000-00005.

79. Public Law 110-233—Genetic Information Nondiscrimination Act of 2008. https://www.govinfo.gov/app/details/PLAW-110publ233. Accessed 19 Aug.

80. Otlowski M, Taylor S, Bombard Y. Genetic discrimination: international perspectives. Ann Rev Genom Hum Genet. 2012;13:433–54. https://doi.org/10.1146/annurev-genom-090711-163800.

81. Joly Y, Burton H, Knoppers BM, Feze IN, Dent T, Pashayan N, et al. Life insurance: genomic stratification and risk classification. Eur J Hum Genet. 2014;22(5):575–9. https://doi.org/10.1038/ejhg.2013.228

82. Muflih S, Al-Husein BA, Karasneh R, Alzoubi KH. Physicians' attitudes and ethical obligations to pharmacogenetic testing. J Multidisc Healthc. 2020;13:249–58. https://doi.org/10.2147/JMDH.S245369.

83. Berkman BE, Hull SC. The "right not to know" in the genomic era: time to break from tradition? Am J Bioeth. 2014;14(3):28–31. https://doi.org/10.1080/15265161.2014.880313.

84. Dheensa S, Fenwick A, Shkedi-rafid S, Crawford G, Lucassen A. Health-care professionals' responsibility to patients' relatives in genetic medicine: a systematic review and synthesis of empirical research. Genet Med. 2016;18(4):290–301. https://doi.org/10.1038/gim.2015.72.

85. Forrest L, Delatycki M, Skene L, et al. Communicating genetic information in families—a review of guidelines and position papers. Eur J Hum Genet. 2007;15:612–8. https://doi.org/10.1038/sj.ejhg.5201822.

86. Prasad K. Role of regulatory agencies in translating pharmacogenetics to the clinics. Clin Cases Miner Bone Metab. 2009;6(1):29–34.

87. FDA. Pharmcogenetics Tests. 21 CFR 862.3364. https://www.fda.gov/medical-devices/in-vitro-diagnostics/direct-consumer-tests#list. Accessed 19 Aug 2022.

88. Direct To Consumer Tests. https://www.fda.gov/medical-devices/in-vitro-diagnostics/direct-consumer-tests. Accessed 8 Apr 2022.

89. Table of Pharmacogenomic Biomarkers in Drug Labeling. https://www.fda.gov/drugs/science-and-research-drugs/table-pharmacogenomic-biomarkers-drug-labeling. Accessed 18 Jan 2022.

90. Office of Human Research Protections. https://www.hhs.gov/ohrp/index.html. Accessed 10 Apr 2022.

91. Zhang G, Zhang Y, Ling Y, Jia J. Web resources for pharmacogenomics. Genom Proteom Bioinform. 2015;13(1):51–4. https://doi.org/10.1016/j.gpb.2015.01.002.

92. Swen JJ, Nijenhuis M, de Boer A, Guchelaar HJ, et al. Pharmacogenetics: from bench to byte—an update of guidelines. Clin Pharmacol Ther. 2011;89:662–73. https://doi.org/10.1038/clpt.2011.34.

93. Relling MV, Klein TE. CPIC: clinical pharmacogenetics implementation consortium of the pharmacogenomics research network. Clin Pharmacol Ther. 2011;89:464–7.

94. Drug Label Annotations. PharmGKB. https://www.pharmgkb.org/labelAnnotations. Accessed 8 Apr 2022.

95. AMP. Advocacy: Position Statements and Letters. https://www.amp.org/advocacy/position-statements-letters/. Accessed 27 Mar 27.

96. AMP Comment to Docket No. FDA-2020-P-0152, Citizen Petition from Hyman, Phelps & McNamara, P.C. on behalf of Coalition to Preserve Access to PGx Information. Submitted May 4, 2020. https://www.amp.org/AMP/assets/File/advocacy/AMP_Response_to_PGx_Citizen_Petition_5-4-2020.pdf?pass=73. Accessed 27 Mar 2022.

97. Moving Beyond Population Averages. A patient centered research agenda advancing personalized medicine. 2020. https://www.personalizedmedicinecoalition.org. Accessed 27 Mar 2022.

Economic Evaluation of Pharmacogenomic Testing

Steve Quinn, Lara Primorac, and Matea Primorac

Abstract

There is a plethora of publications showing that adoption of a PGx screening program would save both money and lives. The economics of an adverse drug reaction (ADR) may vary from country to country; however, the cost of human life is constant. Despite this, there is a not a wide adoption of PGx screening programs. The barriers to entry and economics of pharmacogenomic (PGx) testing are complex and specific for a given institution or in-country healthcare system. When implementing a PGx program, it is important to look closely at the real-world variables that go to make up a cost analysis. In addition to the publicized evidence, this chapter will examine the options available to a healthcare institution when deciding to adopt a PGx program. This will be either a Test Send Out (TSO) program or an in-house Technology Transfer (TT). Given the logistical challenges and the need to minimize operational costs, it is likely most institutions will adopt the TT approach. This chapter will look closely at both the TSO and TT options and act as a guide when considering implementation.

Keywords

Pharmacogenomic (PGx) · Adverse drug reaction (ADR) · Quality-adjusted life years (QALYs) · Cost-benefit analysis (CBA) · Polymerase chain reaction (PCR) · Test send out (TSO) · Technology transfer (TT)

S. Quinn (✉)
Mainz Biomed, Mainz, Germany
e-mail: stevieqman@gmail.com

L. Primorac
Wharton Business School, The University of Pennsylvania, Philadelphia, USA

M. Primorac
School of Economics, Management, Law, Bocconi University, Milan, Italy

1   Introduction

There are a number of decision-analytic models available to assess the health economic benefits of pharmacogenomic (PGx) tests, and they are seen as the most systematic and transparent method for economic evaluation [1]. Nevertheless, the economics of PGx testing is specific for a given institution, complex, and often misunderstood. Given the many variabilities involved, it, therefore, remains significantly underutilized as a tool for driving positive economic and health outcomes for healthcare management.

The most common economic evaluations that can analyze the PGx testing impacts on health are:

- Cost-minimization analysis (CMA), where costs are divided into (1) direct costs of PGx application to the hospital or health services and nonmedical costs (cost to social services related to PGx application) and (2) indirect costs (lost productivity because of mortality and morbidity if PGx is not applied).
- Cost-effectiveness analysis (CEA) compares the cost and potential effects of a PGx. This analysis particularly focuses on procedures' impacts on clinical measures.
- Cost-utility analysis (CUA) focuses mainly on the quality of life rather than the length of life. In other words, this methodology compares the cost of the PGx with health improvements that are expressed in units of both quantity (life years) and quality of life, usually shown as quality-adjusted life years (QALYs).
- Cost-benefit analysis (CBA) compares the cost and benefits of PGx, where both are expressed in monetary units.

The cost of the PGx testing is shown in monetary units, while the outcome on health is usually evaluated as quality-adjusted life years (QALYs), which measures the predictable number of post-PGx testing years of life, particularly the quality of life. On the other hand, CEAs, as was said earlier, compare the effect of PGx on, for example, a number of adverse drug events avoided.

---

2   Documented Evidence

Verbelen and colleagues analyzed 44 economic evaluations of PGx testing and concluded that 57% favored PGx testing [2]. Also, they underlined that comparing differences in cost and health outcomes between standard treatment (ST) and PGx-guided treatment (PGx) is particularly important to calculate the incremental cost-effectiveness ratio (ICER):

$$ICER = (Cost_{PGx} - Cost_{ST})/(Effect_{PGx} - Effect_{ST})$$

If PGx arises at a higher cost but is more effective than ST, the ICER is compared to the willingness-to-pay threshold to define cost-effectiveness. It is usually agreed that if ICERs are up to $30.000–$50.000 per QALY is considered cost-effective [3]. By using a similar concept, Zhu and his colleagues developed a decision analysis model for a hypothetical cohort of 10.000 patients with cardiovascular diseases. In the study, they analyzed three drug–gene pairs (CYP2C19-clopidogrel, CYP2C9/VKORC1-warfarin, and SLCO1B1-statins). According to CUA, costs were analyzed in dollars, while effectiveness was measured in QALYs. The incremental cost-effectiveness ratio (ICER) was used to calculate the outcome of this approach. The authors clearly state that preemptive testing (using PGx-related genetic information at the point of prescribing a drug) is cost-effective in comparison with standard treatment (ICER $86.227/QALY) at the willingness-to-pay threshold of $1000.000/QALY while reactive testing was not (ICER $148.726/QALY) [4].

However, the cost-effectiveness analysis (CEA) of PGx testing is a subject of many debates. Nonetheless, many agree that PGx could be cost-effective, cost-saving, and clinically beneficial. Significantly, nobody argues that objective analysis of a high-quality economic evaluation of benefits related to PGx testing should be a strategic alignment for the future of PGx.

From the perspective of the Dutch Pharmacogenetics Working Group, prevention of drug-related deaths is considered "essential." Therefore, if essential, the main question remains. "Who will be responsible if it is known that certain drug–gene interaction (DGI) could occur, but physicians still do not order the tests, simply because such testing could not be reimbursed?" Recently, van der Wouden and colleagues used a decision-analytic model to calculate the cost-effectiveness of PGx in a case of seven DGIs categorized as "essential." Authors calculated that if all 148.128 patients who used one of seven drugs (clopidogrel, capecitabine, fluorouracil, azathioprine, mercaptopurine, tioguanine, and irinotecan) been tested, the total cost would increase for Euro 21.4 million. However, such an approach would save 419 lives per year, and cost-effectiveness is estimated to be Euro 51.000 per prevented gene–drug-related drug [5].

On the other hand, value-based payment models suggest that the introduction of PGx in routine clinical practice requires innovative financial models and significant organizational changes in the healthcare industry to navigate the application of this technology in routine clinical practice. The price–quality ratio is a key concern for many physicians regarding implementing PGx in clinical practice. In a recently published article, Siamoglou and colleagues proposed that the cost framework for PGx testing should include direct (workforce, necessary equipment, consumables) and indirect costs (maintenance for instruments and laboratory, utility services, laboratory administrative cost). In the end, it is particularly important to calculate the cost of the methodology associated with PGx testing. Based on that, PGx testing will be acceptable or non-acceptable [6].

One of the areas where PGx testing has tremendous potential is, without a doubt, psychiatry, particularly in treating major depressive disorders (MDD) and schizophrenia (SCZ). By analyzing 18 studies, Karemperis et al., concluded that 16 of those favor PGx testing, while in 9 studies, genome-guided interventions were cost-beneficial. However, in addition, PGx testing was less costly than standard treatment [7].

Therefore, it does not surprise recently published cost-utility study using two pharmacoeconomic Markov models shows that screening for CYP2C19 and CYP2D6 in patients with MDD is cost-effective for a willingness-to-pay (WTP) threshold of Euro 75.000 per quality-adjusted life year (QALY) [8].

Considering all written above, United Healthcare became the first insurance company to reimburse PGX testing for antidepressant and antipsychotic medication when certain criteria are met.

A recent study on patients living with HIV, who take abacavir, co-trimoxazole, dapsone, and isoniazid, showed that single- and multiple-PGx testing could reduce the cost of ADR treatment and prevent serious ADR [9]. Kelley et al., by economic simulation, predicted that during the 3-year follow-up period and use of a multigene panel covering 11 PGx genes (14 alleles), the saving in patients with hypertension yields 47% savings [10]. Earlier, it was published that high blood pressure was responsible for about 360.000 deaths in the U.S. and had a $51 billion direct cost to the U.S. healthcare system [11, 12]. Kelley et al., based on 10.000.000 patients with hypertension, figured out that a multipanel-guided therapy would, during the three-year follow-up period, result in net savings of $42.3 billion while the cost for the genetic testing would increase by approximately $2.4 billion.

Timely access to important information related to PGx testing is critical. Several statistical simulation models suggest that preemptive PGx testing in early childhood, in some cases, could achieve savings in health-related costs of up to 50% [13]. Those data are supported by a recent descriptive statistic study showing that out of 108 reviewed publications evaluating 39 drugs, 71% showed PGx-guided treatment to be cost-effective or cost-saving, 20% found it to be not cost-effective, and 9% were ambiguous [14].

3   Implementation

Despite the plethora of available outcome studies, the economics of PGx testing remains specific for a given institution or in-country healthcare system. It is important to look closely at the real-world variables that go to make up a cost analysis when considering adopting a PGx screening regime. Adopting a PGx regime can be broadly categorized as a Test Send Out (TSO) service or in-house Technology Transfer Model.

3.1   Test Send Out (TSO) Model

The source of PGx testing is an important factor when considering the most cost-effective route to implementing a PGx testing regime. There are many specialist laboratories across the world offering a multitude of PGx tests. Healthcare institutions can access these testing services through a Test Send Out (TSO) agreement. In such an agreement, the PGx laboratory provides patient sample collection kits for either EDTA whole blood or buccal swabs. The sample is taken, packaged, and returned to the PGx laboratory, usually using a prepaid envelope. The patient data are collected via a paper and/or electronic secure online test request form. The test request form must include patient consent to the testing as well as consent from the reporting clinician, confirming the test has been explained to the patient. The sample is received in the laboratory, patient data are cross-checked, and the sample is then processed. Results are generated via a secure online portal and can be downloaded by the clinician and also, where legally allowed, by the patient. Costs can vary from $300 to $800 per patient report depending on the methodology employed, genes covered, shipping or postal costs, cost of collection devices, and committed volume of tests. Some tests focus on specific medical specialties such as psychiatry, while others offer tests covering multiple medical specialties. In addition, there may be additional costs for setting up educational programs and the cost to drive clinical adoption. Health system information technology (IT) costs can also add an extra layer of expense especially when there is a need to access patient data prior to testing to set medication alerts. Most commercial companies also offer a Decision Support Tool (DST) that offers easy access to a patient's test results, including genetic information and insights on hundreds of medications based on the patient's genetic profile. The DST can review the patient's current medications for predicted gene–drug interactions, offer gene–drug information, and access data on drug–drug interactions for medications of interest. The DST can often be included in the test price or offered as part of a monthly service charge.

Commercial laboratories based within a country offer their testing services directly to the general public, known as direct-to-consumer genetic tests (DTC-GTs) as well as to medical institutions. DTC-GT laws vary by country and should be researched prior to commencing such services. Many overseas companies offer their testing services via a distributor model in which the testing service is sold directly to the distributor at a fixed price. The distributor then sets a local charge directly either to the patient or to a healthcare institution. In addition, the reporting clinician can also add additional practice fees. Each step of the distribution chain adds an extra layer of expense. Given that most PGx tests are not reimbursed by insurance or by government entities, the end cost to the patient can vary widely from $250 to $1200. This is one of the major reasons why PGx testing is not widely adopted, and the patients feel the test is too expensive.

In many cases, clinicians feel they need to spend too much time explaining the test only to receive a comment that the test is too expensive. As a result, the clinician stops offering the test. Patient education is very important in that it is essential to fully explain the test to the patient and gain consent for testing. This should not be seen as a sales exercise but as a medical consultation to offer the best care possible for the patient.

3.2   In-House Technology Transfer Model

The ideal scenario is for a laboratory to undertake PGx testing in its own laboratory (in-house). The challenge is how to set up an accredited test and implement a PGx testing service. The financial factors to consider are as follows:

1. Staffing requirements
2. Capital equipment
3. Reagents
4. Disposables
5. Curation process
6. Software/licensing fees
7. IT integration
8. Staff training/clinical adoption program
9. Legal/regulatory costs.

3.2.1   Staffing Requirements

Setting up a PGx testing process requires specialist staff with experience in molecular genetic laboratory procedures. Many large institutions have qualified staff in place, so the cost can be apportioned accordingly. The greatest challenge is in understanding and resolving sample reporting challenges. Many off-the-shelf PGx interpretation software packages offer a fully automated reporting feature. However, auto-reporting rates can vary between 95 and 65%, meaning that between 5 and 35% will require manual reporting. It must also be noted that the reporting software is specific for the genes and variants of the chosen assay. Modifying the existing assay to add additional genes or variants is a complex and time-consuming process.

3.2.2   Capital Equipment

Choosing a testing platform is a crucial decision affecting multiple aspects of a PGx program. The laboratory instrumentation or testing platform chosen for PGx analysis will depend upon several variables such as testing volume, the number of variants to be included on the panel, turnaround time, and ongoing clinical development needs. Next-generation sequencing (NGS) platforms utilizing PGx gene panels enable the interrogation of the widest array of clinically useful gene variants with higher discovery power and sensitivity to detect novel or rare variants. However, when the primary consideration is for a cost-effective screening program, then the complexity and expense (reagent costs, capital equipment, instrument maintenance) of NGS can be seen as a disadvantage. In contrast to NGS testing, PCR platforms offer rapid analysis, typically for 1–3 days, with lower reagent costs. Capital costs are also generally lower, with less expense needed for instrument maintenance. A disadvantage is a flexibility to update when new gene variants need to be added. A PCR-based PGx test requires additional assay design and validation which can be expensive and time-consuming. There is also variability in costs depending on the manufacturer and model used. Another factor to consider is the reliability of the instrumentation in terms of mean time between service calls. If the instrument breaks down frequently, then a second backup analyzer will be required, or a more expensive same-day/next-day service contract will be required. All of these factors must be considered to arrive at a final cost per patient result. Additional capital equipment costs include DNA extraction, a spectrophotometer for DNA quality check, autoload system to load samples onto open array plates, a centrifuge, an incubator, a fridge/freezer, a vortexer and balance. The total capital cost to set up a PGx test can vary from $350,000 to over $1,000,000.

3.2.3   Reagents

Reagent costs will vary depending on the instrument of choice and reagent manufacturer. The amount of reagent used will depend on the instrumentation of choice. Smaller PCR instruments typically use 25–50 µl, whereas the larger fully automated PCR instruments can use as little as 1.6 µl. The cost per report per run is the critical factor when considering the final overall cost per patient result. The ratio of control samples to patient samples will determine the final cost. It is common practice to run between 8 and 12 control samples per run. It, therefore, follows that the more patient samples you can include in each assay run, the more cost-effective the process will be. If, for example, the laboratory runs 1 sample with a direct reagent cost of $40 and the control costs are $1000, then the cost per report per run is $1040. If 88 samples are run with eight controls on a 96-well plate, then the cost per report per run is $52. It is clear that the sample volume per day is the key factor. This must also be related to achieving an acceptable turnaround time. Reagent costs should be calculated based on the maximum number of samples that can realistically be achieved from a single reagent container. There inevitably will be a residual volume that cannot be used and is seen as waste. This must be included in any calculation. Another factor to consider is the need to rerun samples because of assay run failure or if duplicate samples are run. Reagent costs for targeted NGS can be significantly higher than PCR.

3.2.4   Disposables

Typical disposable items include, but are not limited to, PCR plate wells, buccal swabs, EDTA blood tubes, and pipette tips. The choice between using buccal swabs and/or EDTA blood tubes will have a significant cost impact, as will the choice of buccal swabs used. Typical EDTA blood tubes cost approximately $0.50 per blood tube, whereas buccal swabs cost between $2 and $9 per swab. When choosing the buccal swab, it is imperative that the appropriate swab is chosen to ensure the quality and quantity of DNA are sufficient to enable PGx assay processing. Additional disposable costs can typically add between $2 and $10 per patient report. These costs can vary country-by-country based on distributor fees and additional import costs.

3.2.5   Curation Process

The curation process undertaken to generate a PGx test report is extremely complex, time-consuming, requiring individuals with vast experience and knowledge [15]. The curation process requires a systematic search of multiple databases by a designated curator with experience in pharmacogenomics literature analysis. The process querries each source and prepares a complete, exhaustive summary of current evidence for individual drugs. This comprehensive summary is then reviewed by a team of pharmacists, pharmacologists, and scientists, all with experience in genetics and/or pharmacogenomics. The whole process is not a one-off process and must be undertaken, albeit on a reduced scale, annually or biannually to keep the reporting database current. Whenever a new drug or gene is added to the testing menu then, a rigorous validation and curation process must be undertaken.

3.2.6   Software/Licensing Fees

Developing bioinformatics to translate PCR or NGS-generated PGx data is a complex process. Taking an off-the-shelf PGx software package is the simplest way to set up an in-house PGx test. PCR PGx assay providers and NGS PGx panel providers will offer interpretation software to enable a PGx report to be generated. At least one commercial PGx laboratory offers an end-to-end solution, including reproducing their own PCR-based PGx test using proprietary assays and generating a patient report through their cloud-based interpretational software solution. Licensing fees for PGx software vary widely from as little as $10 per report to $150 per patient report. The fee depends on the PGx assay run, the volume of tests performed, and the level of support for updating and training.

3.2.7   IT Integration

The utilization of an electronic medical records (EMR) system to manage patient data varies from country to country. Most EMRs do not have the robust data and predictive analytics capabilities to facilitate a PGx program. To facilitate clinical adoption, it is imperative for the hospital system to integrate PGx data analysis into their everyday practice. A successful implementation of PGx provides timely information to clinicians in terms of discrete data results, medication alerts, clinical interpretation of phenotype and genotype data, and CDS on the PGx actionable variants. The cost to implement is extremely variable and requires detailed upfront requirements to be determined so that a cost estimate can be accurately assigned.

3.2.8   Staff Training/Clinical Adoption Program

Clinical adoption of PGx is one of the major barriers to implementing PGx in a hospital system. A study by Eden et al. in 2016 [16] stated of the 212 participants surveyed, 79% felt that it was important to learn about personalized medicine, but only 6% thought that their medical education had adequately prepared them to practice personalized medicine. An earlier study by Stanek et al. [17] undertaken in 2012 involved surveying 10,300 physicians across the USA. 97% agreed PGx is a useful tool; however, only 10% felt they understood how to implement and utilize PGx testing. What is more, only 12.9% of physicians had ordered a test in the previous six months, with 26.4% anticipating ordering a test in the next six months. It is hoped that there has been a considerable shift in PGx knowledge in the last ten years. Indeed, a meta-analysis undertaken by Koufaki et al. [18] in 2021 showed that attitudes and perspectives are improving. In addition, the adoption of PGx seems to vary on a country-by-country basis. In Egypt, both pharmacists and physicians indicated that they obtained a relatively low level of PGx awareness but a rather positive attitude toward the clinical implementation of PGx testing. In Thailand, 46.3% of the respondents of a survey claimed to have poor knowledge, whereas, in Jordan, 73.4% of physicians knew about PGx and pinpointed that they had applied or used PGx in their clinical practice. No matter what the current state of affairs, it is likely that clinical adoption will remain a significant barrier. Overcoming this barrier involves a great deal of investment in PGx training which can be a significant resource drain on any healthcare establishment.

3.2.9 Legal and Regulatory Costs

Acquiring an off-the-shelf bioinformatics package will require the product to be CE-IVDD, and eventually CE-IVDR, for use in Europe. It will be necessary for the acquiring organization to follow local registration requirements before implementation. The cost to a company to acquire CE mark can be considerable. The process involves appointing a notified body and preparing and maintaining a quality management system (QMS). There is likely a requirement for multiple dedicated head counts to maintain this. This cost will no doubt be factored into the end price of any licensing agreement.

4   Can PGx Screening Be Cost-Effective?

There are many ways to assess the cost-effectiveness of PGx testing, including and not limited to cost-utility analysis (CUA), cost-effectiveness analysis (CEA), and cost-minimization analysis (CMA). A study by Berm et al. [19] reviewed 80 studies and concluded that most studies involve CUA or CEA. Prescribing the right drug for the right person at the right time should show a clear economic value. In addition, the benefit to the patient cannot be assessed easily from an economic perspective. This is particularly true in the field of psychiatric medicine, which could lead to quicker patient improvement as well as facilitate an increase in compliance [20]. All of this, in theory, should lead to a more cost-effective prescribing regime. However, there are many considerations, such as the cost of the PGx test, the screening efficiency, and the cost of the alternative medications being prescribed. The other area of discussion regarding cost-effectiveness of PGx testing is in the prevention of adverse drug reactions (ADRs). ADR is covered extensively elsewhere in this book; nevertheless, it is important that we remind ourselves of the burden ADR places on any healthcare system and, more importantly, on human life. The economics of an ADR may vary from country to country; however, the cost of human life is constant.

An impact study was undertaken in 2008 estimated approximately 5% of all hospital admissions are caused by ADRs. In addition, 5% of hospitalized patients will experience an ADR during their hospital stay, with ADRs causing 197,000 deaths annually throughout the EU[20]. However, Bouvy et al. [21] undertook a study of all European epidemiological studies quantifying ADRs between January 1, 2000 and September 3, 2014. Included were studies assessing the number of patients who were admitted to the hospital due to an ADR, studies that assessed the number of patients who developed an ADR during hospitalization, and studies that measured ADRs in the outpatient setting. In total, 47 articles were included in the final review. The median percentage of hospital admissions due to an ADR was 3.5%, based on 22 studies, and the median percentage of patients who experienced an ADR during hospitalization was 10.1%, based on 13 studies.

Data published by Hospital Healthcare Europe [22] in 2020 stated that 17.3% of the EU and UK population would be admitted to hospital every year. If we assume the population of the UK and the EU to be approximately 520 million, then approximately 90 million people will be admitted to hospitals every year. Based on an ADR rate of 10.1% [21], there will be approximately 9 million ADRs due to medications prescribed during a hospital stay per year in Europe alone. Data researched by Bouvy et al. [21] would suggest that approximately 0.25% (or 1 in 400 hospitalized patients) of all patients who are hospitalized due to an ADR will die as a result of an ADR during their stay in a European hospital. This equates to 225,000 patient's deaths per year. To put this in perspective, approximately 245,000 people die from colorectal carcinoma every year in Europe.

How many of these deaths could have been avoided if a PGx screening had been implemented? Due to the many variables involved, this is a very difficult question to answer. The data show that up to 70% of the ADRs could possibly or definitely be avoided [23]. But this does not definitively define that all or most of the deaths could be avoided by adopting a PGx screening program. PGx screening will undoubtedly contribute to safer prescribing practices; however, to what extent is dependent on many variables. Not all PGx tests cover the same genes and alleles; therefore, the range of medications covered will also be variable. In addition, factors such as drug-to-drug interaction, age, and liver and kidney function status also need to be considered.

It is clear in addition to saving lives, the main driver for adopting a PGx screening regime will be the cost to implement versus the costs saved. With so many variables to consider identifying the cost saved is in itself a very difficult task. The level of care required will depend on the nature of the ADR. It may be a prescription change with a higher or lower prescription cost, or it may require intensive care treatment in the emergency room with an associated bed stay. Additional costs to be accounted for are diagnostic and monitoring services, nursing, and treatment care, along with other associated treatment costs.

The cost of hospital services varies significantly on a country-by-country basis. The USA has a much higher cost for services than most other countries around the world. In Europe, higher costs are found in Switzerland and Germany.

Investopedia reports that the average cost in the USA for an MRI scan was between $1119 and $3031. In Australia, the cost averages $215, whereas in Spain, it is as low as $181. The researchers also observed the same trend in prescription drugs. An example is the prescription drug, Avastin, prescribed for oncology patients. The USA has an average price of $3930, whereas the same drug is charged $470 in the U.K.

It must be kept in mind that the cost charged and the actual cost to the hospital are often not the same value. When calculating cost-effectiveness, it is important to use the actual cost to the hospital and not the cost charged to the patient or insurance company. A number of studies have tried to directly measure the cost associated with ADRs. Many studies focus on the length of stay as it relates to bed costs. Here again, the variability of a bed stay is dependent on the country in which the hospitalization occurs. Pirmohamed et al. in 2004 reported the average cost of a bed stays in the UK NHS due to an ADR to be $450 [23]. The average length of stay is 8 days. This would equate to a cost of $3600 for each ADR event requiring hospitalization. If we calculate for inflation, this will equate to $5100 today. In another study undertaken in 2006 by Carrasco-Garrido et al. [24], the cost per ADR was calculated to be $5100. Accounting for inflation, this puts the cost per ADR today at $6250.

How do hospital institutions take this information and calculate if PGx screening is cost-effective? There is no perfect model, and each institution must undertake its own research to calculate whether PGx screening should be adopted. The key considerations are as follows.

1. Which PGx test will be used? Not all PGx tests are the same. Gene and allele coverage will differ. This will determine the medications which can be flagged for screening.
2. Identify internal costs for laboratory and diagnostics services, bed stay, nursing care, administered medications, and other ADR-related costs. Arrive at a cost per ADR and use this to calculate cost-effectiveness.
3. Is the PGx screening program community-based or hospital-based or both? It is extremely difficult to set up and manage a community-based PGx program aimed to reduce PGx-related ADR hospital admissions. It is relatively easier to manage a hospital-based PGx screening program based on patients admitted for a hospital stay or treated through outpatient departments. Setting up a system to flag patients being prescribed a medication with a known PGx component using the hospital EMR system is possible. The costs associated with setting up the EMR to be able to flag the need for a PGx test should be factored into the final cost.
4. What is the true cost per result for the PGx test based on reagent costs, control costs, and disposables used to generate a test result?
5. What is the assumption of the percentage coverage of the PGx test as it relates to ADR-causing medications? It has been shown that 10% of all hospital inpatients experience an ADR[10]. What percentage is assumed to be preventable by incorporating a PGx screening program?

This later point [5] was explored by reviewing 3 ADR-related publications [23-25] in which medications or groups of medications are listed as causative agents for an ADR. Working with a PharmD-qualified individual, a crosswalk of the medications listed was undertaken to estimate the percentage coverage of a commercial PGx test [26]. It must be stressed that the figures are educated estimates and do not necessarily reflect the real-world outcome for any given establishment. The findings indicate that the commercial PGx used in the crosswalk would cover between 25 and 75% of ADR-causing medications. With the above information, it is possible to work up a number of examples to estimate the cost-effectiveness of a PGx program.

5   PGx Financial Modeling

Most countries worldwide operate via direct or indirect government-funded hospital systems. In such institutions, they operate as not-for-profit organizations and are funded centrally by the government. In a very simple model, they are assigned a budget for a particular, fiscal year and are asked to manage the budget. It is therefore in the interest of such organizations to implement programs to help reduce spending. In an attempt to design a guideline to enable a financial modeling exercise for implementing a PGx screening program, the following assumptions have been made.

The model is applicable for hospital inpatient screening as this is the most accessible model for controlling and expediting an efficient screening program. In theory, every patient which is admitted can be checked to see whether the prescription they are to receive has a PGx component and therefore warrants a PGx test before prescription administration. Hospitals operate at 80% bed capacity, with the average bed stay being eight days [22]. Based on this assumption, it is possible to estimate the number of hospital admissions per year based on hospital bed size. For example, a 500-bed hospital running at 80% capacity will have 400 beds occupied at any one time. With an average stay of 8 days, this means there are 18,000 hospital admissions per year $(400 \times (365/8))$. Based on this figure, it is now possible to calculate the number of ADRs expected each year based on an ADR rate of 10% [23]. As such, a 500-bed hospital can expect to see 1800 ADRs per year. If we assume each ADR costs the best case $5100 [23], then the cost of ADRs per year for a 500-bed hospital is $9,180,000 per year. However, if 30% of the ADRs can be avoided by undertaking a PGx screening, then the savings could potentially be $2,754,000 per year. If screening of 50% of the total inpatient population is required to identify the 30% of the preventable ADRs, then the break-even cost of a PGx test is $306. In theory, this could also save 4 or 5 lives.

There are many assumptions in this model, such as assuming that 30% of ADRs with a PGx component will lead to a serious ADR leading to an extended stay in hospital. It also assumes the testing service can be set up in-house, as a Test Send Out model is unlikely to be feasible. The costs associated with the testing and shipping of samples out of the country, along with the legal and regulatory framework, may prove to be problematic. It will therefore be necessary for the hospital laboratory to set up the testing service. In theory, it is possible to be able to offer an in-house test with a cost per reportable of $306. The other major cost is capital equipment. If we assume a capital equipment cost of $750,000 and then assuming a 5-year straight-line depreciation, processing 9000 patient samples per year, then this adds $16.60 to each result. In theory, it is possible to set up an in-house test with a cost per reportable result of under $290.

Given the above assumptions, how can a hospital system implement such a project to prove the above theory? One way is for a definitive ADR study to be undertaken at an acute care hospital. It will be necessary to coordinate education, training, and IT implementation with all relevant departments. It will also take a commercial organization to be willing to offer PGx testing at a significantly lower price to prove out the theory and provide a target cost per reportable to enable real-world calculations.

In conclusion, it is clear that ADRs are costing individual healthcare systems millions of dollars per year. More importantly, the cost of human lives is immense and potentially avoidable. In theory, ADRs are costing a 500-bed hospital almost $3 million per year and will lead to the death of 5 patients per year. In theory, if a PGx screening program is implemented, these cost savings can be realized and potentially lives saved. In addition, the implementation of a hospital-based PGx screening program will inevitably help reduce ADRs in the community as the test is a 'lifetime' test. What is more, additional costs and patient benefits will be seen by prescribing the right patient the right prescription at the right time.

References

1. Peters J, et al. Evidence used in model-based economic evaluations for evaluating pharmaco-genetic and pharmacogenomic tests: a systematic review protocol. BMJ Open. 2015. https://doi.org/10.1136/bmjopen-2015-008465.
2. Verbelen M, Weale ME, Lewis CM. Cost-effectiveness of pharmacogenetic-guided treatment: are we there yet? Pharmacogenomics J. 2017;17(5):395–402. https://doi.org/10.1038/tpj.2017.21.
3. McCabe C, Claxton K, Culyer A. The NICE cost-effectiveness threshold. Pharmacoeconomics. 2008;26:733–44.
4. Zhu Y, Moriarty JP, Swanson KM, et al. A model-based cost-effectiveness analysis of pharma-cogenomic panel testing in cardiovascular disease management: preemptive, reactive, or none? Genet Med. 2021;23:461–70. https://doi.org/10.1038/s41436-020-00995-w.
5. van der Wouden CH, Marck H, Guchelaar H-J, Swen JJ, van den Hout WB. Cost-effectiveness of pharmacogenomics-guided prescribing to prevent gene-drug-related deaths: a decision-analytic model. Front Pharmacol. 2022;13:918493. https://doi.org/10.3389/fphar.2022.918493.
6. Siamoglou S, Karamperis K, Mitropoulou C, Patrinos GP. Costing methods as a means to mea-sure the costs of pharmacogenomics testing. J Appl Lab Med. 2020;5(5):1005–16. https://doi.org/10.1093/jalm/jfaa113.
7. Karamperis K, Koromina M, Papantoniou P, et al. Economic evaluation in psychiatric phar-macogenomics: a systematic review. Pharmacogenomics J. 2021;21:533–41. https://doi.org/10.1038/s41397-021-00249-1.

8. Carta A, Del Zompo M, Meloni A, et al. Cost-utility analysis of pharmacogenetic testing based on CYP2C19 or CYP2D6 in major depressive disorder: assessing the drivers of different cost-effectiveness levels from an Italian societal perspective. Clin Drug Investig. 2022;42:733–46. https://doi.org/10.1007/s40261-022-01182-2.
9. Turongkaravee S, Praditsitthikorn N, Ngamprasertchai T, Jittikoon J, Mahasirimongkol S, Sukasem C, Udomsinprasert W, Wu O, Chaikledkaew U. Economic evaluation of multiple-pharmacogenes testing for the prevention of adverse drug reactions in people living with HIV. ClinicoEcon Outcomes Res. 2022;14:447–63. https://doi.org/10.2147/CEOR.S366906.
10. Kelley EF, Snyder EM, Alkhatib NS, Snyder SC, Sprissler R, Olson TP, Akre MK, Abraham I. Economic evaluation of a pharmacogenomic multi-gene panel test to optimize anti-hypertension therapy: simulation study. J Med Econ. 2018;21(12):1246–53. https://doi.org/10.1080/13696998.2018.1531011.
11. Kearney PM, Whelton M, Reynolds K, et al. Global burden of hypertension: analysis of worldwide data. Lancet. 2005;365:217–23.
12. Cohen JD. Hypertension epidemiology and economic burden: refining risk assessment to lower costs. Manag Care. 2009;18:51–8.
13. Khromykh A. Cost-effectiveness and utility of preemptive pharmacogenomic testing in infants. Master's thesis, Harvard Extension School. 2017.
14. Morris AS, Alsaidi TA, Verbyla A, Cruz A, Macfarlane C, Bauer J, Patel NJ. Cost effectiveness of pharmacogenetic testing for drugs with clinical pharmacogenetics implementation consortium (CPIC) guidelines: a systematic review. Clin Pharmacol Ther. 2022;112(6):1318–28.
15. OneOme Inc medication data curation white paper. A systematic approach to implementing and reporting of complex pharmacogenomic data.
16. Eden C, et al. Medical student preparedness for an era of personalized medicine: findings from one US medical school. PubMed. 2016;13(2):129–41.
17. Stanek E, et al. Adoption of pharmacogenomic testing by US physicians: results of a nation-wide survey. Clin Pharmacol Therapy. 2012. https://doi.org/10.1038/clpt.2011.306. Epub.
18. Koufaki M, et al. Adoption of pharmacogenomic testing: a marketing perspective. Front Pharmacol. 2021.
19. Berm E, et al. Economic evaluations of pharmacogenetic and pharmacogenomic screening tests: a systematic review. Second update of the literature. PLOS One. 2016. https://doi.org/10.1371/journal.pone.0146262.
20. European Commission. Proposal for a regulation amending, as regards pharmacovigilance of medicinal products for human use. Regulation (EC) No 726/2004. Impact assessment. 2008.
21. Bouvy J, et al. Epidemiology of adverse drug reactions in Europe: a review of recent observational studies. Drug Saf. 2015;38(5):437–53. 2015. Europe PMC.
22. https://hospitalhealthcare.com/latest-issue-2017/hospitals-in-europe-healthcare-data-8/.
23. Pirmohamed M, et al. Adverse drug reactions as cause of admission to hospital prospective analysis of 18,820 patients. BMJ. 2004;2004(329):15–9.
24. Carrasco-Garrido P, et al. Trends of adverse drug reactions related hospitalizations in Spain (2001–2006). BMC Health Serv Res. 2010;10:287.
25. Schurig M, et al. Adverse drug reactions (ADR) and emergencies. The prevalence of suspected ADR in four emergency departments in Germany. Dtsch Arztebl Int. 2018;115:251–8. https://doi.org/10.3238/arztebl.2018.0251.
26. Oneome Inc internal study. Data on file.

Role of Public Data Bases for Pharmacogenomics

Bernard Esquivel and Kandace Schuft

Abstract

Integration of pharmacogenomics into clinical practice will enhance patient care and patient outcomes resulting in increasing efficacy and decreasing the risk of adverse effects. Several public, online pharmacogenetics and pharmacogenomic databases available via subscription have been created to aid providers with clinical decision-making. The complexity behind pharmacogenomics is broad, making the genotype–phenotype interpretations (hence clinical recommendations) vary from database to database. Most of databases utilize different but scientifically valid and accepted methodologies, which is why some recommendations and conclusions may eventually differ. The Pharmacogenomic community has acknowledged and agreed that, to avoid possible clinical discrepancies, databases standardization and harmonization should be the next milestone to achieve.

Keywords

Pharmacogenetics · Database · CPIC · FDA · DPWG · PharmGKB

The original version of the chapter has been revised: The correct author's name Bernard Esquivel has been updated. A correction to this chapter can be found at
https://doi.org/10.1007/978-3-031-45903-0_26

B. Esquivel (✉)
GenXys Health Care Systems Inc., Vancouver, BC, Canada
e-mail: bernard.esquivel@genxys.com

B. Esquivel · B. Esquivel
Personalized Medicine Latin American Association, Mexico City, Mexico

K. Schuft
Wolters Kluwer, Hudson, OH, USA
e-mail: kandace.schuft@wolterskluwer.com

1   Introduction

Resources are needed to evaluate literature and provide clinical guidance for the increasing amount of pharmacogenomic information. Several public, online pharmacogenetics databases are available to assist with clinical decision-making. In addition to the multiple public databases, there are pharmacogenetic databases available via subscription. Educational opportunities are needed to increase awareness and understanding. This need is growing to educate patients and providers, as personalized medicine, and specifically pharmacogenomics is frequently mentioned. The online databases include not only regulatory databases but also pharmacogenomic referential databases. As pharmacogenomic resources are developed and more readily available, clinicians are more likely to integrate pharmacogenomics into clinical practice with accessible information. The integration of pharmacogenomics into clinical practice will enhance patient care and patient outcomes when personalizing a patient's medication therapy, increasing efficacy and decreasing the risk of adverse effects.

2   Regulatory Databases

To realize a clinically viable application of pharmacogenomics at the point of care, it is imperative to establish an appropriate regulatory environment. A robust, standardized, and consistent regulatory framework, which aligns with academic and scientific guidelines, has emerged as a paramount requirement in the advancement of pharmacogenomics. Prasad [1] Initial strides have been made in the realm of pharmacogenomics, as evidenced by the establishment of the "Table of Pharmacogenomics Associations" by the U.S. Food and Drug Administration (FDA) and the "Guideline on Good Pharmacogenomic Practice" issued by the European Medicines Agency (EMA). In regulatory contexts, the EMA's guideline, in conjunction with the International Conference on Harmonization (ICH E15), delineates pharmacogenomics as the investigation into DNA and RNA variations and their correlation with drug reactions. Concurrently, The Council for International Organizations of Medical Sciences (CIOMS VII) characterizes it as the utilization of genomic methodologies to determine disease predisposition, the process of drug discovery, understanding pharmacological activities, drug distribution, and predicting therapeutic outcomes. The ICH delineates Pharmacogenetics, a sub-domain of pharmacogenomics, as the examination of DNA sequence variations and their implications on drug reactions. In contrast, CIOMS VII views it as the analysis of individual DNA sequence differences associated with drug metabolism (pharmacokinetics) or drug efficacy (pharmacodynamics) impacting clinical outcomes [2].

The approach adopted by the European Medicines Agency (EMA) aims to amplify awareness among healthcare practitioners. This is accomplished by incorporating pharmacogenomic details into drug labeling and by offering explicit guidance on the rationale, timing, and methods to acquire individual patient pharmacogenomic data. Such measures are designed to bolster the application of pharmacogenomics (PGx) in guiding drug therapies [3]. As per The Pharmacogenomics Knowledgebase (PharmGKB), the European Medicines Agency (EMA) provides distinct pharmacogenomic guidelines for 140 drugs. In evaluating the degree of the pharmacogenetic intervention indicated on each label, PharmGKB categorizes them into four separate tiers: "Mandatory Testing", "Advisable Testing", "Action-oriented PGx", and "Informational PGx" [4]. The FDA has actively demonstrated its endorsement of pharmacogenomics (PGx) advancements in drug creation, evaluation, and authorization. They have released a series of guidelines for the pharmaceutical industry, suggesting the integration of PGx details in the labeling of "Human Prescription Medications and Biological Products" [5].

The Tables of Pharmacogenetic Associations are subdivided into three sections:

- *"Section 1: Pharmacogenetic Associations for which the Data Support Therapeutic Management Recommendations,*
- *Section 2: Pharmacogenetic Associations for which the Data Indicate a Potential Impact on Safety or Response, and*
- *Section 3: Pharmacogenetic Associations for which the Data Demonstrate a Potential Impact on Pharmacokinetic Properties Only."*

The FDA also states on their website that specific information regarding therapeutic management is provided for some pharmacogenetic associations listed in the table. However, most of the associations listed have not been evaluated regarding the impact of genetic testing on clinical outcomes, such as improved therapeutic effectiveness or increased risk of specific adverse events [5].

The FDA's regulatory landscape for pharmacogenetics is built on a framework that includes analytical validation, clinical validation, and clinical utility.

Analytical validation entails the assurance that the assay is precise, consistent, and replicable. For the attainment of analytical validation, producers of pharmacogenetic assays need to manifest that their evaluations can persistently yield trustworthy outcomes. This necessitates the appraisal of the test's fidelity, exactitude, selectivity, and susceptibility. Additionally, it requires the examination of the test's competency in identifying genetic discrepancies within an individual's DNA.

Clinical validation necessitates the proof that the examination can precisely foretell an individual's drug response or discern individuals potentially susceptible to detrimental reactions. Clinical validation predominantly engages in orchestrating clinical investigations to vouch for the test's efficacy and safety. These studies could entail juxtaposing the outcomes of pharmacogenetic evaluations with tangible clinical results, such as therapeutic reactions or unanticipated incidents.

Clinical utility emphasizes the corroboration that implementing the test translates to enhanced patient results. In order to verify clinical utility, pharmacogenetic test manufacturers are compelled to submit evidence suggesting that their test's deployment corresponds to ameliorated patient outcomes, encompassing factors like diminished hospital stays, augmented life quality, or abridged healthcare expenditures.

The approval procedure for pharmacogenetic tests adopted by the FDA generally integrates elements of analytical validation, clinical validation, and clinical utility assessments. To grant approval for use, the FDA mandates clinical research to attest to the safety and effectiveness of pharmacogenetic tests. These investigations could encompass pharmacokinetic evaluations, focusing on the drug's concentration trajectory in the system, and pharmacodynamic assessments, gauging the physiological impact of the drug.

Under the Federal Food, Drug, and Cosmetic Act (FD&C Act), the FDA categorizes pharmacogenetic tests as in vitro diagnostic devices (IVDs). The regulation of these tests is executed by the *FDA's Center for Devices and Radiological Health (CDRH)*, following the directives set by the Medical Device Amendments of 1976.

A significant hurdle that the FDA confronts in the domain of pharmacogenetics is the swift technological evolution. The continuous discovery of novel genetic markers and the accelerated development of new assays pose challenges in maintaining regulatory currency with these technological strides. Further complicating the regulatory landscape is the prevailing non-uniformity in pharmacogenetics, making it intricate for the FDA to ascertain the reliability and effectiveness of these tests.

In a bid to tackle these obstacles, the FDA has constituted specialized working committees tasked with framing guidelines for the evolution and oversight of pharmacogenetic evaluations. Concurrently, the FDA is channeling efforts to refine its advisory framework concerning the clinical relevance of pharmacogenetic tests. This ensures their judicious application, maximizing patient advantages derived from their deployment.

The "Pharmacogenomic Biomarkers in Drug Labeling" segment on the FDA's official web portal serves as a pivotal resource, elucidating the role and clinical implications of pharmacogenomic biomarkers within the realm of drug therapy. The following are ten representative instances of pharmacogenomic biomarkers that have been incorporated into drug labels [5]:

"*CYP2C19*": This biomarker plays a role in the metabolic pathway of the antiplatelet medication, clopidogrel. Individuals exhibiting diminished CYP2C19 function might experience a suboptimal therapeutic response to clopidogrel, potentially elevating their susceptibility to cardiovascular complications.

"*HLA-B57:01*": This genetic marker is linked to a heightened probability of experiencing severe hypersensitivity reactions when exposed to the antiretroviral medication, abacavir. Prior to initiating therapy with abacavir, a genetic screening for HLA-B5701 is advocated.

"*UGT1A1*": Participating in the metabolic processes of the chemotherapy agent, irinotecan, this biomarker, when under expressed, can elevate a patient's vulnerability to certain toxic effects, such as neutropenia and diarrhea. It's suggested to conduct a genetic assessment for UGT1A1 prior to commencing treatment with irinotecan.

"*TPMT*": Integral to the metabolism of the immunosuppressive medication, azathioprine, a deficient TPMT activity can heighten the risk of adverse effects, notably myelosuppression. Prior to introducing azathioprine therapy, it is recommended to perform a genetic test for TPMT.

"*CYP2D6*": This biomarker is instrumental in metabolizing an array of medications, spanning from antidepressants and antipsychotics to opioids. Individuals with compromised CYP2D6 function may face an elevated risk of untoward drug responses or therapeutic inadequacy. For medications predominantly metabolized by CYP2D6, a preliminary genetic screening for this biomarker is suggested.

"*HLA-B1502*": This genetic marker correlates with an augmented risk of conditions like Stevens–Johnson syndrome and toxic epidermal necrolysis in patients administered the antiepileptic agent, carbamazepine. Especially for patients of Asian lineage, a genetic evaluation for HLA-B1502 is advised before initiating carbamazepine therapy.

"*VKORC1*": This genetic marker has a role in the metabolic process of the anticoagulant medication, warfarin. Individuals exhibiting diminished VKORC1 function might necessitate a reduced dosage of warfarin to attain the targeted anticoagulative outcome.

"*NAT2*": Playing a role in the metabolism of the antitubercular agent, isoniazid, a diminished NAT2 activity can escalate a patient's susceptibility to certain toxic manifestations, notably hepatotoxicity and peripheral neuropathy. Before embarking on isoniazid therapy, a genetic evaluation for NAT2 is suggested.

"*CYP3A4/5*": These genetic indicators participate in the metabolic pathways of a diverse range of medications, encompassing statins, calcium channel inhibitors, and immunosuppressive agents. Patients with compromised CYP3A4/5 function may necessitate adjusted, typically decreased, dosages of these drugs to secure the anticipated therapeutic results.

"*SLCO1B1*": This biomarker is instrumental in the liver's assimilation of the cholesterol-reducing medication, simvastatin. Individuals with reduced SLCO1B1 function might face a heightened risk of conditions like myopathy or rhabdomyolysis, especially when administered elevated dosages of simvastatin. A preliminary genetic screening for SLCO1B1 is recommended before introducing simvastatin therapy.

The instances cited underscore the pivotal role that pharmacogenomic data plays within drug labels, empowering healthcare professionals to make judicious therapeutic choices, taking into consideration a patient's unique genetic makeup.

To encapsulate, the "Pharmacogenomic Biomarkers in Drug Labeling" segment on the FDA's online portal stands as a vital repository, shedding light on pharmacogenomics and its interplay in drug therapy. Integrating pharmacogenomic specifics into drug labels equips healthcare professionals with pivotal information, allowing for tailored therapeutic choices rooted in a patient's genomic composition. This repository meticulously catalogs pharmacogenomic biomarkers present in drug labels and elucidates their clinical relevance, rendering it an indispensable tool for both healthcare practitioners and researchers.

In this context, the FDA assumes an indispensable role in overseeing the inception and application of pharmacogenetic diagnostic tools and correlated products. The regulatory model employed by the FDA concerning pharmacogenetics is anchored in the core tenets of analytical validation, clinical validation, and clinical utility. Despite the intricacies inherent in pharmacogenetics oversight, the FDA remains committed to refining its guidelines and sculpting best practices, all with an aim to ascertain the reliability and efficiency of these diagnostic instruments.

3   Pharmacogenomics Specific Databases

3.1   The Clinical Pharmacogenetics Implementation Consortium

Nowadays, the Clinical Pharmacogenomics Implementation Consortium (CPIC) is one of the most well-known and trusted international entities within the pharmacogenomics ecosystem. CPIC guidelines are gaining increased traction, specifically in the clinical space, as an evidence-implementation threshold [7].

The CPIC, or Clinical Pharmacogenetics Implementation Consortium, is a global assembly comprising devoted volunteers and a specialized team. Their primary objective is to bolster the utilization of pharmacogenetic assessments in patient-oriented medical care.

In its inception in 2009, CPIC was conceived as a collaborative endeavor between PharmGKB and the Pharmacogenomics Research Network (PGRN). The guidelines delineated by CPIC have secured a place in PubMed under the category of clinical guidelines. These directives have garnered endorsements from esteemed institutions, namely the American Society of Hospital Pharmacists (ASHP) and the American Society of Clinical Pharmacology and Therapeutics (ASCPT). Furthermore, they are cited in reputable databases such as ClinGen and PharmGKB [8].

The Clinical Pharmacogenetics Implementation Consortium (CPIC) employs a structured system to categorize evidence that correlates genotype with phenotype. The summarized evidence from the literature, integrated within each guideline supplement, is systematically ranked as high, moderate, or weak. The definitions for these ranks are [9]:

- **High**: This refers to evidence stemming from consistent results procured from methodically sound and well-executed studies.
- **Moderate**: Such evidence is adequate for discerning effects. However, its potency might be diminished due to factors such as the limited number of studies, their quality, their consistency, the evidence's relevance to standard practice, or the evidence's indirect character.
- **Weak**: Here, the evidence does not sufficiently address the health outcomes, mainly due to limitations in study numbers, flaws in their design or

execution, existing gaps in the sequential evidence, or an absence of requisite information.

In the context of gene/drug associations, CPIC has outlined specific levels, amalgamating CPIC Level, Clinical Context, Level of Evidence, and Strength of Recommendation:

1. **A**: It is imperative to incorporate genetic information when prescribing the related drug. The overwhelming majority of evidence, whether high or moderate, advocates for a modification in prescription practices. At least one action suggesting a change in prescription is deemed moderate or strong.
2. **A/B**: An initial review suggests that the conclusive CPIC level might fall under A or B. A comprehensive evidence review is essential to determine evidence strength, but the prescription's actionability based on this preliminary data seems probable. An in-depth review by a specialized guideline group is needed to pinpoint the strength of the recommendation.
3. **B**: Genetic data could influence the prescription of the concerned drug, mainly because alternative dosing or therapies are likely just as effective and safe as non-genetically influenced dosing. The majority of the evidence, though weak, has minimal conflicting data. At least one optional action advocating a change in prescription is proposed.
4. **B/C**: An initial review suggests that the final CPIC level might be B or C. The clarity on prescription modifications based on genetic data remains vague without a further evidence review. A specialized guideline group must review thoroughly to determine the recommendation's strength.
5. **C**: Various published studies, exhibiting different evidence levels and some with a foundational rationale, do not recommend any changes in prescribing practices. This is either because genetic-based dosing does not present a significant difference, alternatives are ambiguous or potentially less effective or more harmful, or the limited nature of published studies provides unclear clinical actions. This category is particularly relevant for genes highlighted in other CPIC guidelines or those often part of clinical or direct-to-consumer tests. There are varying levels of evidence, but no changes in prescribing practices are recommended.
6. **C/D**: An initial review suggests that the CPIC level might be C or D. The levels of evidence may vary, but no alterations in prescribing actions are proposed.
7. **D**: With limited published studies, unclear clinical actions, minimal mechanistic foundation, predominantly weak evidence, or significant conflicting data, this level suggests that if the genes are not extensively tested clinically, evaluations are not required. Evidence levels can differ, but no changes in prescribing practices are recommended.

The CPIC has reviewed up to 2020 more than 400 gene–drug pairs and has published recommendations on 106 gene–drug pairs with sufficient evidence for at least one prescribing action in 24 published guidelines [10].

3.2 Dutch Pharmacogenetics Working Group

The Dutch Pharmacogenetics Working Group (DPWG), initiated in 2005, operates under the auspices of the Royal Dutch Pharmacist's Association (KNMP). The DPWG represents a multidisciplinary ensemble, boasting participation from professionals spanning multiple disciplines, including clinical pharmacy, medicine, pharmacology, chemistry, epidemiology, and toxicology. Financial support for the DPWG's operations and endeavors is provided by the KNMP [11].

The Dutch Pharmacogenetics Working Group (DPWG) has delineated several primary objectives:

• The formulation of therapeutic recommendations grounded in pharmacogenetic principles, particularly with respect to dosing.
• Augmenting the capabilities of both prescribers and pharmacists by seamlessly embedding these guidelines into digital drug prescription and medication surveillance platforms.

In 2013, a collaborative venture was undertaken between PharmGKB and the DPWG to publicize the recommendations derived from these investigations. The most current versions of these guidelines for the majority of drugs can now be accessed via the official KNMP website (https://www.knmp.nl/patientenzorg/med icatiebewaking/farmacogenetica/pharmacogenetics-1/pharmacogenetics).

In the quest to amass relevant data for each medicinal agent, the DPWG embarked on comprehensive literature searches. The bibliographies of the shortlisted articles were meticulously examined for any additional pertinent resources. If a European Public Assessment Report contained specific references to gene–drug interactions, manufacturers were approached to furnish more in-depth insights. Notably, the DPWG's assessment process purposely omitted in vitro studies, literature reviews, and investigations that employed non-human subjects.

Upon analyzing each sourced article, the group ascertained the degree of evidence supporting the observed gene–drug interaction and the clinical implications thereof—whether in the form of potential adverse reactions, diminished therapeutic efficacy, or other clinically significant outcomes stemming from the gene–drug dynamic.

To provide clarity on the robustness of the evidence procured, the DPWG instituted a five-tiered grading system. This scale extends from 0, indicative of minimal supporting evidence, to 4, signifying compelling evidence [11].

3.3   Canadian Pharmacogenomics Network for Drug Safety

The Canadian Pharmacogenomics Network for Drug Safety (CPNDS) stands as an integrated consortium, combining efforts from multiple centers with a primary focus on active surveillance and pharmacogenomics. Incepted in 2004, its overarching aim is to elucidate the genetic determinants and underlying mechanisms that govern drug response phenotypes. Further, it strives to design advanced pharmacogenetic tools tailored for clinical implementation, thereby optimizing drug safety and effectiveness for both pediatric and adult populations.

Comprising its core are a plethora of esteemed scientists and on-ground clinicians, hailing not just from diverse provinces of Canada but also from global institutions. It thrives as a multidisciplinary consortium, embracing varied expertise and perspectives. Financial scaffolding for the CPNDS is generously provided by an array of provincial and federal entities. Among these benefactors are the Canadian Institutes of Health Research, Genome Canada, Genome British Columbia, the Michael Smith Foundation for Health Research, the Canada Foundation for Innovation, and the Provincial Health Service Authority [12].

The CPNDS adheres to a rigorous guideline development protocol that aligns with the benchmarks delineated by the Appraisal of Guidelines Research and Evaluation Enterprise (AGREE). The foundation of this process is rooted in a meticulous literature exploration, subsequently subjected to in-depth evidence evaluation. During designated collaborative sessions, the guideline development committee formulates clinical practice recommendations. These preliminary guidelines undergo a multi-level scrutiny, commencing with an intra-committee assessment, succeeded by external audits encompassing subject-matter specialists and the prospective user demographic.

The quantification of the scientific evidence's robustness mirrors a methodology akin to the Grading of Recommendations Assessment, Development, and Evaluation (GRADE) consortium's recommendations [12]:

++++ *Consistent, generalizable.* Conclusions drawn are robust, with the likelihood of alterations due to future studies being minimal.

+++ *Consistent, but limited quantity, quality or generalizability.* Prevailing evidence supports overarching conclusions, albeit with modulated assurance. Anticipated subsequent research may significantly bolster this conviction.

++ Inconsistent or insufficient quantity/quality, encouraging. Prevailing insights neither offer a clear directive nor are they absolute, but they exude promise.

+ *Inconsistent or insufficient quantity/quality, discouraging.* Current evidence neither lays down a definitive path nor instills optimism.

During collaborative workshop sessions, the recommendation development committee crafts clinical practice directives. Each of these directives is endowed with an evidence-backed potency rating. This potency is contingent on the evidence's strength, the equilibrium between genotype-informed treatment's advantages and disadvantages, and potential disparities in patients' individualized inclinations and values. A potent directive (level A) is one that most well-informed clinicians and patients would concur with. In contrast, a moderate directive (level B) would necessitate personalized consultations, factoring in the unique characteristics, desires, and values intrinsic to every patient. Level C directives primarily advocate the deployment of a genetic assay within a research milieu.

3.4   French National Network (Réseau) of Pharmacogenetics

The French National Network of Pharmacogenetics (Réseau National de Pharmacogénétique or RNPGx) comprises a substantial membership, extending across France and spilling into other Francophone territories. With roughly 30 active members, the majority are professionals deeply rooted in the hospital pharmacogenetics sphere.

The RNPGx has a structured approach toward pharmacogenetic variants, categorizing them based on their evidence of functionality. This classification trifurcates into: established, likely, or potential functional significance. Notably, only those variants that display established or likely functional relevance are deemed worthy of testing consideration.

Delving deeper into their methodology, RNPGx furnishes pharmacogenetic testing recommendations based on a tiered system. This hierarchy, built on the utility and importance of the test, classifies them as: indispensable, recommended, or potentially beneficial [13].

3.5   Swiss Group of Pharmacogenomics and Personalized Therapy

Established in February 2016 as a division within the Swiss Society of Clinical Pharmacology and Toxicology, the Swiss Group of Pharmacogenomics and Personalized Therapy (SPT) came into existence. Internationally recognized for its scientific contributions and collaborations, the SPT operates as Switzerland's main representative linked to the European Society of Pharmacogenomics and Personalized Therapy.

Citing the official records from the SPT's webpage, their mission is multifaceted. Primarily, they are committed to championing the cause of pharmacogenomics and personalized medicine within Swiss borders. Concurrently, they work to enhance both clinicians' and patients' grasp and application of pharmacogenomics. Furthermore, they aim to offer a balanced and independent perspective on pharmacogenomics and personalized medicine to a diverse group, from regulators and the public to various other interested parties. Adding another feather to their cap, they ardently support scientific endeavors in this rapidly evolving domain.

Among the various accomplishments of the Swiss Group of Pharmacogenomics and Personalized Therapy, a standout has been their role in advancing the integration of pharmacogenomics into the reimbursement structure in Switzerland.

Notably, from the year 2017 onward, pharmacogenetic evaluations have been assimilated into the Swiss Federal list of analyses. This list delineates the rates for laboratory evaluations and sets the conditions that dictate the coverage of these analyses under Switzerland's obligatory basic health insurance scheme. To be deemed appropriate for this coverage, a few prerequisites are established [14]:

1. *The pharmacogenetic assessment should be geared towards addressing the medical repercussions of a disease. To put it succinctly, the outcome of this test should be instrumental in deciding the course of the patient's care.*
2. *Reimbursements are granted only when the pharmacogenetic test is aligned with a drug that is presently deemed suitable for the patient or one that the patient is actively receiving.*
3. *It's pertinent to note that proactive evaluations—meaning pharmacogenetic tests conducted for drugs not currently indicated for a particular patient—do not fall under the ambit of the prevailing coverage criteria.*

In addition, there are important limitations regarding the prescription of pharmacogenetic tests:

- *"Only certain pharmacogenetic tests can be prescribed by any physician, independent of the specialization. These tests are defined in a list provided and maintained by the Swiss Society of Clinical Pharmacology and Toxicology (SSCPT). This list currently includes the following gene-drug pairs*
  - *Abacavir: HLA-B*57:01*
  - *Carbamazepine: HLA-A*31:01, HLA-B*15:02*
  - *Thiopurines (azathioprine, 6-mercaptopurine): TPMT*
  - *Fluoropyrimidines (5-fluorouracil, capecitabine): DPYD*
  - *Irinotecan: UGT1A1*28."*

4 Referential Databases

4.1 National Institutes of Health

The National Institutes of Health (NIH), representing a conglomerate of research components, stands as the globe's premier institution for biomedical research. Senator Claude Pepper, discerning the pivotal role of computerized data processing in the realm of biomedical studies, championed the legislation leading to the inception of the National Center for Biotechnology Information (NCBI) on November 4, 1988. This center was strategically nestled within the National Library of Medicine (NLM) at NIH due to NLM's adeptness in curating and stewarding biomedical databases. Furthermore, the positioning within NIH allowed it to inaugurate an intramural research venture in the computational molecular biology sector [15].

NCBI, serving as a keystone in molecular biology information dissemination, is tasked with pioneering innovative information technologies. These technologies are instrumental in deciphering the intricate molecular and genetic machinations governing health and disease dynamics. Delving deeper into NCBI's mandate, it encompasses the creation of automated infrastructures for cataloging knowledge in molecular biology, biochemistry, and genetics. It is also committed to bolstering the research and medical fraternities' engagement with these databases, orchestrating biotechnological information collection on both domestic and global scales, and spearheading research into avant-garde computer-centric methodologies for scrutinizing biologically pertinent molecules [15].

Parallelly, the National Human Genome Research Institute (NHGRI) acts as the propellant, fostering genomics research undertakings within NIH. Come 1989, NHGRI initiated synergistic engagements with the wider scientific and medical echelons, supporting endeavors probing specific diseases in tandem with NIH counterparts. This consortium thrives on a shared zeal for high-caliber research, pooling resources to transition groundbreaking findings into tangible enhancements in human health [16].

Fast-forward to 2012, NHGRI underwent a seminal restructure, segmenting its Extramural Research Program into four distinct divisions. Additionally, the overseeing offices of policy, outreach, and administration attained divisional stature. This revamp, sanctioned by the U.S. Department of Health and Human Services, was publicly disclosed during the 66th conclave of the National Advisory Council for Human Genome Research. This reshaped configuration caters to NHGRI's broadening scope, transitioning from a concentrated commitment to the Human Genome Project to embracing a plethora of prospects that leverage genomics to revolutionize medicine and elevate human health [16].

4.2   Pharmacogenomics Knowledge Base

Housed within the National Institute of General Medical Sciences at the NIH, the Pharmacogenomics Knowledgebase (PharmGKB) stands as an eminent online repository, amalgamating and categorizing pharmacogenetic information for a vast array of over 650 medications. The database encapsulates over 20,000 pharmacogenetic variants, 3000 + clinical pharmacogenetic annotations, and a substantial collection of 100 dosing guidelines. Users can navigate this data trove by specifying the drug, gene target, or related pharmacological pathway. Furthermore, the platform offers insight into clinical protocols, intricate genotype–phenotype correlations, and an inventory of pharmacogenetic drug labels procured from reputed regulatory bodies including the FDA, EMA, and Japan's Pharmaceuticals and Medical Devices Agency [17].

Funded by the NIH, PharmGKB operates as an information conduit, enlightening users about the intricate interplay between genetic discrepancies and drug responsiveness. The platform meticulously assembles, curates, and propagates information regarding clinically pertinent gene–drug interactions and genotype–phenotype correlations. Within the PharmGKB structure, information is divided into four primary categories: variants, genes, drugs, and diseases or clinical phenotypes. It draws data from renowned external databases. For instance, individual nucleotide polymorphisms (SNPs) bearing rsIDs are extracted from NCBI's SNP database (dbSNP), while gene symbols are attributed to the HUGO Gene Nomenclature Committee (HGNC). The database gleans drug-related data from sources such as PubChem and the WHO's Anatomical Therapeutic Chemical (ATC) classification. Disease and phenotype specifics are adopted from MeSH and SnoMedCT lexicons. It's worth noting that PharmGKB's database is not exhaustive concerning any particular lexicon; the data are progressively integrated based on relevance and demand. Moreover, the in-house scientific curators at PharmGKB possess the autonomy to manually enrich these lexicons or ontologies [17].

The multifaceted composition of PharmGKB, spanning from primary literature to clinical interpretation, underpins the clinical assimilation of pharmacogenomics. This clinical integration encapsulates PGx data from FDA and other international drug labels, fostering collaboration with peer research entities to expedite PGx into clinical practice. Affiliates collaborating with PharmGKB encompass institutions like PharmCAT, PharmVar, CPIC, and ClinGen, among several others [17].

PharmGKB employs a rigorous annotation grading system to assign levels of evidence (LOE) for clinical annotations. An abridged outline of the system [17] includes:

- **Level 1A**: Pertain to variant-drug pairings with specific prescribing guidance in extant clinical guidelines or FDA-endorsed drug labels. At least one supplementary publication, alongside the guideline or drug label, is mandatory.
- **Level 1B**: Concern variant-drug combinations with substantial evidence, albeit devoid of variant-specific prescribing guidance. A minimum of two autonomous publications support these annotations.
- **Level 2A**: These annotations are cataloged within PharmGKB's Tier 1 Very Important Pharmacogenes (VIPs) and signify known pharmacogenes. Supported by no fewer than two discrete publications, these annotations illustrate variant-drug pairings with a moderate evidence foundation.
- **Level 2B**: Unlike the previous category, these annotations fall outside the purview of PharmGKB's Tier 1 VIPs but still denote variant-drug combinations with a moderate degree of evidence.
- **Level 3**: Represents variant-drug pairings with limited supporting evidence, possibly stemming from a solitary study or multiple inconclusive research endeavors.
- **Level 4**: These annotations imply a lack of supportive evidence, suggesting no discernible link between the variant and the drug phenotype.

4.3   Wolters Kluwer

Wolters Kluwer is a global provider of professional information, software solutions, and services for clinicians, nurses, accountants, lawyers, and tax, finance, audit, risk, compliance, and regulatory sectors. There are four global operating divisions and based on strategic customer segments, including Health, Tax and Accounting, Governance, Risk & Compliance, and Legal & Regulatory. Of the four divisions, we will focus on the Health division, which provides trusted clinical technology and evidence-based solutions that engage clinicians, patients, researchers, and students. The health portfolio includes Emmi Patient Engagement, Health Language, Lexicomp, Lippincott, MediSpan, Ovid, POC Advisor, Sentri7, Simplfi 797, UpToDate, and UpToDate Advanced. Among the health portfolios, Lexicomp is the largest provider of pharmacogenomics knowledge [18].

Lexicomp offers drug reference options that tackle critical and challenging areas of drug decision support, accessible at the point of care in an easy-to-use, easily searchable interface in a variety of healthcare settings. The content is evidence-based, meticulously reviewed, and developed from primary sources relied upon by the healthcare community, including primary literature, product labeling, base pharmacology studies, clinical trials, and more. The editorial team synthesizes this critical information into clear, concise information for use at the point of care. The release of new regulatory agency approvals and regulatory, manufacturer, and scientific reports initiates the creation or revision of a referential drug monograph. In addition, medication patient education leaflets and drug interaction information are created and updated to reflect the latest findings, but in language that is patient appropriate [19].

A comprehensive but concise and clear presentation of important pharmacogenomic recommendations and supporting information has been developed and made available in Lexicomp Online. Gene–drug associations covered by a published guideline and actionable pharmacogenomic content in a drug's approved prescribing information are preferentially created, but the intent is to create a comprehensive library of content to cover all potentially relevant gene–drug associations. Publication of content in this format began in early 2017; although, pharmacogenomics content in other formats has been available for many years prior to the development of this concise monograph format. A pharmacogenomic monograph format based on the Lexi-Interact drug interactions monograph was developed. Each monograph contains the following sections: (1) Testing Recommendations, (2) Evidence Ratings, (3) Management, (4) Discussion, and (5) References. Clinical pharmacists with specific pharmacogenomics training and experience author each monograph following a detailed review of available data, and all monographs are reviewed by a separate clinical specialist before publication [20].

5   Conclusion

Pharmacogenomics understanding has been growing exponentially, and databases have played a crucial role by bringing closer to the different stakeholders reliable information, thus fostering acceptance and clinical implementation. The complexity behind pharmacogenomics is broad, making the genotype–phenotype interpretations complex; hence, clinical recommendations may vary from database to database. Most of them utilize different but scientifically valid and accepted methodologies, which is why some recommendations and conclusions may eventually differ. The Pharmacogenomic community has acknowledged and agreed that, in order to avoid possible clinical discrepancies, databases standardization and harmonization should be the next milestone to achieve. In fact, the first steps have been taken, and an active and continued effort toward standardization is in progress within the leading databases, including CPIC and DPWG.

References

1. Prasad K. Role of regulatory agencies in translating pharmacogenetics to the clinics. Clin Cases Miner Bone Metab. 2009;6(1):29–34.
2. European Medicines Agency. https://www.ema.europa.eu/en/good-pharmacogenomic-practice. Accessed 29 Dec 2021.
3. Mendrick DL, Brazell C, Mansfield EA, Pietrusko R, Barilero I, Hackett J, et al. Pharmacogenomics and regulatory decision making: an international perspective. Pharmacogenomics J. 2006;6(3):154–7. https://doi.org/10.1038/sj.tpj.6500364.
4. PHARMGKB. https://www.pharmgkb.org/ (2021). Accessed 27 Dec 2021.
5. US Food and Drug Administratrion. https://www.fda.gov/medical-devices/precision-medicine/table-pharmacogenetic-associations. Accessed Mar 2023.
6. Kim JA, Ceccarelli R, Lu CY. Pharmacogenomic biomarkers in US FDA-approved drug labels (2000–2020). J Pers Med. 2021;11(3):179. https://doi.org/10.3390/jpm11030179.
7. Relling MV, Klein TE, Gammal RS, Whirl-Carrillo M, Hoffman JM, Caudle KE. The clinical pharmacogenetics implementation consortium: 10 years later. Clin Pharmacol Ther. 2020;107(1):171–5. https://doi.org/10.1002/cpt.1651.
8. Clinical Pharmacogenetics Implementations Consortium. https://cpicpgx.org/. Accessed 15 Dec 2021.
9. Valdes R, Payne DA, Linder MW. Laboratory analysis and application of pharmacogenetics to clinical practice. Washington, DC: National Academy of Clinical Biochemistry; 2010.
10. Abdullah-Koolmees H, van Keulen AM, Nijenhuis M, Deneer VHM. Pharmacogenetics guidelines: overview and comparison of the DPWG, CPIC, CPNDS, and RNPGx guidelines. Front Pharmacol. 2021;11: 595219. https://doi.org/10.3389/fphar.2020.595219.
11. Koninklijke Nederlandse Maatschappij ter bevordering der Pharmacie. https://www.knmp.nl/patientenzorg/medicatiebewaking/farmacogenetica/pharmacogenetics-1/pharmacogenetics. Accessed 3 Dec 2021.
12. Canadian Pharmacogenomics Network for Drug Safety. http://cpnds.ubc.ca/. Accessed 12 Dec 2021.
13. Picard N, Boyer JC, Etienne-Grimaldi MC, Barin-Le Guellec C, Thomas F, Loriot MA. French national network of pharmacogenetics (RNPGx). Pharmacogenetics-based personalized therapy: levels of evidence and recommendations from the french network of pharmacogenetics (RNPGx). Therapie. 2017;72(2):185–192. https://doi.org/10.1016/j.therap.2016.09.014.

14. Swiss Society of Clinical Pharmacology and Toxicology. https://clinpharm.ch/en/pharmacog enetics_spt/swiss_group_of_personalised_therapy_and_pharmacogenomics. Accessed 30 Dec 2021.
15. National Center for Biotechnology Information (NCBI) U.S. National library of medicine. https://www.ncbi.nlm.nih.gov/. Accessed 5 Jan 2022
16. National Institutes of Health (NIH). National Human Genome Research Institute (NHGRI). https://www.nih.gov/about-nih/what-we-do/nih-almanac/national-human-genome-research-institute-nhgri. Accessed 5 Jan 2022.
17. Whirl-Carrillo M, Huddart R, Gong L, Sangkuhl K, Thorn CF, Whaley R, Klein TE. An evidence-based framework for evaluating pharmacogenomics knowledge for personalized medicine. Clin Pharmacol Ther. 2021;110(3):563–572. https://doi.org/10.1002/cpt.2350
18. Wolters Kluwer. https://www.wolterskluwer.com/en. Accessed 5 Jan 2022.
19. Wolters Kluwer. https://www.wolterskluwer.com/en/solutions/lexicomp. (2022). Accessed 5 Jan 2022.
20. Schuft K, Warren S, Haque N, Isley S, Stout S, Streetman D. The integration of CPIC guidelines into a referential drug information database. Poster presented at: Clinical Pharmacogenetics Implementation Consortium (CPIC) Meeting; 2019 June 6-7; Memphis, Tennessee, USA.

Pharmacogenomics Education

Ana Petrović, Kristina Bojanić, Lucija Kuna, Dragan Primorac,
Lidija Bach-Rojecky, and Martina Smolić

Abstract

In this chapter, we discuss current teaching practice in pharmacogenomics
education. While there is an abundance of published data regarding scientific progress in pharmacogenomics, pharmacogenomics education has not been
proportionally progressive. Pharmacogenomics is fundamental for precision
(personalized) medicine; however, studies show a lack of knowledge and appropriate education among healthcare professionals and students. Here, we focus
on the most important publications regarding history, guidelines, and progress

A. Petrović · K. Bojanić · L. Kuna · M. Smolić (✉)
Department of Pharmacology and Biochemistry, Josip Juraj Strossmayer University of Osijek
Faculty of Dental Medicine and Health Osijek, Osijek, Croatia
e-mail: martina.smolic@fdmz.hr

A. Petrović · M. Smolić
Department of Pharmacology, Josip Juraj Strossmayer University of Osijek Faculty of Medicine
Osijek, Osijek, Croatia

K. Bojanić
Department of Biophysics and Radiology, Josip Juraj Strossmayer University of Osijek Faculty of
Medicine Osijek, Osijek, Croatia

Department of Radiology, Health Center Osijek, Osijek, Croatia

D. Primorac
St. Catherine Specialty Hospital, Zagreb, Croatia

University of Split School of Medicine, Split, Croatia

Josip Juraj Strossmayer University of Osijek Faculty of Medicine, Osijek, Croatia

University of Rijeka School of Medicine, Rijeka, Croatia

Josip Juraj Strossmayer University of Osijek Faculty of Dental Medicine and Health, Osijek,
Croatia

made in the integration of pharmacogenomics into healthcare education programs and curricula design. Finally, we briefly discuss the current status and main issues of pharmacogenomics implementation in clinical practice.

Keywords

Pharmacogenomics • Education • Study programs • Medical schools • Pharmacy schools

1   Introduction

This chapter is divided into three sections. In the first section, we discuss the history and importance of pharmacogenomics, followed by the most important call for action and publications at the beginning of the pharmacogenomics integration into healthcare professionals' education programs. In 2005, Gurwitz et al. launched one of the earliest pharmacogenomics education initiatives with recommendations to incorporate pharmacogenomics into universities curricula [1]. In the second section, we examine and evaluate progress made regarding pharmacogenomics education. We discuss current pharmacogenomics integration in pharmacology curricula, as well as independent mandatory and elective subjects, teaching hours, educational tools, and pharmacogenomics education at the graduate and postgraduate level (postgraduate specialists' and Ph.D. programs). We also provide data obtained from studies that surveyed students and their awareness and knowledge of pharmacogenomics. Finally, in the third section, we discuss the implementation of pharmacogenomics into clinical practice, The Clinical Pharmacogenetics Implementation Consortium (CPIC) guidelines, and healthcare professionals' opinions and issues regarding pharmacogenomics knowledge.

2   History and Importance of Pharmacogenomic Education

Over a century ago, in 1902, to explain observed differences in drug response, a foresightful English physician Archibald Garrod [2] concluded that no two individuals are identical. He wrote: *"If it is, indeed, the case that in alkaptonuria and the other conditions mentioned we are dealing with individualities of metabolism*

Eberly College of Science, Penn State University, 517 Thomas St, State College, PA 16803, USA

The Henry C. Lee College of Criminal Justice and Forensic Sciences, University of New Haven, West Haven, CT, USA

Medical School REGIOMED, 96450 Coburg, Germany

L. Bach-Rojecky
Department of Pharmacology, University of Zagreb Faculty of Pharmacy and Biochemistry, Zagreb, Croatia

and not with the results of morbid processes, the thought naturally presents itself that these are merely extreme examples of variations in chemical behavior which are probably everywhere present in minor degrees and that just as no two individuals of a species are absolutely identical in bodily structure neither are their chemical processes carried out on exactly the same lines ... and if we pass to differences presumably chemical in their basis idiosyncrasies as regards drugs and the various degrees of natural immunity against infection are only less marked in individual human beings and in the several races of mankind than in distinct genera, and species of animals."

However, more than half a century later, in the 1950s, interindividual differences in drug response were found to be due to the types of "chemical behavior" anticipated by English physician Sir Archibald Garrod. It was discovered that people who developed apnea after being given succinylcholine were low in the enzyme butyrylcholinesterase, which is required for succinylcholine hydrolysis [3]. Price Evans et al. established that patients who developed peripheral neuritis after taking isoniazid lacked the N-acetyl transferase activity required for the isoniazid excretion [4]. Ten percent of African Americans who received the antimalarial drug primaquine developed hemolytic anemia. Sensitivity was associated with glucose-6-phosphate dehydrogenase deficiency [5]. Glucose-6-phosphate dehydrogenase is required for the synthesis of reduced glutathione in red blood cells, which protects cells from oxidative stress. When exposed to free radical metabolites of primaquine, deficient individuals had hemolysis.

Overall, these groundbreaking early discoveries contributed to the identification of the genetic background of various drug responses and provided the framework for a new scientific discipline of medical research.

In 1959, Friedrich Vogel introduced the term "pharmacogenetics" to explain the abovementioned phenotypic differences in drug metabolism and medication response [6]. By the end of the 1950s, the originally utilized term pharmacogenetics had become commonplace for some drug therapies [7].

Following little advances in the 1960s and 1970s, improved analytical methods, more extensive drug development programs, and human gene cloning led in a considerably better comprehension of the genetic basis of phenotypic diversity in the 1980s [7]. Since the sequencing of the human genome in 2003, pharmacogenetics has evolved rapidly. Hundreds of thousands of genetic variants across the genome have been examined in genome-wide association (GWA) studies over the past two decades for their association with treatment response. This has led to the identification of numerous significant polymorphisms that result in variability in both therapeutic and adverse clinical outcomes [8].

As a result, the term "pharmacogenomics", coined in 1997, has been used alongside pharmacogenetics [9]. Both terms are now often used interchangeably, while pharmacogenomics, as a broader discipline, integrates new gene profiling technologies, proteomics, and bioinformatics, and raises awareness that drug response may be influenced by more than one genetic variant.

Personalized medicine and stratified medicine are related to pharmacogenetics; however, they are wider categories that include nongenetic elements as well [7].

Therefore, pharmacogenetics is fundamental to the goal of personalized medicine to provide medical treatment tailored to an individual's genetic background [10].

The prerequisite for more efficient implementation of pharmacogenomics into routine clinical practice is certainly related to the appropriate level of education, from those involved in sample analysis (e.g., clinical chemists, medical biochemists), to those responsible for results interpretation and their translation into a clinical decision. Inadequate knowledge regarding the interpretation of pharmacogenetic tests and the consequent treatment decisions was identified by a preliminary study conducted in the summer of 2004. The results were presented at the 3rd Annual International Society of Pharmacogenomics (ISP) Meeting. Until then, only a few medical institutions in Europe and the USA have integrated pharmacogenomics into their basic pharmacology curriculum. The need for regulated pharmacogenomics education programs for medical doctors, pharmacists, and other healthcare professionals, like nurses and medical biochemists, has been recognized field [1].

One of the earliest initiatives for pharmacogenomics education was launched with the publication of Gurwitz et al. in 2005 [1]. The paper contained documents "Background Statement" and "Recommendations and Call for Action" addressed to Deans of Education at Pharmaceutical, Medical, and Health Schools globally. The authors suggested introducing of pharmacogenomics into the core curriculum of pharmacology, which is mandatory course in every study program in the biomedicine field. The authors advised at least 4 h, and ideally 8 h, of pharmacogenomics training to be included in the basic curriculum. Also, more intensive education for study programs in pharmaceutical, biological sciences, and public health institutions was proposed, without specifying the number of hours [1].

3   Current Pharmacogenomic Education at University

The Completion of the Human Genome Project in 2003 significantly advanced research and discovery of novel pharmacogenomics biomarkers, but despite these revolutionary discoveries, there is discrepancy between slow but propulsive incorporation and implementation of genomic biomarkers into clinical practice and low degree of pharmacogenomics education for healthcare professionals. Although medical professionals recognize the importance of PGx testing for optimizing patient's therapy, they are careful when it comes to interpretation of the PGx testing results, largely due to inadequate knowledge in the field [11].

As already mentioned, Gurwitz et al. [1] were first to address this issue and attempted to engage the deans of medical, pharmacy, and health sciences schools in pharmacogenomics education.

In 2019, a multicenter study from six continents (Europe, Asia, Africa, North America, South America, and Australia and Oceania) included 248 university schools of medicine, pharmacy, nursing, or other health professions to assess improvement in pharmacogenomics education and to make additional recommendations. Variables analyzed were pharmacogenomics subject type, amount of teaching hours at graduate and postgraduate level, educational tools, further plans for education implementation, use of biomarkers, integration with other scientific areas, progress made since implementation, etc. [11].

Among all study programs, 13.4% reported no pharmacogenomic education, while about half of the programs, mainly M.D., pharmacy, and nursing programs, reported pharmacogenomic education as a part of the pharmacology curricula. Independent elective pharmacogenomics subjects were reported by nearly 20% of the responding institutions, followed by independent mandatory subjects (about 10%). Significantly fewer institutions reported pharmacogenomics teaching as part of human genetics, clinical biochemistry, and other non-specified subjects. Pharmacogenomics teaching as a part of the pharmacology curricula was reported by approximately 55% of the programs from Europe, 53% from Asia, 85% from Africa, 12% from North America, and 36% from Australia and Oceania. 30 PhD programs offer PGx education, where 43.3% were medical doctors, 30.0% pharmacy, 23.3% graduate schools in faculties of medicine or life sciences, and 3.3% laboratory medicine [11]. Analysis in southeastern Europe showed that pharmacogenomics is taught in 23% of postgraduate programs (PhD, MSc, medical specialties studies), in 12.5% as a standalone course, and in 87.5% as a part of other modules or courses.

Teaching hours comparison showed 63% of the programs offer at least the minimum of those recommended by the 2005 ISP, with pharmacy schools reporting greater integration than medical schools in the USA [11].

Research papers were indicated as a main teaching tool (70%), followed by internet data bases and textbooks. Results regarding biomarkers use in education were in line with the 2005 ISP recommendations, with most frequently taught *CYP* genes (*CYP2D6, CYP2C19, CYP2C*), *VKORC1, TPMT, UGT1A1, ABC* transporter genes). These results correlated with biomarkers' PharmGKB level of evidence [11]. The main limitation of this study was the low response rate, possibly providing a less accurate representation of the global pharmacogenomics education.

However, the authors concluded that the majority of the 2005 ISP recommendations and issues have been implemented or at least progressively improved. They also highlighted potential areas for further progress, indicating that most curricula are still offered by most programs as a minimum of those recommended and should be increased with a focus on the medical doctor and nursing programs. Also, some pharmacogenes with the highest level of evidence (1A) and prescription recommendations are being overlooked (including some that are currently commonly used in clinical practice); therefore, education should enrich pharmacogenomic markers (at least eight per program), with an emphasis on those with high levels of evidence.

A minority of surveyed institutions integrated pharmacogenomics with other "omics", suggesting the need for further development of the curricula regarding epigenomics, metabolomics, and bioinformatics. Finally, Kuželički et al. highly suggest the introduction of pharmacogenomics education for biomedical Ph.D. programs internationally since the majority of the universities surveyed do not report available Ph.D. programs in pharmacogenomics. Graduates in these programs are the most likely to be recruited by biomedical research institutes, private sector firms, and the fast-developing e-health sector [11].

Similar studies reported that 82% of medical schools from North America [12] and 84% of medical schools from Great Britain incorporated pharmacogenomics education into their study programs [13]. In comparison, 89% of the US schools and colleges of pharmacy included pharmacogenomics in their pharmacology curricula and 21% reported independent pharmacogenomics subjects [14]. Among 22 medical schools in the US surveyed in one recent study, most include some pharmacogenomics content in their curricula to a variable extent. Even though most respondents believe that healthcare professionals do not possess an appropriate level of knowledge in pharmacogenomics, only a few institutions plan to increase the extent of pharmacogenomics instruction [15]. Similarly, southeast European countries indicated significant variations in pharmacogenomics teaching, even between universities in the same countries. However, it was mostly reported as part of pharmacology or other subjects curricula in variable amounts [16].

In Croatia, during the last decade, pharmacogenomics' knowledge is progressively incorporated into health study programs (medicine, pharmacy, medicinal biochemistry, nursing) at undergraduate, graduate, and postgraduate levels (specialist and doctoral studies). Commonly, a varying number of hours is incorporated in core pharmacology curricula, with additional 15–30 h of teaching through elective courses. Recently, a 5-year specialist study program in medicinal genetics was introduced, for medical doctors with incorporated theoretical and practical teaching in pharmacogenomics. Learning outcomes related to pharmacogenetics include, among others: understanding the principles of pharmacogenetics, drug metabolism (pharmacokinetics, pharmacodynamics); the impact of genetic variation on drug efficacy; interpretation of pharmacogenetic tests to modify treatment and knowledge of the principles of personalized medicine; and understanding the application of pharmacogenetics and personalized medicine in the treatment of genetic diseases.

The development of new study programs, together with revisions of actual ones, takes a lot of effort and is a time-consuming task (usually takes several years) that cannot timely follow propulsive changes in sciences such as pharmacogenetics. Therefore, academic teachers should be up to date with the most recent scientific knowledge to update lectures and offer their students scientific-grounded information in the field.

On the other hand, targeted and focused lifelong education programs, in the forms of webinars, seminars, short courses, etc., provide opportunities to communicate the latest knowledge in pharmacogenomics to health professionals.

Also, there is an increasing number of data sources related to pharmacogenetics, from scientific journals and books, educational materials, handbooks, online sources, etc. Several important freely available sources of accurate and applicable information related to pharmacogenomics are websites of Pharmacogenomics Knowledge Resource (PharmGKB) and The Clinical Pharmacogenetics Implementation Consortium (CPIC). The PharmGKB is an interactive tool providing a user-friendly search and browse the knowledgebase by genes, variants, drugs, diseases, and pathways [17]. CPIC creates and posts peer-reviewed, evidence-based, updatable, and detailed gene/drug clinical practice guidelines freely available to the scientific community and clinicians [18].

A recent cross-sectional study conducted in India in 2021 examined medical student's pharmacogenomics knowledge regarding genomic polymorphisms, enzymes, and transporters influencing therapeutic response, availability of pharmacogenomics tests. Participants were primarily aware and supportive of incorporating further education for precision medicine [19]. Similar results and conclusions were obtained from recent studies regarding medical and pharmacy students and graduates' opinions and knowledge of pharmacogenomics [20, 21]. Studies highlight the need for improving knowledge about pharmacogenomics and pharmacogenetics among students as a prerequisite to easier implementation of pharmacogenomics testing in clinical practice.

4   Current Status of Pharmacogenomics Implementation in Clinical Practice

In 2015, president Obama launched Precision Medicine Initiative, representing a public health commitment to infrastructure building, incorporating and sharing information from a first nationwide cohort of one million volunteers to advance personalized medicine applications [22].

Multicentric research in the USA published in 2017 analyzed common methods for integrating pharmacogenomics advances into clinical practice. Results were obtained across six different studies within the National Human Genome Research Institute (NHGRI)-funded network termed IGNITE (Implementing GeNomics In pracTicE) [23]. Three main issues were recognized. The first one was to highlight the importance of incorporating genomics into the electronic health record of the health system (EHR). Techniques for data warehousing were employed in some projects to complete the integration. The second major difficulty was to improve doctor's education and attitudes about pharmacogenomics. To address this issue, all teams created instructional materials and had seminars and communication aimed toward doctors interested in genomics. The third difficulty was including patients in genetic medicine research. Using the media to raise awareness, actively including patients in implementation (e.g., a patient advisory board), and training patients to be active participants in their healthcare decisions were some of the strategies used to overcome this obstacle [23, 24].

At the same time, in 2017, results of a survey on healthcare professional's pharmacogenetic knowledge working within seven European countries (Austria, Greece, Italy, the Netherlands, Slovenia, Spain, and the United Kingdom) as potential implementation locations of the European pharmacogenomics clinical implementation project Ubiquitous Pharmacogenomics (U-PGx) were published [25]. In preparation for a controlled clinical study [PREPARE], a 29-question survey was distributed aiming to investigate present pharmacogenetic knowledge at the implementation locations. Overall favorable attitude and interest in pharmacogenomic testing was evident. However, ambiguity arose due to a lack of personal experience and pharmacogenomics application and interpretation expertise. The authors concluded that standardized education and training programs might be helpful in ensuring that pharmacogenomics is implemented uniformly across Europe.

The European Commission's Horizon-2020 program has supported the abovementioned Ubiquitous Pharmacogenomics (U-PGx) Consortium to address the incorporation of pharmacogenomic testing in medical care. In a prospective, block-randomized, controlled human trials, preemptive genotyping of a panel of therapeutically relevant biomarkers was deployed across medical facilities in seven European nations (PREemptive Pharmacogenomic testing for prevention of Adverse drug REactions [PREPARE]). This initiative was unique and distinctive in its multigene, multidrug, multicenter, multiethnic, and multi-healthcare system strategy [26].

The absence of professional guidance for the utilization of pharmacogenetic tests results in change regarding the usage or dose of drugs has been one of the biggest challenges when incorporating pharmacogenetic data into regular clinical treatment. The CPIC was formed as a joint project of the Pharmacogenomics Knowledgebase (PharmGKB, http://www.pharmgkb.org) and the National Institutes of Health (NIH) to improve the translation of research discoveries into clinical actions for gene/drug pairings that have a lot of evidence [27].

CPIC has identified around 480 gene–drug interactions so far [28]. Eighty-three of these, including 22 genes and 63 medications, have prescription recommendations and are hallmarked with the highest level of evidence. Although these 63 medications are a minority of authorized pharmaceuticals, they account for a significant share of prescribed drugs [29], with 35–65 percent of the population having been exposed to at least one prescription drug with a pharmacogenetics indication [30].

Despite the abovementioned, implementation of pharmacogenetics into clinical practice has been unexpectedly subtle and slow. Major challenges identified regarding its clinical applicability were concerns about clinical validity and cost-effectiveness, infrastructure and data administration, ethical and regulatory difficulties, and lack of knowledge and education of health professionals [31].

Following acknowledgment of these challenges, Mayo Clinic published "Considerations when applying pharmacogenomics to your practice" in 2021, providing help for many practitioners struggling with ordering, interpreting, and applying pharmacogenomics in clinical practice, due to inadequate pharmacogenomic education [32].

References

1. Gurwitz D, Lunshof JE, Dedoussis G, Flordellis CS, Fuhr U, Kirchheiner J, et al. Pharmacogenomics education: international society of pharmacogenomics recommendations for medical, pharmaceutical, and health schools deans of education. Pharmacogenom J. 2005;5(4):221–5. https://doi.org/10.1038/sj.tpj.6500312.
2. Garrod AE. About Alkaptonuria. Med Chir Trans. 1902;85:69–78.
3. Evans FT, Gray PW, lehmann H, Silk E. Sensitivity to succinylcholine in relation to serum-cholinesterase. Lancet. 1952;1(6721):1229–1230. https://doi.org/10.1016/s0140-6736(52)920 59-x.
4. Evans DA, Manley KA, Mckusick VA. Genetic control of isoniazid metabolism in man. Br Med J. 1960;2(5197):485–91. https://doi.org/10.1136/bmj.2.5197.485.
5. Alving AS, Carson PE, Flanagan CL, Ickes CE. Enzymatic deficiency in primaquine-sensitive erythrocytes. Science. 1956;124(3220):484–5. https://doi.org/10.1126/science.124. 3220.484-a.
6. Vogel, F. Moderne Probleme der Humangenetik; 1959. https://doi.org/10.1007/978-3-642-947 44-5_2.
7. Daly AK. Pharmacogenetics: a general review on progress to date. Br Med Bull. 2017;124(1):65–79. https://doi.org/10.1093/bmb/ldx035.
8. Uffelmann E, Huang QQ, Munung NS, de Vries J, Okada Y, Martin AR, et al. Genome-wide association studies. Nat Rev Methods Primers. 2021;1:59. https://doi.org/10.1038/s43586-021-00056-9.
9. Marshall A. Laying the foundations for personalized medicines. Nat Biotechnol. 1997;15(10):954–7. https://doi.org/10.1038/nbt1097-954.
10. Auwerx C, Sadler MC, Reymond A, Kutalik Z. From pharmacogenetics to pharmaco-omics: milestones and future directions. HGG Adv. 2022;3(2):100100. https://doi.org/10.1016/j.xhgg. 2022.100100.
11. Karas Kuželički N, Prodan Žitnik I, Gurwitz D, Llerena A, Cascorbi I, Siest S, et al., Pharmacogenomics Education Working Group (PGxEWG), European Society of Pharmacogenomics and Personalized Therapy (ESPT). Pharmacogenomics education in medical and pharmacy schools: conclusions of a global survey. Pharmacogenomics. 2019;20(9):643–657. https://doi.org/10.2217/pgs-2019-0009.
12. Green JS, O'Brien TJ, Chiappinelli VA, Harralson AF. Pharmacogenomics instruction in US and Canadian medical schools: implications for personalized medicine. Pharmacogenomics. 2010;11(9):1331–40. https://doi.org/10.2217/pgs.10.122.
13. Higgs JE, Andrews J, Gurwitz D, Payne K, Newman W. Pharmacogenetics education in British medical schools. Genomic Med. 2008;2(3–4):101–5. https://doi.org/10.1007/s11568-009-9032-6.
14. Murphy JE, Green JS, Adams LA, Squire RB, Kuo GM, McKay A. Pharmacogenomics in the curricula of colleges and schools of pharmacy in the United States. Am J Pharm Educ. 2010;74(1):7. https://doi.org/10.5688/aj740107.
15. Basyouni D, Shatnawi A. Pharmacogenomics instruction depth, extent, and perception in US Medical Curricula. J Med Educ Curric Dev. 2020;7:2382120520930772. https://doi.org/10. 1177/2382120520930772.
16. Pisanu C, Tsermpini EE, Mavroidi E, Katsila T, Patrinos GP, Squassina A. Assessment of the pharmacogenomics educational environment in Southeast Europe. Public Health Genomics. 2014;17(5–6):272–9. https://doi.org/10.1159/000366461.
17. Thorn CF, Klein TE, Altman RB. PharmGKB: the pharmacogenomics knowledge base. Methods Mol Biol. 2013;1015:311–20. https://doi.org/10.1007/978-1-62703-435-7_20.
18. Relling MV, Klein TE. CPIC: clinical pharmacogenetics implementation consortium of the pharmacogenomics research network. Clin Pharmacol Ther. 2011;89(3):464–7. https://doi.org/10.1038/clpt.2010.279.

19. Agrawal M, Kirtania L, Jha A, Hishikar R. Students' knowledge and views on pharmacoge-nomic education in the medical curriculum. Indian J Pharmacol. 2021;53(1):19–24. https://doi.org/10.4103/ijp.IJP_495_19.
20. Yehya A, Matalgah L. Toward interprofessional education of pharmacogenomics: an inter-disciplinary assessment. Pharmacology. 2021;106(9–10):534–41. https://doi.org/10.1159/000517385.
21. Jarrar Y, Musleh R, Ghanim M, AbuKhader I, Jarrar Q. Assessment of the need for phar-macogenomics education among pharmacists in the West Bank of Palestine. Int J Clin Pract. 2021;75(9):e14435. https://doi.org/10.1111/ijcp.14435.
22. Collins FS, Varmus H. A new initiative on precision medicine. N Engl J Med. 2015;372(9):793–5. https://doi.org/10.1056/NEJMp1500523.
23. Weitzel KW, Alexander M, Bernhardt BA, Calman N, Carey DJ, Cavallari LH, et al. The IGNITE network: a model for genomic medicine implementation and research. BMC Med Genomics. 2016;9:1. https://doi.org/10.1186/s12920-015-0162-5.
24. Sperber NR, Carpenter JS, Cavallari LH, J Damschroder L, Cooper-DeHoff RM, Denny JC, et al. Challenges and strategies for implementing genomic services in diverse settings: experiences from the Implementing GeNomics In pracTicE (IGNITE) network. BMC Med Genomics. 2017;10(1):35. https://doi.org/10.1186/s12920-017-0273-2.
25. Just KS, Steffens M, Swen JJ, Patrinos GP, Guchelaar HJ, Stingl JC. Medical education in pharmacogenomics-results from a survey on pharmacogenetic knowledge in healthcare pro-fessionals within the European pharmacogenomics clinical implementation project ubiquitous pharmacogenomics (U-PGx). Eur J Clin Pharmacol. 2017;73(10):1247–52. https://doi.org/10.1007/s00228-017-2292-5.
26. van der Wouden CH, Cambon-Thomsen A, Cecchin E, Cheung KC, Dávila-Fajardo CL, Deneer VH, et al. Implementing pharmacogenomics in Europe: design and implemen-tation strategy of the ubiquitous pharmacogenomics consortium. Clin Pharmacol Ther. 2017;101(3):341–58 (Erratum in: Clin Pharmacol Ther 2017;102(1):152). https://doi.org/10.1002/cpt.602.
27. Relling MV, Klein TE, Gammal RS, Whirl-Carrillo M, Hoffman JM, Caudle KE. The clin-ical pharmacogenetics implementation consortium: 10 years later. Clin Pharmacol Ther. 2020;107(1):171–5. https://doi.org/10.1002/cpt.1651.
28. Genes-Drugs—CPIC. https://cpicpgx.org/genes-drugs. Accessed 18 Apr 2022.
29. Alshabeeb MA, Deneer VHM, Khan A, Asselbergs FW. Use of pharmacogenetic drugs by the Dutch population. Front Genet. 2019;10:567. https://doi.org/10.3389/fgene.2019.00567.
30. Krebs K, Milani L. Translating pharmacogenomics into clinical decisions: do not let the per-fect be the enemy of the good. Hum Genomics. 2019;13(1):39. https://doi.org/10.1186/s40246-019-0229-z.
31. Klein ME, Parvez MM, Shin JG. Clinical implementation of pharmacogenomics for person-alized precision medicine: barriers and solutions. J Pharm Sci. 2017;106(9):2368–79. https://doi.org/10.1016/j.xphs.2017.04.051.
32. Nicholson WT, Formea CM, Matey ET, Wright JA, Giri J, Moyer AM. Considerations when applying pharmacogenomics to your practice. Mayo Clin Proc. 2021;96(1):218–30. https://doi.org/10.1016/j.mayocp.2020.03.011.

Pharmacogenomics of Drug Safety

Sonja Vukadin, Ana Petrović, Dragan Primorac, and Martina Smolić

Abstract

In this chapter, we discuss the impact of genetic variation on drug metabolism and risk of certain serious adverse events that are otherwise unpredictable and generally rarely occur. There is an abundance of published data throughout the years, of which some are contradictory and sometimes can be misleading for clinicians. In this chapter, we mention a list of drugs for which the Clinical Pharmacogenetics Implementation Consortium (CPIC) published guidelines for their dosing regimens depending on the phenotype of their metabolizing enzymes. In addition, CPIC provides recommendations on usage of drugs in which there

S. Vukadin · A. Petrović · M. Smolić (✉)
Department of Pharmacology and Biochemistry, Josip Juraj Strossmayer University of Osijek Faculty of Dental Medicine and Health Osijek, Osijek, Croatia
e-mail: martina.smolic@fdmz.hr

Department of Pharmacology , Josip Juraj Strossmayer University of Osijek Faculty of Medicine Osijek, Osijek, Croatia

D. Primorac
St. Catherine Specialty Hospital, Zagreb, Croatia

School of Medicine, University of Split, Split, Croatia

Josip Juraj Strossmayer University of Osijek Faculty of Medicine, Osijek, Croatia

University of Rijeka School of Medicine, Rijeka, Croatia

Josip Juraj Strossmayer University of Osijek Faculty of Dental Medicine and Health, Osijek, Croatia

Eberly College of Science, 517 Thomas St, State College, Penn State University, University Park, PA 16803, USA

The Henry C. Lee College of Criminal Justice and Forensic Sciences, University of New Haven, West Haven, CT, USA

Medical School REGIOMED, 96450 Coburg, Germany

is risk of idiosyncratic adverse events that are associated with certain genetic predispositions which can be detected by pharmacogenetic testing before the drug is introduced. For each drug, we briefly discuss its background and clinical implications of pharmacogenetic testing. Finally, for each drug, we list up to date recommendations for their dosing.

Keywords

Pharmacogenomics • Guidelines • Drug reactions • Adverse drug reactions

---

1   Introduction

This chapter is divided into two sections. In the first section, we list and discuss biomarkers related to medicines whose pharmacokinetics and pharmacodynamics can significantly be influenced by certain genetic polymorphisms. Proteins affected by those polymorphisms are mostly different hepatic cytochrome P450 isoenzymes and some other proteins involved in pharmacokinetic and pharmacodynamic processes, consequently leading to clinically significant variations in drug plasma concentrations which determine drug therapeutic or adverse effects. In the second section, we discuss genomic biomarkers associated with drug-induced toxicity risk status for medicines with idiosyncratic reactions related to specific genetic polymorphisms, most commonly human leukocyte antigen (HLA) variations but also some other.

---

2   Drugs and Biomarkers Related to Pharmacokinetics and/or Pharmacodynamics

2.1   Atazanavir

Atazanavir is a drug indicated for the treatment of human immunodeficiency virus (HIV)-1 infection. Atazanavir acts as a HIV protease inhibitor affecting the replication of the virus and lowering the amount of HIV in infected patients. Along with few other enzymes, HIV protease is one of the main components of HIV virus involved in its replication cycle, therefore an important target for anti-HIV drug development. However, due to its off-target effects such as inhibition of a specific hepatic uridine diphosphate glucuronosyltransferase UGT1A1, enzyme which mediates glucuronidation of bilirubin, it can cause unconjugated bilirubin accumulation and jaundice, requiring treatment cessation [1].

Genetic variations involved in UGT1A1 coding can greatly influence metabolism of atazanavir causing higher plasma drug concentrations and increasing the risk for hyperbilirubinemia. Variant alleles which result in phenotypes with decreased function of UGT1A1 are *UGT1A1**28 and *37. Based on *UGT1A1* genotype, patients can be identified as extensive, intermediate, and poor metabolizers. Poor metabolizers have severely decreased function of UGT1A1 enzyme and include individuals carrying two decreased function alleles *28/*28; *28/*37; *37/*37, while intermediate metabolizers carry at least one functional allele or increased function allele (*36) and decreased function allele, resulting in somewhat decreased UGT1A1 activity. Extensive metabolizers carry two functional alleles or one functional allele and/or increased function allele (*1/*1; *1/*36; *36/*36).

CPIC guidelines state that there is no need to avoid atazanavir in extensive and intermediate metabolizers due to low likelihood of atazanavir related hyperbilirubinemia. Patient who is identified to be extensive or intermediate metabolizers should nevertheless be informed about their low risk of developing jaundice [1].

Poor metabolizers have markedly decreased UGT1A1 activity, high risk for atazanavir-induced hyperbilirubinemia and jaundice and subsequential high likelihood of treatment cessation (at least 20% and as high as 60%). Alternative therapy should be considered [1].

2.2   Atomoxetine

Atomoxetine is used for the treatment of attention deficit hyperactivity disorder (ADHD). Its mechanism of action is selective inhibition of noradrenaline transporter (NAT), but it increases both noradrenergic and dopamine transmission in prefrontal cortex [2]. Atomoxetine is metabolized by CYP2D6 which is coded by highly polymorphic gene. Certain polymorphisms can significantly affect atomoxetine plasma concentrations, with consequent treatment failure or risk of side effects like increased systolic and diastolic blood pressure and heart rate [3].

Activity scores (AS) of *CYP2D6* differ depending on gene variants coding the enzyme. CYP2D6 ultrarapid metabolizer carries two functional alleles: *1/*1xN, *1/*2xN or *2/*2xN (N denotes a number of gene copies). Based on moderate strength evidence, ultrarapid metabolizers are likely to achieve subtherapeutic atomoxetine plasma concentrations leading to increased chance of treatment failure. Carriers of *CYP2D6* *1/*1, *1/*2, *1/*9, *1/*41, *2/*2 diplotypes have *CYP2D6* with AS of 1.5–2.0, while diplotypes *1/*4, *1/*5, *41/*4, *10/*10 code CYP2D6 with AS of 1.0 which is by some laboratories characterized as normal and by other as intermediate metabolizer. For all CYP2D6 phenotypes, the following recommendation applies and it is based on moderate strength evidence: atomoxetine should be introduced at dose 0.5 mg/kg/day and after 3 days should be increased to 1.2 mg/kg/day. A further change in atomoxetine dosing regimen should be performed in case of lack of therapeutic effect with no drug adverse effects observed, but only based on therapeutic drug monitoring by measuring peak plasma concentration 1–2 hours after dose. In such case, dose can be gradually increased do reach 400 ng/mL.

Carriers of the following alleles code *CYP2D6* with AS of 0.5: *4/*10, *4/*41, *5/*9. The resulting phenotype from such combination of allele with decreased and lack of function is intermediate metabolizer. Carriers of two functional alleles (*3/*4, *4/*4, *5/*5, *5/*6) are poor CYP2D6 metabolizers. For both the intermediate and poor metabolizers, CPIC recommends to initiate atomoxetine at dose of 0.5 mg/kg/day and further dose adjustment, if required, should only be performed after obtaining peak plasma concentration (blood sample should be collected from the patient 4 hours after the dose). In case of dose increase, peak plasma concentration should not exceed 400 ng/mL [4].

2.3   Clopidogrel

Clopidogrel is an antiplatelet agent that blocks platelet activation and aggregation by binding to P2Y12 class of ADP receptors on platelets [5]. It is widely used in treatment of acute coronary syndrome and for prevention of cardiovascular and cerebrovascular incidents, ischemia due to peripheral vascular disease and after percutaneous coronary intervention (PCI).

Clopidogrel is a prodrug that is metabolized into active metabolite by CYP2C19. In poor CYP2C19 metabolizers, this activation is insufficient and can result in lack of therapeutic effect. Due to great variability in *CYP2C19* gene and consequently in CYP2C19 activity dose, it is good to perform pharmacogenetic analysis before clopidogrel initiation or shortly afterward. Alternative agents are recommended in order to ensure therapeutic effect in likely intermediate (carriers of *CYP2C19*1/*9, *9/*17, *9/*9* diplotypes), intermediate (**1/*2, *1/*3, *2/ *17, *3/*17*), likely poor (**2/*9, *3/*9*), and poor (**2/*2, *3/*3, *2/*3*) CYP2C19 metabolizers. Good alternatives for clopidogrel are prasugrel and ticagrelor and their standard doses can be used. A standard dose for particular indication is recommended in ultrarapid (*CYP2C19*17/*17*), rapid (*CYP2C19*1/*17*), and normal (*CYP*1/*1*) metabolizers [6].

2.4   Efavirenz

Efavirenz is a non-nucleoside reverse transcriptase inhibitor used for the treatment of HIV-1 infections. It is metabolized into inactive metabolites in liver by CYP2B6 and partially by CYP2A6. It was discovered that late-onset efavirenz neurotoxicity syndrome (LENS), a serious side effect of this drug, is associated with its high plasma levels [7]. Significantly elevated efavirenz plasma levels are measured in CYP2B6 slow metabolizers and therefore identification of carriers of *CYP2B6* gene polymorphisms affecting its metabolic activity is clinically important.

According to the CYP2B6 level of activity, metabolizers are divided into five different phenotypes: UM—ultrarapid metabolizers (carriers of **4/*4, *22/*22* or **4/*22* diplotype), RM—rapid metabolizers (RM, **1/*4* or **1/*22*), NM—normal metabolizers (**1/*1*), IM—intermediate (**1/*6, *1/*18, *4/*6, *4/*18, *6/*22* or **18/*22*) and PM—poor (**6/*6, *18/*18* or **6/*18*) metabolizers. Given the risk of severe adverse effect on central nervous system (CNS), the Clinical Pharmacogenetics Implementation Consortium (CPIC) in their clinical guidelines recommend standard starting dose of efavirenz (600 mg daily) for ultrarapid, rapid, and normal CYP2B6 metabolizers. These recommendations are based on strong supporting evidence. Reduced dosing (400 mg daily) is recommended in intermediate and poor CYP2B6 metabolizers in order to prevent adverse effects on CNS. These recommendations can be applied on adult patients and pediatric population with body weight ≥ 40 kg [8].

2.5   Fluoropyrimidines

The fluoropyrimidines are a group of cytotoxic drugs that include 5-fluorouracil and capecitabine, indicated for treatment of various types of neoplasms, such as breast, gastrointestinal, and other cancers. Capecitabine is a prodrug of 5-fluorouracil. These drugs have narrow therapeutic window and high pharmacokinetic variability between individuals, which make it challenging for a physician to achieve efficacious, yet tolerable and non-toxic doses. Severe and sometimes fatal adverse effects of fluoropyrimidines include neurotoxicity, neutropenia, severe gastrointestinal disorders, and hand-foot syndrome.

Enzyme responsible for 5-fluorouracil catabolism is dihydropyrimidine dehydrogenase (DPD) which makes plasma concentrations and drug metabolism susceptible to genetic variations of DPYD, a gene which encodes DPD. These genetic variants result in phenotype with decreased function of DPD and increased risk of 5-fluorouracil accumulation and toxicity. Depending on *DPYD* genotype, phenotype can be described as DPD normal metabolizer, DPD intermediate metabolizer, or DPD poor metabolizer with variant enzyme activity and risk of drug toxicity.

According to CPIC, normal metabolizers which carry two normal function alleles have normal DPD activity and "normal" risk of toxicity require no special change to drug dose. Intermediate metabolizers, which carry one normal function allele and one no function/one decreased function allele, or two decreased function alleles may have decreased DPD activity and enhanced risk for severe adverse reactions, therefore reducing starting dose based on activity score followed by therapeutic drug monitoring or routine evaluation of toxicity is recommended [9].

DPD poor metabolizers, those with two no function alleles or one no function and one decreased function allele have complete enzyme deficiency, increased toxicity risk, and require avoidance of fluoropyrimidines if alternative drug can be used [9].

2.6   Non-steroidal Anti-inflammatory drugs

Non-steroidal anti-inflammatory drugs (NSAIDs) are group of drugs used for the treatment of pain, inflammatory diseases, and as antipyretics. Their mechanism of action is based on inhibition of one or both isoforms of cyclooxygenase enzymes—COX1 and COX2 and therefore they inhibit prostaglandin synthesis from arachidonic acid. Based on their selectivity, we divide them into two groups: non-selective NSAIDs (e.g., diclofenac, ibuprofen, indomethacin, mefenamic acid, meloxicam, piroxicam, naproxen) and selective COX2 inhibitors (celecoxib, rofecoxib, valdecoxib) [10].

Major concern, especially with long-term or frequent use, is their potential to cause serious side effects: GI irritation, peptic ulcer disease, GI bleeding, or bleeding from other sites, renal failure, fluid retention, and hypertension.

NSAIDs are predominantly metabolized by liver enzyme CYP2C9 and its variations in metabolic activity can significantly influence drug plasma concentrations. Based on *CYP2C9* diplotypes, there are three different phenotypes of CYP2C9 and an additional one of indeterminate level of activity. Notably, irrespective of *CYP2C9* polymorphisms, these drugs should be used with caution, with lowest effective dose and for the shortest possible duration depending on the condition being treated. Standard doses as per SPC of celecoxib, flurbiprofen, lornoxicam, and ibuprofen can safely be prescribed to normal (*1/*1) and intermediate (*1/*2) CYP2C9 metabolizers. As for intermediate metabolizers, carriers of either *1/*3 or *2/*2 diplotypes, the lowest recommended dose should be prescribed. If required, dose can be increased gradually to maximum recommended or tolerated dose. In poor metabolizers (*2/*3, *3/*3), 25–50% of the lowest recommended starting dose should be used and cautiously increased to 25–50% of the maximum recommended dose, as required. Alternatively, a different drug which is not metabolized by CYP2C9 (aspirin, ketorolac, naproxen, and sulindac) should be used. There are no particular recommendations for intermediate (*1/*7, *1/*10, *7/*10, *1/*57) CYP2C9 metabolizers.

The following are the guidelines for dosing of meloxicam based on *CYP2C9* gene analysis. Normal and intermediate CYP2C9 metabolizers can safely be prescribed standard doses as per SPC. In intermediate metabolizers, 50% of the lowest recommended starting dose should be prescribed and cautiously increased to 50% of the maximum recommended dose, as required. Alternatively, a different drug which is not metabolized by CYP2C9 (aspirin, ketorolac, naproxen, and sulindac) can be prescribed. Poor CYP2C9 metabolizers should not use meloxicam, but an alternative agent which is not significantly affected by *CYP2C9* polymorphism. No specific recommendation is given for intermediate metabolizers.

CPIC guidelines for piroxicam and tenoxicam, based on *CYP2C9* gene analysis, are as follows. Normal and intermediate metabolizers can safely be prescribed standard doses. Intermediate and poor metabolizers should use an alternative agent which is not significantly affected by *CYP2C9* polymorphism. No specific recommendation is given for indeterminate CYP2C9 metabolizers [11].

2.7   Ondansetron and Tropisetron

Ondansetron and tropisetron are antiemetics commonly used in treatment of chemotherapy or radiotherapy-induced nausea and vomiting. They act both centrally and peripherally by blocking serotonin 5-HT3 receptors (5-HT3R). Centrally, they inhibit 5-HT3R in chemoreceptor trigger zone, which is exposed to emetic substances. Peripherally, they block 5-HT3 receptors on vagus nerve endings, which are activated after gastrointestinal mucosa is damaged by chemotherapeutics or radiotherapy [12]. Both drugs can cause several non-serious adverse events, such as headache, xerostomia, and constipation, but are also associated with QT interval prolongation. As with other drugs that can cause the same ECG changes, the main concern is development of *torsades de pointes* and sudden cardiac death. For that reason, ECG should be monitored, especially in people with electrolyte disbalance such as ones suffering from recurrent or prolonged vomiting. In addition, they should not be combined with other drugs that can cause QT prolongation because of additive effect [12].

Ondansetron and tropisetron are metabolized by hepatic CYP2D6 enzyme, whose AS depends on polymorphisms of *CYP2D6*. There are four different CYP2D6 phenotypes depending on their AS.

Ultrarapid metabolizers have AS of >2.0 and are carriers of double functional alleles (*1/*1xN, *1/*2xN, *2/*2N). Because they extensively metabolize both drugs and are less likely to benefit from ondansetron and tropisetron therapy, a different agent which undergoes different metabolic pathway should be used, i.e., granisetron [13]. Globally, majority of population have CYP2D6 AS of 2.0 to 1.0 and are normal metabolizers. Examples of their CYP2D6 diplotypes are *1/*1, *1/*2, *1/*4, *1/*5, *1/*9, *1/*41, *2/*2, and *41/*41. Based on strong evidence, CPIC recommends a standard dose of either of the two drugs. For the remaining two CYP2D6 phenotypes (intermediate and poor metabolizers), there are very limited data and CPIC has no special recommendation regarding the dosing, therefore a standard dose as per Summary of Product Characteristics should be used. Examples of gene alleles coding CYP2D6 with AS of 0.5 (intermediate metabolizer) are *4/*10, *4/*41, *5/*9, CYP2D6 with AS of 0 (poor metabolizer) are *3/*4, *4/*4, *5/*5, *5/*6 [13].

2.8 Opioid Analgetics

Opioids are analgetics and are used in treatment of moderate to severe pain. They can be used in acute setting or as chronic therapy. There are different types of opioids, strong opioids like morphine, oxycodone, fentanyl, or hydromorphone and weak opioids like codeine and tramadol. Even at therapeutic doses, opioids cause side effects like constipation and sedation, but supratherapeutic plasma concentrations can be lethal due to respiratory depression.

CPIC published clinical guidelines for dosing of codeine, tramadol, and hydrocodone based on CYP2D6 phenotype [14]. Codeine is metabolized into its active metabolite, morphine, therefore it needs to be avoided in patients who are ultrarapid CYP2D6 metabolizers (*1/*1xN, *1/*2xN, *2/*2xN) due to risk of severe adverse reactions. If an opioid is still required, neither tramadol should be used because its metabolite O-desmethyl-tramadol binds with high affinity to opioid μ receptor and also achieves pharmacological effect. Tramadol is metabolized into O-desmethyl-tramadol via CYP2D6. Due to lack of evidence, no recommendation is given about hydrocodone dosing in ultrarapid metabolizers.

Normal CYP2D6 metabolizers (*1/*10 *1/*41, *1/*9 *10/*41 × 3 *1/*1, *1/ *2 *2 × 2/*10) should be prescribed standard doses of codeine or tramadol or hydrocodone for their age and body weight.

Intermediate CYP2D6 metabolizers (*4/*10 *4/*41, *10/*10 *10/*41 *41/ *41, *1/*5) can be prescribed standard doses of either tramadol, codeine, or hydrocodone. However, if either of them does not achieve its expected therapeutic effect, another opioid (not including any of the three) should be used instead.

Poor CYP2D6 metabolizers (*3/*4, *4/*4, *5/*5, *5/*6) should not be prescribed codeine or tramadol because it is unlikely that therapeutic effect will be achieved. If opioid therapy is required, a different agent should be used. Hydrocodone can be used in poor CYP2D6 metabolizers, at the standard dose for age and body weight. If there is lack of therapeutic effect, a different opioid should be used, but not tramadol or codeine.

Due to insufficient evidence, CPIC has no special recommendations for opioid dosing and usage in intermediate CYP2D6 metabolizers (*1/*22, *1/*25, *22/*25) [15].

2.9   Phenytoin

Phenytoin is an epileptic drug used for the treatment of many different types of epilepsy. Although many new antiepileptic drugs emerged over time, phenytoin is still widely present and commonly used in clinical practice. Its pharmacological effect is based on blockade of voltage-gated sodium channels and thereby phenytoin inhibits the propagation of action potentials in neurons. The main challenge in dosing of this drug is its narrow therapeutic window, and therefore, there is a high risk of adverse events or inefficient treatment. Many different factors influence interindividual variations in plasma drug concentration, and among them is variation in CYP2C9 gene which codes the enzyme which predominantly metabolizes this drug. Adverse reactions related to higher phenytoin plasma concentrations are signs of neurotoxicity like nystagmus, tremor, slurred speech, ataxia, and nausea or more serious events like seizures and coma at very high concentrations [16]. With intravenous administration, there is a risk of bradycardia, hypotension, and asystole due to its effect on sodium channels, and therefore, it should be applied as a slow intravenous infusion of no more than 50 mg/min [16].

Apart from adverse events arising from supratherapeutic drug concentrations, phenytoin can cause idiosyncratic reactions which are both unpredictable and dose independent [17]. Idiosyncratic drug reactions associated with phenytoin use are skin eruptions of different severity, from maculopapular rash to severe cutaneous adverse drug reactions (SCARs) like Stevens-Johnson syndrome (SJS), toxic epidermal necrolysis (TEN), drug reaction with eosinophilia, and systemic symptoms (DRESS) and hypersensitivity syndrome (HSS). Genetic marker of an increased risk for the onset of SJS and TEN after exposure to phenytoin is HLA B*15:02 allele.

Due to clinical significance of *CYP2C9* polymorphisms and *HLA B*15:02* allele, CPIC incorporated them in their clinical guidelines regarding phenytoin usage and dosing [18], as follows:

If the patient is *HLA B*15:02* positive, phenytoin should be avoided. However, if the patient is already taking phenytoin for more than three months the drug can be continued with caution. Namely, SJS and TEN most frequently appear within the first four weeks of exposure to phenytoin.

If the patient is *HLA B*15:02* negative and normal (**1/*1*) or intermediate (activity score 1.5, **1/*2*) CYP2C9 metabolizer, a standard initial dose of phenytoin should be used. Therapeutic drug monitoring should be employed and subsequent doses adjusted accordingly.

If the patient is *HLA B*15:02* negative and intermediate (activity score 1.0, **1/*3, *2/*2*) CYP2C9 metabolizer, a standard initial dose of phenytoin should be used, but maintenance dose should be 25% lower than usual. Therapeutic drug monitoring should be employed and subsequent doses adjusted accordingly.

If the patient is *HLA B*15:02* negative and poor (**2/*3, *3/*3*) CYP2C9 metabolizer, a standard initial dose of phenytoin should be used, but maintenance dose should be 50% lower than usual. Therapeutic drug monitoring should be employed and subsequent doses adjusted accordingly.

2.10   Selective Serotonin Reuptake Inhibitors

Selective serotonin reuptake inhibitors (SSRIs) are a group of medications used for the treatment of depression, anxiety and several other psychiatric disorders. Nowadays, this is one of the most commonly prescribed group of medicines. As the name suggests, these drugs inhibit serotonin reuptake in synaptic cleft and thereby increase serotonin-mediated signal transmission. These drugs can cause different adverse events, such as nausea and other gastrointestinal symptoms, insomnia, sexual dysfunction, xerostomia, changes in body weight [19]. More serious side effects are the onset of serotonin syndrome or cardiac arrhythmias due to QT interval elongation. CPIC published dosing recommendations with regards to CYP2D6 for paroxetine, citalopram, escitalopram, and sertraline. There are two hepatic enzymes implicated in metabolism of SSRIs, paroxetine and fluvoxamine are metabolized via CYP2D6, while citalopram and escitalopram are metabolized via CYP2C19. Both paroxetine and fluvoxamine are metabolized into less pharmacologically active compounds, therefore ultrarapid metabolizers (carriers of two or more functional alleles) should not be prescribed paroxetine (this recommendation is based on strong evidence). For the use of fluvoxamine at present there is no sufficient data to support any recommendation. Individuals who are either extensive or intermediate CYP2D6 metabolizers can be prescribed standard doses of both medications. Even though there is no sufficient data to support strong recommendation for the use of either of the two drugs in poor CYP2D6 metabolizers, CPIC suggests choosing a different agent that is not primarily metabolized by the same isoenzyme, or if these drugs are absolutely indicated then dose reduction by 50% and 25–50% for paroxetine and fluvoxamine, respectively should be done.

Metabolism of citalopram, escitalopram, and sertraline mainly depends in CYP2C19 and its different activity scores can significantly alter plasma drug concentrations and have clinical implications. Depending on AS, CYP2C19 can be classified as ultrarapid, extensive, intermediate, and poor metabolizers. Individuals who are extensive or intermediate metabolizers can be prescribed standard doses of either of three drugs. Such recommendation is based on strong evidence. Patients who are found to be ultrarapid CYP2C19 metabolizers should not be prescribed citalopram or escitalopram, preferably not even fluvoxamine, but rather a drug that is not primarily metabolized via this enzyme. In poor CYP2C19 metabolizers, it is again preferable to choose an alternative agent, this time because of increased risk of adverse events. But in case one of the three drugs are prescribed, their dose should be reduced by 50%, e.g., for citalopram, it should not exceed 20 mg/day [20].

2.11   Simvastatin

Simvastatin is a 3-hydroxy-3-methyl-glutaryl-coenzyme A (HMG-CoA) reductase inhibitor and one of the most commonly prescribed statins, a cholesterol reduction agent used in dyslipidemia. Statins are relatively safe due to their wide therapeutic index and severe adverse reaction induced by statins are relatively rare. The most common adverse effect which can range from mild to severe caused by simvastatin, along with other statins, is skeletal muscle toxicity. Muscle disorders induced by statins include myalgia with no muscle degradation, myopathy with some muscle degradation, and rhabdomyolysis with severe damage to the muscle tissue and renal injury. These adverse effects, even in mild cases, are potentially harmful due to the fact that patients with myalgia decide to discontinue their statin treatment which increases risk for cardiovascular disorders [21].

Specific genetic polymorphisms have been linked to statin-induced muscle damage. Specific single nucleotide polymorphisms (SNP) of *SLCO1B1*, a gene encoding transporter protein SLCO1B1, lead to transporter deficiency and decreased clearance of the drug, therefore increasing systemic exposure and risk of toxic effects of simvastatin. A genetic variant commonly found is c.521T>C, rs4149056, contained within *SLCO1B1*5, *15, and *17 genotypes.

Based on a genotype at rs4149056, CPIC identifies normal function (homozygous wild type or normal) phenotype, carrying two normal function alleles (*1a/*1a, *1a/*1b, *1b/*1b), intermediate function (heterozygous) phenotype, carrying one normal function allele, and one decreased function allele (*1a/*5, *1a/*15, *1a/*17, *1b/*5, *1b/*15, *1b/*17) and low function phenotype (homozygous variant or mutant), carrying two decreased function alleles (*5/*5, *5/*15, *5/*17, *15/*15, *15/*17, *17/*17) [22].

Due to high myopathy risk in low function allele carriers, CPIC recommends prescribing a lower dose, alternative statin (pravastatin/rosuvastatin), and regular creatine kinase evaluations. The same is recommended for intermediate function phenotypes due to their intermediate myopathy risk. Individuals with normal function require no special dose adjustments; starting dose should be prescribed and adjusted depending on the disease that is being treated [23].

2.11.1 Tacrolimus

Tacrolimus is an immunosuppressive drug indicated for prevention and treatment of post-transplant rejection in solid organ and hematopoietic cells transplantation and graft-versus-host disease (GVHD). By binding to a cytoplasmic protein receptor FK binding protein 12 in T lymphocytes and forming a complex that binds to calcineurin, tacrolimus acts as a calcineurin inhibitor (CNI) which results in inhibition of T-cell lymphocyte activation and suppression of immune response. Due to its narrow therapeutic index and high pharmacokinetic variability between individuals, it usually requires therapeutic drug monitoring [24].

Tacrolimus is predominantly metabolized by CYP3A family of enzymes, specifically CYP3A4 and CYP3A5, thus its metabolism and concentration in blood is highly influenced by variations of its coding gene.

Most common variant alleles for CYP3A5 are *CYP3A5*3*, *6*, and *7* which can result in loss of enzyme function. Based on *CYP3A5* diplotype, patients can be identified as extensive, intermediate, and poor metabolizers. Extensive metabolizers (CYP3A5 expressors) carry two functional alleles (*1/*1), intermediate metabolizers (also CYP3A5 expressors) carry one functional and one nonfunctional allele (*1/*3, *1/*6, *1/*7), while poor metabolizers (CYP3A5 non-expressors) carry two nonfunctional alleles (*3/*3, *6/*6, *7/*7, *3/*6, *3/*7, *6/*7).

CPIC Guidelines for *CYP3A5* genotype and tacrolimus dosing differ from other CYP enzyme variations and dosing recommendations, in such way that an extensive metabolizer, usually classified as "normal" and requiring no changes to the drug dosing, in case of tacrolimus requires increase of starting dose 1.5–2 times of the standard starting dose. Therapeutic recommendations for intermediate metabolizer are the same as for extensive metabolizers, while only poor metabolizers require standard dosing due to increased possibility of achieving target plasma concentrations.

Therapeutic drug monitoring for dose adjustments is recommended in all three phenotypes.

2.11.2 Tamoxifen

Tamoxifen is selective estrogen receptor modulator used in treatment of hormone receptor positive breast cancer. It can also be used in chemoprevention of hormone receptor positive breast cancer in persons with high risk of disease [25]. Tamoxifen inhibits estrogen receptors in breast tissue, but acts as estrogen receptor agonist in endometrium and bone. Tamoxifen is known to cause certain side effects, of which most serious are venous thromboembolic events and an increased risk of endometrial cancer [26]. Other, less serious, but side effects that are affecting quality of life which are menopause-like symptoms and neurotoxicity with tremor, ataxia, and vertigo.

Tamoxifen is metabolized by hepatic P450 enzymes, of which genetic variations in gene coding CYP2D6 can impact on therapeutic outcome in patients treated with tamoxifen, some studies show. CYP2D6 enzyme metabolizes tamoxifen into two metabolites which exhibit stronger antiestrogenic effect than tamoxifen itself, therefore reduced AS of CYP2D6 leads to potential failure to prevent hormone receptor positive breast cancer. Apart from genetic variations, concomitant use of CYP2D6 inhibitors also impacts tamoxifen therapeutic effect [27].

As regards to CYP2D6 phenotypes, as mentioned earlier, there are 4 of them: ultrarapid, normal, intermediate, and poor metabolizers. For each of them, activity scores and examples of gene variants are mentioned earlier. Dosage recommendations as per CPIC are: based on strong evidence, individuals with ultrarapid and normal CYP2D6 metabolism rate should avoid concomitant use of drugs that are moderate and strong inhibitors of CYP2D6 and should be prescribed standard dose of tamoxifen, which is 20 mg/day. Individuals with CYP2D6 AS of 1.0 (with or without *10 allele) and 0.5 should rather be prescribed a different medication, i.e., for post-menopausal women, an aromatase inhibitor (anastrozole) can be used and in premenopausal a combination of ovarian suppression and aromatase inhibitor are an option [27]. Both this alternative approaches are superior to tamoxifen in preventing hormone receptor positive breast cancer, as reported by the Early Breast Cancer Trialists' Collaborative Group (EBCTCG) [28]. In cases when aromatase inhibitors are contraindicated, tamoxifen can be used, but a higher dosage is required, i.e., 40 mg/day. In addition, concomitant use of CYP2D6 inhibitors should be avoided. Individuals who are poor, CYP2D6 metabolizers have AS of 0 and should not be prescribed tamoxifen, but rather one of the alternatives as mentioned earlier. Moreover, prescriber should be aware that in case tamoxifen is the only option in a given case, even the highest FDA-approved dose of 40 mg/day still does not ensure therapeutic concentrations and this is supported by strong evidence [27].

2.11.3 Thiopurines

Thiopurines are a group of purine antimetabolites commonly used for their immunosuppressive and cytotoxic effects in treatment of autoimmune diseases such as rheumatoid arthritis and inflammatory bowel diseases, acute and chronic hematologic neoplasms, and as an anti-rejection drug after organ transplant. This group of drugs includes 6-mercaptopurine (6-MP), 6-thioguanine (6-TG), and a prodrug of 6-MP, azathioprine (AZA). Due to their inhibition of DNA and RNA synthesis as an underlying mechanism of immunosuppression and cytotoxicity, overexposure to these drugs can lead to serious and life-threatening hematopoietic toxicity, resulting in myelosuppression, severe anemia, and thrombocytopenia [14, 29].

Two important enzymes are involved in catabolism of thiopurines and their active metabolites—thiopurine methyltransferase (TPMT) and Nudix hydrolase-15 (NUDT15). Genetic variations in the TPMT and NUDT15 coding genes decrease metabolism and increase plasma concentrations of thiopurines or their cytotoxic metabolites, therefore causing their accumulation and increased risk of drug-induced toxicity.

CPIC in their guidelines recommends therapeutic doses based on *TPMT* and *NUDT15* genotypes [30]. Diplotypes with two nonfunctional alleles are categorized as poor metabolizers. Individual carrying two normal alleles is identified as normal metabolizer, while intermediate metabolizer is an individual with one normal function allele plus no function allele. Phenotype can also be presented as possible intermediate metabolizer in carriers of diplotypes with one uncertain function allele and one no function allele.

TPMT and NUDT15 normal metabolizers have lower concentrations of metabolites and average risk of myelosuppression, requiring standard starting doses of thiopurines. For intermediate and possible intermediate metabolizers, reduced starting dose (up to 80% of normal dose) is recommended, but it can vary and may not even be necessary depending on the amount of the starting dose which is different for each indication. TPMT and NUDT15 poor metabolizers have very high concentrations of metabolites with increased risk of hematopoietic toxicity and require drastically reduced doses in malignant conditions, while alternative non-thiopurine therapy is recommended for nonmalignant indications. In all individuals treated with thiopurine drugs evaluation and dose adjustment depending on the risk of myelosuppression is recommended [30].

2.12   Tricyclic Antidepressants

Tricyclic antidepressants (TCAs) are group of drugs that were primarily introduced into clinical practice for the treatment of depression, but are nowadays also used for other indications, such as treatment of neuropathic pain or prevention of migraine attacks. They proved to be very useful in controlling the symptoms of depression, but their use can often be limited due to side effects. The mechanism of therapeutic effect is an increase in serotoninergic and noradrenergic transmission in central nervous system by inhibition of serotonin and noradrenalin reuptake. But in addition, it is non-selective and also inhibits muscarinic, alpha 1 adrenergic, histamine H1, and serotonin receptors which results in side effects such as dry mouth, difficulty urinating, orthostatic hypotension, drowsiness, sexual dysfunction, and weight gain. Metabolism of TCAs is highly influenced by hepatic enzymes CYP2D6 and CYP2C19. As mentioned earlier, both genes encoding them are highly polymorphic and therefore their variants significantly impact metabolic activity of both enzymes.

Based on their chemical structure, TCAs are divided into tertiary amines: amitriptyline, imipramine, trimipramine, doxepin, and clomipramine and secondary amines: desipramine and nortriptyline.

CPIC published clinical guidelines for TCA usage based on different CYP2D6 and CYP2C19 phenotypes. Based on strong supporting evidence, individuals who are CYP2D6 normal metabolizers (*1/*1, *1/*2, *2/*2, *1/*9, *1/*41, *41/*41,

1/*5, *1/*4) can safely be prescribed standard TCA doses for the treatment of depression. A 25% dose reduction should be employed for intermediate CYP2D6 metabolizers (**4/*41, *5/*9, *4/*10*) due to higher expected plasma concentrations. In order to further reduce the risk of adverse events, any increase in dose should be guided by the results of therapeutic drug monitoring. In poor metabolizers (**4/*4, (*4/*4) × N, *3/*4, *5/*5, *5/*6*), initial dose reduction should be 50% from standard dose recommended for treatment of depressive illness. TCAs should preferably be avoided in ultrarapid CYP2D6 metabolizers ((**1/*1*) × N, (**1/*2*) × N, (**2/*2*) × N) due to lack of clinical efficacy with use of standard doses. However, if TCAs are going to be used, it is recommended to try with higher doses which should adequately be monitored to avoid toxic plasma concentrations.

If CYP2C19 phenotype is determined, dosing recommendations for TCAs that are tertiary amines (as listed above) are as follows. Based on strong supporting evidence, both normal and intermediate CYP2C19 metabolizers can be prescribed standard doses. On the other hand, tertiary amines should be avoided in ultrarapid, rapid, and poor metabolizers. Alternatively, secondary amines can be used. In cases when tertiary amines are required, therapeutic drug monitoring should guide dosing.

In cases when both *CYP2D6* and *CYP2C19* are analyzed, decision about TCA usage should be guided by the results of both analyses.

When TCAs are used for the treatment of neuropathic pain, lower doses are used and no dose adjustment is required, however, if higher doses are prescribed, clinician should be vigilant about possible adverse events [31].

2.13 Voriconazole

Voriconazole is an antifungal agent used for the prevention of mycotic infections in immunosuppressed individuals and for the treatment of invasive aspergillosis, systemic infections with *Candida species*, *Scedosporium apiospermum*, and *Fusarium species*. It is a very useful medication but potentially can cause serious CNS toxicity and ophthalmic damage when its plasma concentration reaches supratherapeutic levels [32]. Voriconazole is metabolized into inactive metabolites mainly by CYP2C19 and to lesser extent by CYP3A4. Because it has a narrow therapeutic window, even small variations in plasma concentration can have serious adverse effects on patient outcome [33]. *CYP2C19* is a highly polymorphic gene which results in different level of metabolic activity exhibited by its protein product. The most common gene variants are *CYP2C19*1, *2, *3,* and **17*. Based on different *CYP2C19* diplotypes, CYP2C19 enzyme has five different phenotypes. CPIC published clinical guidelines for voriconazole dosing based on different phenotypes. Standard dose as per Summary of Product Characteristics (SPC) can safely be prescribed to individuals who are normal (**1/*1*) or intermediate (**1/*2, *1/*3, *2/*17*) CYP2C19 metabolizers. Voriconazole should be avoided in patients who are ultrarapid (**17/*17*) and rapid (**1/*17*) CYP2C19 metabolizers. In poor metabolizers (*2/*2, *2/*3, *3/*3), voriconazole should be avoided and an alternative agent should be used, such as isavuconazole, liposomal amphotericin B, or posaconazole. If voriconazole must be used, lower initial dose should be started and plasma concentrations closely monitored [22].

2.14 Warfarin

Warfarin is an oral anticoagulant which inhibits the synthesis of vitamin K-dependent clotting factors II, VII, IX, and X and proteins C and S. Although its dosing can be very challenging due to narrow therapeutic index, it remained one of the most commonly used anticoagulants in clinical practice. The advent of newer, safer alternative oral anticoagulants did not completely eliminate its use, moreover, it is still the only therapeutic option for valvular atrial fibrillation (atrial fibrillation associated with moderate or severe mitral stenosis or with metallic prosthetic heart valve) [34]. Warfarin is metabolized by hepatic CYP2C9, a common metabolic pathway for many medications and food ingredients which leads to many interactions and changes in warfarin plasma concentrations impacting its pharmacological effect. International normalized ratio (INR) is a measure of warfarin effect, the most common therapeutic target is INR 2–3, but it varies depending on the indication. Subtherapeutic INR increases the risk of thromboembolic events, whereas supratherapeutic INR increases the risk of hemorrhagic events. In fact, there are several causes of interindividual variation in warfarin plasma drug concentration and genetic variation of CYP2C9 is one of them. There are significant differences in the distribution of certain gene variants among different ethnic groups and geographic territories. Namely, CYP2C9*2 and *3 are the two polymorphisms associated with poor enzyme activity but are only characteristic for people of European and East Asian ancestry. On the other hand, in African American population, gene alleles associated with reduced enzyme activity are CYP2C9*5, *6, *8, and *11. This should be kept in mind when testing different racial or ethnical groups because the majority of FDA-approved tests do not analyze for all the CYP2C9 polymorphisms and therefore the results can be misleading in some populations.

Another factor influencing warfarin anticoagulant effect is variation in its protein target, vitamin K epoxide reductase complex 1 (VKORC1). Polymorphisms in VKORC1 determine individual sensitivity to warfarin, so that carriers of polymorphism 1639A/A or A/G are much more sensitive to its effect and require lower doses in comparison to carriers of 1639 G/G.

Dosing recommendations from CPIC is based on CYP2C9 phenotype, so that in carriers of CYP2C9*5, *6, *8, *11 alleles, the initial dose should be reduced by 15–30%. Carriers of alleles *2 or *3 should receive a standard dose based on validated published pharmacogenetic algorithms (e.g., International Warfarin Pharmacogenetics Consortium Dosing Algorithm, available online on CPIC official web page). As regards to VKORC1 genotype, dosing should be determined by the validated published pharmacogenetic algorithms which already include different VKORC1 variants into dose calculation. Additional variations in two genes, *CYP4F2*3* and *CYP2C cluster* (rs12777823) affect dosing requirements, but slightly. If an individual is of African American ancestry and carries *CYP2C cluster* (rs12777823), his initial dose should be reduced by 10–25% from what is calculated by a validated pharmacogenetic algorithm. There is no need for dose adjustment in carriers who are non-African descents. In carriers of *CYP4F2*3* of non-African ancestry, initial dose should be increased by 5–10% of the calculated, while no dosage adjustment is required for African descents [35, 36].

3   Drugs and Genomic Biomarkers Associated with Drug-Induced Toxicity Risk Status

3.1   Abacavir

Abacavir is a guanosine analog used for the treatment of HIV-1 infection. It acts as a nucleoside reverse transcriptase inhibitor, interfering with HIV RNA-dependent DNA polymerase and inhibiting replication of the virus. Abacavir is usually well tolerated, however hypersensitivity reactions (HSR) have been reported in approximately 5–8% of the patients in the first few weeks of treatment, including rash, pyrexia, nausea, vomiting, fatigue, and cough. In some cases, severe and sometimes fatal hypersensitivity reactions can occur. HSR requires immediate cessation of abacavir [37].

There is a strong association between these adverse effects and *HLA* gene polymorphism. A variant allele *HLA-B*57:01* has been identified as a genetic marker for abacavir-induced HSR risk assessment. Presence of at least one *57:01 allele is considered positive on a genotyping test and presents high risk of hypersensitivity.

Due to severity of these adverse reactions, *HLA-B*57:01* screening is recommended in all patients before starting abacavir treatment by CPIC, FDA, EMA, and the US Department of Health and Human Services.

CPIC in their guidelines state that non-carriers of *HLA-B*57:01* are reported as negative and have a very low risk of hypersensitivity reactions. This phenotype is present in approximately 94% of the patients, carries low risk of hypersensitivity reactions and standard dose of abacavir can be administered. Adverse reactions can be clinically present in patients with no genetic predisposition. If patient had hypersensitivity reactions related to abacavir, treatment should be discontinued and an alternative agent should be considered [38].

Carriers of *HLA-B*57:01* (approximately 6% of patients) with presence of at least one *57:01 allele are considered positive, exert a markedly higher risk of abacavir-induced hypersensitivity, therefore abacavir is contraindicated and other treatment should be selected [39].

3.2 Allopurinol

Allopurinol is an urate-lowering drug used in disorders caused by hyperuricemia, such as gout and uric acid nephrolithiasis, as well as for hyperuricemia in tumor lysis syndrome following chemotherapeutic treatments. Allopurinol and its active metabolite act as inhibitors of xanthine oxidase therefore preventing the breakdown of purines to uric acid. It is recommended as a first-line pharmacologic approach in gout. However, its use has been linked to severe cutaneous adverse reactions (SCAR), including Stevens-Johnson syndrome and toxic epidermal necrolysis [40].

There is a strong association between these adverse effects and a specific human leukocyte antigen (*HLA*) gene polymorphism. Human leukocyte antigen-B (HLA-B) variant allele *HLA-B**58:01, most commonly found in some Asian subpopulations, has been identified as a genetic marker for allopurinol-induced SCAR risk assessment. There is substantial evidence associating *HLA-B**58:01 genotype with phenotypic variability. The American College of Rheumatology (ACR) recommend that *HLA-B**58:01 screening should be considered before starting allopurinol in patients of Southeast-Asian descent and African Americans [41].

Current guidelines of CPIC state that allopurinol is contraindicated for carriers of *HLA-B**58:01 due to their significantly higher risk of allopurinol-induced SCAR and that alternative therapeutic options should be considered. Non-carriers of *HLA-B**58:01 have low or reduced risk of allopurinol-related adverse reactions, thus the use of allopurinol per standard dosing guidelines is recommended. Due to high negative predictive value of allele, specifically in individuals of Asian descent, genotype screening could be a valuable tool for reducing risk and incidence for allopurinol-induced SCAR. However, testing negative for *HLA-B**58:01 does not completely eliminate the risk for SCAR and several non-genetic factors such as renal dysfunction have been associated with allopurinol-induced hypersensitivity [42].

3.3 Aminoglycoside

Aminoglycosides are a group of antibiotics that include gentamicin, amikacin, tobramycin, neomycin, and others. They are valuable for their broad-spectrum activity demonstrating effectiveness in aerobic bacterial infections, including multi-drug resistant Gram-negative bacteria and mycobacteria. The mechanism of their bactericidal effect is inhibition of protein synthesis in a prokaryotic cell by binding to the bacterial ribosomal RNA. The significant adverse effect of aminoglycosides is nephrotoxicity and ototoxicity (both vestibulotoxicity and cochleotoxicity) with subsequent aminoglycoside-induced hearing loss (AIHL) [43].

These adverse reactions are usually dose-dependent and associated with high-dose treatment with aminoglycoside antibiotics for a longer period. However, a genetic predisposition appears to have a role in some individuals with AIHL.

Higher incidence and increased risk of AIHL has been linked to *MT-RNR1* gene polymorphism. *MT-RNR1* is a gene responsible for encoding human ribosomal RNA (rRNA) subunit, a mitochondrial homologue to prokaryotic rRNA subunit.

Mutations in mitochondrial genome are highly linked to hearing disorders, thus high doses of the drug lead to ototoxicity regardless of genetic predisposition. However, some of *MT-RNR1* genetic variations, such as m.1095T>C, m.1494C>T and m.1555A>G, cause human rRNA subunit to resemble bacterial more closely causing the mitochondria of cochlear cells to be more susceptible to toxic effects of aminoglycosides [38].

CPIC identify m.1095T>C, m.1494C>T and m.1555A>G variations of *MT-RNR* as a genotype with increased risk for AIHL [43]. For these individuals, aminoglycoside antibiotics are considered relatively contraindicated, meaning that avoidance of aminoglycoside antibiotics is recommended in patients with these variants. Exemptions are cases when the severity of infection and unavailability of alternative therapies outweigh the risk of ototoxicity. If no alternative therapy is available or effective, frequent evaluation for hearing loss and precautions, such as administration of the lowest effective dose for shortest possible duration, therapeutic drug monitoring and regular renal function evaluation is recommended.

For individuals with variants associated with average (m.827A>G) or uncertain risk of hearing loss, standard doses for the shortest possible duration with monitoring and evaluation of hearing loss are recommended [43].

3.4   Carbamazepine and Oxcarbazepine

Carbamazepine is used to treat epileptic disorders, bipolar disorder, and trigeminal neuralgia, as well as schizophrenia and alcohol withdrawal syndrome. It suppresses neuron excitability, mainly by modulating the activity of voltage-gated sodium channels resulting in decreased synaptic transmission. Most common serious side effects include agranulocytosis, aplastic anemia, central nervous system depression, kidney and liver toxicity, and carbamazepine-induced severe dermatologic reactions. SJS, TEN, DRESS, and maculopapular exanthema (MPE) have all been reported with carbamazepine use.

Oxcarbazepine is an analog of carbamazepine. Due to its similar chemical structure and properties, oxcarbazepine therapeutic indications, as well as adverse reactions overlap with those of carbamazepine. Thus, in patients with genetic predisposition to carbamazepine-related hypersensitivity reactions, oxcarbazepine use is also considered to be contraindicated and alternative therapeutic options should be found [44].

These adverse effects have been associated with specific *HLA* gene polymorphisms. The variant allele *HLA-B**15:02 and *HLA-A**31:01 have been identified as genetic markers for risk assessment for these severe adverse reactions.

Food and Drug Administration (FDA) recommends genetic testing in patients before initiating carbamazepine treatment. CPIC state that in patients tested positive for either *HLA-B**15:02 or *HLA-A**31:01 alleles with no previous use of carbamazepine (carbamazepine-naïve patients) and if alternative agents are available, carbamazepine should not be used due to higher risk for SJS, toxic epidermal necrolysis, DRESS, and maculopapular exanthema development. Patients who tested negative for *HLA-B**15:02 or *HLA-A**31:01 have average risk of these adverse events and carbamazepine should be used per standard dosing guidelines and monitoring, as well as patients who have previously used carbamazepine consistently for periods longer than 3 months with no adverse reactions [45].

3.5   Halogenated Volatile Anesthetics and Depolarizing Muscle Relaxants

General anesthesia can be induced by numerous agents. Potent volatile anesthetics, which include halothane, sevoflurane, enflurane, isoflurane, methoxyflurane, and desflurane, are commonly used inhalation agents for inducing general anesthesia. Although extensively researched and regularly used, their mechanism of action still remains unclear [46].

Depolarizing muscle relaxants such as succinylcholine, which cause sustained depolarization of the muscular membrane leading to muscle relaxation, are also commonly used in anesthesiology for patients undergoing intubation.

Malignant hyperthermia (MH), a rare, life-threatening disorder of skeletal muscles is a hereditary acute pharmacogenetic disorder that manifests as hypermetabolic response to these anesthetics and muscle relaxants in susceptible individuals. Pathophysiological mechanisms involved in this disorder are depletion of adenosine triphosphate (ATP) in muscle contraction which increases consumption of oxygen, carbon dioxide and heat production, causing disruption of muscle cell integrity and uncontrolled release of myoglobin, creatinine kinase, and potassium into the blood.

Several genes' mutations have been linked to malignant hyperthermia in response to these anesthetics and succinylcholine, most importantly *RYR1* and *CACNA1S* genes [46].

RYR1 gene encodes the ryanodine receptor isoform 1 protein (RYR1), a subunit of calcium channel in the sarcoplasmic reticulum membrane which is involved in triggering muscle contraction. *CACNA1S* gene encodes a protein located in sarcolemma, a subunit of the dihydropyridine receptor which acts as a voltage-sensor and activates RYR1 channels.

Pathogenic variants of both genes are autosomal dominantly inherited. However, primary locus for the MH susceptibility trait is *RYR1*, found in approximately 70% of individuals with malignant hyperthermia susceptibility. List of 50 variants have been identified and are considered as genetic markers for MH susceptibility [47].

CPIC Guidelines regarding the use of potent volatile anesthetic agents and succinylcholine in the context of *RYR1* or *CACNA1S* genotypes state that in individuals with one of the 50 variants identified as diagnostic mutations potent volatile anesthetics as well as succinylcholine are considered relatively contraindicated.

Uncertain susceptibility in individuals with none of the 50 variants identified does not eliminate the possibility of MH susceptibility [47].

3.6   Rasburicase

Rasburicase is a recombinant urate oxidase enzyme and is used in treatment hyperuricemia in tumor lysis syndrome caused by chemotherapy in hematologic malignancies and solid tumors. Rasburicase metabolizes uric acid to allantoin and hydrogen peroxide [48].

According to FDA, EMA and Japan's Pharmaceuticals and Medical Devices Agency, it is contraindicated in individuals with glucose-6-phospate dehydrogenase (G6PD) deficiency. G6PD is an enzyme involved in pentose phosphate pathway and also production of reduced nicotinamide dinucleotide phosphate (NADPH) which is important protective factor in oxidative stress. In erythrocytes, G6PD is one of the only two enzymes producing NADPH in erythrocytes and therefore is crucial in protecting them from oxidative stress. G6PD-deficient cells have depleted levels of NADPH which makes them susceptible to oxidative stress and drug-induced lysis. G6PD gene is located on the X chromosome. Rasburicase breaks down uric acid to hydrogen peroxide and leads to increased oxidative stress to which G6PD-deficiant cells are prone, and therefore have greater risk of rasburicase-induced hemolysis and methemoglobinemia, a serious disorder which can lead to severe neurologic, respiratory, and cardiac dysfunction [48].

CPIC guidelines provide therapeutic recommendations that are based on G6PD genotype with assigned phenotype. Normal phenotype with mild or no enzyme deficiency in males carrying a non-deficient allele or a female carrying two non-deficient alleles have low risk of hemolytic anemia and rasburicase can be used in treatment. Individuals carrying a deficient allele (in males) and two deficient alleles (in females) have deficient G6PD with or without CNSHA (chronic non-spherocytic hemolytic anemia) phenotype, and enzyme activity can range from <10 to 60% of normal G6PD activity to severe deficiency (< 10% activity), usually associated with CNHSA. Deficient or deficient with CNSHA individuals are at high risk of hemolytic anemia, therefore rasburicase is contraindicated and alternative therapy should be considered [48].

3.7   Ribavirin and Pegylated Interferon-α

Combination of ribavirin (RBV) and pegylated interferon-α (PEG-IFN-α or PEG-IFN 2a and 2b) is the mainstay of treatment of hepatitis C virus (HCV) type 1 infection, along with more recently developed HCV protease inhibitors. Success of the treatment is measured by sustained virologic response (SVR) defined as undetectable viral RNA in serum 12–24 weeks post-treatment [49].

There have been several genome wide association studies which associate IFNL3 genetic variation with response to RBV and PEG-IFN-α treatment.

IFNL3 gene, or *IL28B* encodes antiviral, antiproliferative, and immunomodulatory interferon-λ 3. Genetic variants associated with treatment response are located near the *IFNL3* gene on chromosome 19. Most commonly tested SNPs are rs12979860 and rs809991 [50].

Successful responses genotypes (CC for rs12979860 and TT for rs8099917) have approximately twofold increase in SVR. These alleles vary greatly among different populations which explain the differences in SVRs and treatment efficiency worldwide. This correlation and its mechanisms remain poorly understood.

Based on rs12979860 genotype, phenotype can be described as favorable response and unfavorable response. Individuals carrying two favorable response alleles (CC) have higher SVR likelihood to PEG-IFN-α and RBV therapy. Individuals with at least one unfavorable response allele (CT or TT) have lower SVR rate with this therapy.

CPIC Guidelines for use of PEG-IFN-α–containing regimens based on *IFNL3* genotype implicate 70% chance of SVR after 48 weeks of PEG-IFNα and RBV-based therapy and approximately 90% chance for SVR after 24–48 weeks of treatment with addition of protease inhibitor to therapy in favorable response genotype. Unfavorable response phenotype individuals have approximately 30% chance of SVR after 48 weeks of PEG-IFN-α and RBV treatment and 60% chance when protease inhibitor is added to therapy [50].

Considering the cost of the treatment, significant adverse reactions and variability of favorable response rates, a prognostic factor such as *IFNL3* genotype is valuable for clinicians and patients when deciding for a specific anti-HCV treatment [50].

4   Conclusion

Considering the frequency and severity of adverse drug reactions, often requiring hospitalization, but also cost and effectiveness ratio of some drugs, sometimes varying greatly due to genetic polymorphisms, there is an urgent need to implement available pharmacogenomic guidelines in clinical practice and for further research to ensure safe, effective, and individualized approach to each patient.

References

1. Gammal RS, Court MH, Haidar CE, Iwuchukwu OF, Gaur AH, Alvarellos M, et al. Clinical pharmacogenetics implementation consortium (CPIC) Guideline for UGT1A1 and atazanavir prescribing. Clin Pharmacol Ther. 2016;99(4):363–9. https://doi.org/10.1002/cpt.269.
2. Bymaster FP, Katner JS, Nelson DL, Hemrick-Luecke SK, Threlkeld PG, Heiligenstein JH, et al. Atomoxetine increases extracellular levels of norepinephrine and dopamine in prefrontal cortex of rat: a potential mechanism for efficacy in attention deficit/hyperactivity disorder. Neuropsychopharmacology. 2002;27(5):699–711. https://doi.org/10.1016/S0893-133 X(02)00346-9.

3. Cortese S, Adamo N, Del Giovane C, Mohr-Jensen C, Hayes AJ, Carucci S, et al. Comparative efficacy and tolerability of medications for attention-deficit hyperactivity disorder in children, adolescents, and adults: a systematic review and network meta-analysis. Lancet Psychiatry. 2018;5(9):727–38. https://doi.org/10.1016/S2215-0366(18)30269-4.

4. Brown JT, Bishop JR, Sangkuhl K, Nurmi EL, Mueller DJ, Dinh JC, et al. Clinical pharmacogenetics implementation consortium guideline for cytochrome P450 (CYP)2D6 genotype and atomoxetine therapy. Clin Pharmacol Ther. 2019;106(1):94–102. https://doi.org/10.1002/cpt.1409.

5. Dragan P, Wolfgang H, editors. Pharmacogenetics in clinical practice: experience with 55 commonly used drugs. Zagreb, Hamburg, Philadelphia: St. Catherine Specialty Hospital, Republic of Croatia; 2021.

6. Scott SA, Sangkuhl K, Stein CM, Hulot JS, Mega JL, Roden DM, et al. Clinical pharmacogenetics implementation consortium guidelines for CYP2C19 genotype and clopidogrel therapy: 2013 update. Clin Pharmacol Ther. 2013;94(3):317–23. https://doi.org/10.1038/clpt.2013.105.

7. van Rensburg R, Nightingale S, Brey N, Albertyn CH, Kellermann TA, Taljaard JJ, et al. Pharmacogenetics of the late-onset efavirenz neurotoxicity syndrome (LENS). Clin Infect Dis. 2021. https://doi.org/10.1093/cid/ciab961.

8. Desta Z, Gammal RS, Gong L, Whirl-Carrillo M, Gaur AH, Sukasem C, et al. Clinical pharmacogenetics implementation consortium (CPIC) guideline for CYP2B6 and efavirenz-containing antiretroviral therapy. Clin Pharmacol Ther. 2019;106(4):726–33. https://doi.org/10.1002/cpt.911.

9. Amstutz U, Henricks LM, Offer SM, Barbarino J, Schellens JHM, Swen JJ, et al. Clinical pharmacogenetics implementation consortium (CPIC) Guideline for dihydropyrimidine dehydrogenase genotype and fluoropyrimidine dosing: 2017 update. Clin Pharmacol Ther. 2018;103(2):210–6.

10. Ghlichloo I, Gerriets V. Nonsteroidal anti-inflammatory drugs (NSAIDs). Treasure Island (FL): StatPearls Publishing; 2021. Available from: https://www.ncbi.nlm.nih.gov/books/NBK 547742/. Accessed on 15 Jan 2022.

11. Theken KN, Lee CR, Gong L, Caudle KE, Formea CM, Gaedigk A, et al. Clinical pharmacogenetics implementation consortium guideline (CPIC) for CYP2C9 and nonsteroidal anti-inflammatory drugs. Clin Pharmacol Ther. 2020;108(2):191–200. https://doi.org/10.1002/cpt.1830.

12. Griddine A, Bush JS. Ondansetron. Treasure Island (FL): StatPearls Publishing; 2021. Available from: https://www.ncbi.nlm.nih.gov/books/NBK499839/. Accessed on 15 Jan 2022.

13. Bell GC, Caudle KE, Whirl-Carrillo M, Gordon RJ, Hikino K, Prows CA, et al. Clinical pharmacogenetics implementation consortium (CPIC) guideline for CYP2D6 genotype and use of ondansetron and tropisetron. Clin Pharmacol Ther. 2017;102(2):213–8. https://doi.org/10.1002/cpt.598.

14. Mohammadi O, Kassim TA. Azathioprine 2021. Available from: https://www.ncbi.nlm.nih.gov/books/NBK542190/. Accessed on 15 Jan 2022.

15. Crews KR, Monte AA, Huddart R, Caudle KE, Kharasch ED, Gaedigk A, et al. Clinical pharmacogenetics implementation consortium guideline for CYP2D6, OPRM1, and COMT genotypes and select opioid therapy. Clin Pharmacol Ther. 2021;110(4):888–96. https://doi.org/10.1002/cpt.2149.

16. Iorga A, Horowitz BZ. Phenytoin toxicity. Treasure Island, Florida: StatPearls Publishing LLC; 2021. Available from: https://www.ncbi.nlm.nih.gov/books/NBK482444/. Accessed on 15 Jan 2022.

17. Ahmed AF, Sukasem C, Sabbah MA, Musa NF, Mohamed Noor DA, Daud NAA. Genetic determinants in. J Pers Med. 2021;11(5). https://doi.org/10.3390/jpm11050383.

18. Karnes JH, Rettie AE, Somogyi AA, Huddart R, Fohner AE, Formea CM, et al. Clinical pharmacogenetics implementation consortium (CPIC) guideline for CYP2C9 and HLA-B genotypes and phenytoin dosing: 2020 update. Clin Pharmacol Ther. 2021;109(2):302–9. https://doi.org/10.1002/cpt.2008.

19. Dording CM, Mischoulon D, Petersen TJ, Kornbluh R, Gordon J, Nierenberg AA, et al. The pharmacologic management of SSRI-induced side effects: a survey of psychiatrists. Ann Clin Psychiatry. 2002;14(3):143–7. https://doi.org/10.1023/a:1021137118956.doi:10.1002/cpt.147.
20. Hicks JK, Bishop JR, Sangkuhl K, Müller DJ, Ji Y, Leckband SG, et al. Clinical pharmacogenetics implementation consortium (CPIC) guideline for CYP2D6 and CYP2C19 genotypes and dosing of selective serotonin reuptake inhibitors. Clin Pharmacol Ther. 2015;98(2):127–34.
21. Talreja O, Kerndt CC, Cassagnol M. Simvastatin. StatPearls Publishing LLC; 2021. Available from: https://www.ncbi.nlm.nih.gov/books/NBK532919/. Accessed on 15 Jan 2022.
22. Moriyama B, Obeng AO, Barbarino J, Penzak SR, Henning SA, Scott SA, et al. Clinical pharmacogenetics implementation consortium (CPIC) guidelines for CYP2C19 and voriconazole therapy. Clin Pharmacol Ther. 2017;102(1):45–51. https://doi.org/10.1002/cpt.583.
23. Ramsey LB, Johnson SG, Caudle KE, Haidar CE, Voora D, Wilke RA, et al. The clinical pharmacogenetics implementation consortium guideline for SLCO1B1 and simvastatin-induced myopathy: 2014 update. Clin Pharmacol Ther. 2014;96(4):423–8. https://doi.org/10.1038/clpt.2014.125.
24. Birdwell KA, Decker B, Barbarino JM, Peterson JF, Stein CM, Sadee W, et al. Clinical pharmacogenetics implementation consortium (CPIC) guidelines for CYP3A5 genotype and tacrolimus dosing. Clin Pharmacol Ther. 2015;98(1):19–24. https://doi.org/10.1002/cpt.113.
25. Suemasu T, Shimomura A, Shimizu C, Hashimoto K, Kitagawa D. Regarding the appropriate target and duration of chemoprevention in breast cancer. J Clin Oncol. 2021;39(26):2965–6. https://doi.org/10.1200/JCO.21.01060.
26. Pather K, Augustine TN. Tamoxifen induces hypercoagulation and alterations in ERα and ERβ dependent on breast cancer sub-phenotype ex vivo. Sci Rep. 2020;10(1):19256. https://doi.org/10.1038/s41598-020-75779-y.
27. Goetz MP, Sangkuhl K, Guchelaar HJ, Schwab M, Province M, Whirl-Carrillo M, et al. Clinical pharmacogenetics implementation consortium (CPIC) Guideline for CYP2D6 and tamoxifen therapy. Clin Pharmacol Ther. 2018;103(5):770–7. https://doi.org/10.1002/cpt.1007.
28. (EBCTCG) EBCTCG. Aromatase inhibitors versus tamoxifen in early breast cancer: patient-level meta-analysis of the randomised trials. Lancet. 2015;386(10001):1341–52. https://doi.org/10.1016/S0140-6736(15)61074-1.
29. Sharma H, Wadhwa R. Mercaptopurine. In: StatPearls [Internet]. Treasure Island (FL): StatPearls Publishing; 2022. [Updated 23 May 2022]. Available from: https://www.ncbi.nlm.nih.gov/books/NBK557620/. Accessed on 15 Jan 2022.
30. Relling MV, Schwab M, Whirl-Carrillo M, Suarez-Kurtz G, Pui CH, Stein CM, et al. Clinical pharmacogenetics implementation consortium guideline for thiopurine dosing based on TPMT and NUDT15 genotypes: 2018 Update. Clin Pharmacol Ther. 2019;105(5):1095–105. https://doi.org/10.1002/cpt.1304.
31. Hicks JK, Sangkuhl K, Swen JJ, Ellingrod VL, Müller DJ, Shimoda K, et al. Clinical pharmacogenetics implementation consortium guideline (CPIC) for CYP2D6 and CYP2C19 genotypes and dosing of tricyclic antidepressants: 2016 update. Clin Pharmacol Ther. 2017;102(1):37–44. https://doi.org/10.1002/cpt.597.
32. Orssaud C, Guillemain R, Lillo Le Louet A. Toxic optic neuropathy due to voriconazole: possible potentiation by reduction of CYP2C19 activity. Eur Rev Med Pharmacol Sci. 2021;25(24):7823–8. https://doi.org/10.26355/eurrev_202112_27628.
33. Mafuru M, Wu S, Mayala H, Msengwa Z, Phillip A, Mgone C. Analysis of combined effect of CYP2C19 genetic polymorphism and proton pump inhibitors coadministration on trough concentration of voriconazole. Pharmgenomics Pers Med. 2021;14:1379–89. https://doi.org/10.2147/PGPM.S329662.
34. Heidenreich PA, Estes NAM, Fonarow GC, Jurgens CY, Kittleson MM, Marine JE, et al. 2020 Update to the 2016 ACC/AHA clinical performance and quality measures for adults with atrial fibrillation or atrial flutter: a report of the American College of Cardiology/American Heart Association task force on performance measures. J Am Coll Cardiol. 2021;77(3):326–41. https://doi.org/10.1016/j.jacc.2020.08.037.

35. Johnson JA, Caudle KE, Gong L, Whirl-Carrillo M, Stein CM, Scott SA, et al. Clinical pharmacogenetics implementation consortium (CPIC) guideline for pharmacogenetics-guided warfarin dosing: 2017 update. Clin Pharmacol Ther. 2017;102(3):397–404. https://doi.org/10.1002/cpt.668.

36. Johnson JA, Gong L, Whirl-Carrillo M, Gage BF, Scott SA, Stein CM, et al. Clinical pharmacogenetics implementation consortium guidelines for CYP2C9 and VKORC1 genotypes and warfarin dosing. Clin Pharmacol Ther. 2011;90(4):625–9. https://doi.org/10.1038/clpt.2011.185.

37. Fernandez JV, Munir A. Abacavir. In: StatPearls [Internet]. Treasure Island (FL): StatPearls Publishing; 2022. [Updated 1 May 2022]. Available from: https://www.ncbi.nlm.nih.gov/books/NBK537117/. Accessed on 15 Jan 2022.

38. Prasun P, Ginevic I, Oishi K. Mitochondrial dysfunction in nonalcoholic fatty liver disease and alcohol related liver disease. Transl Gastroenterol Hepatol. 2021;6:4. https://doi.org/10.21037/tgh-20-125.

39. Martin MA, Hoffman JM, Freimuth RR, Klein TE, Dong BJ, Pirmohamed M, et al. Clinical pharmacogenetics implementation consortium guidelines for HLA-B genotype and abacavir dosing: 2014 update. Clin Pharmacol Ther. 2014;95(5):499–500. https://doi.org/10.1038/clpt.2014.38.

40. Pacher P, Nivorozhkin A, Szabó C. Therapeutic effects of xanthine oxidase inhibitors: renaissance half a century after the discovery of allopurinol. Pharmacol Rev. 2006;58(1):87–114.

41. Khanna D, Fitzgerald JD, Khanna PP, Bae S, Singh MK, Neogi T, et al. American College of Rheumatology guidelines for management of gout. Part 1: Systematic nonpharmacologic and pharmacologic therapeutic approaches to hyperuricemia. Arthritis Care Res (Hoboken). 2012;64(10):1431–46. https://doi.org/10.1002/acr.21772.

42. Hershfield MS, Callaghan JT, Tassaneeyakul W, Mushiroda T, Thorn CF, Klein TE, et al. Clinical pharmacogenetics implementation consortium guidelines for human leukocyte antigen-B genotype and allopurinol dosing. Clin Pharmacol Ther. 2013;93(2):153–8. https://doi.org/10.1038/clpt.2012.209.

43. McDermott JH, Wolf J, Hoshitsuki K, Huddart R, Caudle KE, Whirl-Carrillo M, et al. Clinical pharmacogenetics implementation consortium guideline for the use of aminoglycosides based on MT-RNR1 Genotype. Clin Pharmacol Ther. 2022;111(2):366–72. https://doi.org/10.1002/cpt.2309.

44. Maan JS, Duong TVH, Saadabadi A. Carbamazepine. StatPearls Publishing LLC; 2021. Available from: https://www.ncbi.nlm.nih.gov/books/NBK482455/. Accessed on 15 Jan 2022.

45. Leckband SG, Kelsoe JR, Dunnenberger HM, George AL, Tran E, Berger R, et al. Clinical pharmacogenetics implementation consortium guidelines for HLA-B genotype and carbamazepine dosing. Clin Pharmacol Ther. 2013;94(3):324–8. https://doi.org/10.1038/clpt.2013.103.

46. Bach-Rojecky L, Vađunec D, Lozić M, Žunić K, Špoljar GG, Ćutura T, et al. Challenges in anesthesia personalization: resolving the pharmacogenomic puzzle. Per Med. 2019;16(6):511–25. https://doi.org/10.1002/cpt.1319.

47. Gonsalves SG, Dirksen RT, Sangkuhl K, Pulk R, Alvarellos M, Vo T, et al. Clinical pharmacogenetics implementation consortium (CPIC) guideline for the use of potent volatile anesthetic agents and succinylcholine in the context of RYR1 or CACNA1S genotypes. Clin Pharmacol Ther. 2019;105(6):1338–44.

48. Relling MV, McDonagh EM, Chang T, Caudle KE, McLeod HL, Haidar CE, et al. Clinical pharmacogenetics implementation consortium (CPIC) guidelines for rasburicase therapy in the context of G6PD deficiency genotype. Clin Pharmacol Ther. 2014;96(2):169–74. https://doi.org/10.1038/clpt.2014.97.

49. Tsubota A, Fujise K, Namiki Y, Tada N. Peginterferon and ribavirin treatment for hepatitis C virus infection. World J Gastroenterol. 2011;17(4):419–32. https://doi.org/10.3748/wjg.v17.i4.419.
50. Muir AJ, Gong L, Johnson SG, Lee MT, Williams MS, Klein TE, et al. Clinical pharmacogenetics implementation consortium (CPIC) guidelines for IFNL3 (IL28B) genotype and PEG interferon-α-based regimens. Clin Pharmacol Ther. 2014;95(2):141–6. https://doi.org/10.1038/clpt.2013.203.

Pharmacogenomics in Drug Research and Development

Damir Erceg

Abstract

Pharmacogenomics (PGx), transcriptomics, proteinomics, epigenomics, and metabolomics are rapidly advanced -omics and potential tools for identifying biomarkers to guide treatment and novel mechanisms of diseases. Pharmacogenomics is looking at variants in the DNA, epigenomics examines heritable changes non-DNA related, but lead to alteration of gene expression. Transcriptomics studies gene expression including the complete mRNA transcript in a cell or tissue. A well-phenotyped patient together with advanced technologies (high-throughput screening, artificial intelligence), bioinformatics, and statistical tools will help us to better understand molecular mechanisms involved in diseases onset and progression. This is a base for selecting and stratifying a therapeutic approach and bringing personalized medicine into everyday clinical practice. Multi-omics are powerful and useful tools for identifying new biomarkers to guide novel mechanisms of diseases as well as new treatments. The central place in the -omics repertoire during drug research and development is reserved for pharmacogenomics.

Keywords

Pharmacogenomics • Translational medicine • Precision medicine • Drug research • Drug development

D. Erceg (✉)
"Srebrnjak" Children S Hospital, Zagreb, Croatia
e-mail: derceg@bolnicasrebrnjak.hr

Josip Juraj Strossmayer University of Osijek Faculty of Dental Medicine and Health, Osijek, Croatia

Catholic University of Croatia, Zagreb, Croatia

"St. Catherine" Hospital, Zagreb, Croatia

Josip Juraj Strossmayer University of Osijek Medical School, Osijek, Croatia

© The Author(s), under exclusive license to Springer Nature Switzerland AG 2023   439
D. Primorac et al. (eds.), *Pharmacogenomics in Clinical Practice*,
https://doi.org/10.1007/978-3-031-45903-0_24

1   History of Drug Discovery and Development

The long history of drug discovery dates back to the old times. Drugs were used in ancient times as remedies as well as an important part of spiritual and religious healing. From that time until the late 1800s, they were derived from herbs, animal products, and minerals. Drugs were discovered as a result of trial and error experimentations, and observations of human and animal reactions as a consequence of ingesting such products [1].

The modern drug discovery can be divided into three main periods [2]. The first one started in the nineteenth century when the drug discovery was based on the serendipity in medicinal chemistry. The second period was characterized by the discovery of antibiotics and other new structures. This period started in the early twentieth century. Various drugs were examined, but mostly they were used for symptomatic treatment rather than completely curing the diseases.

The natural products and their active ingredients (exactly synthetic versions) were the basis for drug discovery in the early 1930s. Another name for the synthetic version of active ingredients is a new chemical entity (NCE). According to regulatory requirements, NCE has to go through many steps and prove that it is safe and effective. Behind time (in the late 1970s), the knowledge of molecular biology led to the development of recombinant products and started a new period in drug discovery. The biotech industry became reality. These discoveries of new structures along with new scientific methods such as molecular modeling, combinatorial chemistry, and automated high-throughput screening (HTS) are enabling fast advances in the drug discovery process. At a beginning of the twenty-first century was announced a third period where new technologies such as different -omics expanded and enabled the approval of biopharmaceutical drugs. The important place in medical practice for many years was occupied by small molecules developed as therapeutic agents.

In the USA, at beginning of twenty century, approximately one-third of total mortality was related to three common causes: tuberculosis, pneumonia, and diarrhea [3]. Today, they are preventable and treatable, and rare as causes of death, excluding pneumonia. The chance of dying from these pathophysiological conditions was 1 in 11 in the 1940s. The odds were down by 2000 to 1 in 25. Now, only pneumonia was in the top ten causes of mortality, and leading places were occupied by complex diseases such as cardiovascular diseases and different types of cancer. The improved sanitation and vaccinations certainly played a role in the increase in life expectancy, but the availability of drugs to control different pathophysiological conditions and diseases such as cancer, infection, hypertension, hyperlipidemia also contributed to the increase in life expectancy and made a clear improvement in public health [3]. The life expectancy increased from less than 50 years in 1900 to more than 70 years in 2000, much more in the last a 100 years than from A.D. to 1900.

2   A New Approach to Drug Development Versus Conventional Approach

The pharmaceutical industry at the end of the twentieth century faced several challenges. Some of them are relatively low productivity and failure to introduce new drugs to the market. Investors were constantly demanding that pharmaceutical companies deliver new drugs with novel mechanisms of action. Additional pressure in the form of price control came from state governments, insurance companies, and other institutions that manage health care [4].

Medications are a major pillar in the treatment of acute and chronic diseases. The response to drugs can be variable, so in 40–70% of patients drugs show a lack of effectiveness or harmful effects. Genetic variability has been reported as the cause in 15–95% of such cases [5, 6]. It has been a long way to try to define the cause of disease at the molecular level, from Mendel's discovery of the gene in 1865 to the completion of the Human Genome Project (HGP) in 2003 [7]. This created the basis for the development of personalized medicine, a new approach in clinical medicine, in which pharmacogenomics plays a key role.

Although the terms pharmacogenetics and pharmacogenomics are often confused and used interchangeably, there are differences. Pharmacogenetics usually refers to the effect of a single gene on the action of a drug. Successful drug development requires knowledge of the fate of the drug in the body (pharmacokinetics), and the way the drug acts in the body (pharmacodynamics). Pharmacogenomics is the science that studies the effect of genomic variants on drug action. Its contribution to the discovery and development of drugs is expressed in the following [8]:

- increasing the number of new therapeutic targets,
- elimination of unsuitable candidates and therapeutic targets in the earlier stages of drug development,
- accelerating clinical development and enabling the design of studies showing better efficacy and safety of drugs, and
- optimizing risk and welfare profiles in target populations.

The development of pharmacogenomics has opened the possibility of adopting a new paradigm in drug development. Figure 1 presents a sales model (green line) of a classic drug that loses market share over time due to different reasons (adverse effects, insufficient efficacy, the emergence of competing drugs, and ultimately the emergence of drugs with a pharmacogenomic test). In addition to the classic model, there is a model (blue line) of drug sales with a pharmacogenomic test, which does not lose market due to the paradigm shift, but after a certain number of years of sales, the year reaches a stable level.

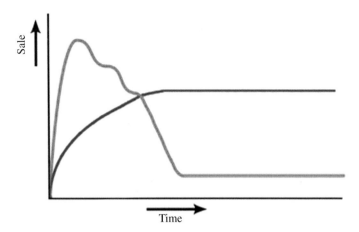

Fig. 1 Sales model of classic drug (green line) and drug with PGx test (blue line)

2.1   Changing Paradigm in Drug Development—Astra Zeneca Case

The main goal of the pharma industry is to develop safe and effective drugs. Thousands of new molecules are tested annually, but only a few become new drugs that are approved for use by regulators and appear on the market. Research and development in the pharma industry are accompanied by a large number of NCEs that fail at different stages of drug development, thus contributing to the low productivity of research and development. In 2011, Astra Zeneca decided to make changes in its strategic approach to research and development. The goal was to raise productivity, which in the period 2005–2010 fell below the average of the pharmaceutical industry. The revision of the strategy was based on the 5R framework and included the right: target, tissue, safety, patient, and market potential [9]. The new development strategy had a solid biological approach in the selection of targets and patients, based on pharmacogenomic research. In 2016, Astra Zeneca increased its NCE development success rate from 4 to 19%, suggesting that precision medicine can improve the drug development process [9]. Among the new disciplines, disease genetics and pharmacogenomics occupy a central place. The main processes in the development of new forms of treatment are the identification and characterization of the target of treatment and both the evaluation and optimization of pharmacokinetics, pharmacodynamics, efficacy, and safety of the drug.

3   Impact of New Technologies on the Drug Discovery and Development

Human diseases are heterogeneous and complex, often with limiting diagnostic and therapeutic methods. Personalized medicine tries to design therapeutic interventions based on the individual patient's condition. In patients with breast cancer, trastuzumab is effective therapy only in patients with HER2 overexpression. A diagnostic test that determines HER2 overexpression is a pre-requisite before starting with trastuzumab treatment.

Furthermore, there are examples of limiting drug efficacy due to a lack of "precision mechanism". Thus, statins are only effective in 5% of the population [10]. Many research efforts (e.g., GWAS studies) are trying to identify genetic variations related to the disease. However, genomic variations are not responsible for all disease occurrences. The existing gap between genomics and phenotypes can be bridged by other -omics, such as transcriptomics, epigenomics, proteomics, and metabolomics [11, 12].

3.1   Genomics

Genomics is the study of all sets of genes, their structure, function, and expression. The term was coined by Thomas Roderick in 1986. Pharmacogenomics (PGx) is the study of how a person's genome influences on response to medications. There are four main areas of genomics: functional genomics, structural genomics, epigenomics, and environmental genomics [13]. The first three are in the current interest of PGx.

The most studied in PGx is functional genomics. It explores the effect of gene variations on functions or levels of expression. Both the genome and the transcriptome are the focus of functional genomics. Epigenomics explores reversible modifications affected by gene expressions without changing the DNA sequence. Finally, structural genomics assesses the 3D structures of proteins. It makes modeling interactions with environmental compounds possible using molecular dynamic simulations. This may be a promising PGx area. PGx studies generate a very large amount of information commonly referred as to "Big Data", and specific methodologies have to be applied for the analysis of such data. It generally consists of the following steps: collection, processing, analysis, and interpretation (including clinical translation).

Pharmacogenomics studies genetic variations in metabolizing enzymes, drug transporters, and other proteins which can affect individual responses to drugs in terms of therapeutic and adverse effects. The DNA testing that includes genetic variations related to the risk of adverse response or drug response is PGx testing.

3.2   Transcriptomics

The term transcriptome was the first time used by Auffray as a description of the entire set of transcripts [14]. Transcriptomics is the study of the transcriptome that covers all types of transcripts, including microRNAs (miRNAs), messenger RNAs (mRNAs), and different types of long non-coding RNAs (lncRNAs). Modern transcriptomics is rapidly expanding our understanding of the relationships between the transcriptome and the phenotype across a wide range of living entities. It uses HTS methods to analyze the expression of multiple transcripts in different pathological or physiological conditions.

Transcriptomics technologies are the techniques used to study an organism's transcriptome. The information is recorded in the DNA of its genome and expressed through transcription. Here, mRNA serves as a transient intermediary molecule in the information network, while non-coding RNAs perform additional diverse functions. A transcriptome captures a snapshot in time of the total transcripts present in a cell.

The development of new techniques is enabling a fast advancement of transcriptomics. This is visible in the following example explained by Love et al. [15]:

- the first attempt at capturing a partial human transcriptome was published in 1991 and reported 609 mRNA sequences,
- two human transcriptomes composed of millions of transcript-derived sequences covering 16,000 genes were published in 2008,
- transcriptomes had been published for a hundred individuals in 2015.

The development of new techniques made the previous ones obsolete. This explosion in transcriptomics led to routinely generated transcriptomes of different cells, tissue, or diseases states.

The study of RNA transcripts is based on two main principles: RNA sequencing (RNA Seq) and microarray. RNA Seq is the sequencing of individual transcripts. Microarray is the hybridization of transcripts to an ordered array of nucleotide probes.

Microarray quantifies a set of predetermined sequences, which uses high-throughput sequencing to capture all sequences. RNA microarrays are typically prepared with a library of transcripts of known origin (representative tags for a known complement of genes). Thus, the current human RNA arrays contain approximately 60,000 probes, representative of a majority of known RNA species from the 20,000 or so human genes [16]. These are then interrogated with RNA (typically reverse transcribed into cDNA) from two different samples, labeled with different dyes (commonly green and red dyes). This allows the relative abundance (in one sample versus the other) of each RNA transcript to be assessed. Experiments of this type are routinely used to determine which RNAs are upregulated or downregulated in a disease sample versus a normal sample. This information is highly variable because transcriptions level can be potentially influenced by different factors.

3.3   Proteomics

Proteins are polymers of amino acids with important roles in living cells. Berzelius introduced the term protein in 1938. The level and activity of cellular proteins are regulated by internal and external changes. The first protein studies started with the introduction of two-dimensional gel and mapping of proteins from E. coli in 1975. Many proteins could be separated and visualized but they could not be identified till the early 1990s. Marc Wilkins introduced the terms proteome and proteomics [17]. Proteome represents all proteins in a living organism, while changes in proteome describe living dynamics. Proteomics is the large-scale study of proteins and enables the identification and understanding of their composition, structure, and activity. Many of the functions of the protein are related to other proteins, and proteomics identifies the type of interaction.

According to protein response, proteomics can be divided into the following groups [18]:

- structural proteomics enables an understanding of the structural complexities of functional proteins and their three-dimensional shape. Mainly used methods for structure determination are X-ray crystallography and NMR spectroscopy;
- expression proteomics is used to study the qualitative and quantitative expression of total proteins under two different conditions (the normal cell and abnormal cell). The protein expressional changes can be determined by 2D gel electrophoresis and the mass spectrometry technique (MS);
- functional proteomics determines the protein functions, and their role in larger complexes, and identifies the interacting protein partners.

The modifications in the protein expression such as stress or drug effects will change the protein pattern and cause the presence or absence of a protein or gradual variation in abundance. The main goal of proteomics is not only to pinpoint the whole of the proteins in a cell but also to generate a complete three-dimensional map of the cell indicating their exact location. Furthermore, proteomics analyzes and compares protein expression profiles, and determines where and in which ratio and under what condition proteins are expressed. It shows the observed protein changes to the causal effects.

Understanding the structure, function, and modification of each protein and the complexities of protein–protein interactions will be critical for developing the most effective diagnostic techniques and disease treatments in the future.

The various MS-based platforms, including different types of proteomics, are involved in the modern drug discovery process. The enormous progress in MS instrumentation enabled identification of the thousands of proteins per experiment. In the complex drug discovery pipeline, the various MS-based proteomics approaches extend beyond the common objective of drug-target discovery, enabling the study of drug-target interaction (selectivity and specificity), drug activity (efficacy, resistance, toxicity), and elucidating the mechanism of action of a new drug [19].

Proteomics is the method that has a high impact on the economy of the pharmaceutical industry via biomarker discovery, follow-up of patients, evaluation of drug efficacy in the treated samples, and also the capacity for the joint to the other large-scale methods as like bioinformatics.

3.4 Metabolomics

Metabolomics is a comprehensive and quantitative analysis of all sets of metabolites present in cells, tissues, body fluids, and whole organisms under different conditions (normal and altered states promoted by pathophysiological conditions or other types of modulation (drugs, environmental factors, etc.). Metabolome as a term was the first time reported in the scientific literature in 1998 when Olivier was describing changes in metabolites concentrations as consequences of genes deletion or overexpression [20]. Alterations in metabolite concentrations are results from disease processes, gene function, drug effects, or toxicity.

4 Artificial Intelligence in Drug Discovery and Development

Different networks and tools incorporated in a system based on technology with the possibility to mimic human intelligence is the short description of artificial intelligence (AI). It was developed into a hot topic in medicine. The pharmaceutical industry is making efforts to approach AI to reduce research and development costs, speed up the drug discovery process, reduce failure rates in the clinical phases of drug development, and finally produce better medicines.

The beginning of AI represents a summer workshop titled "The Dartmouth Summer Research Project on Artificial Intelligence" held in 1956 in Dartmouth, UK. A few biomedical AI systems were developed during the 1970s. There are many changes in subsequent years in the early 1990s, such as exponential growth in high-performance computing, Internet communication, clouds apps, big data, etc. An especially important date was in 1997 when IBM's supercomputer Deep Blue won against Gary Kasparov in chess. At that moment, AI gained the attention of the world public. The accelerated development of machine learning algorithms and an enormous quantity of data collected in the drug discovery and development process led to the evolution of AI-based start-up companies dedicated to drug research. There are new AI-biopharmaceutical associations declared in the last few years, such as Pfizer and IBM Watson, Bayer, Sanofi and Excentia, Roche and Owkin, Astra Zeneca, and Jansen and Benevolent AI [21, 22].

Machine learning (ML) and deep learning (DL) algorithms have been implemented in several drug discovery processes such as physiochemical activity, peptide synthesis, ligand-based virtual screening, structure-based virtual screening, toxicity prediction, drug monitoring and release, pharmacophore modeling, quantitative structure–activity relationship, drug repositioning, and polypharmacology [23].

4.1   Machine Learning

AI is an umbrella term that describes computers' possibility to behave human performance, while machine learning is a subset of AI where data and different algorithms like decision tree (DT), Naïve Bayes, hidden Markov models (HMM), and others are coupled in the system to imitate the way that humans learn.

ML has been introduced as a useful tool in drug discovery since the late 1990s. This technique can be divided into two groups of techniques: supervised and unsupervised learning [24]. Unsupervised learning is a method used for exploratory purposes, while supervised learning serves to develop a training model to predict the future.

4.2   Deep Learning

The high demand for exploring and analyzing big data enabled the development of algorithms like DL. A huge success of DL in a wide range of applications such as speech recognition, natural language processing, computer vision, computer games, and self-driving cars. In summary, DL is changing our everyday life. According to Gartner-selected top ten technology trends of 2018, DL-represented AI technologies were ranked at the top position [25]. Over the past decade, there has been a remarkable increase in the amount of available compound activity and biomedical data owing to the emergence of new experimental techniques such as HTS, parallel synthesis, among others [26, 27]. The first wave of applications of DL in pharmaceutical research has emerged in recent years, and its utility has gone beyond bioactivity predictions and has shown promise in addressing diverse problems in drug discovery. Examples will be discussed covering bioactivity prediction, de novo molecular design, synthesis prediction, and biological-image analysis.

The application of DL in drug discovery can be divided into three main different categories [28]: drug properties prediction, de novo drug design, and drug-target interaction (DTI) prediction.

5   Biomarkers in Drug Discovery and Development

Biomarkers are essential in the drug discovery and development process [29]. In 2005, the US Food and Drug Administration (FDA) and National Institute of Health (NIH) were formed a joint task force to forge common definitions and to make them publicly available through a continuously updated online document—the "Biomarkers, EndpointS, and other Tools" (BEST) resource [30].

Biomarkers are defined as an objectively measured and evaluated characteristic that serves as an indicator of biological and pathogenic processes or responses to an intervention or exposure [31]. Biomarkers should be distinct from a clinical outcome assessment (COA) (direct measures of how a person feels, functions, or survives). This difference between biomarkers and COAs is important because COAs measure outcomes that are directly important to the patients and can be used to meet standards for regulatory approval of therapeutics, whereas biomarkers serve a variety of purposes, one of which is to link measurement to a prediction of COAs [29]. Only validated biomarkers can serve as a basis for regulatory approval.

5.1   Types of Biomarkers

There are seven different types of biomarkers [30]:

– risk/safety biomarkers,
– monitoring biomarkers,
– diagnostic biomarkers,
– prognostic biomarkers,
– predictive biomarkers,
– susceptibility biomarkers,
– pharmacodynamic/response biomarkers.

Safety/risk biomarkers

Safety/risk biomarkers are indicators of toxicity [32]. They are measured before and after exposure of potential to with above-mentioned variant has increased risk for the serious and fatal reaction of the toxic agent. The good safety marker will signal the development of toxicity before any irreversible organ changes. In some cases, treatment interruptions or dose modification are adequate procedures to escape toxic injury. Good examples of typical safety biomarkers are hepatic aminotransferases and bilirubin as indicators of hepatotoxic potential as well as serum creatinine in monitoring nephrotoxicity [33, 34]. Also, the presence of some genetic variants such as *HLA-B**1502 may be used as a safety biomarker before starting therapy with the antiepileptic drug carbamazepine [35]. The patient with positive findings has an increased risk of serious and fatal skin reactions [35]. During clinical drug development, around 40% of the drug development attrition of NMEs is related to safety (20% clinical adverse events, 20% preclinical toxicology) compared to 22% failing because of lack of efficacy [36]. Biomarkers for toxicity in animals and man, therefore, merit greater attention.

Safety biomarkers should be used so early that onset during dose escalation in early clinical trials can allow dosing to be reduced or stopped before clinically significant adverse effects occur. Furthermore, they should be so specific that the target organ indicated is accurate and erroneous signals from unrelated organs do not interfere with toxicity identification. In the end, safety biomarkers should be so sensitive that low doses causing toxicity can be detected so that high doses potentially irreversible injury is not caused.

Zabka et al. in their article presented patterns of safety biomarkers use in 20 member companies of IQ DruSafe as well as their criteria and aspirations for future implementation [37]. About 65% or a majority of companies reported using safety biomarkers in investigational new drug submissions, but not so frequently. There are the following reasons:

– missing suitable safety markers,
– drug development programs did not need safety markers,
– the lack of resources or capability to use safety biomarkers, and
– use of safety biomarkers mainly in the pre-candidate selection.

Diagnostic biomarkers

The diagnostic biomarker is used to detect or confirm the presence of a disease or condition of interest or to identify individuals with a subtype of the disease [38].

The presence of disease or subtype of disease can be detected or confirmed by diagnostic biomarkers. An example of diagnostic biomarkers is a sweat chloride as a tool to detect cystic fibrosis (CF) [39]. Also, mutations of cystic fibrosis transmembrane conductance regulator (*CFTR*) may be used as a diagnostic biomarker in CF clinical trials [40]. Diagnostic biomarkers have two important characteristics: -sensitivity to detect all patients with disease as positive and -specificity -to detect all patients without disease as negative.

Diagnostic biomarkers sometimes have an important role in the classification of disease and could serve as prognostic or predictive biomarkers [40]. An example of prognostic markers is various genetic markers that can predict the recurrence of particular types of cancer. Predictive markers could predict responders of specific treatment. Other very important characteristics of good tests are positive predictive value (PPV) and negative predictive value (NPV). PPV and NPV are indicators of sensitivity and specificity. The choice of test depends on its intention. If the prevalence of the disease is very low in the population, it is impossible to have high PPV. Also, in the opposite case, a very high prevalence in the population will be difficult followed by low NPV.

Acceptable trade-offs among performance characteristics such as sensitivity, specificity, PPV, and NPV will depend on the relative potential of false-positive and false-negative results [40]. The diagnostic test is intended for screening an asymptomatic healthy population where the prevalence of the target disease is very low, tests with high specificity and PPV are necessary to avoid a large number of false-positive results. This type of results may trigger unnecessary medical interventions and possibly psychological suffering. In contrast, if a test is used for diagnostic purposes, then greater emphasis might be placed on a test's sensitivity and NPV. Besides clinical performance, suitable analytical characteristics could be necessary before a biomarker test can be accepted as a diagnostic tool. For example, qualified sites and operators running the same diagnostic biomarker test should obtain highly concordant results. A poor analytical performance will decrease the clinical performance of the diagnostic test [40].

Prognostic biomarkers

A biomarker that informs about the disease, medical condition, or outcome of interest (disease progression, recurrence of disease, death) is a prognostic marker. Mutations of genes (e.g., BReast CAncer gene 1 (*BRCA 1*) and (*BRCA 2*)) may serve to assess the likelihood of second breast cancer in the evaluation of women with breast cancer [41]. Another example of the prognostic marker is plasma fibrinogen, to select patients in clinical trials with chronic obstructive pulmonary disease (COPD) [42]. This is an indicator of increased risk for exacerbation and mortality [43].

A prognostic biomarker can assess the likelihood of future clinical events in some population, or individuals with some disease or medical condition.

Tumor size and presence of metastasis are traditional oncologic biomarkers used for prognostic purposes. Patients with previous heart attack, diabetes, cholesterol, or elevated LDL are examples of risk biomarkers for another heart attack. Patients with concomitant diseases like hypertension, and diabetes have a higher risk for future coronary heart disease events. The prognostic biomarker predicts an increased likelihood of an event without the influence of therapeutic intervention. In clinical trials, prognostic biomarkers are often used to identify patients with an increased likelihood of disease progression or a particular clinical event. It is necessary to distinguish prognostic and susceptibility/risk biomarkers. The last one can be applied to subjects without apparent disease.

The clinical endpoint, time-to-event, or event rate are usually measured to assess medical intervention in clinical trials. The prognostic markers can be often used to identify patients with particular clinical events or disease progression. Also, the prognostic markers are used in the drug development process as part of the enrichment strategy [44]. Similarly, the risk biomarkers are used for the enrichment of prevention trials population. The treatment effect in clinical trials depends on a planned number of events or a planned size of the effect. The clinical trials can be enriched by the patients who have a higher possibility to experience an event. Also, the statistical power of such a trial is increased.

Monitoring biomarkers

Monitoring biomarkers are serially measured over time to assess disease progression or the occurrence of a new disease [45]. They have a very important application in medical care. Blood pressure is repeatedly monitored in a hypertensive patient treated with antihypertensive drugs. The safety of human research participants depends on monitoring biomarkers. Thus, the possible toxic liver drug is monitored through repeated measurement of liver function tests [45].

Predictive biomarkers

Predictive biomarkers are used to identify individuals with a higher likelihood of response or lack of response to a particular therapy, and allow the identification of patients most likely to benefit from a given treatment, thus sparing other patients from the toxicities of ineffective therapies [46]. Examples of predictive biomarkers are *BRCA1* and 2 mutations when evaluating women with platinum-sensitive ovarian cancer, to identify patients likely to respond to Poly (ADP-ribose) polymerase (PARP) inhibitors [46]. Also, some *CFTR* mutations can predict patients are more likely to respond to particular treatments in clinical trials with cystic fibrosis [39].

A prognostic biomarker informs about a disease outcome (e.g., death, disease progression, or disease recurrence) independent of treatment received. A biomarker is predictive if the treatment effect (experimental compared with control) is different for biomarker-positive patients compared with biomarker-negative patients.

Some biomarkers could be both predictive and prognostic. Predictive and prognostic biomarkers cannot be distinguished when only patients who have received a particular therapy are studied [47].

Susceptibility biomarkers

The risk or susceptibility biomarkers are a useful tool in the search for a subject more responsive (susceptible) to specific exposure of treatment in comparison with less responsive or less susceptible subjects [48]. Two important applications of risk biomarkers are in cancer treatment in personalized medicine and the prediction of toxic effects during the drug development process.

Personalized medicine is based on the identification of different biomarkers that can distinguish patients with good prognoses or cancer patients who are unlikely to respond to therapy.

Pharmacodynamic biomarkers

The goal of the new drug development process is to demonstrate the efficacy and safety of medicinal products intended to use in some patient populations. Many scientists use PD biomarkers to explore the pathophysiology of different diseases in the search for new biological targets and therapeutic agents. Pharmacodynamic or response biomarkers have a different role in the drug development process. PD biomarkers have a broad repertoire of use in a preclinical, clinical, and regulatory parts of the drug development process [49, 50]. They can serve as molecular indicators of pharmacological response or target effects. Furthermore, the lead compounds from preclinical studies can be selected based on preclinical data using PD biomarkers. Measurements of PD biomarkers provide essential data for early go/no go decisions.

The small proportion of PD biomarkers reached a status of validated surrogate endpoint. Their role in confirmatory clinical trials is priceless and serves as proof of concept. The new space for PD or response biomarkers represents the concept of biosimilarity [50]. No clinically meaningful difference between reference and biosimilar products can be proven based on clinical pharmacology data where pharmacokinetic (PK) and pharmacodynamics (PD) data are critical parts of evidence for biosimilarity.

These biomarkers have various roles in regulatory submission through the following fields:

- verification of drug response,
- quantitative measuring of pharmacological response,
- discovery and confirmation of mechanisms of drug action, and as
- indicators of health benefits.

6 Pharmacogenomics—the Central Place of Personalized Medicine

Pharmacogenomics is a central part of personalized medicine that connects genomic variations and patients' responses to drug therapy. Figure 2 (reuse with permission from publisher Springer Nature) represents the impact of pharmacogenomics on drug discovery and the drug development process [51].

The role of pharmacogenomics is twofold today. It is reflected in the fact of successful development of new personalized drugs in the pharmaceutical industry, while doctors are increasingly using its postulates in their daily work, looking for the right medicine in the right dose based on genetic information.

Regulatory agencies early recognized the role of pharmacogenomics in drug development. The Food and Drug Administration (FDA), the Japanese regulatory authority, the Pharmaceutical and Medical Devices Agency (PMDA), and the European Medical Agency (EMA) have been emphasizing the importance of identifying genetic polymorphisms since the first guidelines for industry on drug metabolism/interaction during development and allow safe dosing and approval of medications. The introduction of pharmacogenomic testing during drug development significantly increases the likelihood of drug development used by most patients without the occurrence of serious side effects [51].

6.1 History of Pharmacogenomics

The first observation related to pharmacogenomics returns us to ancient times. Pythagoras was reported about 510 before Christ in a village Crotonia in southern Italy that eating fava beans can be dangerous. One in three males in Sardinia and southern Italy has mentioned a pathophysiological disorder known today as

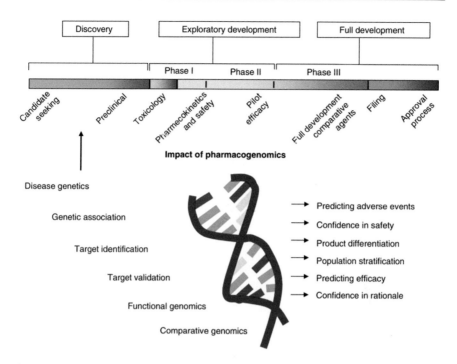

Fig. 2 Impact of PGx on drug research and development

favism [52]. This is an X-linked trait based on glucose-6-phosphate dehydrogenase (G6PD) deficiency. Pythagoras had warned about cramping and severe abdominal pain as a symptom of the hemolytic crisis. A deficiency of 80–95% of the G6PD enzyme leads to hemolytic anemia, but a complete shortage of enzyme G6PD is incompatible with life [52].

Treating someone based on their body type or other constitutional factors, as is the practice in ancient Ayurveda, Chinese, Tibetan, and Iranian traditional medicine systems, incorporates genetic features into treatment considerations [53]. Many centuries later, the advent of PGx as a science and tool in drug development was first announced by Motulsky in 1957, coining the term pharmacogenetics [54].

The first pieces of evidence of genetic-based pharmacokinetics were in subsequent years a twin study of dicumarol PK and individual dosing in anesthesia adapted by patient's signs and symptoms [53].

6.2   Pharmacogenomics in Drug Discovery

Research and development in the pharmaceutical industry have received a significant impetus with advances in genome sequencing technology. New molecular models have been developed with adequate computer and IT support [55, 56].

Furthermore, advances in sequencing technology have enabled pharmaceutical companies to develop sophisticated molecular models, with adequate computer and information support [56].

The probability of finding a cure with the help of genomic data and computer support is twice as high compared to the old methods [57]. Genomics can help identify new targets for drugs as well as accelerate drug development processes, and predict drug responses based on personalized responses during clinical trials [58]. Researchers are increasingly interested in detecting and validating tests for possible clinical use.

The first step is to associate genes with the disease, then scientists from different fields of the investigation come together to obtain a molecule that they can modify to treat the disease [59]. Advances in genomics affect the development of new drugs because we better characterize the disease and the pharmacokinetics and pharmacodynamics of the new drug [54]. Targets that are successful during the validation process are more likely to be genetically confirmed [60, 61]. However, to date, there is a small proportion of targets with genetic data. This is important because genetically validated drugs result in cost reductions [60, 61]. The candidate drug is more likely to correct the biochemical defect by increasing the chance of being placed on the market [57, 58].

A better understanding of genomics saves time and lowers the cost of clinical drug development, as well as reduces side effects of a new drug by optimizing the risk–benefit ratio [62]. Human genomics provides key information and clinical evidence in drug discovery and development and allows for an easier and safer transition to multiple stages of the process. This allows scientists to select the most suitable patients for a clinical study, with the best chance of success and reliability of the drug development process [60]. Researchers are entering a new era of precision medicine in which research, technology, and new policies for patients, researchers, and service providers are united [62].

6.3   Pharmacogenomics in Early Clinical Development

PGx has important roles in drug development from drug discovery to the end of the development process [53]. Also, some PGx discoveries are related to post-marketing studies. The early phase of drug development is important because it is the first application of a drug in humans. This phase of drug development is characterized by many challenges regarding safety and efficacy parameters, outcome measures, doses used in clinical development, the population involved in clinical studies, as well as a limited number of clinical trial participants due to ethical and economic requests [63].

Also, genetic variants can affect drug transporters and metabolism. PK parameters are studied in vitro and in vivo before the first application in humans. Thus, detection of some genetic variants in *HLA* by in vitro tests enables the prediction of different types of reactions such as allergic or idiosyncratic. Also, the PD property of a drug can be affected by genetic polymorphisms. Some patients could be excluded from clinical trials due to potential toxicity or being at risk of adverse drug reactions. Adverse event profiles can help to identify new drug targets. Thus, some adverse drug reactions undesirable in one project can be beneficial in another one.

PGx approach is especially useful in Phase II studies (about 70% positive results) versus 19% positive results in Phase I according to O'Donnell and Studler [63]. The same authors concluded that Phase I is likely too early, and Phase III may be so late to incorporate PGx studies in drug development. The title of the article suggests the answer (Is there a sweet spot in phase II?) [63].

An illustrative example is using *KRAS* mutation in colon cancer. Anti-EGF receptor (EGFR) drug cetuximab was first approved in 2004, but it was not known till labeled changes in 2009 that patients with mutated *KRAS* have no benefit from the addition of anti-EGFR therapy. Retrospectively, the total number of patients included in Phase III trials was 5657, but only 3287 patients had a *KRAS* result, and of those, 651 *KRAS*-mutant patients received anti-EGFR monoclonal antibody therapy, inappropriately [64]. As a consequence, early incorporation of *KRAS* status in the treatment anti-EGFR therapy saved money, and fewer patients would receive the ineffective drug. Thus, labeling justifies the necessity of *KRAS* testing.

The number of studies using randomization in Phase II is increasing which is a good opportunity to incorporate pharmacogenomics markers and evaluate whether are they predictive for treatment response or prognostic for disease. PGx factors can explain some answers in disease heterogeneity in oncology, but other factors such as drug resistance, interindividual variability, excretory organ functions, comorbidity, and compliance are other responsible causes [53]. In randomized discontinuation trials (RDTs) design, all patients are initially treated with the same drug, and then only patients who respond continue therapy. Also, stable diseases enable randomization against a placebo [63]. Without the incorporation of PGx in RTD and other randomized phase II trials, many reasons for variability can remain unanswered.

6.4   PGx-Dose Recommendations, Guidelines, and Drug Labeling

The field of PGx is developing rapidly. The first PGx dose recommendations for antidepressant and psychiatric drugs were published in 2001, even before the first human genome was sequenced [65, 66]. An increase in available evidence and the ambition to implement PGx in clinical practice has led to the need for more comprehensive dosing guidelines and genotyping strategies. In 2005, the Dutch Pharmacogenetics Working Group (DPWG) was formed to develop evidence-based PGx guidelines. In 2011, the Clinical Pharmacogenomics Implementation Consortium (CPIC) was founded. Currently, CPIC and the DPWG combined have issued PGx dose recommendations covering more than 50 drugs and more than 20 genes [67, 68, 69].

Kim et al. assessed US FDA approval of new drugs labeled with PGx information from 2000 to 2020 [70]. According to regulatory authorities, PGx information is clinically actionable, if they are categorized as "actionable PGx", "required genetic testing" or "recommended genetic testing" [71, 72]. PGx was assigned as "informative PGx" if they lack actionability and their label by PharmGKB only describes the role of the variant in drug metabolism or states the dose adjustment are not necessary [73].

The annual proportion of new drug approvals with PGx labeling has increased approximately three times during mentioned period (10.3% vs. 28.2%) [70]. The most prominent drugs with PGx labeling are cancer drugs (75.5%). Clinically actionable information was often observed in cancer drugs in comparison with other therapeutic areas. These results suggest more opportunities for including PGx in non-cancer therapeutic areas [73].

6.5   Companion Diagnostic

The merge between molecular diagnostic and personalized medicine led us to the development of companion diagnostic. The companion diagnostic (CDx) is a test that provides information regarding the effective and safe use of medicinal products. This type of medical device is targeted drug treatment, highly tailored, and useful in everyday practice to determine the suitability of a drug for a particular patient.

The first CDx associated with drug development was HercepTest, based on the predictive biomarker HER2 protein, approved by the FDA in 1998 for detection and treatment of metastatic breast cancer.

According to Valle et al., the total number of FDA-approved CDx tests to March 2021 was 44 [74]. Majority of them, 53%, were approved in the last 5 years, but 47% in the period from 1998 till 2015. Only two tests were approved for indications not related to cancer. The test gives vital information and is a prerequisite for drug use. CDx is regulatory approved for use only as part of the licensing of the drug. Information about a companion diagnostic is a part of the therapeutic product labeling.

There are different types of companion diagnostics intended for the following applications:

– screening and detection; tests for detection of aggressive types of cancers,
– prognosis; the test can predict a course of diseases,
– monitoring; test examines appropriate drug dosing and effectiveness (e.g., *VKORC1* and *CYP2C9* genotype for warfarin dosing),
– recurrence; the test can evaluate the risk for recurrence of disease (e.g., recurrence of different type of cancer), and
– theranostics; this type of test combines therapeutics and diagnostics (e.g., Her2/neu); this test is an indicator of the patient's response to a particular treatment.

In some cases that are necessary to repurpose existing drugs to get more information in favor of better stratified CDx. Some examples like the antiplatelet drug clopidogrel could be illustrative. This prodrug is mainly metabolized by CYP2C19. The highly polymorphic enzyme with variant *CYP2C19*2* (phenotype of poor metabolizer) reduces activation of clopidogrel. This variant has a different frequency from 25 to 30% in the European population to 70% in the Asian population [74]. Clinical trials are mainly commenced in the USA and Europe. The lack of diversity of subjects involved in clinical trials limits poor metabolizers and CDx potential for population not presented in clinical trials. This is the most common variant with loss of function led to an increase in the risk of ADRs in the Asian population, especially expressed in patients related to stent placement or balloon angioplasty. FDA issued a clopidogrel label warning based on this data [75]. This illustrative example expressed the importance of CDx design, test sensitivity, and the significance of CDx's early role in drug development. Advancement in CDx approvals is a result of a better understanding of the pathological condition and the mechanism of action of companion drugs.

Further improvements in CDx approvals should come from a better understanding of both the pathology in question and the companion drug's mechanism of action.

References

1. Ng R. History of drug discovery and development. In: Ng T, editor. Drugs: from discovery to approval. Wiley; 2005. p. 392–99. https://doi.org/10.1002/0471722804.app1.
2. Pina AS, Hussain A, Roque ACA. A historic1al overview of drug discovery. Meth Mol Biol. 2009;572:3–12. https://doi.org/10.1007/978-1-60761-244-5_1.
3. UCI School of Pharmacy & Pharmaceutical Sciences. A short history of drug discovery. https://pharmsci.uci.edu/programs/a-short-history-of-drug-discovery/. Accessed 1 Mar 2022.
4. Murphy MP. Pharmacogenomics: a new paradigm for drug development. Drug Discov World. 2000;1:23–32.
5. Davis BH, Limdi NA. Translational pharmacogenomics: discovery, evidence synthesis and delivery of race-conscious medicine. Clin Pharmacol Ther. 2021;110:909–25. https://doi.org/10.1002/cpt.2357.
6. Cacabelos R, Naidoo V, Corzo L, Cacabelos N, Carril JC. Genophenotypic factors and pharmacogenomics in adverse drug reactions. Int J Mol Sci. 2021;22(24):13302. https://doi.org/10.3390/ijms222413302.
7. Hood L, Rowen L. The Human Genome Project: big science transforms biology and medicine. Genome Med. 2013;5:79. https://doi.org/10.1186/gm483.
8. Yin O, Vandell A. Incorporating pharmacogenomics in drug development: a perspective from industry. In: Lam YWF, SA Scott, editors. Pharmacogenomics, challenges, and opportunities therapeutic implementation. Academic Press; 2019. p. 81–101.
9. Morgan P, Brown DG, Lennard S, Anderton MJ, Barrett JC, Eriksson U, et al. Impact of a five-dimensional framework on R&D productivity at AstraZeneca. Nat Rev Drug Discov. 2018;17(3):167–81. https://doi.org/10.1038/nrd.2017.244.
10. Schork NJ. Personalized medicine: time for one-person trials. Nature. 2015;520(7549):609–11.
11. Li S, Todor A, Luo R. Blood transcriptomics and metabolomics for personalized medicine. Comput Struct Biotechnol J. 2015;31(14):1–7. https://doi.org/10.1016/j.csbj.2015.10.005.

12. Beger RD, Dunn W, Schmidt MA, Gross SS, Kirwan JA, et al. Metabolomics enables precision medicine: "A White Paper, Community Perspective". Metabolomics. 2016;12(10):149. https://doi.org/10.1007/s11306-016-1094-6.
13. Barrot CC, Woillard JB, Picard N. Big data in pharmacogenomics: current applications, perspectives, and pitfalls. Pharmacogenomics. 2019;20(8):609–20. https://doi.org/10.2217/pgs-2018-0184 (PMID: 31190620).
14. Piétu G, Mariage-Samson R, Fayein NA, Matingou C, Eveno E, Houlgatte R, et al. The Genexpress IMAGE knowledge base of the human brain transcriptome: a prototype integrated resource for functional and computational genomics. Genome Res. 1999;9:195–209.
15. Lowe R, Shirley N, Bleackley M, Dolan S, Shafee T. Transcriptomics technologies. PLoS Comput Biol. 2017;13(5):e1005457. https://doi.org/10.1371/journal.pcbi.1005457.
16. Barmada MM, Whitcomb DC. Integrative systems biology: implications for the understanding of human disease. Elsevier; 2009. https://doi.org/10.1016/b978-0-12-374419-7.00010-x.
17. KhalKhal E, Rezaei-Tavirani M, Rostamii-Nejad M. Pharmaceutical advances and proteomics researches. Iran J Pharm Res. 2019;18(Suppl1):51–67. https://doi.org/10.22037/ijpr.2020.112 440.13758.
18. Al-Amrani S, Al-Jabri Z, Al-Zaabi A, Alshekaili J, Al-Khabori M. Proteomics: concepts and applications in human medicine. World J Biol Chem. 2021;12(5):57–69. https://doi.org/10. 4331/wjbc.v12.i5.57.
19. Savino R, Paduano S, Preiano M, Terracciano R. The proteomics big challenge for biomarkers and new drug-targets discovery. Int J Mol Sci. 2012;13(11): 13926–48. https://doi.org/10.3390/ijms131113926.
20. Oliver SG, Winson MK, Kell DB, Baganz F. Systematic functional analysis of the yeast genome. Trends Biotechnol. 1998;16:373–8. https://doi.org/10.1016/S0167-7799(98)01214-1.
21. Agrawal P. Artificial intelligence in drug discovery and development. J Pharmacovigil. 2018;6:e173. https://doi.org/10.4172/2329-6887.1000e173.
22. Paul D, Sanap G, Shenoy S, Kalyane D, Kalia K, Tekade RK. Artificial intelligence in drug discovery and development. Drug Discov Today. 2021;26(1):80–93. https://doi.org/10.1016/j.drudis.2020.10.010.
23. Gupta R, Srivastava D, Sahu M, Tiwari S, Ambasta RK, Kumar P. Artificial intelligence to deep learning: machine intelligence approach for drug discovery. Mol Divers. 2021;25(3):1315–60. https://doi.org/10.1007/s11030-021-10217-3.
24. Vamathevan J, Clark D, Czodrowski P, Dunham I, Ferran E, Lee G, et al. Applications of machine learning in drug discovery and development. Nat Rev Drug Discov. 2019;18(6):463–477. https://doi.org/10.1038/s41573-019-0024-5.
25. Chen H, Engkvist O, Wang Y, Olivecrona M, Blaschke T. The rise of deep learning in drug discovery. Drug Discov Today. 2018;23(6):1241–50. https://doi.org/10.1016/j.drudis.2018. 01.039.
26. Top Strategic Technology Trends for 2018. http://www.gartner.com/technology/research/top-10-technology-trends/. Accessed 1 Apr 2022.
27. Kim S, Thiessen PA, Bolton EE, Chen JFG, Gindulyte A, Han L, et al. PubChem substance and compound databases. Nucl Acids Res. 2016;44(D1):D1202–13.
28. Fooladi, H. Review: deep learning. In: Fooladi H, editor. Drug discovery. Hosein Fooladi; 2018. https://hfooladi.github.io/posts/2018/10/Review-Deep-Learning-In-Drug-Discovery/. Accessed 1 Apr 2022.
29. Califf RM. Biomarker definitions and their applications. Exp Biol Med. 2018;243(3):213–221. https://doi.org/10.1177/1535370217750088.
30. FDA-NIH Biomarker Working Group. BEST (Biomarkers, EndpointS, and other tools) resource (Internet). Silver Spring (MD): Food and Drug Administration (US). Diagnostic Biomarker; 2016 (Updated 2020 Nov 16). https://www.ncbi.nlm.nih.gov/books/NBK402285/. Accessed 1 Apr 2022 (Co-published by National Institutes of Health (US), Bethesda (MD)).
31. Kraus VB. Biomarkers as drug development tools: discovery, validation, qualification, and use. Nat Rev Rheumatol. 2018;14:354–62. https://doi.org/10.1038/s41584-018-0005-9.

32. FDA-NIH Biomarker Working Group. BEST (Biomarkers, EndpointS, and other Tools) Resource (Internet). Silver Spring (MD): Food and Drug Administration (US); 2016. Available from: https://www.ncbi.nlm.nih.gov/books/NBK326791/. Accessed 1 Apr 2022 (Co-published by National Institutes of Health (US), Bethesda (MD)).

33. Senior JR. Evolution of the food and drug administration approach to liver safety for new drugs: current status and challenges. Drug Saf. 2014;37(Suppl 1):S9-17. https://doi.org/10.1007/s40264-014-0182-7.

34. Wasung ME, Chawla LS, Madero M. Biomarkers of renal function, which and when? Clin Chim Acta. 2015;438:350–7. https://doi.org/10.1016/j.cca.2014.08.039.

35. Chung WH, Hung SI, Hong HS, Hsih MS, Yang LC, Ho HC, et al. Medical genetics: a marker for Stevens-Johnson syndrome. Nature. 2004;428(6982):486. https://doi.org/10.1038/428486a.

36. Betton GR. Biomarkers efficacy and safety. https://www.europeanpharmaceuticalreview.com/issue/issue-3-2005/. Accessed 1 Apr 2022.

37. Zabka TS, Burkhardt J, Reagan WJ, Gautier J, Glaab WE, Guffroy M, et al. The use of emerging safety biomarkers in nonclinical and clinical safety assessment—the current and future state: an IQ DruSafe industry survey. Regul Toxicol Pharmacol. 2021;120:104857. https://doi.org/10.1016/j.yrtph.2020.104857.

38. Farrell PM, Rosenstein BJ, White TB, Accurso FJ, Castellani C, Cutting GR, et al. Cystic Fibrosis Foundation. Guidelines for diagnosis of cystic fibrosis in newborns through older adults: Cystic Fibrosis Foundation consensus report. J Pediatr. 2008;153(2): S4–S14. https://doi.org/10.1016/j.jpeds.2008.05.005.

39. Davies JC, Wainwright CE, Canny GJ, Chilvers MA, Howenstine MS, Munck A, et al. VX08-770-103 (ENVISION) Study Group. Efficacy and safety of ivacaftor in patients aged 6 to 11 years with cystic fibrosis with a G551D mutation. Am J Respir Crit Care Med. 2013;187(11):1219–25. https://doi.org/10.1164/rccm.201301-0153OC.

40. FDA-NIH Biomarker Working Group. BEST (Biomarkers, EndpointS, and other Tools) Resource (Internet). Silver Spring (MD): Food and Drug Administration (US). Diagnostic Biomarker. 2016 (Updated 2020 Nov 16). https://www.ncbi.nlm.nih.gov/books/NBK402285/ (Co-published by National Institutes of Health (US), Bethesda (MD)).

41. Basu NN, Ingham S, Hodson J, Lalloo F, Bulman M, Howell A, et al. Risk of contralateral breast cancer in BRCA1 and BRCA2 mutation carriers: a 30-year semi-prospective analysis. Fam Cancer. 2015;14(4):531–8. https://doi.org/10.1007/s10689-015-9825-9.

42. U.S. Food and Drug Administration. Guidance for industry: qualification of biomarker-plasma fibrinogen in studies examining exacerbations and/or all-cause mortality in patients with chronic obstructive pulmonary disease. 2016. http://www.fda.gov/downloads/Drugs/GuidanceComplianceRegulatoryInformation/Guidances/UCM453496.pdf. Accessed 1 Apr 2022.

43. Miller BE, Tal-Singer R, Rennard SI, Furtwaengler A, Leidy N, Lowings M, et al. Plasma fibrinogen qualification as a drug development tool in chronic obstructive pulmonary disease. Perspective of the chronic obstructive pulmonary disease biomarker qualification consortium. Am J Respir Crit Care Med. 2016;193(6):607–13. https://doi.org/10.1164/rccm.201509-1722PP.

44. U.S. Food and Drug Administration. Draft guidance for industry: enrichment strategies for clinical trials to support approval of human drugs and biological products. 2012. https://www.fda.gov/downloads/drugs/guidancecomplianceregulatoryinformation/guidances/ucm332181.pdf. Accessed 1 Mar 2022.

45. FDA-NIH Biomarker Working Group. BEST (biomarkers, EndpointS, and other tools) resource (Internet). Silver Spring (MD): Food and Drug Administration (US). Monitoring Biomarker. 2016 (Updated 2021 Jan 25). https://www.ncbi.nlm.nih.gov/books/NBK402282/ (Co-published by National Institutes of Health (US), Bethesda (MD)).

46. FDA-NIH Biomarker Working Group. BEST (biomarkers, EndpointS, and other tools) resource (Internet). Silver Spring (MD): Food and Drug Administration (US). Predictive Biomarker. 2016. https://www.ncbi.nlm.nih.gov/books/NBK402283/ (Co-published by National Institutes of Health (US), Bethesda (MD)).

47. FDA-NIH Biomarker Working Group. BEST (biomarkers, EndpointS, and other tools) resource (Internet). Silver Spring (MD): Food and Drug Administration (US). Understanding Prognostic versus Predictive Biomarkers. 2016. https://www.ncbi.nlm.nih.gov/books/NBK402 284/ (Co-published by National Institutes of Health (US), Bethesda (MD)).
48. FDA-NIH Biomarker Working Group. BEST (biomarkers, EndpointS, and other tools) resource (Internet). Silver Spring (MD): Food and Drug Administration (US). Susceptibility/ Risk Biomarker. 2016 (Updated 2020 Aug 27). https://www.ncbi.nlm.nih.gov/books/NBK402 288/ (Co-published by National Institutes of Health (US), Bethesda (MD)).
49. FDA-NIH Biomarker Working Group. BEST (biomarkers, EndpointS, and other tools) resource (Internet). Silver Spring (MD): Food and Drug Administration (US). Response Biomarker. 2016 (Updated 2021 Sep 17). https://www.ncbi.nlm.nih.gov/books/NBK402286/ (Co-published by National Institutes of Health (US), Bethesda (MD)).
50. Wang YC, Strauss DG, Huang SM. Use of pharmacodynamic/response biomarkers for therapeutic biologics regulatory submissions. Biomark Med. 2019;13(10):805–9. https://doi.org/10.2217/bmm-2019-0197.
51. Penny MA, McHale D. Pharmacogenomics and the drug discovery pipeline. Am J Pharmacogenom. 2005;5:53–62. https://doi.org/10.2165/00129785-200505010-00005.
52. Favism MJ. A brief history from the—"abstain from beans" of Pythagoras to the present. Arch Hell Med. 2012;29:258–63.
53. Burt T, Dhillon S. Pharmacogenomics in early-phase clinical development. Pharmacogenomics. 2013;14(9):1085–97. https://doi.org/10.2217/pgs.13.81.
54. Motulsky AG. Drug reactions enzymes, and biochemical genetics. J Am Med Assoc. 1957;165(7):835–7. https://doi.org/10.1001/jama.1957.72980250010016.
55. Oates JT, Lopez D. Pharmacogenetics: an important part of drug development with a focus on its application. Int J Biomed Investig. 2018;1:111. https://doi.org/10.31531/25814745.100 0111.
56. Kuznetsov V, Lee HK, Maurer-Stroh S, Molnar MJ, Pongor S, Eisenhaber B, et al. How bioinformatics influences health informatics: usage of biomolecular sequences, expression profiles and automated microscopic image analyses for clinical needs and public health. Health Inf Sci Syst. 2013;1:2. https://doi.org/10.1186/2047-2501-1-2.
57. Sliwoski G, Kothiwale S, Meiler J, Lowe EW. Computational methods in drug discovery. Pharmacol Rev. 2014;66:334–95. https://doi.org/10.1124/pr.112.007336.
58. Kraljevic S, Stambrook PJ, Pavelic K. Accelerating drug discovery. EMBO Rep. 2004;5:837–42. https://doi.org/10.1038/sj.embor.7400236.
59. Hughes JP, Rees S, Kalindjian SB, Philpott KL. Principles of early drug discovery. Br J Pharmacol. 2011;162: 1239–1249. https://doi.org/10.1111/j.1476-5381.2010.01127.x.
60. Cully M. Target validation: genetic information adds supporting weight. Nat Rev Drug Discov. 2015;14:525. https://doi.org/10.1038/nrd4692.
61. Thomsen SK, Gloyn AL. Human genetics as a model for target validation: finding new therapies for diabetes. Diabetologia. 2017;60:960–70. https://doi.org/10.1007/s00125-017-4270-y.
62. Ahmed S, Zhou Z, Zhou J, Chen SQ. Pharmacogenomics of drug metabolizing enzymes and transporters: relevance to precision medicine. Genom Proteom Bioinform. 2016;14:298–313. https://doi.org/10.1016/j.gpb.2016.03.008.
63. O'Donnell PH, Stadler WM. Pharmacogenomics in early-phase oncology clinical trials: is there a sweet spot in phase II? Clin Cancer Res. 2012;18(10):2809–16. https://doi.org/10.1158/1078-0432.CCR-11-2445.
64. Bardelli A, Siena S. Molecular mechanisms of resistance to cetuximab and panitumumab in colorectal cancer. J Clin Oncol. 2010;28(7):1254–61. https://doi.org/10.1200/jco.2009.24.6116.
65. van der Lee M, Kriek M, Guchelaar HJ, Swen JJ. Technologies for Pharmacogenomics: a review. Genes. 2020;11(12):1456. https://doi.org/10.3390/genes11121456.
66. Kirchheiner J, Brøsen K, Dahl ML, Gram LF, Kasper S, Roots I, et al. CYP2D6 and CYP2C19 genotype-based dose recommendations for antidepressants: a first step towards

subpopulation-specific dosages. Acta Psychiatr Scand. 2001;104:173–92. https://doi.org/10. 1034/j.1600-0447.2001.00299.x.

67. Dutch Pharmacogenetics Working group. Pharmacogenetics Guidelines; Royal Dutch Pharmacists Association (KNMP Kennisbank): The Hague, The Netherlands, 2020. https://www. knmp.nl/dossiers/farmacogenetica. Accessed 1 Mar 2022.

68. Clinical Pharmacogenetics Implementation Consortium. CPIC-guidelines. https://cpicpgx. org/. Accessed 1 Mar 2022.

69. Primorac D, Höppner W, editors. Pharmacogenetics in clinical practice/Pharmakogenetik in der klinischen Praxis/Farmakogenetika u kliničkoj praksi. Zagreb: St. Catherine Specialty Hospital, International Society for Applied Biological Sciences; 2022.

70. Kim JA, Ceccarelli R, Lu CY. Pharmacogenomic biomarkers in US FDA-approved drug labels (2000–2020). J Pers Med. 2021;11(3):179. https://doi.org/10.3390/jpm11030179.

71. US Food and Drug Administration Table of Pharmacogenomic Biomarkers in Drug Labeling. https://www.fda.gov/drugs/science-and-research-drugs/table-pharmacogenomic-biomarkers-drug-labeling. Accessed 31 Mar 2022.

72. Ehmann F, Caneva L, Papaluca M. EMA initiatives, and perspectives on pharmacogenomics. Br J Clin Pharmacol. 2014;77:612–7. https://doi.org/10.1111/bcp.12319.

73. PharmGKB Drug Label Information and Legend. https://www.pharmgkb.org/page/drugLabel Legend. Accessed 1 Mar 2022.

74. Valla V, Alzabin S, Koukoura A, Lewis A, Nielsen AA, Vassiliadis E. Companion diagnostics: state of the art and new regulations. Biomark Insights. 2021;16:11772719211047764. https:// doi.org/10.1177/11772719211047763.FDA.

75. FDA drug safety communication: reduced effectiveness of Plavix (clopidogrel) in patients who are poor metabolizers of the drug. 2017. https://www.fda.gov/drugs/postmarket-drug-safety-information-patients-and-providers/fda-drug-safety-communication-reduced-effective ness-plavix-clopidogrel-patients-who-are-poor. Accessed 1 Apr 2022.

Future Perspectives of Pharmacogenomics

Wolfgang Höppner, Lidija Bach-Rojecky, and Dragan Primorac

Abstract

This chapter summarizes how far pharmacogenomics has come since its inception 22 years ago, the challenges it faces as complexity increases, and how new technologies are opening opportunities to become true precision medicine in future. However, it also describes the need to make primary care physicians familiar with these advances and empower them to use the opportunities for the benefit of both the patient and the healthcare system.

W. Höppner (✉)
Bioglobe GmbH, Hamburg, Germany
e-mail: hoeppner@bioglobe.net

L. Bach-Rojecky
University of Zagreb Faculty of Pharmacy and Biochemistry, 10000 Zagreb, Croatia

D. Primorac
St. Catherine Specialty Hospital, 10000 Zagreb, Croatia

St. Catherine Specialty Hospital, 49210 Zabok, Croatia

University of Split School of Medicine, 21000 Split, Croatia

Josip Juraj Strossmayer University of Osijek Faculty of Medicine, 31000 Osijek, Croatia

University of Rijeka School of Medicine, 51000 Rijeka, Croatia

Josip Juraj Strossmayer University of Osijek Faculty of Dental Medicine and Health, 31000 Osijek, Croatia

Eberly College of Science, State College Penn State University, 17 Thomas St, PA 16803, USA

The Henry C. Lee College of Criminal Justice and Forensic Sciences, University of New Haven, West Haven, CT, USA

Medical School Regiomed, 96450 Coburg, Germany

International Center For Applied Biological Sciences, Zagreb 10000, Croatia

Keywords

Personalized medicine • Drug–gene association • SNV panel • Next-generation sequencing • Whole-exome sequencing • Genotype

1 Pharmacogenomics and Precision Medicine

Pharmacogenomics (PGx) is an interdisciplinary field of medicine in which human genetics and pharmacology meet almost all clinical disciplines. The first PGx dosing recommendations for antidepressants and psychotropic drugs were published in 2001 [1]. This was before the complete sequencing of the first human genome was available. Since then, increasing attention has been paid to the mechanisms that lead to interindividual differences in treatment response with the same drug. The goal is to understand the relationships that lead to these differences and to use PGx to contribute to the emergence of precision medicine or personalized medicine. In future, the individual patient should be offered the best possible therapy according to the current state of science and technology and with careful consideration of his/her characteristics, including genetics.

The cause of interindividual variability is complex and influenced by several factors, including personal characteristics (e.g., age, gender, body mass index), clinical factors (e.g., renal, or hepatic dysfunction, concomitant medication, illnesses), environmental and lifestyle factors (e.g., air pollution, smoking, diet, stimulants, dietary supplements), among which genetics plays a significant role.

2 Increasing Complexity in Pharmacogenomics

Genes that encode drug absorption, distribution, metabolism, and excretion (ADME) were the focus of the first PGx studies more than two decades ago. Clinically relevant changes in therapeutic action or adverse side effects were attributed to pairs of ADME genes and drugs of interest. This approach was also referred to as "companion diagnostics" since it was usually the association between a gene for a metabolic enzyme or transporter and an active drug that was the basis for assessing clinical efficacy. The genotype determines whether the patient should be classified as a slow or fast metabolizer for a drug, and how dose adjustment can achieve the targeted therapeutic window at which the desired effect occurs. If a genotype is present that is associated with severe adverse drug reactions (ADR) or treatment failure that cannot be influenced by dose modification, switching to another agent is suggested.

Meanwhile, many drugs are affected by several different genes of the ADME system. Thus, future PGx will need to screen multiple gene variants to predict their impact more reliably on the pharmacokinetics of a drug.

If the changes in the ADME genes lead to a low drug level (fast metabolism or slow transport to the target), the therapeutic efficacy may be reduced, or the desired effect may even fail (therapy failure). In a case when a genetic variant leads to an increased drug level (slow metabolism, fast transport to the target), this often leads to ADRs or an excessive pharmacodynamic effect on the target (referred to as on-target type ADR or "type A"). One example is the occurrence of bleeding during therapy with warfarin. Genetic variants of the target protein can alter the effect of the drug. Therefore, for some drugs, analysis of the gene encoding the target is required (e.g., VKORC1 in therapy with warfarin).

Thus, future PGx must consider not only the influence of genetic variants in ADME genes that affect pharmacokinetics but also the genetic variants of the target associated with the on-target pharmacodynamic effect and the genetic variants of off-target genes that may lead to off-target adverse effects. By taking these genetic conditions into account, it is hoped to reduce ADRs.

3   Advancement of Technology in Pharmacogenomics

Certain genes that metabolize most drugs and only the most frequent variants are analyzed in contemporary clinical practice. Genes encoding cytochrome P450 (CYP) enzymes involved in phase I of drug metabolism are involved in the most exploitable drug–gene associations.

To assess genetic influences on the therapeutic effects of the drug as well as ADRs, two types of genetic variants are predominantly studied in PGx to date: single base exchanges (single-nucleotide variants—SNVs) and copy number variations (CNVs). Depending on the type of genetic change, the variants lead to a greater or lesser effect on drug metabolism or target effect. For some genes, deletions or amplifications of complete gene copies play a role. These changes lead to a particularly large effect on the metabolism of the drug.

3.1   Application of SNV Arrays in Pharmacogenomics

Sanger-based sequencing techniques, which were aimed to detect and identify "novel" SNV, and single SNV arrays were employed for variant identification at the time when the first PGx guideline was introduced.

SNV panel testing is the most common approach, where preselected SNVs assembled according to the actual clinical guidelines in PGx practice are analyzed, using commercially available microarray platforms. Moreover, customer-specific arrays can be assembled for specific issues. Almost all array technologies employ PCR technology and synthesis on nanospheres or beads, using fluorescence or chemiluminescence detection to determine which variant is present at the targeted site [2–4]. Another technology is mass spectrometry, which relies on the mass differences between wild-type and mutant nucleotides [5].

This approach with preselected gene variants has some advantages, like fast results and low cost, but there is no chance to discover rare or not yet-known variants with these methods. The claim of future PGx to precision medicine or personalized medicine can therefore only be fulfilled to a limited extent.

3.2   State of the Art: Next-Generation Sequencing

A wide spectrum of structural changes in DNA is known from human genetic diagnostics, which lead to functional changes and are thus of great importance for the clarification of diseases. In the last 10 years, next-generation sequencing (NGS) has become established as a high-throughput technology. It is now well-standardized and cost-effective and is increasingly displacing Sanger sequencing from molecular genetics laboratories. It is proving to be versatile, and cost-effective [6, 7]. To date, this technology has been little used in PGx. In contrast to SNV panels that cover a limited set of selected variants, sequencing data cover the whole exome or genome. This technological advancement will improve PGx in future.

NGS technologies are capable of sequencing reads of 100–200 bp at high throughput. Thus, a complete genome can be sequenced within a few hours. Variants are identified based on deviations from the reference genome. There are 3 approaches into which NGS can be divided: 1. targeted parallel sequencing of a region or group of genes of interest, 2. sequencing the coding regions (1–2%) of the genome (whole-exome sequencing, WES), and 3. sequencing both coding and noncoding regions (whole-genome sequencing, WGS) [6, 7]. As compared to SNP panel testing, processing a large amount of data is the greater challenge of NGS, while the cost is comparable.

3.3   Advantage to Use NGS in Pharmacogenomics

NGS has become a standard procedure in clinical diagnostics and research. In 2014, Londin et al. [8] compared NGS with more widely available array technology and reported that the NGS technique provided false-negative results due to poorer coverage. As reviewed by van der Lee et al. [9] in 2020, subsequent studies revealed a difference in concordance of array technology of 94% for exome sequencing (WES—whole-exome sequencing) and 96% for genome sequencing (WGS—whole-genome sequencing) [10, 11].

While WES cannot detect relevant variants if they are in the intronic or intergenic regions, WGS has an expanded coverage that includes intronic regions. Of course, it is advantageous that previously unknown, very rare variants can be discovered as "private SNVs" by WES or WGS. Because of these advantages, a broader implementation of NGS in routine diagnostics will be a key benefit in terms of personalized medicine.

4   Long-Read Sequencing—Opportunity for Future Pharmacogenomics

All methods discussed so far have the disadvantage that they cannot clearly resolve complex genetic loci, such as tandem repeats. Also, it is hardly possible to unambiguously determine the phasing of haplotypes. However, genotyping of genes for CYP enzymes would be of great importance [12, 13].

These problems are overcome by the recently available long-read sequencing. Instead of using read lengths of 100–400 bp, read lengths of up to 45 kb can be achieved for individual DNA strands. This then allows clear haplotype phasing to be performed. In PGx, the problem of high sequence homologies in gene families or pseudogenes with high homologies can also be solved [14]. For example, 57 members of the CYP enzyme gene family have homologies as high as 98%. 12 of these CYP genes are involved in drug biotransformation and are thus diagnostically relevant. Nevertheless, few long-read sequencing studies have been performed on pharmacogenes. The most thoroughly studied complex locus is the *CYP2D6* gene, which contains not only SNVs but also structural variants.

---

5   Modern Approaches to Data Analysis in Pharmacogenomics

5.1   Evaluation of Known SNVs in Known Genes

The applications of NGS technology for PGx allow all known drug genes to be evaluated and all positions considered to have an influence on the drug's effect to be tested. To aid CNV calling, bioinformatic tools have been developed for NGS [15]. However, the SNV analysis yields many variants that contribute nothing to the question. One can filter these results. However, if the patient shows an altered drug response with no relevant SNVs found, re-evaluation of the data can reveal possibly new pharmacogentically relevant variants.

5.2   Variants with Unknown Effect

Rare variants which are associated with drug effect, but have not previously been analyzed, should be deposited in a common PGx database that stores rare variants found in patients who showed an interaction. Over time, new variants emerge as relevant because they are reported multiple times with similar effects [16, 17]. This approach has worked well for NGS data in human genetics. It is also possible to use in silico predictions to explore whether the variant affects the activity of the protein, thereby altering the pharmacological effect of the drug.

5.3   Pharmacogenomics and Disease Genes

In addition, variants can be found that predict disease. Complex examples include genes that are both pharmacogenes and disease-causing genes. The gene coding for ryanodine receptor *RYR1* has been associated with increased risk for development of malignant hyperthermia (MH), which could classify it as a disease gene, and as such, it is listed in the American College of Medical Genetics and Genomics guidelines [18]. However, in susceptible patients, MH could be triggered by administration of halogenated inhalational anesthetics and muscle relaxant suxamethonium, which could classify *RYR1* as a pharmacogene [19].

6   Continuing Education and Guidelines for Primary Care

PGx is used even less in primary care than in inpatient settings. There is a lack of knowledge about the importance of pharmacogenetics, PGx testing, interpretation of results, and logistical reasons for not using pharmacogenetic analysis [20]. Poor drug tolerability due to adverse effects leads to lower compliance and nonadherence, resulting in lack of treatment success. Instead, costs increase because prescribed medications are not taken [21]. Serious adverse drug reactions are estimated to account for 6.5% of hospital admissions [22]. The clinical and financial consequences of adverse drug reactions are high. More efficient routine screening for possible genetic limitations in drug tolerance would save patients suffering and the healthcare system costs. As the population ages, the proportion of multimorbid patients will increase. To prevent polypharmacy, physicians working in primary care should be intensively trained in the use of pharmacogenetics.

6.1   Guidelines

Pharmacogenetics made rapid scientific and clinical progress. However, translation into clinical application to date has been limited. Initially, a major obstacle to implementation was the lack of clear guidelines for the interpretation and application of PGx test results. Of the many expert groups that addressed this problem, the Dutch Pharmacogenetics Working Group (DPWG) and the Clinical Pharmacogenetics Implementation Consortium (CPIC) are the best known. The guidelines developed by these organizations are based on systematic literature reviews. They are intended to make it easier for physicians and pharmacists to take pharmacogenetic knowledge into account when prescribing.

The National Institutes of Health has established the PharmGKB as a resource that collects, curates, and makes available knowledge on clinically actionable gene–drug associations and genotype–phenotype relationships, as indicated on the PharmGKB website (https://www.pharmgkb.org/). In addition, PharmGKB manages comments on clinical guidelines produced by the Dutch Pharmacogenetics Working Group (DPWG) [23], the Clinical Pharmacogenetic Implementation

Consortium (CPIC) [24], and other professional societies such as the Canadian Pharmacogenomics Network for Drug Safety (CPNDS) and the French National Network of Pharmacogenetics (RNPGx).

The PharmGKB resource is available online for all interested parties. It is free of charge and user-friendly. To date, 763 medicines with variant annotations are available and 200 PGx association guidelines have been developed with actionable PGx recommendations for clinical practice [25]. Most of these actionable drug–gene associations involve genes encoding enzymes that degrade drugs (~66%). A smaller number of drug–gene associations involve transporter genes involved in the distribution of drugs in and out of cells, and less than one-third involve genes that affect drug pharmacodynamics. ~5% encode drug targets, and ~26% encode other protein targets related to drug action. These include genes encoding human leukocyte antigens that can cause severe hypersensitivity.

6.2   Recommendations from FDA

The US Food & Drug Administration (FDA) has published on its website a list of drugs for which the clinical utility of pharmacogenetic diagnostics has been established (61 drugs) and a list of drugs for which research data indicate a potential impact on safety or response (33 drugs) [26]. In addition, there are pharmacogenetic associations for which the data suggest a potential impact on pharmacokinetic properties (25 drugs). There is a strong overlap between the CPIC and DPWG guidelines and the FDA recommendations.

References

1. Kirchheiner J, Brøsen K, Dahl ML, Gram LF, Kasper S, Roots I, et al. CYP2D6 and CYP2C19 genotype-based dose recommendations for antidepressants: a first step towards subpopulation-specific dosages. Acta Psychiatr Scand. 2001;104:173–92. https://doi.org/10.1034/j.1600-0447.2001.00299.x.
2. VeraCode® ADME Core Panel Assay Guide—Illumina. Available online: https://support.illumina.com/downloads/veracode_adme_core_panel_assay_guide_15007510.html. Accessed 12 Apr 2022.
3. Arbitrio M, Di Martino MT, Scionti F, Agapito G, Guzzi PH, Cannataro M, et al. DMET™ (Drug Metabolism Enzymes and Transporters): a pharmacogenomic platform for precision medicine. Oncotarget. 2016;7:54028–50. https://doi.org/10.18632/oncotarget.9927.
4. ThermoFisher Scientific. Pharmacoscan Assay. Available online: https://www.thermofisher.com/order/catalog/product/903010TS. Accessed 10 Apr 2022.
5. Gabriel S, Ziaugra L, Tabbaa D. SNP genotyping using the Sequenom mass array iPLEX platform. Curr Protoc Hum Genet. 2:2–12. (2009). https://doi.org/10.1002/0471142905.hg0212s60.
6. Levy SE, Myers RM. Advancements in next-generation sequencing. Annu Rev Genom Hum Genet. 2016;17:95–115. https://doi.org/10.1146/annurev-genom-083115-022413.
7. Slatko BE, Gardner AF, Ausubel FM. Overview of next-generation sequencing technologies. Curr Protoc Mol Biol. 2018;122: e59. https://doi.org/10.1002/cpmb.59.

8. Londin ER, Clark P, Sponziello M, Kricka LJ, Fortina P, Park JY. Performance of exome sequencing for pharmacogenomics. Pers Med. 2014;12:109–15. https://doi.org/10.2217/PME. 14.77.
9. der Lee V, Kriek M, Guchelaar H-J, Swen JJ. Technologies for pharmacogenomics: a review. Genes. 2020;11:1456. https://doi.org/10.3390/genes11121456
10. Yang W, Wu G, Broeckel U, Smith CA, Turner V, Haidar CE, et al. Comparison of genome sequencing and clinical genotyping for pharmacogenetics. Clin Pharmacol Ther. 2016;100:380–8. https://doi.org/10.1002/cpt.411.
11. Rasmussen-Torvik LJ, Almoguera B, Doheny KF, Freimuth RR, Gordon AS, Hakonarson H, et al. Concordance between research sequencing and clinical pharmacogenetic genotyping in the eMERGE-PGx Study. J Mol Diagn. 2017;19:561–6. https://doi.org/10.1016/j.jmoldx.2017. 04.002.
12. Qiao W, Yang Y, Sebra R, Mendiratta G, Gaedigk A, Desnick RJ, Scott SA. Long-read single molecule real-time full gene sequencing of cytochrome P450–2D6. Hum Mutat. 2016;37:315–23. https://doi.org/10.1002/humu.22936.
13. Buermans HP, Vossen RH, Anvar SY, Allard WG, Guchelaar HJ, White SJ, et al. Flexible and Scalable Full-Length CYP2D6 Long Amplicon PacBio Sequencing. Hum Mutat. 2017;38:310–6. https://doi.org/10.1002/humu.23166.
14. Jin Y, Wang J, Bachtiar M, Chong SS, Lee CGL. Architecture of polymorphisms in the human genome reveals functionally important and positively selected variants in immune response and drug transporter genes. Hum Genom. 2018;12:43. https://doi.org/10.1186/s40246-018-0175-1.
15. Fromer M, Moran JL, Chambert K, Banks E, Bergen SE, Ruderfer DM, et al. Discovery and statistical genotyping of copy-number variation from whole-exome sequencing depth. Am J Hum Genet. 2012;91:597–607. https://doi.org/10.1016/j.ajhg.2012.08.005.
16. Drogemoller BI, Wright GE, Warnich L. Considerations for rare variants in drug metabolism genes and the clinical implications. Expert Opin Drug Metab Toxicol. 2014;10:873–84. https://doi.org/10.1517/17425255.2014.903239.
17. Ingelman-Sundberg M, Mkrtchian S, Zhou Y, Lauschke VM. Integrating rare genetic variants into pharmacogenetic drug response predictions. Hum Genom. 2018;12:26. https://doi.org/10.1186/s40246-018-0157-3.
18. Kalia SS, Adelman K, Bale SJ, Chung WK, Eng C, Evans JP et al. Recommendations for reporting of secondary findings in clinical exome and genome sequencing, 2016 update (ACMG SF v2.0): A policy statement of the American college of medical genetics and genomics. Genet Med. 2017;19:249–255. https://doi.org/10.1038/gim.2016.190.
19. Gonsalves SG, Dirksen RT, Sangkuhl K, Pulk R, Alvarellos M, Vo T, et al. Clinical pharmacogenetics implementation consortium (CPIC) guideline for the use of potent volatile anesthetic agents and succinylcholine in the context of RYR1 or CACNA1S genotypes. Clin Pharmacol Ther. 2019;105:1338–44. https://doi.org/10.1002/cpt.1319.
20. Rollinson V, Turner R, Pirmohamed M. Pharmacogenomics for primary care: an overview. Genes. 2020;11:1337. https://doi.org/10.3390/genes11111337.
21. Wei MY, Ito MK, Cohen JD, Brinton EA, Jacobson TA. Predictors of statin adherence, switching, and discontinuation in the usage survey: understanding the use of statins in America and gaps in patient education. J Clin Lipidol. 2013;7:472–83. https://doi.org/10.1016/j.jacl.2013. 03.001.
22. Pirmohamed M, James S, Meakin S, Green C, Scott AK, Walley TJ, et al. Adverse drug reactions as cause of admission to hospital: prospective analysis of 18 820 patients. BMJ. 2004;329:15–9. https://doi.org/10.1136/bmj.329.7456.15.
23. Dutch Pharmacogenetics Working Group. Pharmacogenetics Guidelines; Royal Dutch Pharmacists Association (KNMP Kennisbank). Available at https://www.knmp.nl/dossiers/farmac ogenetica. Accessed 10 Apr 2022.
24. Clinical Pharmacogenetics Implementation Consortium. CPIC-guidelines. Available online: https://cpicpgx.org/. Accessed 17 July 2023.

25. Pharmacogenomics Knowledge Base (PharmGKB). Clinical guideline annotations. https://www.pharmgkb.org/guidelineAnnotations. Accessed 17 July 2023.
26. Food and Drug Administration (FDA). Table of pharmacogenetic associations. Available online: https://www.fda.gov/medical-devices/precision-medicine/table-pharmacogenetic-associations. Accessed 18 July 2023.

Correction to: Role of Public Data Bases for Pharmacogenomics

Bernard Esquivel and Kandace Schuft

Correction to:
Chapter 21 in: D. Primorac et al. (eds.), *Pharmacogenomics in Clinical Practice*,
https://doi.org/10.1007/978-3-031-45903-0_21

In the original version of the book, the author's name Bernard Esquivel has been updated in Chapter 21. The book and the chapter have been updated with the change.

The updated version of this chapter can be found at
https://doi.org/10.1007/978-3-031-45903-0_21

Appendix

Overview of Pharmacogenes with Significance to Clinical Practice

ABCB1, also known as multi-drug resistance protein 1 (MDRP1, or P-gp), is one of forty-nine members in the superfamily of human adenosine triphosphate (ATP)-binding cassette (ABC) transporters that encode transporter and channel proteins. These proteins function as efflux pumps and eliminate substrates from the systemic circulation at the urine-facing side of the brush border membrane of proximal tubules in the kidney and via biliary excretion. Current clinical considerations for P-gp are related to its role in multi-drug resistance and drug-drug interactions, derived primarily from its broad substrate specificity and variable intrinsic and drug-induced expression.

ABCC4, also known as multi-drug resistance protein 4 (MDRP4), is one of forty-nine putative members in the superfamily of human adenosine triphosphate (ATP)-binding cassette (ABC) transporters that encode transporter and channel proteins that function as efflux pumps. This family member plays a role in cellular detoxification as pump organic anions. Some gene variants may be associated with lower plasma concentrations of substrate drugs, like tenofovir, methotrexate, and thiopurines.

ABCG2, ABC subfamily G, isoform 2 (ABCG2) is a gene encoding the breast cancer resistance protein (BCRP), which is an ATP-binding cassette (ABC) efflux transporter, that plays a role in substrate drugs response. BCRP substrates include endogenous and naturally occurring polar molecules, like conjugated organic ions and chemotherapeutics. Genetic variations have been associated with resistance to chemotherapy, including tyrosine kinase inhibitors.

ACEx—This gene encodes an angiotensin-converting enzyme (ACE), which plays an important role in pathways that contribute to the regulation of blood pressure and is the target of a major class of antihypertensive drugs, ACE inhibitors.

ADD1—This gene encodes for adducins—a family of cytoskeletal proteins. Diseases associated with *ADD1* include, among others, hypertension. *ADD1* variants are associated with diuretic drugs action.

ADORA2A—This gene encodes for the adenosine A2a receptor. It plays a role in many biological functions, such as cardiac rhythm and circulation, cerebral and renal blood flow, immune function, pain regulation, and sleep. It has been implicated in pathophysiological conditions such as inflammatory diseases and neurodegenerative disorders. It is associated with the action of caffeine and other methylxanthine drugs.

ADRB1—This gene codes for beta-1-adrenoreceptors—the G-protein-coupled receptors expressed in cardiac, renal, vascular, and adipose tissues. It is associated with the action of beta1 receptor agonists (dobutamine) and antagonists (metoprolol and carvedilol).

ADRB2—Beta-2-adrenergic receptor, a member of the G-protein-coupled receptor superfamily, is encoded by this gene. Different polymorphic forms, point mutations, and/or downregulation are associated with nocturnal asthma, obesity, type 2 diabetes, and cardiovascular disease. Certain polymorphisms are associated with the action of agonists (salbutamol) and antagonists of beta2-adrenoreceptors (carvedilol and propranolol).

AGXT—This gene, expressed only in the liver, encodes protein alanine—glyoxylate and serine—pyruvate aminotransferases involved in glyoxylate detoxification in peroxisomes. Mutations in this gene have been associated with type I primary hyperoxaluria. Testing for *AGXT* gene mutation is required before initiating therapy with lumasiran in primary hyperoxaluria type I.

ALK—The anaplastic lymphoma kinase (ALK) gene encodes a tyrosine kinase receptor belonging to the insulin receptor superfamily. This oncogene is overexpressed in more than 16 different malignancies, including neuroblastoma. Targeted inhibitors of ALK are discovered, like crizotinib and ceritinib.

ANKK1—This gene encodes for the protein "ankyrin repeat and kinase domain containing 1" which belongs to the Ser/Thr protein kinase family and protein kinase superfamily involved in signal transduction pathways. Diseases associated with *ANKK1* include impulse control disorder and alexithymia. It relates to antipsychotic drugs (clozapine, olanzapine, and risperidone) actions.

APOE—The protein encoded by this gene is a major apoprotein of the chylomicron. It binds to a specific liver and peripheral cell receptor and is essential for the normal catabolism of triglyceride-rich lipoproteins. Mutations in this gene result in familial dysbetalipoproteinemia or type III hyperlipoproteinemia. Certain polymorphisms are associated with statin drug (atorvastatin) efficacy.

BCHE—This gene encodes a cholinesterase enzyme, a member of the type-B carboxylesterase/lipase family of proteins. It contributes to the inactivation of the neurotransmitter acetylcholine and degrades neurotoxic organophosphate esters. It is also involved in the metabolism of drugs like cocaine, heroin, and aspirin. Some gene mutations in humans are associated with prolonged apnea after the application of the muscle relaxant drug succinylcholine.

BRAF—This oncogene (B-Raf Proto-Oncogene, Serine/Threonine Kinase) encodes a protein belonging to the RAF family of serine/threonine protein kinases, which plays a role in regulating cell division, differentiation, and secretion. *BRAF* mutations, especially the most prevalent activating V600E, are found to be recurrent in many cancers (like melanoma, non-Hodgkin lymphoma, and colorectal cancer) and are correlated with poor prognosis. Testing to mutations is required before initiating therapy with BRAF inhibitors, like vemurafenib and dabrafenib.

CACNA1S— This gene encodes one of the five subunits of the slowly inactivating L-type voltage-dependent calcium channel in skeletal muscle cells. Mutations in this gene have been associated with malignant hyperthermia susceptibility after the application of halogenated volatile anesthetics and succinylcholine.

CBR3—Carbonyl reductase 3, which catalyzes the reduction of many biologically and pharmacologically active carbonyl compounds to their corresponding alcohols, is encoded by this gene. Some variants are associated with an increased risk of cardiac damage after anthracycline drugs exposure.

CD19—This gene (CD19 molecule) encodes a member of the immunoglobulin gene superfamily, which functions as coreceptor for the B-cell antigen receptor complex on B-lymphocytes. This protein is a target of chimeric antigen receptor (CAR) T-cells used in the treatment of lymphoblastic leukemia.

CD30 (TNFRSF8)—The protein encoded by this gene is a member of the TNF-receptor superfamily. This receptor is expressed only by activated T and B cells. It serves as a positive regulator of apoptosis and limits the proliferative potential of autoreactive CD8 effector T cells and protect the body against autoimmunity. It may play a role in the regulation of cellular growth and transformation of activated lymphoblasts. Testing for *CD30* is required before initiating therapy with brentuximab in Hodgkin lymphoma, among other indications.

CES1—This gene encodes a member of the large carboxylesterase family, responsible for the hydrolysis or transesterification of various xenobiotics, such as cocaine and heroin, and endogenous substrates with ester, thioester, or amide bonds. Variations in the gene are associated with efficacy of anticoagulant drug clopidogrel.

CETP—The protein encoded by this gene transfers cholesteryl ester from high-density lipoprotein to other lipoproteins in plasma. Defects in this gene are a cause of hyperalphalipoproteinemia 1. Gene variants can affect statin drugs' actions.

CFTR—This gene encodes a member of the ATP-binding cassette (ABC) transporter superfamily. The encoded protein is a chloride channel and controls ion and water secretion and absorption in epithelial tissues. Mutations in this gene cause cystic fibrosis and predict the efficacy of ivacaftor.

COMT—Enzyme catechol-O-methyltransferase is a product of this gene. It catalyzes the transfer of a methyl group from S-adenosylmethionine to catecholamines, including the neurotransmitters dopamine, epinephrine, norepinephrine, and catechol drugs, used in the treatment of hypertension, asthma, and Parkinson's disease. Diseases associated with COMT include schizophrenia and panic disorder 1.

CPS1—The mitochondrial enzyme carbamoyl-phosphate synthase 1 encoded by this gene catalyzes the synthesis of carbamoyl phosphate from ammonia and bicarbonate, the first committed step of the urea cycle. This is important for the elimination of excess urea from cells. Gene mutations are associated with the susceptibility to pulmonary hypertension development and the risk of hyperammonemia during the treatment with the antiseizure drug valproate.

CRHR1—This gene encodes a G-protein-coupled receptor that binds neuropeptides of the corticotropin-releasing hormone family. It plays a significant role in the regulation of the hypothalamic–pituitary–adrenal pathway. The encoded protein is essential for signal transduction pathways that regulate diverse physiological processes, including stress, reproduction, immune response, and obesity. Diseases associated with *CRHR1* include anxiety and irritable bowel syndrome. It is associated with the pharmacological actions of antidepressants and corticosteroids.

CRHR2—The protein encoded by this gene belongs to the G-protein-coupled receptor 2 family, and the subfamily of corticotropin-releasing hormone receptors. Diseases associated with *CRHR2* include eating disorders and irritable bowel syndrome. Some variants are associated with beta2-adrenoreceptor agonists' action.

CYB5R(1–4)—The NADH-cytochrome b5 reductase is encoded by these genes. It includes a membrane-bound form in somatic cells and a soluble form in erythrocytes. Gene mutations causing enzyme deficiency are associated with susceptibility to methemoglobinemia/sulfhemoglobinemia when metoclopramide is administered.

CYB5R—This gene encodes cytochrome b5-related proteins (known as NADH-cytochrome b5 reductases). These enzymes catalyze the desaturation and elongation of fatty acids, cholesterol biosynthesis, and methemoglobin reduction in erythrocytes. Some polymorphisms may increase the risk of methemoglobinemia and/or sulfhemoglobinemia when treated with metoclopramide.

CYP2B6—This gene encodes a member of the cytochrome P450 superfamily (CYP450) of enzymes that catalyze many reactions involved in drug metabolism and synthesis of cholesterol, steroids, and other lipids. CYP2B6 localizes to the endoplasmic reticulum and metabolizes some xenobiotics, such as the anti-cancer drugs cyclophosphamide and ifosfamide, antiviral drugs efavirenz, and nevirapine. Certain polymorphisms increase the risk of toxicity after application of substrate drugs.

CYP2C19—Enzymes in the CYP2C subfamily account for approximately 20% of cytochrome P450 in the adult liver. The cytochrome P450, family 2, subfamily C, polypeptide 19 (CYP2C19) enzyme contributes to the metabolism of many clinically relevant drugs such as antidepressants, benzodiazepines, mephenytoin, proton pump inhibitors, and the antiplatelet prodrug clopidogrel. Polymorphisms in this gene may affect the efficacy and safety of these drugs.

CYP2C8—Cytochrome P450, family 2, subfamily C, polypeptide 8 (CYP2C8) is a phase I metabolizing enzyme that plays an integral role in the biotransformation of structurally diverse xenobiotics and endogenous compounds. CYP2C8 is responsible for the biotransformation of 5% of currently used drugs that undergo phase I hepatic metabolism (ibuprofen, diclofenac, statins, opioids, etc.).

CYP2C9—This gene encodes for a phase I drug-metabolizing cytochrome P450 (CYP450) enzyme isoform that oxidizes xenobiotic and endogenous compounds. CYP2C9 is primarily expressed in the liver and is responsible for the metabolic clearance of up to 15–20% of all drugs, like nonsteroidal anti-inflammatory drugs, statins, and warfarin. Gene variants may significantly affect substrate drugs' efficacy and safety.

CYP2D6—The protein, encoded by this gene, localizes to the endoplasmic reticulum and metabolizes almost 25% of commonly prescribed drugs, like antidepressants, antipsychotics, analgesics, antitussives, beta-adrenergic blocking agents, antiarrhythmics, and antiemetics. The gene is highly polymorphic, and certain polymorphisms significantly change drugs' pharmacological actions.

CYP3A4 and *CYP3A5*—CYP3A4 and CYP3A5, encoded by the same-named genes, are the predominant cytochrome P450 enzymes expressed in the human liver, with CYP3A4 thought to dominate in Whites and CYP3A5 in Blacks/African Americans. The two share specificities for substrates. CYP3A4 is responsible for the metabolism of approximately 50–60% of drugs. Multiple polymorphisms are identified within these genes however, only some are associated with changes in substrate drugs' pharmacological action.

CYP4F2—This gene encodes for the enzyme CYP4F2, predominately expressed in the liver and kidneys, which regulates the bioavailability of vitamin E and vitamin K, a cofactor that is critical to coagulation. Variations in *CYP4F2* that affect the bioavailability of vitamin K also affect the dosing of vitamin K antagonists such as warfarin or acenocoumarol.

DMD—This gene (Dystrophin) encodes a protein, a component of the dystrophin-glycoprotein complex, which bridges the inner cytoskeleton and the extracellular matrix. Deletions, duplications, and point mutations may cause Duchenne muscular dystrophy, Becker muscular dystrophy or cardiomyopathy. Testing for mutation of this gene is required before initiating therapy with antisense oligonucleotides, like casimersen and vitolarsen for Duchenne muscular dystrophy.

DPYD—This gene encodes for dihydropyrimidine dehydrogenase, an enzyme involved in the breakdown of pyrimidines uracil and thymine. The gene mutations resulting in the enzyme deficiency manifest with excess quantities of pyrimidines and are also associated with fluoropyrimidine drugs (5-fluorouracil, capecitabine) accumulation, and their increased toxicities.

DRD2—The dopamine D2 receptor (DRD2), one of five dopamine receptors isoforms, shows high expression in both the pituitary gland and the central nervous system. Variants of the *DRD2* gene are risk factors for alcoholism and cocaine, nicotine and opioid dependence, mood disorders, schizophrenia, and movement disorders. DRD2 variants have been associated with the efficacy of several antipsychotic drugs.

EGFR—This gene encodes a member of the protein kinase superfamily, which is activated by epidermal growth factor (EGF). Because of its overexpression in the human epithelial malignancies, mutations can be used as predictive markers for the treatment of cancer. There are targeted therapies, involving tyrosine kinase inhibitors (like gefitinib and erlotinib) and monoclonal antibodies (cetuximab and panitumumab).

ESR1/2—widely distributed estrogen receptor, encoded by this gene, localizes in the cell nucleus and regulates the transcription of many estrogen-inducible genes that play a role in growth, metabolism, sexual development, gestation, and other reproductive functions. It plays a key role in breast cancer, endometrial cancer, and osteoporosis, and some polymorphisms may influence pharmacological action of estrogen receptor modulators and antiestrogens.

ERRB2—This gene, also known as *HER2*, encodes a member of the epidermal growth factor (EGF) receptor family. This receptor is amplified and/or overexpressed in 20–30% of invasive breast carcinomas. It has an important diagnostic pharmacogene for cancer pharmacogenomics. Metastatic HER2-positive breast cancer is now commonly treated with HER2-targeted therapy, such as trastuzumab. *ERBB2* activating mutations have clinical importance in HER2-negative breast cancer because mutated receptors are sensitive to the tyrosine kinase inhibitor neratinib.

F5—Factor V is an essential coagulation cofactor that enhances thrombin activation by factor Xa. A genetic variant of *F5* (Factor V Leiden (FVL) polymorphism) is associated with the risk of venous thromboembolism (VTE). The risk of VTE is greater among individuals with FVL, particularly among smokers and women using oral contraceptives or estrogen hormone replacement therapy.

FGFR2—This gene encodes fibroblast growth factor receptor, a tyrosine-protein kinase receptor which plays an essential role in the regulation of embryonic development, cell proliferation, differentiation, and migration. Amplification of the receptors was observed in lung and breast cancers, while coding mutations and deletions were seen in many cancers. Kinase inhibitors infigratinib and erdafitinib are used only in patients with confirmed *FGFR2* gene alterations.

FKBP5—The protein encoded by this gene is a member of the immunophilin protein family and plays a role in immunoregulation and basic cellular processes involving protein folding and trafficking. Some gene variants are associated with antidepressant drugs action.

FLT3—This gene (Fms Related Receptor Tyrosine Kinase 3) encodes a class III receptor tyrosine kinase that regulates hematopoiesis. The constitutive activation of this receptor because of gene mutations is associated with acute myeloid leukemia (AML) and acute lymphoblastic leukemia. Gene mutations must be confirmed before initiation of therapy with midostaurin and gilteritinib in AML patients.

GAA—This gene encodes lysosomal alpha-glucosidase, essential for the lysosomal degradation of glycogen to glucose. Defects in this gene are the cause of an autosomal recessive disorder glycogen storage disease II, also known as Pompe's disease, characterized by glycogen accumulation in various tissues. Gene testing is required before initiating long-term alpha-glucosidase replacement therapy.

G6PD—Glucose-6-phosphate dehydrogenase (G6PD), encoded by the same-named gene, mediates the production of NADPH and ribose-5-phosphate. This gen is one of the first associated with variable drug response. G6PD deficiency may result in increased risks of adverse reactions to many drugs, including primaquine, chloroquine, dapsone, rasburicase, and some antidiabetics.

GBA—This gene encodes the enzyme that catalyzes the hydrolysis of glucocerebroside to glucose and ceramide in the lysosome. Mutations in this gene cause Gaucher disease, a lysosomal storage disease characterized by an accumulation of glucocerebrosides. Velaglucerase alfa—a recombinant form of glucocerebrosidase—is indicated as a long-term enzyme replacement therapy in Gaucher disease Type 1.

GRIK4—This gene encodes a protein that belongs to the glutamate gated ionic channel family. Glutamate functions as the major excitatory neurotransmitter in the central nervous system. Diseases associated with *GRIK4* polymorphisms include bipolar disorder and depersonalization disorder. Certain gene variants are associated with antidepressant drugs action.

GRK5—This gene encodes a member of the guanine nucleotide-binding protein (G-protein)-coupled receptor kinase subfamily of the Ser/Thr protein kinase family. The protein phosphorylates the activated forms of G-protein-coupled receptors, thus initiating their deactivation. Diseases associated with *GRK5* include systolic heart failure and asthma. Gene variants have been related to the action of beta-adrenoreceptor antagonists.

HLA-A—HLA-A locus located at human chromosome 6p21.3 encodes a group of human leukocyte antigens (HLA). HLA is a major histocompatibility complex (MHC) antigen. MHC Class I molecules such as HLA-A are expressed in nearly all cells and play a central role in the immune system by presenting peptides derived from the endoplasmic reticulum lumen to be recognized by cytotoxic T cells. More than 6000 HLA-A alleles have been described. HLA-A is ranked among the genes in humans with the fastest-evolving coding sequence. This level of variation on MHC Class I is the primary cause of transplant rejection, and some variants are connected with the toxicity of carbamazepine and allopurinol.

HLA-B—The human leukocyte antigen B (*HLA-B*) gene, along with *HLA-A* and *HLA-C*, encodes cell surface molecules responsible for the presentation of endogenous peptides to CD8+ T-cells. Hundreds of alleles of the HLA-B gene are identified. Some allelic variants are associated with an increased risk of the development of some diseases, like ankylosing spondylitis, rheumatoid arthritis, and psoriatic arthritis. Also, certain alleles are associated with the increased risk of life-threatening skin reactions (Steven-Johnson syndrome/toxic epidermal necrolysis) during therapy with antiseizure drugs (carbamazepine, phenytoin, and lamotrigine), allopurinol, and antiviral drug abacavir.

HLA-DPB1—This gene in humans encodes HLA class II histocompatibility antigen, DP (W2) beta chain. It plays a central role in the immune system by presenting peptides derived from extracellular proteins. Class II molecules are expressed in antigen-presenting cells and are connected with the risk of asthma associated with aspirin therapy.

HLA-DQA1—Major histocompatibility complex, class II, DQ alpha 1 is a human gene presented on the short arm of chromosome 6. The protein encoded by this gene is one of two proteins required to form the DQ heterodimer, a cell surface receptor essential to the function of the immune system. Typing for certain polymorphisms is routinely done for bone marrow transplantation.

HLA-DRB1—This gene encodes HLA class II histocompatibility antigen, DRB1 beta chain. Some *DRB1* alleles are associated with risk of rheumatoid arthritis and the risk of antiviral drug nevirapine-induced adverse reactions.

HMGCR—This gene encodes the 3-hydroxy-3-methylglutaryl coenzyme A (HMG-CoA) reductase enzyme which catalyzes the NADP-dependent conversion of HMG-CoA to mevalonate in the rate-limiting step of cholesterol biosynthesis in hepatocytes. Inhibition of this enzyme is the primary mechanism of action of statin drugs. Some haplotypes are associated with therapeutic responses to statins.

HPRT1—This gene encodes hypoxanthine-guanine phosphoribosyltransferase (HGPRT). HGPRT catalyzes the conversion of hypoxanthine to inosine monophosphate and guanine to guanosine monophosphate. Thus, it plays a central role in the generation of purine nucleotides. Mycophenolic acid is an inhibitor of inosine monophosphate dehydrogenase and should be avoided in patients with rare hereditary deficiency of HGPRT, such as Lesch-Nyhan and Kelley-Seegmiller syndromes.

HTR1A—This gene encodes the serotonin 1A receptor (or 5-HT1A receptor), expressed in the brain, spleen, and neonatal kidney. Its activation in the brain mediates hyperpolarisation and reduction of the firing rate of the postsynaptic neuron. Some variants are connected with antidepressant drugs efficacy.

HTR2A—This gene encodes the 5-HT2A receptor for serotonin. This receptor is widely distributed and affects neural activity, perception, cognition, and mood, among other functions. It is one of the molecular targets for antipsychotic drugs. Mutations in this gene are associated with susceptibility to schizophrenia and obsessive-compulsive disorder and are also associated with response to the antidepressant drug citalopram in patients with major depressive disorder.

HTR2C—5-HT2C receptor, encoded by the same-named gene, is a G-protein-coupled receptor that is coupled to Gq/G11 and mediates excitatory neurotransmission. Gene variants correlate with susceptibility to some conditions, including substance use disorders, obesity, depression, and anxiety-related conditions. Certain polymorphisms are connected with the risk of weight gain when using antipsychotic drugs (like risperidone, olanzapine, and clozapine).

IDH1—This gene encodes enzyme isocitrate dehydrogenases. It catalyzes the oxidative decarboxylation of isocitrate to 2-oxoglutarate. *IDH1* mutations have been observed in sarcomas, hematologic malignancies, colon cancer, and brain cancer. Testing for *IDH1* mutation is required before initiating therapy with ivosidenib, an enzyme inhibitor indicated for the treatment of acute myeloid leukemia.

IFNL3—Interferon lambda 3 encodes the IFNL3 protein. This gene, along with genes interleukin 28A (IL28A) and interleukin 29 (IL29), forms a cytokine gene cluster on a chromosomal region mapped to 19q13. Viral infection can induce the expression of the cytokines encoded by the three genes. Diseases associated with *IFNL3* include hepatitis C and cryoglobulinemia. Certain polymorphisms predict the therapeutic response to interferon therapy in patients with HCV infection.

IFNL4—This gene is a polymorphic pseudogene that, in some humans, encodes the interferon (IFN) lambda 4 protein. Diseases associated with *IFNL4* include hepatitis C, while the therapeutic response to interferon therapy is associated with particular gene variants.

ITPA—This gene encodes inosine triphosphate pyrophosphatase (ITP), an enzyme that hydrolyzes inosine triphosphate and deoxyinosine triphosphate to the monophosphate nucleotide and diphosphate. Gene variants predicting reduced ITPase activity are associated with decreased risk of ribavirin-induced anemia, increased risk of thrombocytopenia, lower ribavirin concentrations, and reduced relapse risk following interferon-based therapy for hepatitis C.

KIF6—This gene (Kinesin Family Member 6) encodes kinesin, a member of a family of molecular motors which are involved in the intracellular transport of protein complexes, membrane organelles, and mRNA along microtubules. Certain gene variants are associated with the risk of heart disease and the efficacy of statin drugs treatment.

KIT—KIT Proto-Oncogene, Receptor Tyrosine Kinase encodes a receptor tyrosine kinase activated by cytokine stem cell factor. It plays a role in the proliferation, differentiation, migration, and apoptosis of many cell types. Mutations in this gene are associated with gastrointestinal stromal tumors, melanoma, and leukemias. Determination of specific mutations is required before imatinib use in the treatment of gastrointestinal stromal tumors.

LDLR—This gene belongs to a family of the low-density lipoprotein (LDL) receptor genes. It is highly expressed in bronchial epithelial cells, adrenal gland, and cortex. The encoded LDL-receptor protein mediates the endocytosis of the cholesterol-rich LDL into the cells. Mutations in the gene are known to cause familial hypercholesterolemia. Some gene variants are associated with the efficacy of statin drugs.

LEP—This gene encodes leptin that is secreted by white adipocytes and plays a major role in the regulation of energy homeostasis. Mutations in this gene and its regulatory regions cause severe obesity with hypogonadism and are also associated with type 2 diabetes mellitus development. Testing for *LEP* gene mutation is required before therapy with metreleptin in patients with congenital or acquired generalized lipodystrophy.

LPA—The protein encoded by this gene is a serine proteinase that inhibits the activity of tissue-type plasminogen activator I. Certain genotypes are associated with increased risks of familial hyperlipidemia and coronary artery disease in patients on statin drugs therapy.

MC4R—The protein encoded by this gene is a member of the melanocortin receptor family. It interacts with adrenocorticotropic and MSH hormones. MC4 receptors are involved in feeding behavior, the regulation of metabolism, sexual behavior, and male erectile function.

MET—This oncogene encodes mesenchymal epithelial transition (MET), a receptor tyrosine kinase activated by hepatocyte growth factor. Regulates many physiological processes including proliferation, scattering, morphogenesis, and survival. Its amplification and resulting overexpression have been reported in several cancers, like glioblastomas and childhood hepatocellular carcinoma. Testing for a specific alteration is required before initiating therapy with capmatinib and tepotinib in metastatic non-small cell lung cancer.

MTHFR—This gene encodes the enzyme methylenetetrahydrofolate reductase (MTHFR), which plays a key role in folate metabolism. It catalyzes the conversion of 5,10-methylenetetrahydrofolate to 5-methyltetrahydrofolate, a co-substrate for homocysteine remethylation to methionine. Genetic variation in this gene influences susceptibility to occlusive vascular disease, neural tube defects, colon cancer, and acute leukemia. Mutations in this gene are associated with methylenetetrahydrofolate reductase deficiency. Mutations are also connected with the risk of nephrotoxicity in patients treated with cisplatin and doxorubicin.

MT-RNR1—This gene encodes mitochondrially encoded 12S ribosomal RNA (12S or 12S rRNA), which is responsible for regulating insulin sensitivity and metabolic homeostasis. Mutations in the *MT-RNR1* gene may be associated with hearing loss and aminoglycoside antibiotic-induced ototoxic effects.

NLRP3—NLR Family Pyrin Domain Containing 3 gene encodes for a pyrin-like protein, a component of the NLRP3 inflammasome, which plays a role in innate immunity and inflammation. Spontaneous mutations activate inflammasome, which results in secretion of IL-1β, an important mediator of the systemic inflammation and manifestations of neonatal-onset multisystem inflammatory disease. Testing is required before using IL-1 β antagonist anakinra in the treatment of cryopyrin-associated periodic syndromes.

NAT2—This gene encodes an enzyme N-acetyltransferase 2 that functions to both activate and deactivate arylamine and hydrazine drugs and carcinogens. Polymorphisms in this gene are associated with a higher risk of cancer and pharmacological activity of multiple drugs, like anti-infective agents.

NEDD4L—This gene encodes a member of the Nedd4 family of HECT domain E3 ubiquitin ligases which transfer ubiquitin from E2 ubiquitin-conjugating enzymes to protein substrates, thus targeting specific proteins for lysosomal degradation. The encoded protein mediates the ubiquitination of multiple target substrates and plays a critical role in epithelial sodium transport by regulating the cell surface expression of the epithelial sodium channel. Single nucleotide polymorphisms in this gene may be associated with essential hypertension and response to treatment to some diuretic drugs.

NQO1—This gene is a member of the NAD(P)H dehydrogenase family and encodes a cytoplasmic 2-electron reductase. Mutations in this gene have been associated with tardive dyskinesia, an increased risk of hematotoxicity after exposure to benzene, and susceptibility to various forms of cancer. NQO1 catalyzes the reduction of a range of substrates, particularly quinones. Variations in the gene may lead to resistance to chemotherapeutics.

NT5C2—This gene encodes a hydrolase that plays an important role in cellular purine metabolism by acting primarily on inosine 5′-monophosphate and other purine nucleotides. This gene, when mutated to be over-active, has been linked to chemotherapy resistance in relapsed T-cell acute lymphoblastic leukemia.

NTRK—The Neurotrophic Tyrosine Receptor Kinase gene family contains three members, namely *NTRK1*, *NTRK2*, and *NTRK3*, which produce TRKA, TRKB, and TRKC proteins, respectively. These proteins help regulate cell signaling and function in healthy tissues. Rearrangements in the *NTRK* genes can be found in a broad range of solid tumor types, including non-small cell lung, etc. Testing of gene fusion is required before initiating therapy with entrectinib and larotrectinib in non-small cell lung cancer carcinoma.

NUDT15—This gene encodes an enzyme that belongs to the Nudix hydrolase superfamily. Members of this superfamily catalyze the hydrolysis of nucleo side diphosphates, which are a result of oxidative damage, and can induce base mispairing during DNA replication, causing transversions. The enzyme is a negative regulator of thiopurine activation and toxicity. Mutations in this gene result in poor metabolism of thiopurines and are associated with thiopurine-induced myelotoxicity.

OPRM1—This gene encodes one of at least three isoforms of opioid receptors in humans; the mu-opioid receptor (MOR). The MOR is the principal target of endogenous opioid peptides and opioid analgesic drugs. Certain polymorphisms are connected with the efficacy of opioid analgesic drugs, while others have been linked with increased risks of heart arrest and respiratory depression when using antidepressants, antipsychotics, and benzodiazepine derivatives.

PDGFRA—This oncogene (platelet-derived growth factor receptor alpha) encodes a cell surface tyrosine kinase receptor for members of the platelet-derived growth factor family, which have roles in the regulation of embryonic development, angiogenesis, cell proliferation, and differentiation. Mutations are commonly mutated in GI tract tumors and are a hallmark of gastrointestinal stromal tumors. Some mutations are associated with resistance to the tyrosine kinase inhibitor, imatinib.

PDL-1 (or *CD-274*)—This oncogene a programmed death-ligand 1 encodes an immune inhibitory receptor ligand that is expressed by T cells and B cells and various types of tumor cells. It plays a critical role in the inhibition of the anti-tumor immune response in the tumor microenvironment. Its expression is prognostic in many types of human malignancies, including colon cancer and renal cell carcinoma. Testing is required before initiating therapy with PDL-1 inhibitors, like avelumab, atezolizumab, and pembrolizumab.

PIK3CA—This oncogene encodes phosphoinositide 3-kinases (PI 3-Ks), a family of lipid kinases. This enzyme participates in cellular signaling triggered by various growth factors, thus mediating cell growth, proliferation, motility, and survival. *PIK3CA* is important in a number of cancers, including breast cancer.

PTGFR—The protein encoded by this gene is a member of the G-protein-coupled receptor family. It is a receptor for prostaglandin F2-alpha (PGF2-alpha) and may also be involved in modulating intraocular pressure and smooth muscle contraction in the uterus. Diseases associated with *PTGFR* include ocular hyperemia and ocular hypertension. Certain genotypes are associated with the efficacy of prostaglandin analog latanoprost in the treatment of glaucoma.

PTGS1—This is one of two genes encoding similar enzymes that catalyze the conversion of arachidonate to prostaglandin. The encoded protein regulates angiogenesis in endothelial cells and is inhibited by nonsteroidal anti-inflammatory drugs. The protein may promote cell proliferation during tumor progression. Disease associated with *PTGS1* includes gastric ulcer and is related to aspirin therapy resistance.

RAS—A family of genes (include *KRAS*, *HRAS*, and *NRAS*) that encode proteins involved in cell signaling pathways that control cell growth and death. Mutations in the Ras family of proto-oncogenes are very common, being found in 20–30% of all human tumors. For example, testing for certain *KRAS* mutations is required to exclude patients due to lack of benefit.

ROS1—This proto-oncogene, highly expressed in a variety of tumor cell lines, belongs to the subfamily of tyrosine kinase insulin receptor genes. It is frequently involved in genetic rearrangement in a variety of human cancers. Testing is required before initiating therapy with kinase inhibitor crizotinib in patients with non-small cell lung cancer.

RYR1—This gene encodes the ryanodine receptor isoform 1, a calcium channel expressed in skeletal muscle. It plays a critical role in calcium release and muscle contraction and is the primary locus for malignant hyperthermia susceptibility, a hypermetabolic condition associated by volatile anesthetics (e.g., desflurane, enflurane, halothane, and sevoflurane) and muscle relaxant drug succinylchloride.

SCN1A—This gene encodes for voltage-dependent sodium channels which regulate sodium exchange between intracellular and extracellular spaces and are essential for the generation and propagation of action potentials in excitable tissues (muscle cells and neurons). Allelic variants are associated with generalized epilepsy, febrile seizures, and epileptic encephalopathy, as well as response to some antiseizure drugs.

SERPINC1—The protein encoded by this gene, antithrombin III, is a plasma protease inhibitor and a member of the serpin superfamily. This protein inhibits thrombin as well as other activated serine proteases of the coagulation system. Numerous mutations have been identified, many of which are known to cause antithrombin-III deficiency which constitutes a strong risk factor for thrombosis. Certain gene variants are associated with an increased risk of thrombocytopenia with cytostatic drugs.

SLC6A4—This gene encodes an integral membrane protein that transports the neurotransmitter serotonin from the synaptic cleft into presynaptic neurons. A repeat length polymorphism in the promoter of this gene has been shown to affect the rate of serotonin uptake. Diseases associated with *SLC6A4* include obsessive-compulsive disorder and anxiety, while certain variants can influence the action of antidepressant drugs.

SLCO1B1—The solute carrier organic anion transporter family member 1B1 gene encodes for a membrane-bound sodium-independent organic anion transporter protein (OATP1B1) that is involved in the active cellular influx of many endogenous substrates, such as bile acids, xenobiotic compounds, and a wide panel of pharmaceutical compounds, like statins. OATP1B1-dependent transport is an important step in mediating drug hepatic clearance.

SOD2—This gene is a member of the iron/manganese superoxide dismutase family. It encodes a mitochondrial protein that binds to the superoxide byproducts of oxidative phosphorylation and converts them to hydrogen peroxide and diatomic oxygen. Mutations in this gene have been associated with idiopathic cardiomyopathy, premature aging, sporadic motor neuron disease, and cancer. Certain polymorphisms are connected with the risk of heroin dependence and the efficacy of cyclophosphamide.

SMN2—This gene (survival of motor neuron 2) is part of 500 kb inverted duplication on chromosome 5q13. Diseases associated with *SMN2* include spinal muscular atrophy, Type I and II. Testing of mutations in chromosome 5q is required before initiating therapy with risdiplam, a survival of SMN2 splicing modifier in patients with spinal muscular atrophy.

TNF—This gene encodes a multifunctional proinflammatory cytokine that belongs to the tumor necrosis factor (TNF) superfamily. This cytokine has been implicated in a variety of diseases, including autoimmune diseases, insulin resistance, psoriasis, etc. Certain gene variants have been associated with anti-TNF drugs (etanercept, infliximab) efficacy.

TPMT—This gene encodes thiopurine S-methyltransferase which catalyzes the S-methylation of thiopurine drugs (such as 6-mercaptopurine and azathioprine), aromatic and heterocyclic sulfhydryl compounds. *TPMT* variation can lead to thiopurine toxicity, especially myelotoxicity.

TYMS—This gene encodes thymidylate synthase that catalyzes the methylation of deoxyuridylate to deoxythymidylate. It maintains the dTMP (thymidine-5-prime monophosphate) pool critical for DNA replication and repair. Polymorphisms in this gene may be associated with the etiology of neoplasia and response to chemotherapy since it is the primary site of action for 5-fluorouracil, 5-fluoro-2-prime-deoxyuridine, and some folate analogs.

UGT1A1—This gene encodes a UDP-glucuronosyltransferase, an enzyme of the glucuronidation pathway that transforms small lipophilic molecules, such as steroids, bilirubin, hormones, and drugs, into water-soluble, excretable metabolites. UGT1A1 is the sole enzyme responsible for the glucuronidation of bilirubin and SN-38, the active metabolite of irinotecan.

UGT2B15—This gene encodes a glycosyltransferase that is involved in the metabolism and elimination of toxic compounds, both endogenous and of exogenous origin. This gene plays a role in the regulation of estrogens and androgens.

VDR—This gene encodes the vitamin D receptor (VDR), which binds the active form of vitamin D (1,25-dihydroxyvitamin D3). Due to the pleiotropic effect, the 1,25 dihydroxyvitamin D3- VDR complex exerts, and its genetic variants have been associated with a variety of diseases/phenotypes, including various types of cancer, tuberculosis, asthma, longevity/mortality, insulin-dependent diabetes mellitus, bone mineral density, and hyperparathyroidism. *VDR* expression is reduced in colon cancer and negatively correlates with cancer progression. Given the vast number of genes whose transcription can be upregulated or downregulated by

VDR, one and the same allele may be a risk factor for one trait and a protective one for another.

VKORC1—This gene encodes the catalytic subunit of the vitamin K epoxide reductase complex, which is responsible for the reduction of inactive vitamin K 2,3-epoxide to active vitamin K (a cofactor for gamma-glutamyltransferase). Allelic variations in this gene are associated with vitamin K-dependent clotting factors combined deficiency and increased resistance or sensitivity to warfarin, an inhibitor of vitamin K epoxide reductase.

References

1. GeneCards®: The Human Gene Database. Available at: https://www.genecards.org/.
2. PharmGKB. Available at: https://www.pharmgkb.org/.
3. Clinical Pharmacogenetics Implementation Consortium. Available at: https://cpi cpgx.org.

Index